Michael Zigler DOM Cert VOphthal.

Michael Zigler DOM Cert VOphthal.

Equine
Ophthalmology

Equine
Ophthalmology

Brian C. Gilger, DVM, MS, DACVO

Professor of Ophthalmology
Department of Clinical Sciences
North Carolina State University
Raleigh, North Carolina

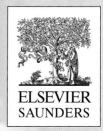

ELSEVIER
SAUNDERS

ELSEVIER
SAUNDERS

11830 Westline Industrial Drive
St. Louis, Missouri 63146

Equine Ophthalmology   ISBN 0-7216-0522-2
Copyright © 2005, Elsevier Inc.

NOTICE

Veterinary Medicine is an ever-changing field. Standard safety precautions must be followed, but as new research and clinical experience broaden our knowledge, changes in treatment and drug therapy may become necessary or appropriate. Readers are advised to check the most current product information provided by the manufacturer of each drug to be administered to verify the recommended dose, the method and duration of administration, and contraindications. It is the responsibility of the licensed prescriber, relying on experience and knowledge of the patient, to determine dosages and the best treatment for each individual patient. Neither the publisher nor the author assumes any liability for any injury and/or damage to persons or property arising from this publication.

International Standard Book Number 0-7216-0522-2

Publishing Director: Linda Duncan
Senior Editor: Liz Fathman
Senior Developmental Editor: Jolynn Gower
Publishing Services Manager: John Rogers
Senior Project Manager: Beth Hayes
Book Designer: Paula Ruckenbrod

Printed in the United States of America

Last digit is the print number: 9 8 7 6 5 4 3 2 1

Contributors

Stacy E. Andrew, DVM, DACVO
Georgia Veterinary Specialists
Atlanta, Georgia
Chapter 4: Diseases of the Cornea and Sclera

Dennis E. Brooks, DVM, PhD, DACVO
Professor, Ophthalmology
College of Veterinary Medicine
University of Florida
Gainesville, Florida
Chapter 8: Equine Glaucoma

Carmen M. H. Colitz, DVM, PhD, DACVO
Assistant Professor
Veterinary Clinical Services
The Ohio State University
Columbus, Ohio
Chapter 12: Ocular Manifestations of Systemic Disease

Tim J. Cutler, DVM, DACVIM, DACVD
Veterinary Ophthalmologist
Animal Eye Specialty Clinics of South Florida
West Palm Beach, Florida
Palm Beach Equine Hospital
Wellington, Florida
Chapter 2: Diseases and Surgery of the Globe and Orbit

Jennifer L. Davis, DVM, DACVIM
Clinical Pharmacology Resident and Doctoral
  Candidate
Molecular and Biomedical Sciences
North Carolina State University
Raleigh, North Carolina
Chapter 12: Ocular Manifestations of Systemic Disease

Ann Dwyer, DVM
Genesse Valley Equine Clinic
Scottsville, New York
Equine Recurrent Uveitis
Chapter 13: Practical Management of Blind Horses

Hartmut Gerhards, Dr. Med. Vet.
Professor
University of Munich
Munich, Bavaria, Germany
Chapter 7: Equine Recurrent Uveitis

Brian C. Gilger, DVM, MS, DACVO
Professor of Ophthalmology
Department of Clinical Sciences
North Carolina State University
Raleigh, North Carolina
*Chapter 3: Diseases of the Eyelids, Conjunctiva,
  and Nasolacrimal Systems*
Chapter 7: Equine Recurrent Uveitis

Steven R. Hollingsworth, DVM, DACVO
Department of Surgical and Radiological Sciences
School of Veterinary Medicine
University of California
Davis, California
Chapter 5: Diseases of the Anterior Uvea

Carolyn Kalsow, PhD
Principal Scientist
Ocular Research Services
Mendon, New York
Chapter 7: Equine Recurrent Uveitis

Mary E. Lassaline, DVM, PhD
Resident, Ophthalmology
College of Veterinary Medicine
University of Florida
Gainesville, Florida
Chapter 8: Equine Glaucoma

**Andy Matthews, BVMcS, PhD, DECEIM,
  FRCVS**
McKenzie, Bryson and Marshall
  Veterinary Surgeons
Kilmarnock
Scotland, United Kingdom
Chapter 4: Diseases of the Cornea and Sclera

**Tammy Miller Michau, DVM, MS,
  DACVD**
Assistant Professor of Ophthalmology
Department of Clinical Sciences
North Carolina State University
Raleigh, North Carolina
*Chapter 1: Equine Ocular Examination: Basic
  and Advanced Diagnostic Techniques*

Paul E. Miller, DVM, DACVO
Clinical Professor of Comparative Ophthalmology
Department of Surgical Sciences
School of Veterinary Medicine
University of Wisconsin–Madison
Madison, Wisconsin
Chapter 10: Equine Vision: Normal and Abnormal

Christopher J. Murphy, DVM, PhD, DACVD
Professor of Comparative Ophthalmology
Department of Surgical Sciences
School of Veterinary Medicine
University of Wisconsin–Madison
Madison, Wisconsin
Chapter 10: Equine Vision: Normal and Abnormal

Franck J. Ollivier, Dr. Med. Vet, PhD
Ophthalmology Resident
Department of Large and Small Animal Clinical
    Sciences
University of Florida
College of Veterinary Medicine
Gainesville, Florida
Chapter 4: Diseases of the Cornea and Sclera

Simon M. Petersen-Jones, DVetMed, PhD, DVOphthal, DECVO, MRCVS
Associate Professor, Comparative Ophthalmology
Department of Small Animal Clinical Sciences
Michigan State University
East Lansing, Michigan
Chapter 11: DNA and Genetic Testing

Riccardo Stoppini, DVM
Equine Ophthalmology Practitioner
Brescia, Italy
*Chapter 3: Diseases of the Eyelids, Conjunctiva,
    and Nasolacrimal Systems*

R. David Whitley, DVM, MS, DACVO
Professor and Department Head
Department of Clinical Sciences
College of Veterinary Medicine
Auburn University
Auburn, Alabama
Chapter 6: Diseases and Surgery of the Lens

David A. Wilkie, DVM, MS, DACVO
Associate Professor
Head, Comparative Ophthalmology
Veterinary Clinical Sciences
The Ohio State University
Columbus, Ohio
Chapter 9: Diseases of the Ocular Posterior Segment

A. Michelle Willis, DVM, DACVO
Animal Vision of Avon
Avon, Connecticut
Chapter 4: Diseases of the Cornea and Sclera

Bettina Wollanke, PD, Dr. Med. Vet.
University of Munich
Munich, Bavaria, Germany
Chapter 7: Equine Recurrent Uveitis

To Elizabeth and Katherine

In memory of my father, James Edward Gilger

Preface

Ocular disease is one of the most common health problems in horses. Although the science of equine ophthalmology has grown tremendously in the past 10 years, our knowledge of these ocular disorders lags behind that of other domestic species. Diagnostic methods and treatments for equine disorders are mostly borrowed from knowledge of the eye diseases of other species. In addition to this lack of specific knowledge, drug availability and cost of medications has limited our ability to systemically treat most equine ocular disorders; especially inflammatory and posterior segment disease. Our understanding of genetic ocular disorders and how to prevent them is also in its infancy. Much research is needed to overcome these obstacles. Unfortunately, we are in a time of shrinking university and private foundation research budgets. It is imperative, therefore, that veterinarians in all clinical settings use their resources wisely, plan appropriate basic and clinical research trials, and, most importantly, share their findings with their colleagues. By not reporting this work, advancement in veterinary ophthalmology will not occur. One objective of this book was to provide a comprehensive basis for the furthering of the science of equine ophthalmology. I encourage those who disagree with opinions in this textbook to perform studies on the subject and to publish their results in refereed journals so that future editions of *Equine Ophthalmology* will include more of this evidence-based information.

Although there are several excellent books available regarding ocular disorders in horses, there is not a comprehensive clinical textbook on equine ophthalmology. The goal of this textbook was to provide a fully referenced, complete guide to the diagnosis and treatment of equine ocular disorders. Over 400 color photographs in 13 chapters also assist in the identification of various ocular diseases, similar to an atlas. The textbook is written by 22 equine experts from around the world. This book has both standard chapters (e.g., examination and diagnostics; diseases organized by anatomical location) and unique chapters (e.g., equine vision). The chapters range from practical (e.g., management of blind horses) to scientific (e.g., genetic testing). Multiple figures, diagrams, tables, and organization of the individual disease sections assist the clinician who needs a quick reference. Extensive text and complete references help those who need in-depth information on the subject.

This is a textbook intended for clinicians and clinical scientists. Anatomy, physiology, embryology, and pathology are not emphasized, except in terms of defining specific disease processes. Sources for anatomy and normal physiology exist (and the reader is encouraged to seek out these sources for more information); however, comprehensive pathology and pathophysiology sources for equine ophthalmic disorders need to be developed.

Finally, the most important goal of this textbook is to help our equine patients by sharing information on diagnoses and treatment of painful and blinding ocular diseases that occur far too frequently in this species.

Acknowledgments

This book could not be possible without the sacrifice and hard work of all the authors, who took time away from their families and professions to contribute. I thank Beth Hayes, Jolynn Gower, and Liz Fathman at Elsevier for their patience and willingness to make this book a reality. In addition, I thank Jacklyn Salmon for all the behind-the-scenes hard work; and Elaine Smith and Melissa Hamman for photography and other support. I thank Drs. Stacy Andrew, Dennis Brooks, Michael Davidson, Claire Latimer, Tammy Miller Michau, Riccardo Stoppini, and David Wilkie for review of manuscripts and for contributing images. I also thank my colleagues at North Carolina State University for their support during the editing of the book. Finally, and most importantly, I thank my wife Elizabeth for her love, support, inspiration, and grace, without which this project, or any other significant endeavors in my life, could not have been accomplished. I also thank our daughter Katherine, whose enthusiasm for life is unparalleled, and to our dogs who kept me company on the couch for months helping me edit this textbook.

Contents

CONTENTS

1 Equine Ocular Examination: Basic and Advanced Diagnostic Techniques

Tammy Miller Michau

The ocular examination of the horse is a challenging but important responsibility, because many equine ocular diseases can result in unsoundness. Understanding normal equine ocular anatomy is integral to performing the examination and detecting abnormalities. The examination techniques, diagnostic procedures, and modalities currently available to veterinarians and veterinary ophthalmologists for use in the equine patient are discussed. Both basic and advanced ophthalmic diagnostic techniques are described. The basic equipment needed for a thorough equine ophthalmic examination is listed in Box 1-1. Examination of the equine eye includes obtaining the history and signalment, inspecting the patient in a well-lighted environment, examining the ocular structures in a darkened environment, and possibly facilitating the examination with restraint, sedation, and local nerve blocks.[1-8]

MEDICAL HISTORY

A thorough medical history relevant to the ocular examination should include signalment, use of the animal (e.g., pet or performance), environment, characterization of the primary complaint, onset and initial clinical signs of the complaint, any treatment and response to that treatment, progression and duration of the complaint, current therapy, concurrent and previous disease, and any additional medications being used. Signalment can provide an important clue as to the cause of many ophthalmic conditions (e.g., congenital stationary night blindness in the Appaloosa, hereditary cataracts in the Morgan). Existing medical therapy can also greatly influence findings on ophthalmic examination. For example, topical atropine has been demonstrated to produce mydriasis for up to 14 days in the horse.[9] Additional information that may prove useful would include a travel history, vaccination history, deworming schedule, presence of nasal discharge, presence of stridor, previous trauma to the head, and whether other horses on the premises have been similarly affected. Further information may be required, depending on the specific complaint.

ANATOMY

Relevant anatomy is covered in detail in subsequent chapters relating to specific anatomic areas. Anatomy directly relevant to the common examination and diagnostic techniques is touched on here. Excellent reviews of equine ocular and head anatomy can be found in other sources,[8,10-15] in addition to those found in subsequent chapters.

Box 1-1   Basic Equipment Needed for General Equine Ophthalmic Examination

- Bright, focal light source: A Finoff transilluminator is ideal (halogen)
- Direct ophthalmoscope
- Sterile fluorescein strips
- Sterile culture swabs
- Kimura spatula, sterile cotton-tipped swabs, No. 10-20 sterile surgical blade—for cytology
- Glass slides
- Sterile eyewash
- Proparacaine (Alcaine)—topical anesthetic
- Tropicamide 1% (Mydriacyl)—short-acting dilating agent
- Sedation: Detomidine hydrochloride, xylazine, butorphanol
- Mepivacaine hydrochloride (Carbocaine) or lidocaine—local nerve blocks
- Graefe fixation forceps
- Open-ended tomcat urinary catheter—for nasolacrimal irrigation

Orbit

The equine orbit is open anteriorly and has a complete bony anterior orbital rim (Fig. 1-1).[8,13,14,16,17] Six bones form the orbit in the horse (lacrimal, zygomatic, frontal, sphenoid, palatine, and temporal).[10] The four bones forming the orbital rim are the frontal, lacrimal, zygomatic, and temporal bones.[8,10,13] The frontal bone forms the prominent dorsal orbital rim and wall and contains the supraorbital fossa. The frontal process of

the zygomatic bone and zygomatic processes of the temporal and frontal bones make up the zygomatic arch.[10] Frontal, lacrimal, sphenoid, and palatine bones contribute to the medial orbital wall.[10] The lacrimal and zygomatic bones contribute to the ventral orbital wall.[10] Arteries, veins, and nerves pass through several foramina (i.e., rostral alar, ethmoidal, orbital, optic, rotundum, supraorbital, caudal palatine, maxillary, and sphenopalatine) that are present in the orbital bones (Fig. 1-2). The orbital foramen is not elongated in the horse, as compared with that in most domestic animals, in which it is referred to as the orbital fissure.[10] The ventral orbital floor is predominantly composed of soft tissues (i.e., fat).[17]

Globe

The equine globe, contained within the orbit, is slightly flattened in the anterior-posterior dimension. In the adult horse, the average horizontal dimension is 48.4 mm, the average vertical dimension is 47.6 mm, and the average anterior-to-posterior axial diameter is 43.7 mm.[2,10] The equine cornea is oval horizontally (Fig. 1-3, A). The horizontal diameter ranges from 28 to 34 mm.[18] The central vertical corneal diameter ranges from 23 to 27 mm.[18] The medial vertical diameter is greater than the lateral vertical diameter.[18] The cornea represents approximately 14% of the total globe surface area and is centrally located to the axis of the globe.[19] Corneal thickness varies, depending on the state of the cornea (in vivo, enucleated, or formalin-fixed) and the type of instrument that was used to perform the measurements (e.g., ultrasound biomicroscope, pachymeter). In a recent study, corneal thickness was reported to be approximately 0.6 mm centrally and 1 mm peripherally.[20]

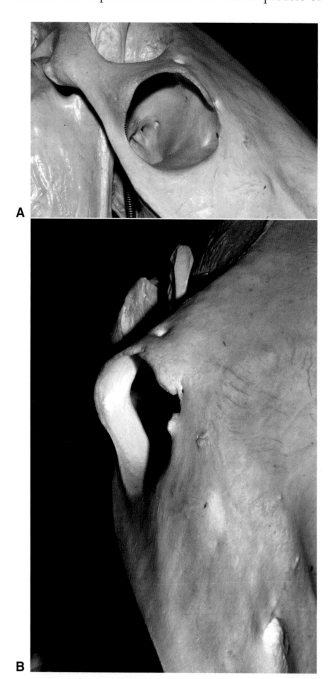

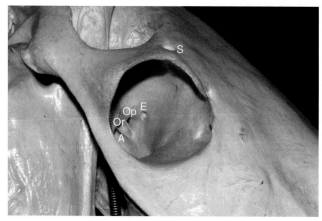

Fig. 1-1 A, Normal external appearance of the orbit in an equine skull viewed from the side. **B,** Normal external appearance of the orbit in an equine skull viewed from the front.

Fig. 1-2 Some of the foramina in the equine orbit are shown. Supraorbital *(S),* ethmoidal *(E),* optic *(Op),* orbital *(Or),* and rostral alar *(A).*

Globe movement results from the yoke action of six extraocular muscles (i.e., medial rectus, lateral rectus, dorsal rectus, ventral rectus, and dorsal and ventral oblique).[10] An extremely powerful retractor bulbi retracts the globe. The blood supply to most of the eye and its associated structures arises from the external ophthalmic artery, a branch of the maxillary artery.[10,21,22] The internal ophthalmic artery anastomoses with branches of the external ophthalmic artery and gives rise to the ciliary artery.[10] Short posterior and long posterior ciliary arteries branch from the ciliary artery. The short posterior ciliary arteries penetrate the sclera close to the optic nerve and supply the retina and choroid.[10] The long posterior ciliary arteries perforate the sclera anterior to the equator, and the lateral and medial arteries can usually be visualized running anteriorly in the sclera at the 3 and 9 o'clock positions.[10]

Eyelids

Additional extrinsic ocular muscles control movement of the thin equine eyelid. Closure of the eyelid results from contraction of the large orbicularis oculi, arranged concentrically around the palpebral fissure.[4,6,10] The levator anguli oculi medialis (corrugator supercilii) creates a notching of the nasal third of the upper eyelid as a result of its insertion (Fig. 1-4).[6] The notching can be pronounced, especially when the horse becomes anxious. The muscles associated with the eye and its adnexa are listed in Table 1-1.[4,16] A prominent fold can be seen on clinical examination, parallel to the lid margin, in the upper and lower eyelids (see Fig. 1-3, A). The upper eyelid is larger and more mobile than the lower eyelid.[4] The palpebral fissure is horizontally oval, and the lateral canthus is more rounded than the medial canthus (Fig. 1-3, A).[4] Numerous eyelashes are present along the lateral two thirds of the upper eyelid, and vibrissae are located dorsonasal to the upper lid and ventral to the lower lid (see Fig. 1-3, A).[6,23] The color of the eyelashes and skin of the eyelids is dependent on the coat color of the horse. A large nictitating membrane, situated in the medial canthus, moves laterally in a horizontal and slightly dorsal action across the globe (see Fig. 1-3, A).[4,6,10] This "third" eyelid is a semilunar fold of conjunctiva enclosing a T-shaped hyaline cartilage. The leading edge is usually partially pigmented but can be devoid of pigment, and the presence or absence of pigment is associated with coat color (see Fig. 1-3, B).

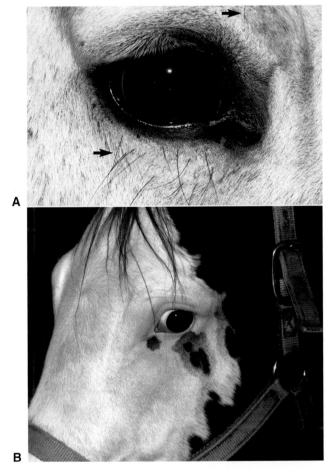

Fig. 1-3 A, Normal external appearance of the equine eye. The horse's palpebral fissure, cornea, and pupil are oval horizontally. The lateral canthus *(L)* is more rounded than the medial canthus *(M)*. There are prominent folds in the upper and lower eyelids. Numerous eyelashes are present along the lateral two thirds of the upper eyelid, and vibrissae are located dorsonasal to the upper lid and ventral to the lower lid *(arrows)*. The leading edge of the third eyelid is usually partially pigmented *(N)*. The lacrimal caruncle *(Lc)* is prominent. **B,** Normal external appearance of the equine eye when eyelid pigment is absent. Note the lack of pigment on the third eyelid, conjunctiva, and sclera as well.

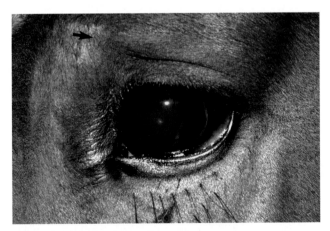

Fig. 1-4 The levator anguli oculi medialis can cause significant dorsal medial eyelid elevation and notching in the horse *(arrow)*. This is more pronounced during anxiety or when the horse is trying to focus on an object that is located to the side of its head.

Table 1-1   Extrinsic Muscles of the Eye and Eyelids

Muscle	Innervation	Function	Origin	Insertion
Globe				
Dorsal rectus	CN III	Upward globe rotation	Around optic foramen	Sclera
Ventral rectus	CN III	Downward globe rotation	Around optic foramen	Sclera
Medial rectus	CN III	Medial globe rotation	Around optic foramen	Sclera
Lateral rectus	CN VI	Lateral globe rotation	Around optic foramen	Sclera
Dorsal oblique	CN IV	Medial and ventral rotation of the dorsal aspect of the globe	Near ethmoidal foramen	Passes between dorsal and lateral rectus
Ventral oblique	CN III	Medial and dorsal rotation of the ventral aspect of the globe	Medial wall of orbit caudal to lacrimal fossa	Sclera near ventral margin of lateral rectus
Rectractor bulbi	CN VI	Globe retraction	Around optic foramen	Sclera posterior to recti
Eyelid				
Levator anguli oculi medialis	Auriculopalpebral branch of CN VII	Assists in upper eyelid elevation	Over root of the zygomatic process	Upper eyelid
Levator anguli oculi lateralis	CN VII	Lateral palpebral fissure lengthening		
Levator palpebrae superioris	CN III	Elevates the upper eyelid	Pterygoid crest	Thin tendon in upper lid
Malaris	CN VII	Depresses the lower eyelid		
Muller's	Sympathetic fibers in ophthalmic branch of CN V	Elevates the upper eyelid		
Orbicularis oculi	Auriculopalpebral branch of CN VII	Closes the palpebral fissure		Skin of the eyelids, medial palpebral ligament
Retractor anguli oculi	CN VII	Draws lateral canthus laterally		

Nasolacrimal System

The relatively large equine lacrimal gland lies just beneath the dorsolateral orbital rim.[13,17] The innervation to this gland is poorly understood but consists of a combination of sympathetic nerve fibers and parasympathetic fibers from the lacrimal branch of cranial nerve (CN) VII.[24] The serous nictitans gland surrounds the base of the third eyelid and is innervated by parasympathetic fibers from CN IX (glossopharyngeal nerve).[10,22] Two lacrimal puncta, located at the margins of both the upper and lower eyelids, are found approximately 8 to 9 mm from the medial canthus (Fig. 1-5).[25] The lower punctum is further from the eyelid margin than the upper punctum.[6] Each punctum is a roughly 2-mm–diameter, horizontal slit in the palpebral conjunctiva.[13,25] A canaliculus leads from each punctum toward the medial canthus, increasing in diameter to 3 or 4 mm and ending in the lacrimal sac, the expanded beginning of the approximately 22- to 30-cm–long nasolacrimal duct.[25] The lacrimal sac is poorly developed in horses.[6] The average diameter of the nasolacrimal duct is 4 to 5 mm.[6] The course of the

nasolacrimal duct follows a line drawn from the medial canthus of the eye to a point just dorsal and rostral to the infraorbital foramen (Fig. 1-5).[25,26] Several dilations or sacculations can occur normally in the duct, with a prominent one being present at the level of the first premolar.[13] The duct terminates in the lower punctum in the skin of the floor of the nostril near the mucocutaneous junction (Fig. 1-6). Horses and mules may have more than one nasal puncta, some of which are usually blind pouches.[6] The anatomy of the nasolacrimal system of the donkey is similar to that of the horse.[27]

Anterior Segment

The anterior chamber volume is approximately 3.04 ± 1.27 ml in the horse.[28] The highly vascular uveal tract is composed of the iris, ciliary body, and the choroid.[10] The iris of most horses is golden to dark brown; but blue, white, and heterochromia iridis may be seen (see Figs. 1-3, *A*, 1-7, and 1-8). Heterochromia iridis more commonly occurs in color-dilute breeds or individuals (e.g., Appaloosa, American Paint horse, palomino).

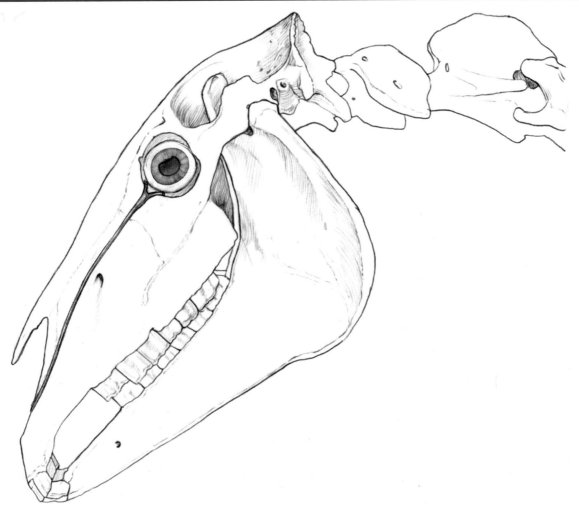

Fig. 1-5 Normal anatomy of the equine nasolacrimal duct. Two upper lacrimal puncta, one in each eyelid, are present along the medial inner eyelid margin. A canaliculus leads from each punctum toward the medial canthus and ends in the lacrimal sac, which is poorly developed in the horse. The lacrimal sac is the expanded beginning of the approximately 22- to 30-cm–long nasolacrimal duct. The course of the nasolacrimal duct follows a line drawn from the medial canthus of the eye to a point just dorsal and rostral to the infraorbital foramen.

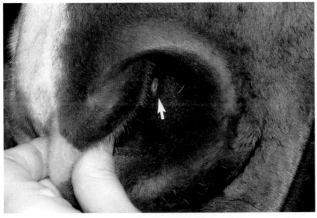

Fig. 1-6 Normally, a single lower punctum of the nasolacrimal system is present and can be located in the skin of the floor of the nostril near the mucocutaneous junction *(arrow)*.

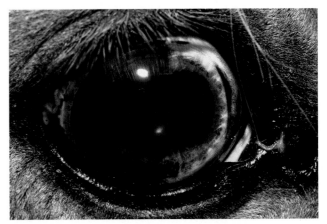

Fig. 1-7 Example of heterochromia iridis in the horse.

A combination of white and blue iridal color with brown corpora nigra is referred to as *walleye*.[2] A white iridal color with brown corpora nigra is referred to as *china eye*. A blue or white iris may turn yellow with inflammation or an elevated systemic bilirubin level (Fig. 1-9). The pupil of the adult horse is horizontally oval and becomes more circular on dilation because of the greater vertical pull of the dilator muscle (see Fig. 1-3, *A*, 1-10).[2] The sympathetically innervated iridal dilator muscle of the horse is less well developed than that of the dog, in contrast to the parasympathetically innervated iridal sphincter muscle, which occupies most of the stroma.[2] The iris is broken down into a central pupillary zone and a peripheral ciliary zone, separated by the collarette (Fig. 1-11).[2] Horses have granula iridica (corpora nigra) arising from the dorsal and, to a lesser extent, the ventral pupillary rim, which may augment the effectiveness of pupillary constriction or even act as a light barrier or "shade" (Fig. 1-11).[2,10] An artery that can be seen passing circumferentially around the iris is a termination of the medial and lateral long posterior ciliary arteries (see Fig. 1-8).[2,10] Each artery forms an incomplete arterial circle at the 12 and 2 o'clock positions.[2] The iridocorneal angle can be directly visualized medially and laterally in the horse (Figs. 1-11 and 1-12).[2,19]

Posterior Segment

The lens in a horse is very large, and normal variations, including prominent lens sutures, commonly occur.[2] Mean vitreous humor volume is 26.15 ± 4.87 ml for the equine eye.[28] Most horses have a triangular fibrous tapetum in the dorsal choroid (Fig. 1-13) that is usually

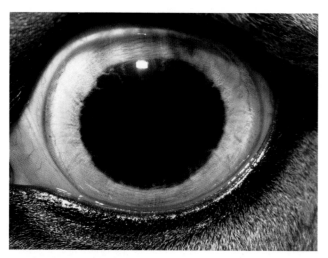

Fig. 1-8 Subalbinotic iris in a horse (walleye). It is easier to visualize the artery passing circumferentially around the peripheral iris in a subalbinotic eye.

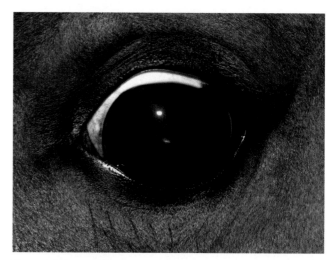

Fig. 1-10 Pupil of the adult horse appears rounder when dilated.

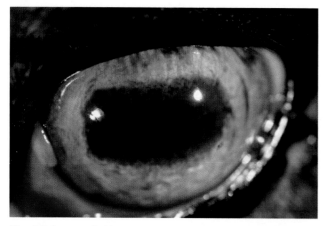

Fig. 1-9 A normally blue or white iris may turn yellow with chronic inflammation or an elevated systemic bilirubin level.

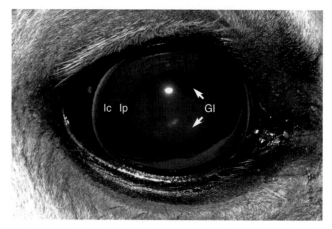

Fig. 1-11 Normal anatomy of the pupil and corpora nigra in a horse. Granula iridica *(GI)* are present on the dorsal and ventral pupillary margins but are normally more prominent on the dorsal margin. The iris can be separated into a pupillary zone *(Ip)* and a more peripheral ciliary zone *(Ic)*.

some variation of green or yellow.[20,29-32] The tapetum may be undeveloped in animals with albinotic or subalbinotic coat colors.[29] End-on choroidal capillaries can be visualized as small dark dots throughout the tapetal fundus (i.e., stars of Winslow) (Fig. 1-13).[29]

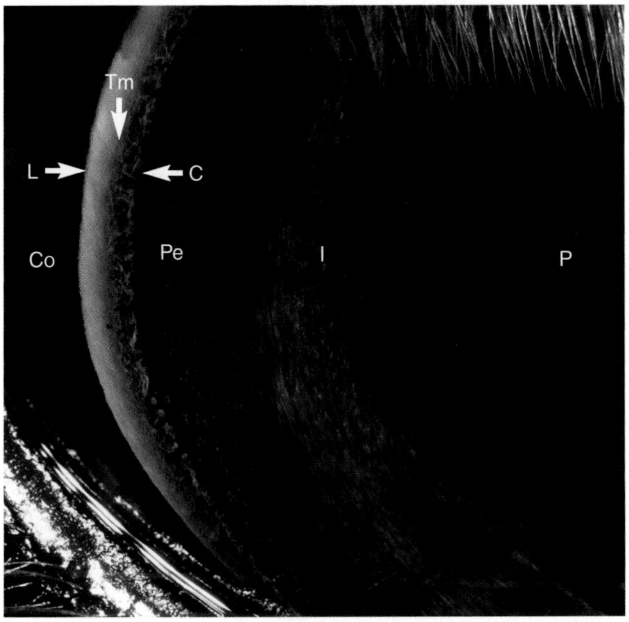

The nontapetal area is usually dark brown, but this melanin in the retinal pigment epithelium (RPE) may be absent, depending on coat and iris coloration (Fig. 1-14).[2] If the pigment is absent, the choroidal vessels can be visualized.

The equine retinal vasculature is paurangiotic, and the vessels arise from the edge of the disc and extend only a short distance.[29,33] The ventral margin of the disc at the 6 o'clock position is less vascular and normally appears slightly whiter in this area. As in other domestic mammals, there is no central retinal artery, and the retinal arterioles arise from chorioretinal arteries.[21] The optic disc is horizontally oval, usually located slightly temporal and ventral in the nontapetal area, and is salmon pink.[29] The equine disc can be differentiated into the optic cup and neuroretinal rim regions, and the cup-to-disc ratio is 0.61.[2]

Periorbital Sinuses

Several sinuses are in close anatomic contact with the orbital bones, the frontal (conchofrontal), maxillary (caudal and rostral), and sphenopalatine (Fig. 1-15).[2,10] Sinus disease involving these sinuses may encroach on the orbit and nasolacrimal duct.[34,35] The frontal sinus is located dorsal and ventral to the orbit.[17] The maxillary sinus is located ventral and nasal to the orbit and separated from the orbit by an extremely thin bony plate.[17]

Fig. 1-12 The attachment of the iridocorneal angle pectinate ligaments to Descemet's membrane (i.e., gray line) can be observed medially and laterally in the adult horse. Pupil *(P)*, iris *(I)*, pectinate ligaments *(Pe)*, attachment of pectinate ligaments to corneal endothelium *(C)*, trabecular meshwork *(Tm)*, limbus *(L)*, and conjunctiva *(Co)*.

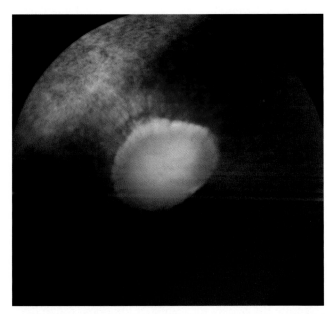

Fig. 1-13 In most horses, a triangular fibrous tapetum in the dorsal choroid can be seen on ophthalmoscopic examination. End-on choroidal capillaries can be visualized as small dark dots throughout the tapetal fundus (i.e., stars of Winslow). The nontapetal area is usually dark brown.

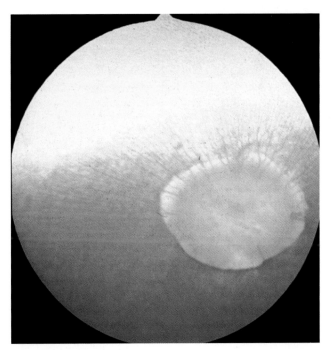

Fig. 1-14 Melanin in the retinal pigment epithelium may be absent, depending on coat and iris coloration. If the pigment is absent, the choroidal vessels can be visualized.

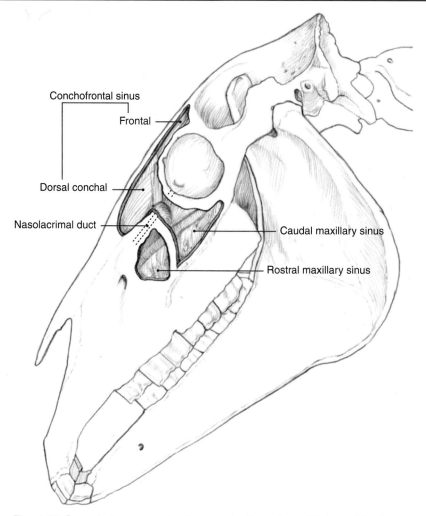

Fig. 1-15 Several sinuses are in close anatomic contact with the orbital bones, including the frontal (conchofrontal), maxillary (caudal and rostral), and sphenopalatine sinuses.

The anterior maxillary sinus can be located just ventral to the intersection of a line between the medial canthus and infraorbital foramen and a perpendicular line from the fourth cheek tooth.[6] Trephination dorsal to a line between the infraorbital foramen and the medial canthus can result in nasolacrimal duct damage.[25] The center of a line between the medial canthus and facial crest indicates the location of the caudal maxillary sinus.[6]

GENERAL OCULAR EXAMINATION

The ocular examination in the horse should proceed in a systematic manner.[2] The general order of steps to be taken in the examination is listed in Box 1-2. Before sedation, an initial examination of the equine eye should take place in a well-lighted area. The area of examination

should be quiet and away from major distractions. Examination of specific components of the eye requires the ability to darken the environment. This can be performed in a darkened stall, or the horse can be placed in stocks in a room in which the lights can be dimmed. For accurate evaluation of the equine pupillary light reflexes, a bright, focal light source and a darkened examination area are often required. The menace response and other subjective vision testing, such as maze testing, in addition to the evaluation of the pupillary light reflex (PLR), should be performed before sedation.

A thorough ocular examination usually requires restraint, tranquilization, regional nerve blocks, and topical anesthesia. Methods of restraint required to examine the ocular structures of the horse range from a halter and lead rope to mechanical restraint in stocks with use of a lip twitch. Use of restraint is dependent on temperament of the horse, availability of equipment,

Box 1-2	General Order of Steps to Take in Equine Ocular Examination

- Medical and ocular history
- Examine horse in its environment (e.g., walking on a lead, loose in a stall or round pen)
- Evaluation for symmetry from the front (globe, orbit, pupils, eyelash direction, ear and lip position)
- Visual testing (menace, dazzle, PLRs)
- Palpebral reflex
- Sedation if required here or at any time during the examination
- Auriculopalpebral nerve block
- Transillumination for gross disease (eyelids, cornea, anterior chamber, iris)
- STT, if indicated (may be performed before auriculopalpebral block)
- Topical fluorescein
- Examination of the eyelids, cornea, anterior chamber, and iris with transillumination and biomicroscopy
- Corneal reflex (may wait until complete corneal exam is performed to avoid iatrogenic damage)
- Topical anesthesia (proparacaine)
- IOP (sedation can affect the IOP)
- Mydriasis (tropicamide)
- Transillumination, retroillumination, and biomicroscopy of the lens and vitreous
- Direct ophthalmoscopy of fundus (± indirect)
- Irrigate nasolacrimal duct if indicated

IOP, Intraocular pressure; PLRs, pupillary light reflexes; STT, Schirmer tear test.

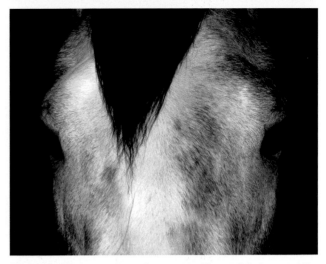

Fig. 1-16 The head (including ears and nostrils), bony orbits, eyelids, globes, and pupils should be examined for symmetry with the examiner positioned in front of the horse.

and comfort level of the handlers and examiner. In addition to manual and mechanical restraint, some form of chemical sedation can be used to smooth the progress of the examination.

Initial Examination

The head, bony orbits, eyelids, globes, and pupils should be examined for symmetry with the examiner positioned in front of the horse (Fig. 1-16) before extensive manipulation, sedation, or blockade of the auriculopalpebral nerve. Comfort may be assessed by evaluation of palpebral fissure size and symmetry, the position of the eyelashes, ocular discharge, and blink rate.[2,4,6] Any type of nasal discharge should also be noted. The upper eyelashes of the healthy horse are nearly perpendicular to the cornea (Fig. 1-17, *A*).[2] A change in the angle between the eyelashes in the cornea may indicate blepharospasm, enophthalmos, exophthalmos, or ptosis (Fig. 1-17, *B*).[2] The globes should also be evaluated for symmetry of size, position, and movement. Apparent changes in globe size

(e.g., buphthalmos, phthisis bulbi) should be differentiated from changes in globe position (e.g., enophthalmos, exophthalmos). Cornea globosa has been reported in the Rocky Mountain horse and may be difficult to distinguish from buphthalmos.[36]

The examiner should then position himself or herself at the side of the horse's head to examine each eye individually. An assistant may be required to elevate the head of a sedated horse to the same level as the examiner's eyes. The examiner may need to use a stool for an extremely tall horse and may need to kneel on the ground for an extremely short horse (e.g., a Miniature horse). Eyelids should be examined for position, movement, and conformation.[2,4,6,8] Attempts to forcefully elevate the upper eyelid should be avoided if an auriculopalpebral nerve block has not yet been performed, and each eye should be examined with minimal handling of the adnexal tissues. The orbit should be examined by observation, palpation of the bony orbital rim, and retropulsion of the globe through a closed eyelid.[2,4,6,8] Forceful manipulation of the eyelid and retropulsion should not be performed if the structural integrity of the cornea or globe may be compromised.

A cranial nerve evaluation (specifically, cranial nerves II, III, IV, V, VI, and VII) is then performed before any sedation is induced. These cranial nerves are assessed through the menace response, pupillary light and dazzle reflexes, globe and eyelid position and mobility, and sensation of ocular and adnexal structures.[2,4] Keratoconjunctivitis sicca may result from loss of the parasympathetic innervation in CN VII to the lacrimal glands. Examination of the cranial nerves is

is a normal response. The brightness of the light is of extreme importance in evaluating the results of this test, especially when opaque media are present. Care should be taken if the light source generates heat, because this can be detected by the horse if the light source is close to the cornea and can also result in blepharospasm.

Palpebral Reflex

Horses normally blink approximately 5 to 25 times per minute at rest.[45] The blink is synchronous between both eyes approximately 30% to 100% of the time.[24,45] Two types of normal blinking occur in the horse at rest, complete and incomplete.[24] Incomplete blinking is most common and consists predominantly of upper eyelid motion downward.[24] Complete blinking is associated with an upward movement of the lower lid to meet the upper lid and is highly variable in occurrence.[24] The blink rate slows when the horse is sedated, anxious, or focused on an object of interest.

The palpebral reflex, tested by touching both the medial and lateral canthi, should result in closure of the eyelid.[41-43] If CN V or CN VII is abnormal or if the eyelids are unable to close (e.g., in cases of buphthalmia or severe trauma and swelling), the blink may be absent or incomplete.

Corneal Reflex

The corneal reflex, tested by touching the unanesthetized cornea with a sterile cotton-tipped swab, should result in closure of the eyelid and retraction of the globe.[41-43] This subcortical reflex occurs in response to a tactile or painful stimulus to the cornea. The afferent pathway of the corneal reflex is via the ophthalmic branch of CN V.[43] The result should be closure of the eyelid and retraction of the globe, mediated by CN VII and CN VI, respectively.[43] If CN V or CN VII is abnormal or if the eyelids are unable to close (e.g., in cases of buphthalmia or severe trauma and swelling), the blink may be absent or incomplete.

Sympathetic Nervous System

The sympathetic nervous system controls dilation of the pupils and other motor functions of the eyes and face. Sympathetic visceral efferent nerves originate in the first three to four thoracic segments, course through the thorax and cervical region, and eventually synapse in the cranial cervical ganglion, which lies beneath the atlas in the wall of the guttural pouch.[41-43] Postganglionic

fibers proceed rostrally between the tympanic bulla and petrous temporal bone.[41-43] Damage to sympathetic innervation to the head may result in Horner's syndrome (miosis, ptosis, enophthalmos, increased sweating on the face and ear of the affected side, ipsilateral distention of facial blood vessels, and ipsilateral hyperemia of the conjunctiva and nasal mucosa).[46-50] The clinical findings of Horner's syndrome in the horse are more subtle and difficult to detect than those in small animals.[1] A mild ptosis is the most consistent finding.[1] Miosis occurs inconsistently and may be subtle.[1,43] Enophthalmos is difficult to appreciate clinically.[1] Unilateral cutaneous facial and cervical hyperthermia, as well as excessive ipsilateral facial sweating (unique to the horse), can also occur.[1] Causes of Horner's syndrome reported in the horse include jugular vein and carotid artery injections, cervicothoracic spinal cord injury, cervical abscesses, guttural pouch disease or surgery, neoplasia or trauma of the neck and thorax, trauma to the vagosympathetic trunk, middle ear disease, traumatic lesions of the basisphenoid area, polyneuritis equi syndrome, equine protozoal myelitis of the cervical spinal cord, esophageal rupture, and trauma to the neck and thorax.[2,43,46-51]

Localization of the neuroanatomic lesion resulting in Horner's syndrome can be difficult. Lesions in the descending brainstem pathways, spinal cord, cord segments T1 to T3, sympathetic cell bodies, segmental ventral roots of T1 to T3, and the cervical sympathetic trunk are considered to be preganglionic.[47] Lesions associated with the cranial cervical ganglion and any of the sympathetic axons coursing to the eye are postganglionic.[47] Pharmaceutical testing for Horner's syndrome has been described elsewhere.[43] Mydriasis occurs more rapidly and extensively in the affected eye after topical application of 10% phenylephrine. The pattern of sweating may be helpful in localizing the lesion in horses. Postganglionic lesions usually exhibit a sharp demarcation of sweating at the level of the atlas.[42] Sweating may extend to the level of the axis (C2 to C3) in preganglionic lesions.[42] Facial nerve paralysis and laryngeal hemiplegia can also be found if there has been damage to adjacent neurologic structures with postganglionic lesions.[43]

Examination for Strabismus and Nystagmus

Disorders of cranial nerves III, IV, and VI, which innervate the extraocular muscles, result in abnormal position or movement of the globe. Characteristic forms of strabismus described for each of these nerves (see Table 1-2) should be present when the head is held in various positions.[42] Normal vestibular nystagmus as the head is moved from side to side requires intact cranial nerves III, IV, and VI, as well as a normal vestibular system (CN VIII). Spontaneous nystagmus when the head is in a normal position or positional nystagmus when the head is moved to another position indicates vestibular disease.[43] The character of the nystagmus may help to distinguish peripheral disease from central disease involving CN VIII. Nystagmus associated with peripheral disorders is usually horizontal or rotary, and the fast phase (directed away from the side of the lesion) remains constant despite changing the position of the head.[43] Nystagmus associated with central lesions can be horizontal, vertical, or rotary, and the fast phase is not consistent in presence or direction.[43] Visual accommodation that masks signs of a head tilt can occur within days in acute vestibular disease.[42] Blindfolding the horse may exacerbate clinical signs compensated for by vision, and blindness may interfere with visual compensation of nystagmus.[42]

Summary

In summary, the thorough ocular examination of the horse should proceed in a systematic manner (with some inherent variation between examiners) (Table 1-3). During the ocular examination, evaluation for the presence or absence of the problems listed in Table 1-3 and their associated differential diagnoses should be performed.

Table 1-3	Guidelines for the Ocular Examination	
What to Evaluate	**Lesion**	**Significance**
Globe (Whole Eyeball)		
Size	Enlarged	Possible chronic glaucoma; vision loss; pain; poor prognosis
	Small	Chronic uveitis, trauma; vision loss, sign of ERU; poor prognosis
Movement	No ocular mobility in one area (strabismus)	May be normal; horses have limited ocular motility
		May indicate neurologic abnormalities, CN III palsy (perform complete CN and neurologic examination)
Position	One or both eyes sunken in	May indicate that the eye(s) are smaller than normal (phthisis); may indicate chronic trauma/uveitis
		Age and emaciation may cause orbital fat atrophy; reversible with proper nutrition in cases of emaciation
	One or both eyes protruded	Space-occupying mass in the orbit—commonly associated with orbital masses—may be primary tumor or chronic inflammation or neoplasm of the sinuses. Skull radiographs and CT are recommended.
Eyelids and Periocular Structures		
Position	Drooping, lowered	Possible neurologic deficit, such as facial nerve palsy, Horner's syndrome; check guttural pouch, etc.
	Elevated, retracted	Associated with scarring of eyelid (cicatricial). Some mass lesions may be surgically corrected in some cases.
Movement	No eyelid mobility	Possible neurologic deficit, such as facial nerve palsy
Sensation	Decreased sensation	Damage to cranial nerve V; check also corneal and facial sensation; prognosis depends on source and location of lesion.
Mass lesion	Pedunculated, fleshy mass	Most commonly SCC; good prognosis for treatment if lesion is small (<1 cm). Most commonly periocular sarcoids; most are slowly growing; poor prognosis; frequent recurrence
	Smooth, nonulcerated, firm mass	
Alopecia	Normal skin	Probably normal if mild
	Ulcerated skin	Associated with self trauma; locate source of irritation (e.g., allergy, foreign body, other ocular pain)
Third Eyelid		
Position	Elevated	Usually associated with pain
		If depigmented, may appear elevated
Movement	Not able to retract/manually elevate	Associated with adhesions from previous trauma/injury
		Masses in third eyelid gland or base of third eyelid
Mass lesion	Fleshy, pedunculated mass	SCC most common on the leading edge of the third eyelid; may extend to surrounding conjunctiva (good prognosis if small)

Table 1-3	Guidelines for the Ocular Examination—cont'd	
What to Evaluate	**Lesion**	**Significance**
	Smooth, subconjunctival mass (soft and fluctuant)	Most likely prolapsed orbital fat is at the base of the third eyelid (usually only a cosmetic defect and does not alter vision).
Cornea		
Opacities	Gray or white, nonpainful	Corneal scar; not likely to progress (size, location, and density determine significance)
	Crystalline	Lipid infiltrate; may be associated with long-term steroid use, chronic inflammation (ERU), or metabolic abnormalities (e.g., Cushing's syndrome) (size, location, and density determine significance)
	Linear opacities	Corneal striae may be secondary to blunt trauma or chronic glaucoma.
Surface irregularities	Thickening	Corneal edema (bluish white) or cellular infiltrate (creamy white, yellow) usually indicates a chronic problem; and size, location, and density determine significance.
	Thinning/crater	Current or previous deep corneal ulcer; stain with fluorescein to see if active
	Punctate lesions	Most commonly associated with herpes virus keratitis (commonly recurrent) or early fungal infections (both have guarded prognosis)
Infiltration	Yellow-white or creamy (cellular) infiltration	Stromal abscess (dense yellow infiltrate with vascularization) or immune-mediated keratitis (mild vascularization and infiltrate)
	Vascular infiltration	Infected, progressive corneal ulcer if fluorescein-positive
Large branching vessels = superficial irritant (e.g., foreign body, superficial keratitis)
Straight short vessels = deep irritation (stromal abscess, uveitis, endophthalmitis)
Fluorescein retention	Uniformly green	Superficial corneal ulcer
	Only margins are green	Possible descemetocele or corneal laceration if associated with surface irregularities
Conjunctiva		
Inflammation	Hyperemic, palpebral, or bulbar conjunctiva	May be normal in excited or recently transported horses
Can be associated with bacterial or irritative conjunctivitis
With blepharospasm, commonly associated with corneal ulceration
Mass lesion	Raised, fleshy, pedunculated mass	Most commonly SCC
	Vascular mass	Possible granulation tissue or vascular tumors
Foreign body		Usually associated with significant discomfort; commonly located beneath the third eyelid or ventral conjunctival cul-de-sac
Anterior Chamber of the Eye		
Depth	Shallow	Chronic uveitis, phthisis bulbi
Swollen iris; active inflammation
Iris cysts/focal iris atrophy (especially light-colored irides)
Leakage of aqueous humor from corneal wound
Lens luxation (rare)
	Deep	Chronic glaucoma, posterior lens luxation
Contents	Hazy aqueous humor	Aqueous flare—sign of active uveitis
	Hyphema	Blood in the anterior chamber of the eye—usually secondary to trauma
	Hypopyon	Pus in the anterior chamber—chronic active uveitis, infectious endophthalmitis
	Other structures	Foreign bodies, cysts, etc.
Mass lesion	Pigmented	Uveal melanoma; usually benign masses in gray horses; look elsewhere for cutaneous or GI melanoma.
	White	Probably cellular infiltrate or fibrin; associated with chronic active uveitis
Iris		
Corpora nigra	Enlarged, smooth	Possible corpora nigra cyst or melanoma (ultrasound exam?)
	Small, atrophic	May be normal; if smooth and different from opposite eye, may indicate chronic uveitis (ERU)
Iris color	Darkened	May be normal; most horses have very pigmented irises
	Red	Sign of chronic uveitis
	Blue	Rare sign of active inflammation, hyphema
	White	Normal; usually a color variant in paints, Appaloosa, and other light-colored horses

Continued

Table 1-3   Guidelines for the Ocular Examination—cont'd

What to Evaluate	Lesion	Significance
Iris surface	Smooth/fibrotic	May indicate chronic uveitis
Pupil	Miotic	Exam performed in light that is too bright
	Dilated	Fixed; indicative of posterior synechia and chronic uveitis
	Abnormally shaped	Nonresponsive; retinal, optic nerve abnormality, CN III palsy, atropine administration, iris atrophy
		Congenital abnormalities; dyscoria (rare)
		Posterior synechia
Lens		
Position	Subluxated lens	Edge of lens visible—congenital microphakia, secondary to chronic glaucoma, trauma
	Anterior or posteriorly luxated	Shallow anterior chamber (anterior)
		Deep anterior chamber (posterior)
Opacity	Nuclear cataract	Rarely progresses; may be inherited; size, location, and density determine significance
	Anterior cortical cataract	Usually indicates chronic uveitis or is secondary to trauma; likely to progress; poor prognosis
	Posterior cortical cataract	
	Equatorial cataract	Usually indicates chronic uveitis; can be inherited; may or may not progress; fair prognosis
	Pigment on anterior lens capsule	Usually indicates chronic uveitis or is secondary to trauma; will progress; poor prognosis
		May be incidental or a sign of previous active uveitis (size, location, and density determine significance)
Vitreous		
Clarity/contents	Yellow/orange haze	Sign of previous active uveitis (size, location, and density determine significance)
	Cellular debris	Sign of previous active uveitis (size, location, and density determine significance)
Masses/neoplasms		Rare; poor prognosis
Retina		
Detachment	Partial	Possible chronic uveitis or secondary to trauma; dorsal detachment likely will progress
	Complete	Chronic uveitis, trauma; vision loss; sign of ERU; poor prognosis
Tapetal color	Red streaks	May be normal; usually a color variant in paints, Appaloosa, and other light-colored horses
	Mottled	
	Depigmented (choroidal vasculature visible)	May be normal; usually a color variant in paints, Appaloosa, other light-colored horses
	Hyperreflective	Chorioretinal scar—previous inflammation (size and location, and density determine significance)
Nontapetal color	Multifocal depigmented spots	Incidental finding; may be associated with previous parasite migration
		May be focal coloboma
	Peripapillary depigmentation	Focal (usually at 6 o'clock position); typical coloboma
		Diffuse—chronic chorioretinitis in ERU
	Diffuse depigmentation/hypopigmentation	Severe chorioretinitis; chronic, lower motor neuron disease; retinal detachment; very poor prognosis
		May be normal; usually a color variant in paints, Appaloosa, and other light-colored horses
Vascular attenuation	Focal peripapillary	Focal optic nerve degeneration (size, location, and density determine significance)
	Diffuse	Optic nerve atrophy; poor prognosis
Optic Nerve		
Color	White	Optic nerve atrophy; poor prognosis
	Salmon pink	Normal
	Dark gray	Optic nerve atrophy; poor prognosis
Size	Enlarged	Decreased vision; optic neuritis
	Small	Optic nerve atrophy; poor prognosis
Mass lesion	Focal	Normal vision + older horse—proliferative optic neuropathy—incidental findings
	Entire optic nerve	Decreased vision; exudative optic neuropathy; poor prognosis
		Optic neuritis, papillary edema, neoplasm (all rare and carry a poor prognosis)

ERU, Equine recurrent uveitis, *GI*, gastrointestinal; *SCC*, squamous cell carcinoma.

EXAMINATION OF THE FOAL

A healthy foal's behavior and responses to some aspects of the normal ocular examination can differ dramatically from those of the adult. Foals tend to respond to stimuli with exaggerated movements; however, they may also exhibit cataplexy or somnolence with firm restraint.[52] Because they can move rapidly from one state to the other, this can make the ophthalmic examination challenging and potentially dangerous.

Subconjunctival or episcleral hemorrhage resulting from birth trauma can be present and will resolve over 7 to 10 days as a bruise would (Fig. 1-20).[53] The menace response develops during the first 2 weeks of life and can therefore be normally absent or incomplete during that time.[6,52,54] However, in other reports a positive menace response has been described in all foals tested between 5 days and 19.5 weeks of age[55] and by 9 days of age.[56] The menace response may not develop symmetrically in both eyes.[56] In sick foals, decreased corneal sensation and tear production, as well as lagophthalmos, may be found[2,8,52,57,58]; thus a foal with a corneal ulcer may exhibit only mild or no discomfort, and healing may be delayed. However, healthy foals have even more sensitive corneas than adults.[2,57] The attachment of the iridocorneal angle pectinate ligaments to Descemet's membrane (i.e., gray line), observable only medially and laterally in the adult, may be observable 360 degrees around the limbus in a foal.[55,59]

The foal's pupil has been reported to be round at birth (Fig. 1-21), but it develops the horizontal elliptical shape of the adult pupil by about 5 days.[6,45,52,58,60-62] Foals older than 5 days have an oval pupil.[55,62]

Foals younger than 5 days have also been reported to have a sluggish PLR, but the reflex is present on day 1.[60,61] Foals, like cats, may exhibit mydriasis with a diminished second phase of the normal biphasic PLR as a result of increased sympathetic discharge under stress.[56]

A ventromedial strabismus, evaluated by noting the angle of the pupil in reference to the horizontal palpebral fissure, is also normally present (Fig. 1-22) and reaches a normal adult position by 1 month of age (Fig. 1-23).[52] Persistent pupillary membranes, usually iris to iris, can regress over the first 4 months of life.[59] Although the adult iris is normally brown, tan mottling may be seen in the peripheral irides of foals.[55]

The lens sutures are normally very prominent and should not be mistaken for a cataract.[6,62,63] Marked variation in lens suture patterns have been reported in foals.[55] The sutures are normally an upright Y anteriorly but vary from Y to sawhorse to stellate, with feathering posteriorly.[55] The anterior sutures may be difficult to

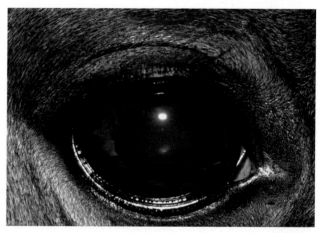

Fig. 1-21 The pupil of a foal is usually round until approximately 2 weeks of age. Tan mottling in the peripheral iris is also visible.

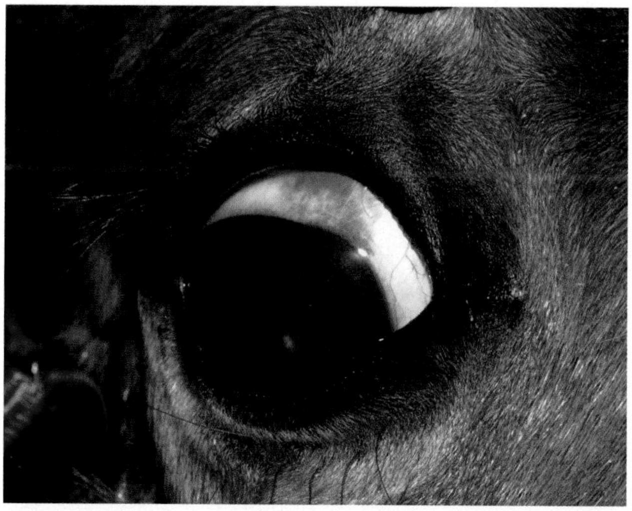

Fig. 1-20 Scleral hemorrhage is frequently present in prenatal foals.

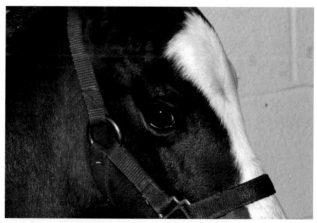

Fig. 1-22 A slight ventral medial strabismus can be seen in a foal. The angle of the pupil is not perfectly parallel to the eyelid margin.

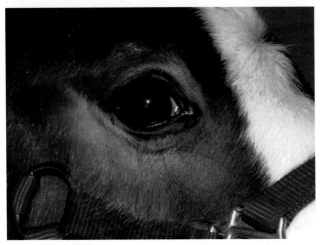

Fig. 1-23 An older foal in which strabismus has resolved. The angle of the pupil is now parallel to the eyelid margin.

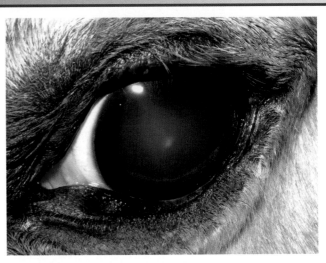

Fig. 1-24 Nuclear sclerosis gives this lens in an aged horse a faint blue appearance.

visualize in Thoroughbred foals.[55] Persistent hyaloid artery remnants may actually contain blood in the newborn, but these remnants generally disappear by 3 to 4 months of age.[53,59]

The tapetal color is highly correlated with coat color and tends toward yellow-green.[55] The optic disc is typically round with smooth margins; and light gray streaks, arcing nasally and temporally away from the optic disc margin in the nontapetal fundus, may be seen. These are thought to represent axon bundles in the nerve fiber layer.[2,55,58] Multifocal subretinal and retinal hemorrhages have also been detected in neonatal foals up to 1 to 2 weeks of age.[64] These hemorrhages are not associated with notable visual deficits, resolve quickly, and are thought to be associated with vascular hypertension and rupture during parturition, especially in larger foals.[64]

EXAMINATION OF THE GERIATRIC HORSE

Examination of the geriatric horse has been recently reviewed.[65] Most of the changes seen in geriatric horses are the result of "normal" aging processes (e.g., supraorbital fat atrophy, vitreal degeneration, focal chorioretinal pigment changes) (see Fig. 1-19). Nuclear sclerosis is a common aging sign found in horses at approximately 7 to 8 years of age.[66] It has also been reported in Grevyi's zebras (Equus grevyi) aged 16 to 25 years.[65] Nuclear sclerosis may appear opaque on transillumination (Fig. 1-24); however, the tapetal reflex and fundus can be visualized. In addition, suture lines and the lens capsule may become slightly more opaque with age.[66]

RESTRAINT AND SEDATION

Many horses can undergo a complete ocular examination without sedation. However, once vision has been assessed and the cranial nerve examination has been performed, sedation, analgesia, and local nerve blocks may be required to complete the ocular examination in some patients. Tranquilization with detomidine hydrochloride (Dormosedan, 0.02 to 0.04 mg/kg, administered intravenously) is preferred, because it provides rapid tranquilization without an excitation phase (either on induction or during recovery) and a steady head position without movement (such as the head "jerks" commonly associated with xylazine or butorphanol tartrate tranquilization). Xylazine (Rompun, Haver-Lockhart, 0.5 to 1.0 mg/kg, administered intravenously) can also be used.[2,4] Butorphanol tartrate (Torbugesic, Bristol Laboratories, 0.01 to 0.02 mg/kg, administered intravenously) may be added for painful procedures or additional restraint.[2,4] Other methods of restraint include the use of stocks and lip twitches. Again, the use of restraint and sedation depends on the temperament of the horse, the availability of equipment, and the comfort level of the handlers and examiner.

REGIONAL NERVE BLOCKS

Two ophthalmic nerves are frequently blocked during the equine ocular examination, the auriculopalpebral/ palpebral branch of the facial nerve (CN VII) and the frontal (supraorbital) branch of the trigeminal nerve (CN V).[67,68] When these nerves are blocked, akinesia and anesthesia, respectively, of the upper eyelid result.

Regional Akinesia

The most common nerve blocked is the palpebral branch of the auriculopalpebral nerve, which innervates the main muscle involved in closing the eyelid, the orbicularis oculi. The strength of this muscle in the horse necessitates its akinesia, especially when painful ocular conditions are present. Akinesia of this muscle is also extremely important in conditions in which the structural integrity of the globe is compromised, because the pressure applied by the muscle during manipulation for examination or during blepharospasm could result in rupture of the globe. Akinesia of the eyelids may be induced for routine eye examination, diagnostic procedures (e.g., corneal cytology and culture), therapy (e.g., subconjunctival injections, placement of a subpalpebral lavage), and standing surgeries.[67,68] More proximal branch blocks are generally preferred and more effective because of the extensive branching of the motor fibers.[38] Auriculopalpebral nerve block alone has been shown to have no effect on tonometry results and should be performed before tonometry for ease of performance of the procedure only.[69]

One to two milliliters of anesthetic is injected with a 25-gauge, ⅝-inch needle, adjacent to the nerve, and the injection site is massaged to facilitate anesthetic diffusion about the nerve.[2,4,38,67,68] Anesthetics most frequently used include lidocaine hydrochloride (Xylocaine) 2%, which has an onset of action of 4 to 6 minutes and a duration of 60 to 90 minutes, and mepivacaine (Carbocaine) 2%, with an onset of action of 3 to 5 minutes and a duration of 90 to 120 minutes.[2,4,38] Procaine or bupivacaine can also be used. Repeated injections of anesthetic may result in a refractory phenomenon, in which higher volumes are required and longer times to akinesia result.[38] The auriculopalpebral nerve block results in paralysis of the orbicularis muscle of the upper eyelid and variable paralysis of the lower eyelid for approximately 1 to 3 hours.[2,4,38] Ptosis, narrowing of the palpebral fissure, and easy manual elevation of the upper eyelid should result.[2,4,38] Sensation to the eyelids remains intact. The duration of anesthesia can be prolonged with the addition of epinephrine.[38]

The auriculopalpebral nerve branches from the main trunk of the facial nerve, where it is protected by the parotid gland for the full length of the caudal border of the ramus of the mandible.[38,43] It then emerges from beneath the gland just caudal to the caudal border of the condyle of the mandible, where it is covered by

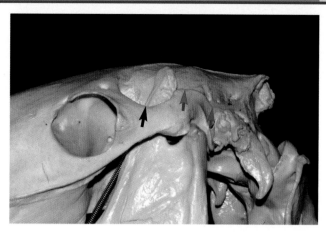

Fig. 1-25 Three sites at which the auriculopalpebral nerve can be blocked: caudal to the posterior ramus of the mandible *(blue arrow)*, dorsal to the highest point of the zygomatic arch *(red arrow)*, and where it lies on the zygomatic arch caudal to the bony process of the frontal bone *(black arrow).*

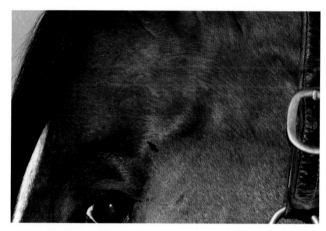

Fig. 1-26 Three sites at which the auriculopalpebral nerve can be blocked: caudal to the posterior ramus of the mandible *(blue arrow)*, dorsal to the highest point of the zygomatic arch *(red arrow)*, and where it lies on the zygomatic arch caudal to the bony process of the frontal bone *(black arrow).*

thin facial muscles and lies close to the rostral auricular artery and vein.[38] The branches then pass rostrally and dorsally to reach their destination. The caudal border of the ramus of the mandible and the zygomatic arch are palpable. The auriculopalpebral nerve can therefore be blocked at three sites (Figs. 1-25 and 1-26).[38,67,68]

- The auriculopalpebral nerve can be blocked subfascially in the depression just anterior to the base of the ear where the caudal border of the coronoid process of the mandible meets the zygomatic process of the temporal bone. At this point, the nerve emerges from the parotid salivary gland and becomes subcutaneous on the lateral aspect of the dorsal tip of the coronoid process (see Figs. 1-25 and 1-26).[38,67,68]

- The palpebral branch of the auriculopalpebral nerve can be blocked just lateral to the highest point of the caudal zygomatic arch where the nerve can actually be "strummed" through the skin by running a finger forcefully over the dorsal border of the bone (see Figs. 1-25 and 1-26).[67,68]

- The palpebral branch of the auriculopalpebral nerve can also be blocked where it lies on the zygomatic arch caudal to the bony process of the frontal bone (see Figs. 1-25 and 1-26).[67,68]

Regional Anesthesia and Analgesia

Sensation to the eyelids is provided by the ophthalmic and maxillary divisions of the trigeminal nerve (CN V) (Figs. 1-27 and 1-28).[38] The frontal, lacrimal, and infratrochlear nerves arise from the ophthalmic branch of CN V; whereas the zygomatic nerve arises from the maxillary branch of CN V.[10,38] The frontal (supraorbital) nerve innervates most of the central upper lid and is the only sensory block normally required for examination.[38] The lacrimal nerve innervates the lateral upper lid.[38] The infratrochlear nerve innervates the area of the medial canthus.[38] The zygomatic nerve innervates most of the lateral lower lid.[38] The nasociliary nerve, a branch of the maxillary branch of CN V, innervates the cornea.[38] Anesthesia of these nerves is sometimes necessary for eyelid and conjunctival biopsies or simple surgeries, as well as subpalpebral lavage placement in the horse. The anesthetics most frequently used are the same as those used for akinesia and include lidocaine hydrochloride (Xylocaine) and mepivacaine (Carbocaine). Infiltration anesthesia is the injection of anesthetic into an area of the lid where surgery is required or where a subpalpebral catheter will be placed. Anesthetic is deposited subcutaneously in a "line block" 8 mm from the lid margin or directly into the area desired.[19] The four main sensory nerve branches can be blocked directly as follows:

- The frontal (supraorbital) nerve is blocked as it emerges from the supraorbital foramen within the frontal bone (Figs. 1-28 and 1-29).[19,38] This foramen can be palpated if the examiner places his or her thumb and middle finger on the lateral cranial and caudal borders of the supraorbital process, respectively. The examiner then moves his or her fingers medially until a widening of the bone is appreciated and then places the index finger down midway between the thumb and middle finger (Fig. 1-30). A depression is usually palpable. This should be in the

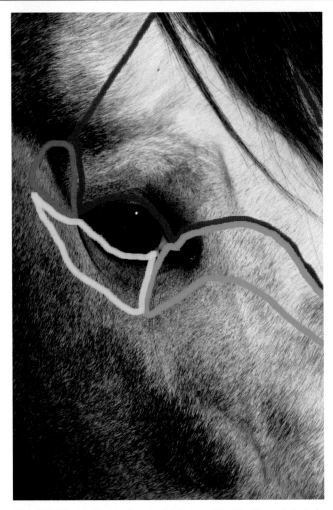

Fig. 1-27 Sensation to the eyelids is provided by the ophthalmic and maxillary divisions of the trigeminal nerve (CN V). The frontal, lacrimal, and infratrochlear nerves arise from the ophthalmic branch of CN V, whereas the zygomatic nerve arises from the maxillary branch of CN V. The approximate areas of sensation that would be blocked with each nerve are indicated as follows: frontal *(blue)*, lacrimal *(red)*, zygomatic *(yellow)*, infratrochlear *(green)*.

immediate area of the foramen. A 25-gauge, ⅝-inch needle is then inserted into or just over the foramen, and 1 to 2 ml of anesthetic is injected (Fig. 1-31). If the needle was passed into the foramen, another 1 to 2 ml is infiltrated subcutaneously as the needle is removed. However, injection into the foramen is unnecessary, and excellent results can be obtained with a subconjunctival injection over the foramen. The frontal nerve is mainly sensory, but this block can result in partial upper eyelid akinesia as well.[4]

- The lacrimal nerve can be blocked with a line block along the lateral third of the dorsal orbital rim (Figs. 1-28 and 1-32).

- The zygomatic nerve can be blocked with a line block along the ventrolateral orbital rim (Figs. 1.28 and 1-33).

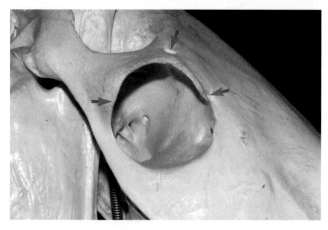

Fig. 1-28 Sensation to the eyelids is provided by the ophthalmic and maxillary divisions of the trigeminal nerve (CN V). The frontal *(blue arrow)*, lacrimal *(red arrow)*, and infratrochlear *(green arrow)* nerves arise from the ophthalmic branch of CN V, whereas the zygomatic *(yellow arrow)* nerve arises from the maxillary branch of CN V.

- The infratrochlear nerve can be blocked as it runs through the trochlear notch located medially on the dorsal orbital rim (Figs. 1-28 and 1-34). The notch can be palpated.

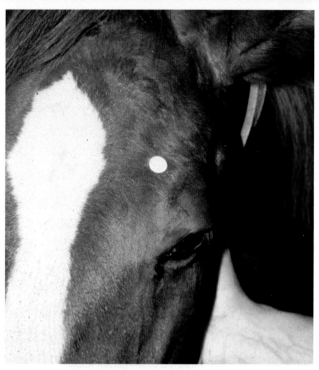

Fig. 1-29 The frontal (supraorbital) nerve is blocked as it emerges from the supraorbital foramen within the frontal bone, as shown on an equine head.

Retrobulbar Block

The retrobulbar nerve block temporarily blocks the optic (CN II) and oculomotor (CN III) nerves, as well as the abducens nerve (CN VI), trochlear nerve (CN IV), and the maxillary and ophthalmic branches of the trigeminal nerve (CN V). Retrobulbar anesthesia can be used as an adjunct to general anesthesia in horses to reduce nystagmus and enophthalmos during corneal and intraocular surgery.[70] It can also be used to perform standing eyelid and corneal surgeries, as well as to perform anterior or posterior chamber paracentesis for diagnostic purposes. Lastly, it can be used for the primary purpose of analgesia (e.g., during the immediate postoperative period after an enucleation). Three methods have been described for retrobulbar anesthesia in the horse and include the four-point block, modified Peterson block, and direct injection into the orbital cone above or below the zygomatic arch.

The site above the zygomatic arch and caudal to the temporal process of the malar bone is preferred because it requires a single injection; is not located near the globe, and if performed properly, avoids the direct location of the optic nerve. The orbital fossa above the dorsal orbital rim and zygomatic arch is clipped and aseptically prepped with povidone-iodine (Betadine) scrub and alcohol. Care must be taken to avoid getting surgical scrub or alcohol on the ocular

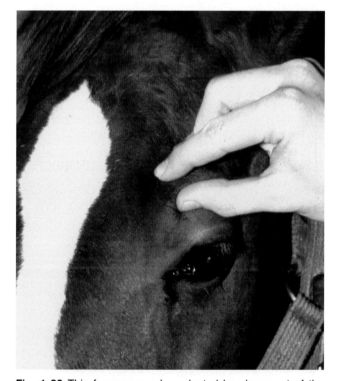

Fig. 1-30 This foramen can be palpated by placement of the thumb and middle finger on the lateral cranial and caudal borders of the supraorbital process, respectively. The examiner then moves his or her fingers medially until a widening of the bone is appreciated and then places the index finger down midway between the thumb and middle finger. A depression is usually palpable. This should be in the immediate area of the foramen.

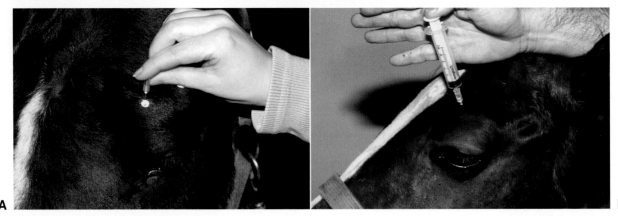

A **B**

Fig. 1-31 A, A 25-gauge, ⅝-inch needle is inserted into or just over the foramen and 1 to 2 ml of anesthetic is injected. **B,** A 25-gauge, ⅝-inch needle can be inserted directly into the foramen. An additional 1 to 2 ml of anesthetic is infiltrated subcutaneously as the needle is removed.

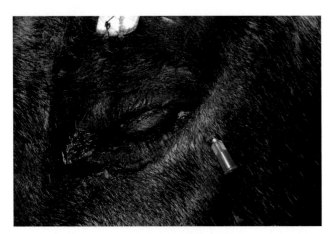

Fig. 1-32 The lacrimal nerve can be blocked by using a line block along the lateral third of the dorsal orbital rim.

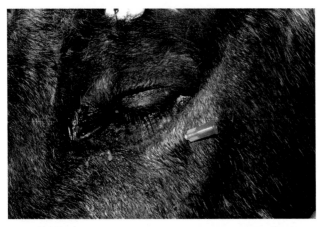

Fig. 1-33 The zygomatic nerve can be blocked with a line block along the ventrolateral orbital rim.

surface because severe irritation and corneal ulceration may develop. A 22-gauge, 2.5-inch spinal needle is placed through the skin perpendicular to the skull, in the orbital fossa, just posterior to the posterior aspect of the dorsal orbital rim (Fig. 1-35). The needle is advanced posterior to the globe until it reaches the retrobulbar orbital cone. When the needle advances to this location, the eye will have a slight dorsal movement as the needle passes through the fascia of the dorsal retrobulbar cone into the retrobulbar space. The needle is advanced until it just passes into the cone, evidenced by the sudden release of the eye back to normal position or a slight "popping" sensation. Once the needle is positioned, 10 to 12 ml of 2% lidocaine hydrochloride is injected into the retrobulbar space. Mepivacaine (Carbocaine) and epinephrine can also be deposited. Aspiration, before injection, should be performed to make sure the needle is not positioned within a blood vessel. During the injection the globe is pushed externally (i.e., slight exophthalmos), indicating an accurate placement of anesthetic. Onset of anesthesia usually occurs within 5 to 10 minutes. The duration of effect is approximately 1 to 2 hours. Ocular sensation, blink reflex, and vision will be compromised during this time. Therefore stall rest and protection of the eye with lubricants are recommended for 2 to 4 hours after anesthesia.

Retrobulbar injections with lidocaine have been performed routinely to provide ocular anesthesia, with and without general anesthesia, for ocular surgery at the North Carolina State University College of Veterinary Medicine for approximately 12 years. From 1996 to 2001, 189 retrobulbar injections were performed. Only two complications were documented. One horse had a hypersensitivity to lidocaine, which resulted in generalized formation of hives and severe retrobulbar swelling after surgery. These lesions resolved with the

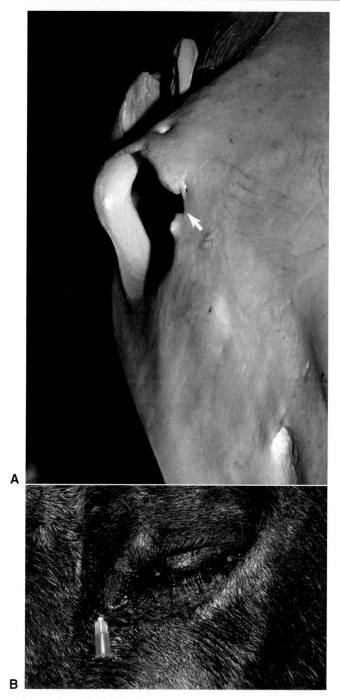

A

B

Fig. 1-34 A, The infratrochlear nerve can be blocked as it runs through the trochlear notch located medially on the dorsal orbital rim on the equine skull *(arrow)*. B, The infratrochlear nerve can be blocked as it runs through the trochlear notch located medially on the dorsal orbital rim. The notch can be palpated.

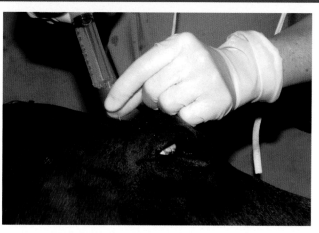

Fig. 1-35 Retrobulbar block. The site above the zygomatic arch and caudal to the temporal process of the malar bone is preferred because it requires a single injection; it is not located near the globe; and if the block is performed properly, the direct location of the optic nerve is avoided. The orbital fossa above the dorsal orbital rim and zygomatic arch is clipped and aseptically prepped. A 22-gauge, 2.5-inch spinal needle is placed through the skin perpendicular to the skull, in the orbital fossa, just posterior to the posterior aspect of the dorsal orbital rim.

The four-point block, a local muscle block, has also been described for retrobulbar anesthesia in the horse (Fig. 1-36).[19] Five to ten milliliters of lidocaine or mepivacaine can be deposited laterally by passing a 20-gauge, 7.5-cm (3-inch) needle through the lateral canthus skin and following the globe posteriorly. Ventrally, the needle passes through the skin or bulbar conjunctiva posteriorly. The needle should be directed slightly nasally to avoid the optic nerve. Nasally, the needle passes through the base of the elevated third eyelid and posteriorly into the orbit. Dorsally, the needle is passed through the center of the upper eyelid following the globe posteriorly. This technique should not be used when intraocular surgery is performed because it may put pressure on the globe.[19] Failure to inject anesthetic into the muscle cone or injecting it in front of the orbital septum may cause the drug to migrate forward under the conjunctiva and cause severe chemosis.[19]

Use of a modified Peterson block has been described in the horse, although it would rarely have application in most types of ocular surgery.[70] This block is specifically designed for cattle but has been modified for the horse. The risk of sudden death described in cattle makes this technique less than desirable, and it is not discussed in detail here.

Although few complications have been seen after retrobulbar and eyelid nerve blocks in horses, rare problems associated with the injections can occur during or after the surgical procedure.[70] Bacteria can be deposited

use of systemic nonsteroidal antiinflammatory and antihistamine medications within 3 days of surgery. In the second horse, a corneal ulcer developed after surgery, likely caused by exposure of the cornea because of poor eyelid function and corneal desensitization.

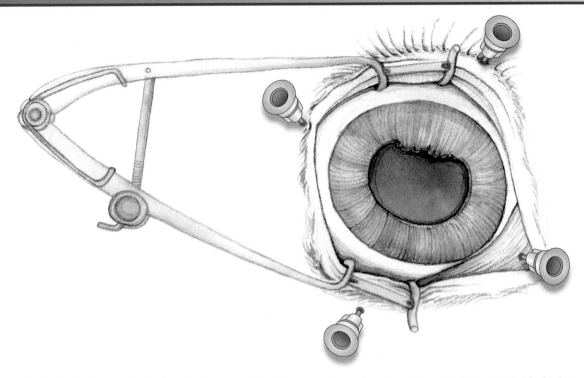

Fig. 1-36 The four-point block, a local muscle block, has also been described for retrobulbar anesthesia in the horse.

in the orbit by the spinal needle if the skin surgical site was not aseptically prepared. This may result in orbital abscess or cellulitis formation. Laceration of the extraocular muscles, optic nerve, sclera, or ophthalmic arteries by the needle is also possible during the injection. Traumatic injury during needle introduction could result in retrobulbar hemorrhage or optic neuritis. An isolated case of oculocardiac reflex elicitation during the block has also been reported.[71] These complications can be mostly avoided by use of appropriate tranquilization, eyelid nerve blocks, antiseptic technique, and added restraint methods to restrict movement by a standing horse. The relatively low complication rate associated with the injection techniques far outweighs the risks associated with general anesthesia in horses.

Orbital Aspiration

Aspiration of a lesion (e.g., mass, fluid) in the equine orbit can be performed for cytology, culture, and histopathologic examination.[38,39] An 18-gauge, 10-cm, slightly curved needle is inserted 1 cm lateral to the lateral canthus and then directed posteriorly in a line parallel to the medial canthus.[2,72] Damage to the globe, orbital vessels, or optic nerve is possible during use of this technique, as in retrobulbar anesthesia. Going behind the globe through the supraorbital fossa is also

an option. Ultrasound-guided fine-needle aspiration, versus blind aspiration, may decrease the risk of injuring orbital structures.

BASIC OPHTHALMIC EXAMINATION AND DIAGNOSTIC PROCEDURES

Schirmer Tear Test

The Schirmer tear test (STT) is the test most commonly used to measure aqueous tear production.[38,39] In the test a filter paper strip is placed in the conjunctival sac, and wetting is then measured in millimeters per 60 seconds. Commercial filter paper strips available include standardized Sno Strips (AKorn) and Color Bar (Eagle Vision, Schering-Plough).[19,38,39] Strips can also be made from Whatmann filter paper (No. 40, 5 × 40 mm with a notch 5 mm from the end).[19,38,39] The Schirmer I, in which no topical anesthesia is used, measures the approximate amount of basal and reflex tearing. The Schirmer II test, performed after the application of topical anesthesia, theoretically only measures basal secretion. Some residual tear volume may make both of these measurements slightly inaccurate. The STT should be performed before manipulation of the eye and orbit during examination to minimize reflex tearing. There are no reports of the effect of an auriculopalpebral nerve block on the STT in horses.

Deficiencies in aqueous tear production have rarely been reported in the horse.[1,73-81] Therefore the STT is not a part of the routine ophthalmic examination in the horse. An STT would be indicated if evidence of CN VII dysfunction (e.g., after trauma, facial paralysis) is observed; if the cornea or conjunctiva appear dry; if tenacious mucoid discharge, corneal vascularization, or persistent corneal ulceration is present; or if an underlying cause cannot be identified. Keratoconjunctivitis sicca is most commonly the result of CN V or VII trauma but has also been reported in cases of fractures of the mandible and stylohyoid bone, locoweed poisoning, eosinophilic dacryoadenitis, and in association with corneal stromal sequestration.[22,73-81]

STT values for healthy horses and foals, sick foals, horses under halothane anesthesia, and horses that have had their third eyelid removed have been reported.[82-85] The effects of age, season, environment, sex, time of day, and placement of strips on STT results in healthy horses and ponies have also been reported.[86] A wide variability between eyes and between the same eye during different times of the day can be found, and this appears to be unrelated to signalment, housing, or season.[86] In general, the STT value in the horse is much greater than that in cats and dogs.[72,82,84] Absorption of tears on the STT strip in horses is not linear; therefore values cannot easily be extrapolated from times when the strip is held in the eye for less than a minute.[65] Healthy horses have been reported to have an STT I range of 11 to greater than 30 mm wetting/min and 15 to 20 mm/30 seconds.[73,82] Both sick and healthy neonatal foals have been reported to have lower STT values than adults.[57,58] STT I values of 14.2 ± 1 mm, 12.8 ± 2.4, and 18.3 ± 2.1 mm wetting/min were reported for sick neonatal foals, healthy neonatal foals, and healthy adult horses, respectively.[58] No differences were noted between sick and healthy foals.[57]

Two comparisons of STT I and STT II values in the horse exist.[81,84] The difference was minimal in one study (i.e., STT I and STT II values of 12.7 ± 9.1 mm wetting/min and 9.9 mm ± 4.25 mm wetting/min).[83] The second study did not reveal a difference between STT I and STT II values.[86] This is in contrast to the dog, in which the STT I value is significantly higher than the STT II value.[87] Stimulation of one eye may result in increased tearing in the contralateral eye and has been reported in horses after removal of the nictitans.[22,83] However, this does not appear to be consistent.[84] Sedation with xylazine does not affect the STT value. However, general inhalant anesthesia with halothane does lower the STT value for up to 3 hours.[84]

Borderline STT measurements (e.g., measurements of 10 to 15 mm wetting/min) should always be repeated. Comparison of tear test results between two eyes should be cautiously interpreted in clinical assessment of decreased tearing.[86] In general, repeatable measurements of less than 10 mm wetting/min should be considered abnormal, in conjunction with clinical signs.[19,22] Evaporative dry eye disorders have not been documented in the horse, although damage to CN VII and resultant inability to blink would contribute to increased evaporation.[22]

Corneoconjunctival Culture and Cytology

The technique for corneoconjunctival culture and cytology is similar to that performed in other species and has been well described in the literature.[38,39] The use of corneal or conjunctival culture and cytology during the ocular examination is of extreme importance in the horse because of the preponderance of infectious causes of ocular disease.[2] Culture and cytology of the ocular surface is indicated in horses with all forms of ulcerative keratitis (e.g., nonhealing, melting, cellular infiltrate); purulent ocular or nasolacrimal discharge; infectious blepharitis or conjunctivitis; and proliferative masses of the cornea, conjunctiva, and nictitans.[1,2] Although the results of microbial culture and cytologic evaluation are usually comparable, discordant results are also possible.[88] Negative results of cytologic evaluation in conjunction with positive microbial culture results may result from inadequate cytologic sampling (e.g., wrong area, not deep enough), the presence of too few microorganisms, and poor staining techniques.[89] Negative results on microbial culture in conjunction with positive cytologic findings may result from inadequate sampling or specimen handling, failure of the microbial culture (e.g., inappropriate media, nutrient-variant *Streptococcus* spp.), and contamination.[89]

Culture

Culture and sensitivity testing can aid in the diagnosis and determination of appropriate antimicrobial therapy in many equine ocular diseases. Specimens for culture should be obtained as early as possible in the examination, before the administration of topical preparations (e.g., proparacaine, fluorescein).[38] Because topical anesthesia is routinely used in the workup of painful ocular disease in the horse, it is important to note that some topical drugs (e.g., proparacaine, tetracaine) have been reported to inhibit organism growth.[90] However, it has also been shown that a single application of proparacaine is unlikely to affect culture results.[91] In reality, some horses are in so much pain that even in the face of sedation and regional nerve blocks, they will not allow the examiner to obtain an appropriate sample without topical anesthesia. Unfortunately, the results of culture, and especially sensitivity testing, are frequently not available in time to affect therapeutic decisions.[38]

Culture of the ocular surface can be performed with sterile moistened, Dacron-tipped swabs or the blunt end of a sterile surgical blade. The Dacron-tipped swab is rubbed or rolled (Fig. 1-37) over the area to be cultured and the blunt end of the surgical blade is used in a scraping motion (Fig. 1-38). The eyelids should be retracted to prevent contamination of the sample, if the eyelids are not the object of the sample collection. Samples should be taken from both the center and the edges of a corneal ulcer.[38] Application of a topical anesthetic can usually be avoided when a Dacron-tipped swab is used but is usually required when a surgical blade is used.[38]

Culture and sensitivity choices should be made on the basis of clinical signs, the ocular tissue being cultured, and the region and environment in which the horse is living. Both aerobic and fungal culture and sensitivity testing are usually indicated for most cases. Anaerobic testing may be indicated in some circumstances, and fungal testing is not required if the region does not indicate it (e.g., Northwestern United States). Fungal pathogens of the equine eye are usually saprophytic fungi that require enriched medium such as Sabouraud dextrose agar or blood agar.[2,38] Fungal or bacterial pathogens can also be so deep within the cornea that a diagnostic sample cannot be obtained, especially in the case of a stromal abscess. Culture of equine herpesvirus-2 (EHV-2) from the cornea has also been reported.[92,93] Viral culture or isolation usually requires that the sample be placed in a sterile saline solution in an Eppendorf tube, but instructions should be obtained directly from the testing laboratory.

Cytology

Cytology is a quick, simple, and indispensable method for characterizing the type of inflammatory (i.e., neutrophilic, lymphocytic, or eosinophilic) process present and may also assist in making a diagnosis (e.g., bacteria or fungal hyphae present).[38] Cytology is indicated in all cases of ulcerative keratitis in the horse. Cytology can provide rapid results that may guide the immediate course of therapy.[94-96]

Tools for collecting cytologic samples include instruments that are also used to obtain samples for culture (i.e., Dacron-tipped swabs, blunt end of a sterile scalpel blade), as well as cytobrushes and spatulas.[2,38] Topical anesthetic, microscope slides, slide stain, and a microscope are also required.[38] A microscope slide alone can be used to perform "impression" cytology. This method is probably not effective in identifying pathologic organisms in the case of corneal disease but may be helpful in situations such as the presence of an ulcerative eyelid mass.

The cotton- or Dacron-tipped swab provides the least traumatic method of retrieving adequate exfoliative samples.[95] This technique is recommended when excessive manipulation is contraindicated (e.g., deep or melting corneal ulceration).[38] Use of a spatula or the blunt end of a scalpel blade is a more precise method of collecting cells from specific areas, and greater numbers of deeper cells can usually be obtained (Fig. 1-39).[38] However, this method may also result in greater damage to the sample and eye.[38] As in the collection of samples for culture, topical anesthetic is probably required with any instrument except the Dacron-tipped swab.[38] The cytobrush has proved to be superior in all cytologic parameters studied when compared with cotton-wool tips and two different spatulas in dogs, cats, sheep, goats, cattle, and horse.[95,97] The large size of the

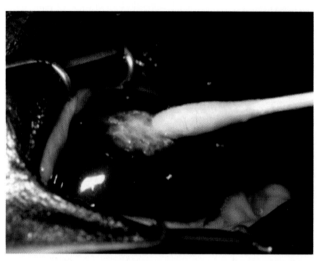

Fig. 1-37 Culture of the ocular surface can be performed with sterile, moistened, Dacron-tipped swabs. The Dacron-tipped swab is rubbed or rolled over the area to be cultured.

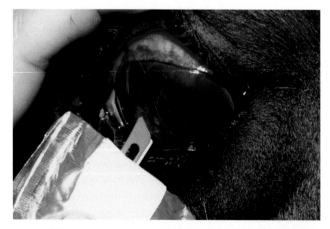

Fig. 1-38 Culture of the ocular surface can be performed with a sterile surgical blade; the blunt end of the surgical blade is used in a scraping motion.

cytobrush is a disadvantage in the eyes of small animals but not in the large equine eye. A cytobrush was used to obtain a cytologic sample in a report in which a *Histoplasma* species was identified in a case of equine keratitis.[97]

Care must be taken with all samples, during collection or transfer to the slides, to prevent cell damage and to gently form a monolayer. The examiner should roll the swab gently, should not "spin" the cytobrush, and should not use excessive force with the blade edge, because this leads to greater cell damage.[95] Commonly used stains include the Gram stain and various Romanowsky-type stains (e.g., Diff-Quik, Wright-Giemsa stain) (Fig. 1-40). The Romanowsky-type stains can be used for quick "screening" in cases of ulcerative keratitis when information is needed to formulate an initial therapeutic plan. The Romanowsky-type stains are generally satisfactory for detection of bacteria, fungal hyphae, yeast bodies, inflammatory cells, and neoplastic cells. The Gram stain is indicated to provide further information about identified bacteria. Fungal hyphae may be difficult to identify on routine staining and may require more specialized stains for fungal elements, which include periodic acid–Schiff (Fig. 1-41) and Gomori's methenamine silver stain (Fig. 1-42).[98] In addition to routine staining, newer tests are becoming available for infectious diseases in the horse; these include the polymerase chain reaction (PCR) and immunofluorescent antibody test for herpes (i.e., EHV-1, EHV-2, EHV-4) and fungal DNA on corneal or conjunctival cytologic and histopathologic specimens (Fig. 1-43).[99-101] The samples should be collected as directed by the testing laboratory, and this usually includes placing the cytologic scraping or biopsy

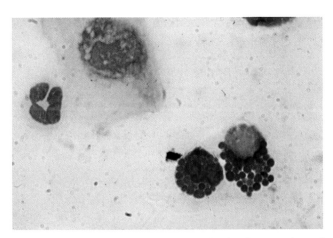

Fig. 1-39 Use of a Kimura spatula (pictured) or the blunt end of a scalpel blade provides a more precise method of collecting cells from specific areas, and greater numbers of deeper cells can usually be obtained.

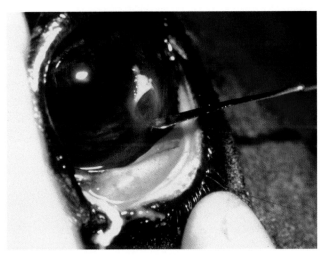

Fig. 1-40 Commonly used stains include the Gram stain and various Romanowsky-type stains (e.g., Diff-Quik, Wright-Giemsa stain). Two equine eosinophils are present on this Wright-Giemsa–stained slide. The equine eosinophil is unique in appearance and is not a routine finding. An epithelial cell and a neutrophil are also seen.

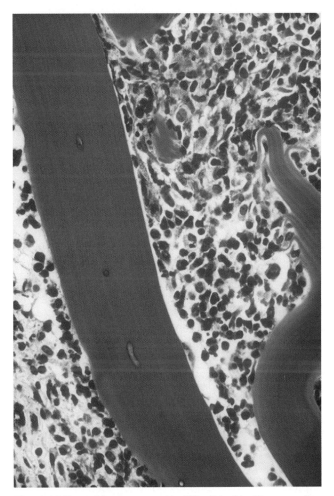

Fig. 1-41 Fungal hyphae may be difficult to identify on routine staining. More specialized stains for fungal elements include periodic acid–Schiff. Descemet's membrane and the epithelium stain a dark pink with periodic acid–Schiff. The fungal hyphae can be seen as clear bodies within Descemet's membrane.

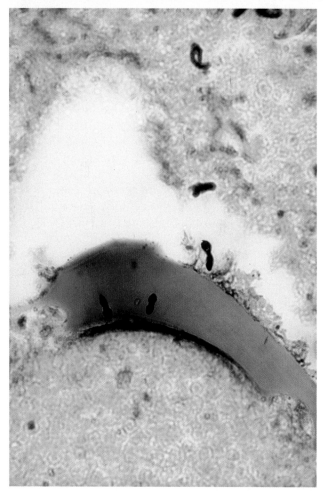

Fig. 1-42 Fungal hyphae may be difficult to identify on routine staining. More specialized stains for fungal elements include Gomori's methenamine silver stain. The cornea stains blue-green and the fungal hyphae stain black or dark brown.

A   F   G   U   Ac   Fc   -   B   Bc

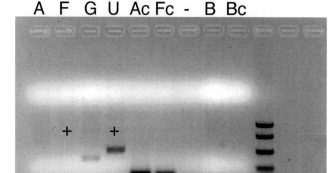

Fig. 1-43 Polymerase chain reaction for fungal DNA.

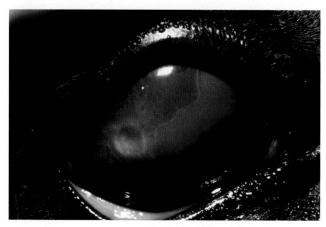

Fig. 1-44 In a corneal ulceration, the hydrophilic fluorescein binds to the corneal stroma, but not to the epithelium or to Descemet's membrane, resulting in a green stain.

specimen in sterile saline solution and freezing it. PCR testing can also be performed on formalin-fixed tissue blocks. Topical fluorescein staining can interfere with test results (i.e., cause false-positive results), and therefore samples for immunofluorescent antibody testing should be collected before fluorescein staining.[38,102]

Ophthalmic Dyes

Sodium Fluorescein

Topical ophthalmic dyes are routinely used in veterinary medicine to aid in the diagnosis of corneal, conjunctival, and nasolacrimal diseases. Commonly used topical ophthalmic dyes include sodium fluorescein, rose bengal, Alcian blue, Trypan blue, and methylene blue.[38,103-105] Sodium fluorescein and rose bengal dyes are the two

most commonly used stains in clinical veterinary ophthalmology.[38,106-108] Indications for the use of topical ophthalmic dyes in the horse include determining the health and integrity of the corneal and conjunctival epithelium and the physiologic flow of the nasolacrimal system. Intravenous sodium fluorescein is used to perform fluorescein angiography and is discussed later.

The most common use for topical sodium fluorescein is in the detection of ulcerative keratitis, but it will also stain conjunctival ulcerations and abrasions. In a corneal ulceration, the hydrophilic fluorescein binds to the corneal stroma, but not to the epithelium or to Descemet's membrane (Fig. 1-44). Small quantities can also pool or diffuse through intact epithelial cell intercellular spaces to reveal weakly staining epithelial microcysts and partial-thickness microerosions.[38,104,109,110] From the stroma, the dye can then readily pass through Descemet's membrane and the corneal endothelium to enter the aqueous humor and can be quantified (e.g., by fluorophotometry).

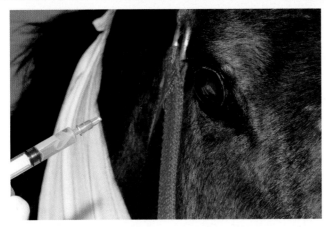

Fig. 1-45 The easiest method of applying topical fluorescein to horses is to place a sterile fluorescein strip in a 3-ml syringe, fill the syringe with sterile eyewash and replace the plunger, and then squirt the solution through the hub of a 25-gauge needle in which the actual needle has been manually broken off.

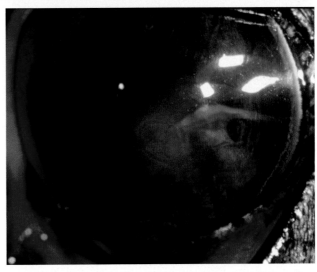

Fig 1-46 Rose bengal stain uptake in an equine corneal ulceration. (Photograph courtesy Dr. Stacy Andrew.)

Fluorescein staining of the cornea is indicated for almost every condition in the horse involving its eye and orbit—including a red or painful eye, discharge from the eye, an obvious corneal irregularity, and history of ocular trauma—and for assessment of physiologic naso-lacrimal function. The possible catastrophic results of not identifying and adequately treating a corneal ulceration in a horse make this test an absolute necessity.

Fluorescein is available as a sterile 0.5% to 2.0% alkaline solution or as a sterile impregnated paper strip.[38,111] The impregnated paper strips should be used for topical application because the solutions have been associated with bacterial contamination.[38,112] Other equipment needed to perform the stain includes sterile eyewash solution and a 3-ml syringe with a 25-gauge needle. The easiest method of applying topical fluorescein to horses is to place a sterile fluorescein strip in a 3-ml syringe, fill the syringe with sterile eyewash and replace the plunger, and then squirt the solution through the hub of a 25-gauge needle in which the actual needle has been manually broken off (Fig. 1-45).[2,19] After application, the eyelids should be closed or the animal should be allowed to blink to distribute the stain evenly across the ocular surfaces.[38] Excess fluorescein can be removed with gentle irrigation, but this may irritate the horse and may not be required. The use of an ultraviolet or blue light, usually available on a direct ophthalmoscope or the slit-lamp biomicroscope, may improve visualization of the stain but is usually not required.[38] False-positive results may occur after the use of proparacaine topical anesthesia or if direct contact between the paper strip and cornea occurs, which may leave a mark that resembles a corneal defect.[19,38]

Fluorescein may also be used to detect the leakage of aqueous humor through the cornea (i.e., Seidel test).[19,38]

The Seidel test can be used to detect full-thickness corneal injuries or to determine whether a corneal suture is leaking. The application of sodium fluorescein without subsequent irrigation results in a high dye concentration in which the dye fluoresces at wavelengths closer to the yellow and orange spectra. With or without gentle pressure on the cornea, aqueous leakage locally dilutes the fluorescein, and the dye fluoresces green.[38]

Rose Bengal

Rose bengal (i.e., dichloro-tetra-iodo-fluorescein) has been used to aid in the diagnosis of preocular tear film disorders, mucin preocular film deficiencies, and superficial corneal epithelial abnormalities in veterinary medicine (Fig. 1-46).[38] It can be used primarily or after sodium fluorescein application. Rose bengal stains dead and degenerating cells and mucus.[104] However, rose bengal has a dose-dependent ability to stain normal cells and this ability is normally blocked by tear film components.[38,103,104] Therefore stain uptake may indicate tear film abnormalities, such as a mucin deficiency, more accurately than cell viability.[38,103,104]

Rose bengal, like sodium fluorescein, is available both as an impregnated paper strip and a solution.[38,106,107] The use of the 0.5% or lower concentrations can minimize the irritation that can be associated with the 1% solution.[38] The dye has also been shown to be toxic to corneal epithelium at routine concentrations.[113] Slit-lamp biomicroscopy may be necessary for adequate visualization of rose bengal stain.[38]

The use of rose bengal would be indicated in the horse in any of the conditions in which corneal or conjunctival ulceration is suspected, but especially when a viral or fungal cause is suspected. Tear film abnormalities have not been extensively studied in the horse.[24] However, rose bengal staining is indicated and has been shown to reveal ocular surface damage in the presence of keratomycosis.[114] Specimens obtained from horses with painful eyes should be stained with both fluorescein and rose bengal because early fungal ulcers may be negative for fluorescein but positive for rose bengal.[24,114]

Nasolacrimal System

The physiologic patency of the nasolacrimal system can be evaluated with topical sodium fluorescein.[38] Fluorescein is applied as previously described and is not rinsed from the eye. Passage of the fluorescein to the lower puncta in the nares (Jones test) is timed and should occur within 5 minutes but may take up to 20 minutes (Fig. 1-47).[19] The required time for passage is influenced by the amount of fluorescein placed, tear production, and length of the individual horse's nasolacrimal system.[19] A positive test result is definitive for a patent nasolacrimal duct but does not prove that both puncta are patent.[19] A negative test result is only suggestive of a problem and may even be normal in the horse because of the large volume capacity of the nasolacrimal duct.[19,25,115] However, the nasolacrimal duct should be irrigated if the dye fails to appear and clinical signs suggest a problem. In addition to failure of passage of fluorescein stain, manual irrigation of the nasolacrimal duct to detect anatomic patency is also indicated in horses that have epiphora (watery ocular discharge) without an obvious cause, mucopurulent ocular or nasal punctal discharge, or dacryohemorrhea.[19,38,116]

The procedure can be performed retrograde (i.e., from the distal nares' opening) or normograde (i.e., from the eyelid puncta).[38] Sedation is usually required to perform either procedure in the horse. Retrograde irrigation through the distal opening to the nasolacrimal duct is easiest to perform (Fig. 1-48) because of the larger size of the opening.[19,116] The size of the lower orifice is variable, but it can usually be cannulated by a number 5-6 polyethylene urinary catheter.[19] Suitable catheters are 4 to 6 Fr canine urinary catheters, 5 Fr feeding tubes, or polyethylene tubing.[19] The largest catheter that will pass through the bony canal in an adult is a number 6 Fr urinary catheter.[19] The tip of the catheter, after it has been coated with lidocaine gel, is inserted into the punctal opening. Digital pressure should be applied to the opening to prevent normograde loss of fluid. A 12- to 20-ml syringe, previously filled with eyewash, is attached, and gentle irrigation of the nasolacrimal duct is performed until fluid exits the upper puncta near the medial canthus of the eye. Sneezing by the horse is common during this procedure and may be violent. A list of supplies needed to perform nasolacrimal duct irrigation can be found in Box 1-3.

If retrograde irrigation is unsuccessful, then normograde irrigation from the upper puncta should be attempted with a lacrimal canula, open-ended tomcat catheter, or teat tube syringe (Fig. 1-49).[19] The puncta in the lower eyelid are usually slightly larger and easier to cannulate than the puncta in the upper eyelid.[19] Gentle pulse pressure may be required to unblock an obstructed duct. Excessive force in the placement of the catheter or during irrigation should be avoided because significant damage to the nasolacrimal duct

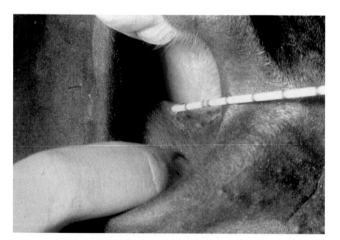

Fig. 1-48 Retrograde irrigation through the distal opening to the nasolacrimal duct is easiest to perform. The tip of the catheter, after it has been coated with lidocaine gel, is inserted into the punctal opening. Digital pressure should be applied to the opening to prevent normograde loss of fluid. The 12-ml syringe, previously filled with eyewash, is attached, and gentle irrigation of the nasolacrimal duct is performed until fluid exits the upper punctum near the medial canthus of the eye.

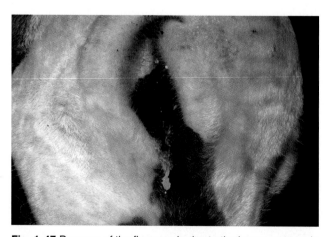

Fig. 1-47 Passage of the fluorescein dye to the lower punctum in the nares (Jones test) is timed and should occur within 5 minutes but may take up to 20 minutes in the horse.

could result.[19] Ducts that are compromised by a foreign body or other anatomic obstruction (e.g., after trauma, mass effect) may not be effectively irrigated.[19,38] Skull radiographs and a contrast dye study (e.g., dacryocystorhinography) should be performed next if the duct cannot be irrigated.

Transillumination and Retroillumination

The technique of direct focal illumination for inspection of the anterior structures of the eye is referred to as transillumination and should be performed both

<table>
<tr><td>**Box 1-3**</td><td>Supplies Needed for Irrigation of the Nasolacrimal Duct</td></tr>
</table>

- Topical anesthetic (proparacaine) for normograde
- Lidocaine gel for retrograde
- Catheters
  - *Normograde:* open-ended tomcat catheter, lacrimal canula, teat tube syringe
  - *Retrograde:* open-ended tomcat catheter, 4-6 Fr polyethylene urinary catheter, 5 Fr feeding tubes, or polyethylene tubing
- A 12- to 20-ml syringe
- Sterile eyewash or balanced salt solution

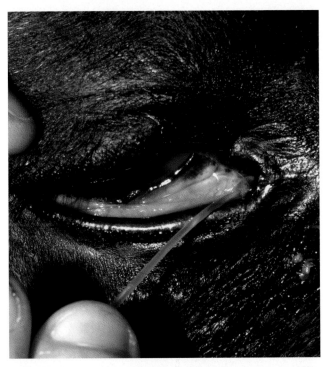

Fig. 1-49 Normograde irrigation from the upper puncta should be attempted if the result of the Jones test is negative and the duct cannot be irrigated from the nasal puncta. Catheterization of the punctum in the lower eyelid is demonstrated.

before and after mydriasis. It can be performed with a Finoff transilluminator (Welch-Allyn), direct ophthalmoscope, slit-lamp biomicroscope, or even a penlight. Retroillumination is performed by viewing the lens and aqueous and vitreous humors through a direct ophthalmoscope (arm's distance away) or biomicroscope.

The Purkinje-Sanson reflexes are three reflections produced by the light source during transillumination (Fig. 1-50).[19] Disease may alter the sharpness and location of these reflexes. The first, largest, and most anterior is the Sanson-Sanson reflex, which originates from the cornea. The second originates from the anterior lens capsule, and the third and most posterior originates from the posterior lens capsule. If a slit-lamp biomicroscope is used, two corneal reflexes are seen from the anterior surface and from the endothelium.[19] The corneal and anterior lens capsule reflex will move in the same direction as a change in the light position; the posterior lens capsule reflex will move in the opposite direction.[19] The images are valuable in determining corneal clarity, the depth of the anterior chamber, and the thickness and position of the lens (after mydriasis) and in locating lesions within the lens.[19]

The anterior structures of the horse's eye (i.e., cornea, iris surface) and the periocular tissues including the eyelids, conjunctiva, sclera, and nictitans should be inspected with transillumination.[19] This inspection can first be performed with a Finoff transilluminator or a direct ophthalmoscope but should be followed by examination with a slit-lamp biomicroscope if one is available. The cornea, anterior chamber, lens, and vitreous should be examined with both transillumination and retroillumination.[19] The corneal examination should be performed with the observer located in front of the eye. Light directed diagonally across the cornea will reveal opacities of the cornea against the dark background of the pupil.[19]

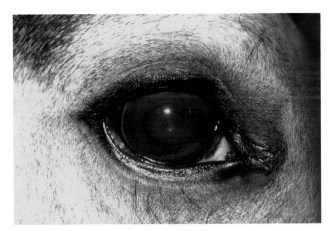

Fig. 1-50 The Purkinje-Sanson reflexes are three reflections produced by the light source during transillumination. The largest is produced by the cornea. The second is produced by the anterior lens capsule. The third is not easily visible and is produced by the posterior lens capsule.

The intraocular portion of the examination is conducted next. With a thin beam (slit) or small circular beam of light from the light source directed at a 45-degree angle to the eye, the anterior chamber depth and clarity are inspected. In a healthy horse, this will not result in any internal reflection of light from the aqueous, and the anterior chamber should appear clear (Fig. 1-51). If solids (e.g., protein, cells) are present in the aqueous, there will be a reflection of light from these particles (i.e., the Tyndall effect) (Fig. 1-51).[19] This turbidity results in visualization of the beam of light traversing the anterior chamber and is referred to as aqueous flare.[19,38] Aqueous flare (and other ocular lesions such as corneal edema, corneal pigment, and conjunctival redness) can be graded on a subjective scale from 1+ to 4+, with 4+ being the greatest degree of severity.

Transillumination of the lens is performed by directing a beam of light at a 45-degree angle into the lens.[19] Normal Y sutures can be visualized with transillumination but not with retroillumination.[19] With transillumination, nuclear sclerosis will appear as a greater translucence with the cortex remaining clear (see Fig. 1-23).[19] On retroillumination, the lens will appear clear with the pupil filled with the tapetal reflex, and a junction "ring" will be seen at the nuclear-cortical junction (Fig. 1-52). Cataracts will appear white on transillumination, and black, if they are not complete (i.e., light can pass around them), when observed on retroillumination (Figs. 1-53 and 1-54).[19] The attachment of the lens zonules can also be seen with transillumination in

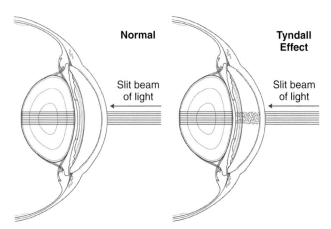

Fig. 1-51 With a thin beam (slit) or small circular beam of light from the light source directed at a 45-degree angle to the eye, the anterior chamber depth and clarity are inspected. In a healthy horse, this will not result in any internal reflection of light from the aqueous, and the anterior chamber should appear clear. If solids (e.g., protein, cells) are present in the aqueous, there will be reflection of light from these particles (i.e., the Tyndall effect). This turbidity results in visualization of the beam of light traversing the anterior chamber and is referred to as aqueous flare.

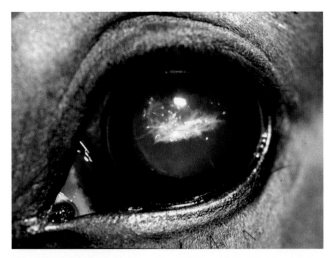

Fig. 1-53 Direct transillumination of a cataract. The lesion appears white.

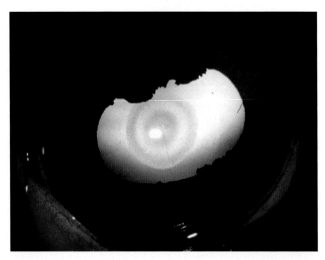

Fig. 1-52 Retroillumination of nuclear sclerosis. The lens appears clear with the pupil filled with the tapetal reflex, and a junction "ring" can be visualized at the nuclear-cortical junction.

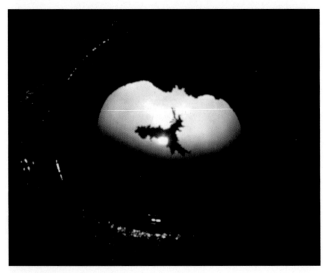

Fig. 1-54 Retroillumination of an incomplete cataract. The lesion appears black.

a well-dilated eye, immediately behind the edge of the pupil.[19]

Transillumination of the vitreous can reveal small posterior polar remnants of the hyaloid artery and areas of light reflection between vitreous planes.[19] Neither can be seen with retroillumination.

Transillumination can also be used to look directly at the fundus of the horse.[19] A light source is held against the examiner's face, and the light is directed into the horse's pupil. The examiner moves forward until the fundus becomes visible. A large fundus area, approximately six times greater than that seen with an ophthalmoscope, can be seen.[19] The entire fundus is not in clear focus but can be seen adequately to screen for disease. Details can then be evaluated with direct ophthalmoscopy. This can be especially useful if the examiner does not have a handheld indirect lens.

The eye is retroilluminated to assess for opacities in the ocular media with a direct ophthalmoscope or other focal light source (e.g., a Finoff transilluminator).[19] Both direct and indirect retroillumination are dependent on reflection of light from the ocular fundus while the observer is focusing on more anterior structures.[19] This technique improves detection of opacities in the cornea, anterior chamber, lens, and vitreous because these opacities reflect, refract, or obstruct returning light.[19] The light is directed into the eye from an arm's distance. Direct retroillumination is performed by placing the objectives in the path of the refracted light, which causes opaque lesions to appear dark against a light background and transparent lesions to appear clear within a dark halo.[19] Indirect retroillumination allows improved detection of transparent lesions by taking advantage of differences between their refractive indices and those of surrounding tissues.[19] Lesions are observed against a darker background because the reflected light is directed away from the objectives.[19] Any noted opacities can be further investigated with the slit-lamp biomicroscope.

Biomicroscopy

The technique of biomicroscopy, in which a slit-lamp binocular microscope with an external, pivoting light source is used, is the same as that described for humans and small animals and has been well described elsewhere.[38,117-120] Slit-lamp biomicroscopy improves visualization and localization of even slight lesions of the cornea, anterior chamber, lens, and anterior vitreous by means of transillumination and retroillumination.[38] It can also be used to assess corneal thickness (i.e., pachymetry), anterior chamber depth, and aqueous flare.[38]

The availability of portable handheld models of the slit-lamp biomicroscope has made the use of this technique in equine ophthalmology easy and efficient. Portable models are available from Clement-Clark, Kowa, Nippon, and Zeiss. The Kowa SL-14 or SL-15 (10× or 16× magnification) is light and powered by a rechargeable battery, and therefore, exceptionally easy to use in examination of a horse (Fig. 1-55). An alternative to a biomicroscope is the slit beam on the direct ophthalmoscope. Very small "slit-lamps" are also made by Zeiss and Welch-Allyn; each resembles a penlight with a magnifier on the end. Although these instruments

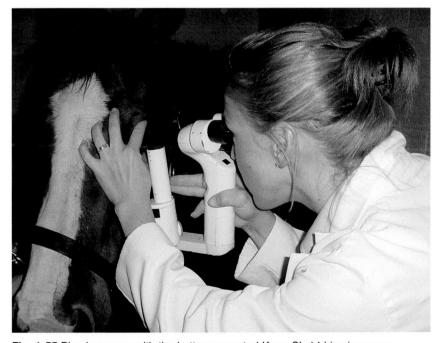

Fig. 1-55 Biomicroscopy with the battery-operated Kowa SL-14 biomicroscope.

are inexpensive and portable, their lack of magnification and illumination limits their usefulness.[38]

The light beam of the biomicroscope should be angled at 20 to 45 degrees from the axis of the microscope; the light beam width, length, orientation, and color can then be modified by a series of diaphragms and filters.[38] The focal distance of the instrument is 7 to 10 cm, and fine focus is achieved by moving either toward or away from the eye within this range.[38]

The initial examination of the horse should proceed with diffuse illumination; a wide, low-intensity slit beam should be used, and the microscope should be defocused from the light.[38] Most portable slit lamps do not have adjustable focus (except by exchange of the oculars), so direct focal illumination is used to achieve the same goal.[38] The surfaces of the eyelids, cornea, conjunctiva, and iris should be inspected. With the use of low magnification, a broad slit beam is focused on the cornea, creating a parallelepiped (i.e., a three-dimensional section) of illuminated tissue.[38] This allows visualization of transparent structures, such as the cornea and lens, in three dimensions. For example, the anterior surface, stroma, and posterior surface of the cornea can be visualized.[38] Nontransparent structures, such as the iris, only yield a magnified two-dimensional view.[38] The slit beam is then narrowed and intensified to reveal a two-dimensional cross-section of the cornea and lens, allowing the examiner to accurately determine lesion depth and axial positioning.[38] This is extremely important in evaluating the depth of corneal lesions, such as stromal ulcerative keratitis and stromal abscesses, in the horse.

Direct and indirect retroillumination are performed by reflecting the slit beam from deeper structures while focusing on more superficial structures.[38] Other techniques that can be performed with slit-lamp biomicroscopy, such as specular reflection, are difficult to impossible in a horse because of continuous slight ocular movements.

Tonometry

The measurement of intraocular pressure (IOP) in the horse has been revolutionized by the development of handheld applanation tonometers that do not require the horse to be in lateral recumbency. Direct tonometry via a manometer is the most accurate but invasive method for recording the IOP and is not practical for clinical use. Indirect tonometry, the measurement of corneal tension, is the technique used to determine IOP in clinical veterinary ophthalmology.[19] Digital tonometry, indentation tonometry, and applanation tonometry are the methods described.[38] Digital tonometry, the estimation of IOP by digital palpation, cannot be considered accurate. Indentation tonometry, commonly performed with a Schiotz tonometer, requires general anesthesia (a lateral position) in the horse and is not practical. However, normal values have been reported for the Schiotz tonometer in the horse and are 14 to 22 mm Hg.[19] Applanation tonometry measures the amount of flattening (area of contact) of the cornea when a weight touches the cornea.[19,38] The force it takes to flatten this portion of the cornea is an estimate of the IOP (Pressure = Force/Area). Accurate measurement of IOP in the standing horse requires use of applanation tonometry (Fig. 1-56).[2,38]

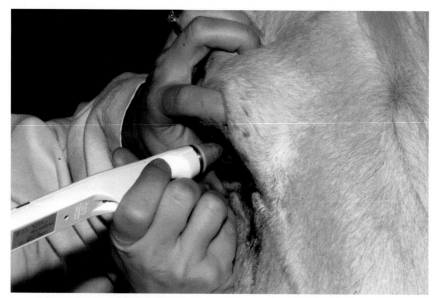

Fig. 1-56 Accurate measurement of intraocular pressure (IOP) in the standing horse requires applanation tonometry.

Tonometry is indicated in horses that have focal or diffuse corneal edema, a red or painful eye, orbital trauma, a history of glaucoma in the opposite eye, or a lens luxation; it is also indicated for follow-up examinations of animals with medically controlled glaucoma.[2,38] Three separate readings with less than 5% standard error are averaged to obtain the IOP in millimeters of mercury.[19,38] If significant corneal disease is present, the most normal part of cornea should be used to take readings.[19] A fibrotic and edematous cornea may result in a falsely elevated IOP.[19]

Horses that require sedation for ocular examination may show dramatic decreases in IOP, as illustrated by one study in which xylazine decreased IOP by 23%.[69] Topical anesthetic is always required. It has been suggested that horses that have not had the auriculopalpebral nerve blocked will have an elevated IOP because of eyelid tension.[19,121] This has not been supported in two other studies.[69,122] IOP in horses without an auriculopalpebral nerve block has been reported as ranging from 24.5 ± 4.0 mm Hg to 28.6 ± 4.8 mm Hg.[123-125] Another report, in horses with an auriculopalpebral block, showed that ketamine and xylazine decreased IOP.[121] IOP in that report was 17.1 ± 3.9 in the left eye (OS) and 18.4 ± 2.2 in the right eye (OD) and was lower than in horses without a block.[121] In another report, the IOP range was 20.5 to 39.8 mm Hg and showed that both acepromazine and xylazine decreased IOP.[124] A combination of xylazine and ketamine had no effect.[121,126] The effect of topical preparations is discussed in Chapter 8 (Equine Glaucoma).

Countertop electronic applanation tonometers may also still be available (e.g., MacKay-Marg [Biotronics], Redding, Calif.; pneumotonometers [Mentor O&O]). The MacKay-Marg tonometer was shown to produce reliable results in comparison with direct tonometry in the dog, rabbit, and horse.[123,127,128] It has been used to study IOP in the horse.[69,122,123,126,129] IOP in one report was 20.6 ± 4.7 mm Hg.[69]

The Tono-Pen (Oculab) is a handheld digital applanation tonometer that is completely portable and highly accurate when the examiner is experienced with using it. However, it has been reported to slightly underestimate IOP (at low, normal, and high values) in the horse.[19] The advantage of the Tono-Pen is that it is battery operated, and therefore the animal's head can be held in any position. The mean equine IOP ranges from 15 to 30 mm Hg, with the IOP of the right and left eyes of a given horse being within 5 to 8 mm Hg of each other.[19,69,122,129] An IOP greater than 30 to 35 mm Hg is usually diagnostic of glaucoma.[2] Average IOP has also been reported for the Miniature horse and the Rocky Mountain horse with cornea globosa and does not differ significantly from values for full-sized horses at 26 mm Hg.[36,130]

The pneumotonograph (Alcon Pneumotonograph; Alcon Laboratories, Fort Worth, Texas) is an applanation tonometer-tonographer that measures IOP via a gas-suspended plunger. Measurements can be permanently recorded on heat-sensitive paper. However, the pneumotonograph may provide falsely elevated pressure readings in the in the horse.[131]

Tonography

Tonography is the use of continuous tonometry to noninvasively estimate the pressure-sensitive facility of conventional aqueous humor outflow.[32,38,129] In theory, the weight of the tonographic probe on the cornea increases both IOP and rate of aqueous humor outflow, without changing the rate of aqueous humor production.[38] The subsequent decline in IOP (decay curve) is measured over 2 to 4 minutes, thereby allowing an estimation of conventional outflow (corneoscleral trabecular outflow).[38] The unconventional outflow (uveoscleral) is pressure independent and thus not estimated by tonography. Uveoscleral outflow in the horse, which appears to be substantial, cannot be measured by tonography.[133] Pneumotonography has been used to establish increased aqueous humor outflow resistance associated with glaucoma in the dog.[132] Tonography has been used in the horse, and the facility of aqueous humor outflow (C-value) is 0.88 ± 0.65 µl/min per mm Hg, which is significantly higher than that reported for the healthy dog and cat (0.24 to 0.27 µl/min per mm Hg).[129,132,134]

Ophthalmoscopy

Ophthalmoscopy is the examination of the ocular fundus (i.e., choroid, retina, and optic nerve) and is an integral part of any ophthalmic or physical examination. There are two common methods of performing ophthalmoscopy in the horse: direct and indirect. Direct ophthalmoscopy can be performed in the horse by means of transillumination as previously described or with the use of a direct ophthalmoscope. Indirect ophthalmoscopy requires the use of a handheld lens. In contrast to examination of small animals, in which indirect ophthalmoscopy is most indicated, direct ophthalmoscopy is very useful in the initial examination of the horse because of the large size of the equine ocular fundus. The instruments and technique for ophthalmoscopy are reviewed in detail elsewhere.[38]

Advantages of the direct ophthalmoscope are its upright image, availability of options such as slit and graticule, ability to alter the dioptric power of the ophthalmoscope, and greater magnification provided.[19,38] Disadvantages include the short working distance to the horse's head, a small field of view, lack of stereopsis, difficulty in examining the peripheral fundus, and greater distortion of the image when the visual axis is not clear.[19,38]

Advantages of indirect ophthalmoscopy include a wider field of view, a safer working distance from the horse's head, potential for stereopsis (i.e., depth perception) if binocular equipment is used, greater view of peripheral fundus, and ability to alter the magnification by changing the diopter strength of the lens being used.[19,38] Disadvantages of indirect ophthalmoscopy include the expense of binocular equipment and the increased difficulty of the technique (i.e., image is inverted and reversed).[19,38]

The fundus can be visualized without mydriasis in the horse, but the presence of mydriasis ensures a thorough examination. The use of a short-acting mydriatic (0.5% or 1% tropicamide) is recommended as previously described. Again, full mydriasis should occur within 10 to 20 minutes and should last for 4 to 6 hours.[37] The menace response, dazzle reflex, resting pupil size, and direct and consensual PLRs in each eye in bright and dim lighting should be evaluated before mydriasis is induced. Tonometry before pharmacologic mydriasis, indicated in small animals, is not absolutely necessary in the horse, unless glaucoma is high on the list of differential diagnoses. Many horses tolerate this part of the examination better after an auriculopalpebral nerve block.

The normal ophthalmoscopic appearance of the fundus of the horse has been well described and is also covered in Chapter 9 (see Fig. 1-13).[29-32] It is dominated by the tapetum fibrosum, which occupies the dorsal two thirds of the posterior segment, and the stars of Winslow. The tapetal color varies from green-yellow (most common) to aquamarine or turquoise.[2,65] Changes in tapetal color intensity from the central to peripheral tapetum have also been described.[65] The tapetum may be undeveloped in animals with albinotic or sub-albinotic coat colors.[2,29] The nontapetal area is usually dark brown, but this melanin in the RPE may be absent, depending on coat and iris coloration.[2] If the pigment is absent, the choroidal vessels can be visualized (see Fig. 1-14). The optic disc is horizontally oval, usually located slightly temporal and ventral in the nontapetal area, and salmon pink.[2,29] Retinal vessels radiate out only a short distance from the optic disc and are usually absent at the ventral disc border.[2,29]

Direct Ophthalmoscopy

Direct ophthalmoscopy is extremely useful for rapid ocular examination in horses, and it can be used to identify most lesions of the equine ocular fundus (Fig. 1-57).[2] The resulting image with a direct ophthalmoscope is upright and magnified several times above normal (7.9) with a millimeter equivalent per dioptric change of 1.33.[38,135] As in small animals, magnification

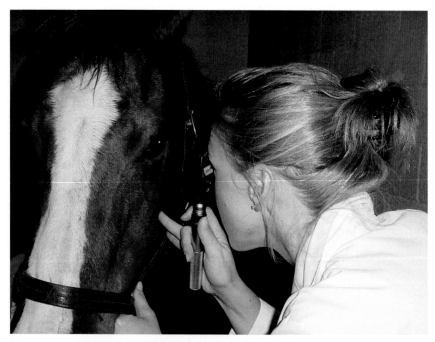

Fig. 1-57 Direct ophthalmoscopy is extremely useful for rapid ocular examination in horses and can be used to identify most lesions of the equine ocular fundus. There is a short working distance to the horse's head.

of the image varies with working distance, and thus lesions should be compared with optic disc diameter rather than by units of measurement.[19,38] The direct ophthalmoscope can also be used to perform direct illumination and retroillumination of structures and media anterior to the fundus.

Direct ophthalmoscopy can be performed with a transilluminator in the horse. The light source should be held against the examiner's face, near the eye, and directed through the horse's pupil. This provides a larger view of the fundus than can be seen with the direct ophthalmoscope, but it is not entirely in focus. This is a quick and useful method to screen for obvious signs of disease.

The direct ophthalmoscope consists of a halogen coaxial optical system and a power source.[38] A series of concave and convex lenses can be rotated through the viewing aperture by means of a dial.[38,136-138] Green or black numbers represent convex or converging lenses, and red numbers represent concave or diverging lenses.[38,136-138] The size, shape, and color of the light beam can be adjusted by a second dial, which produces large and small circles of light, a slit beam of light, a graticule, and two filters.[19,38] The size of the circular spot of white light should be adjusted to the patient's pupil size to minimize light reflections from the corneal surface.[38] The smallest circular spot, as well as the slit beam, can be used to evaluate for aqueous flare. The slit beam also aids in the detection of elevations or depressions in the ocular fundus, and distances can be estimated by changing the dioptric power of the ophthalmoscope.[38] When the retina is in focus at 0 diopters (D), the lesion is elevated if the lesion surface is in focus at a positive diopters setting (i.e., black numbers) and depressed if the lesion surface is in focus at a negative diopter setting (i.e., red numbers).[38] The graticule is a grid that can be used to size the optic disc and estimate the size of fundic lesions.[38] A red-free filter (appears green) is used to evaluate retinal vessels and to differentiate hemorrhage (which appears black) from pigmented lesions (which appear brown).[38] A blue filter can be used to help visualize fluorescein staining.[38]

Most ocular fundi are in focus at 0 to −2 diopters if the examiner's vision is emmetropic, and therefore the ophthalmoscope should initially be set at 0 D.[19,38] The direct ophthalmoscope should be placed against the examiner's brow, using the examiner's dominant eye, the examiner should identify the horse's fundic reflex from a distance of approximately 0.5 to 0.75 m.[19,38] Once the fundic reflex is identified, the examiner moves toward the horse to a point approximately 2 to 3 cm from the eye to visualize the fundus.[19,38] Ophthalmoscopy should then proceed to identification and examination of the optic nerve, retinal vasculature, nontapetal fundus, and tapetal fundus in quadrants.

Available monocular direct ophthalmoscopes include the Heine, Keeler, Propper, Reichert, and Welch Allyn models.[38] Welch Allyn has developed a new monocular indirect ophthalmoscope (PanOptic) that can be used in an undilated pupil and has five times greater magnification than a routine ophthalmoscope.

Indirect Ophthalmoscopy

Monocular or binocular indirect ophthalmoscopy involves the use of a handheld converging lens held near the patient and a light source near the examiner's eye. A larger area of ocular fundus can be visualized with indirect versus direct ophthalmoscopy and may allow the examiner to more easily detect disease.

In binocular indirect ophthalmoscopy, a light source fitted onto a headband and a mirror are used to direct light into the patient's eye; the handheld lens is used to magnify the reflected image; and two prisms are used to split the reflected beam so that it can be directed into both of the examiner's eyes, permitting stereopsis (Fig. 1-58).[38] The light intensity should be adjusted to permit adequate illumination without causing patient discomfort.[38]

In monocular indirect ophthalmoscopy, a handheld light source is used in addition to the handheld lens (Fig. 1-59). The light source should be placed near the examiner's eye near the temple so that both the head and light source function as one unit. A direct ophthalmoscope can be used for indirect ophthalmoscopy, and the dioptric power of the ophthalmoscope should be adjusted to +4 or +6 D.[38]

The handheld lens provides a virtual image (i.e., the image is inverted and reversed) of the patient's fundus. A variety of lenses are available, ranging from +14 to +90 D in strength. The +20-D and +28-D lenses are the most useful in the horse, providing a fundus view of approximately 40 degrees. The quality of the handheld converging lens affects the ease and clarity of the evaluation. The smaller the lens diopters rating, the greater is the fundic magnification.[38] In the horse, lateral magnification has been reported for 14-D (1.18), 20-D (0.79), 30-D (0.51), and 40-D (0.38) lenses.[135] Axial magnification in the horse has also been reported for 14-D (0.38), 20-D (0.84), 30-D (0.35), 40-D (0.19) lenses.[135]

The refractive error of an animal can be semi-qualified during indirect ophthalmoscopy by slowly withdrawing the lens toward the examiner and further from the eye and observing any change in magnification. The fundic image will get larger (myopic) or smaller (hyperopic), or it will remain static (emmetropia).[29]

Binocular indirect ophthalmoscopes are available from Heine, Keeler, Propper, Topcon, Xonix, and Zeiss.

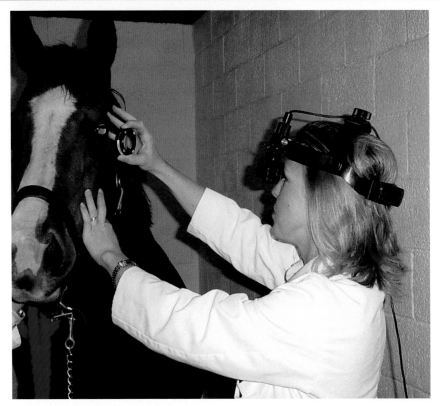

Fig. 1-58 In binocular indirect ophthalmoscopy, a light source fitted onto a headband and a mirror are used to direct light into the patient's eye; the handheld lens magnifies the reflected image, and two prisms split the reflected beam so that it can be directed into both of the examiner's eyes, permitting stereopsis.

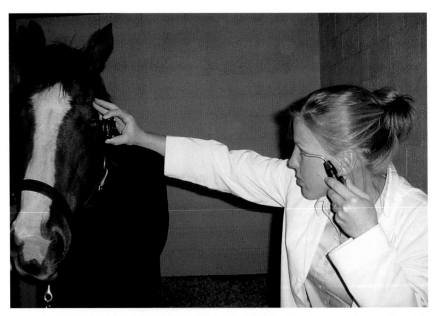

Fig. 1-59 In monocular indirect ophthalmoscopy, a handheld light source is used in addition to the handheld lens. The light source should be placed near the examiner's eye near the temple so that both the head and light source function as one unit.

Commercial monocular indirect ophthalmoscopes are manufactured by Reichert and the American Optical Corporation. In these instruments an internal lens is used to magnify the reflected fundic image.[38] The American Optical Reichert monocular indirect ophthalmoscope is easy to use because it provides an upright image and does not require mydriasis.[19,38]

ADVANCED OPHTHALMIC EXAMINATION AND DIAGNOSTIC PROCEDURES

Aqueous Paracentesis

Aqueous humor fills the anterior segment of the eye and supplies nutrients to the avascular cornea and lens, as well as removing waste products from the interior of the eye. Normal components of the aqueous humor in the horse have been reported.[45] Small amounts of aqueous humor can be aspirated from the anterior chamber for both diagnostic samples and palliative therapy in the horse.[38,139,140] This procedure is relatively quick and simple, but complications are possible.

Aqueous paracentesis can be performed with the horse under general anesthesia or standing with sedation, topical anesthesia, and a retrobulbar block.[38] Short general anesthesia minimizes the risk of injuring an eye with intact vision. The technique is the same as that used in small animals, except that the site for aspiration should be the dorsal to temporal limbus to take advantage of the scleral extension beyond the iris base.[19] The bulbar conjunctiva should be cleaned with dilute Betadine (5%) solution and sterile saline solution or eyewash.[38] The bulbar conjunctiva is grasped with thumb forceps near the site of entry, and a 27- to 30-gauge needle is directed through the limbal cornea or subconjunctival limbus (bevel up) anterior and parallel to the iris (Fig. 1-60).[38] A drilling and tunneling motion will facilitate entry through the sclera and may facilitate rapid formation of a seal after the needle is withdrawn.[38] A small volume, 0.2 to 0.5 ml, of aqueous humor is slowly aspirated, and the needle is withdrawn.[38] A syringe can be attached to the needle when

this is first performed, after the needle is placed into the anterior chamber, or no syringe may be used and the aqueous that fills the hub can be drawn into a capillary tube. The final method is less awkward. Without the syringe, the clinician has greater control over the needle and its position relative to the iris and lens.[141] The tip of the needle should be visualized at all times to avoid lacerating the iris or lens capsule.

Possible complications of aqueous paracentesis include hyphema, anterior lens capsule rupture with subsequent phacoclastic uveitis, endophthalmitis, anterior uveitis, corneal edema associated with endothelial damage, and choroidal edema and hemorrhage.[38] In an attempt to prevent increased release of prostaglandins and uveitis after the procedure, the volume removed should be replaced with an equal amount of sterile normal saline solution or balanced salt solution, especially if more than 0.3 ml has been removed.[38]

Diagnostic procedures that can be with aqueous humor samples in the horse include cytology, culture and sensitivity, protein measurement, antibody titers (e.g., *Leptospira* species), and PCR.[38,142-152] Aqueous paracentesis can also be performed to instill total plasminogen activator into the anterior chamber in cases of postsurgical or traumatic hyphema.

Vitreous Paracentesis

The technique described is the same as that used for small animals, except that previous recommendations have been to place the needle 10 to 15 mm posterior to the limbus in the horse.[19] Because of the dorsal scleral overhang, a greater distance from the limbus is needed with a dorsal site than with a temporal site. However, 10 mm, rather than 15 mm, is probably more appropriate dorsally to avoid introducing the needle through the sensory retina.[18] A 23-gauge needle is inserted through the conjunctiva and sclera, with the object being to pass through the pars plana of the ciliary body (Fig. 1-61). The needle should be directed toward the optic nerve to avoid the lens.

As for the aqueous humor, diagnostic procedures available with vitreous humor samples include culture and sensitivity, cytology, protein measurement, antibody titers, and PCR.[38,151,152] Vitreous paracentesis can also be performed to instill ocular toxic gentamicin for ciliary body ablation in cases of glaucoma and to instill antibiotics in cases of endophthalmitis.

Retinoscopy (Skiascopy)

Retinoscopy, or skiascopy, is the technique to determine the refractive error or dioptric state of the eye.

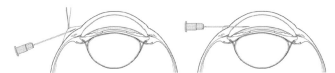

Fig. 1-60 Aqueous paracentesis. The bulbar conjunctiva is grasped with thumb forceps near the site of entry, and a 27- to 30-gauge needle is directed through the limbal cornea or subconjunctival limbus (bevel up) anterior and parallel to the iris, avoiding the lens. A drilling and tunneling motion will facilitate entry through the sclera and may facilitate rapid formation of a seal after the needle is withdrawn.

Retinoscopy is the only clinical means of refraction in veterinary ophthalmology. Commonly used in human ophthalmology, this technique has been used in veterinary medicine to define the normal, pathologic, and surgically induced refractive state of the eyes of the horse.[6,153-163] The instrumentation and technique used can be challenging, and the reader is referred to an article by Davidson for further information.[164]

Light rays projected onto an eye from infinity emerge from an emmetropic eye as parallel rays, from a myopic (near-sighted) eye as converging rays, and from a hyperopic (far-sighted) eye as diverging rays.[153,164] The location at which these emergent light rays form a focal point is called the *far point*.[164] The far point is at infinity, in front of infinity, and beyond infinity for the emmetropic, myopic, and hyperopic eyes, respectively.[153,164]

The retinoscope is either spot or streak, but streak retinoscopes are the most commonly used in veterinary medicine.[164] Both streak and spot retinoscopes are available from Copeland, Heine, Keeler, Propper, Reichert, and Welch Allyn. Plus or minus spherical lenses, available in increments of 0.25 D, are placed between the retinoscope and the horse to quantitate the refractive error of the eye.[164] A simple and inexpensive skiascopy bar or rack contains a series of plus and minus lenses in increments of 0.5 to 1.0 D.[164]

Retinoscopy is performed in a darkened room with a handler restraining the horse's head. Mydriasis is often unnecessary and can even make the technique more difficult, and the limited accommodative ability of the horse makes cycloplegia less important.[164,165] The retinoscope is placed against the examiner's brow, and the examiner is positioned 0.67 m (approximately an arm's length) from the patient's eye.[164] The streak is swept horizontally across the horse's pupil, rotated horizontally, and then swept vertically across the pupil.[164] Finally, a trial lens or skiascopy bar is placed 1 to 2 cm from the patient's cornea, and the process is repeated (Fig. 1-62).[154,164]

As the streak is slowly swept across the pupil, the fundic reflex will move in either the same or the opposite direction, depending on the refractive error of the patient. With no refractive lens, the fundic reflex

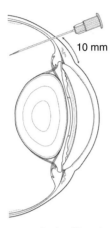

Fig. 1-61 Vitreous paracentesis. The dorsal scleral overhang requires a greater distance from the limbus with a dorsal site than with a temporal site. However, 10 mm, rather than 15 mm, is probably more appropriate dorsally to avoid introducing the needle through the sensory retina. A 23-gauge needle is inserted through the conjunctiva and sclera, with the object being to pass through the pars plana of the ciliary body. The needle should be directed toward the optic nerve to avoid the lens.

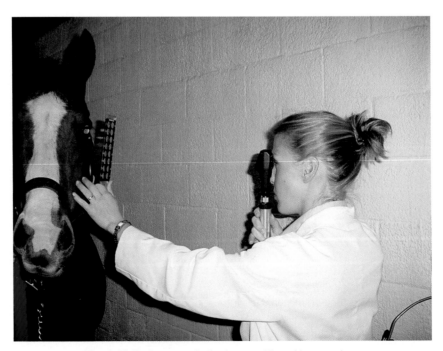

Fig. 1-62 Retinoscopy in the horse with a skiascopy bar.

will move in the same direction as the sweep with emmetropic and hyperopic eyes (a with motion) and in the opposite direction of the sweep with more than 1.5-D myopic eyes (an against motion).[164] If a with motion is observed, plus lenses of increasing dioptric strength are placed in front of the patient's eye until an against motion is observed or neutralization is reached.[164] Neutralization is characterized by a fundic reflex that completely fills the pupil without any noticeable direction of movement.[164] If an against motion is observed, minus lenses of increasing dioptric strength are used to achieve neutrality.[164] At a working distance of 0.67 m, a +1.5-D lens is needed to achieve neutralization with an emmetropic eye; therefore the refractive error of an eye is determined by subtracting 1.5 D from the gross refraction needed to achieve neutrality.[164]

Retinoscopy may allow selection of intraocular lens implants in horses and assist with evaluation of performance problems in working animals. However, refractive error has an unknown effect on horses and is discussed further in Chapter 10 (Equine Vision). In healthy horses refractive error has been reported to range from –3 to +3 D.[160,161] However, most appear to be within 1 D of emmetropia.[153,154,159] The aphakic equine eye, after cataract surgery, has been reported to be hyperopic (+9.94 D).[158] An intraocular lens implant with a refractive power of 25 D resulted in an improvement to only +8 D hyperopia.[158] Astigmatism, a state of unequal refraction along the different meridians of the eye (i.e., vertical vs horizontal), has not been reported in horses.[162,163] Variation in the reported refractive error in horses can be explained by the technique used, the skill of the examiner, the sample size, and accommodative state of the animal.[153]

Fluorescein Angiography

Fluorescein angiography is the dynamic recording of dye, after intravenous administration, as it passes through the retinal and choroidal circulation (Fig. 1-63).[166] It can be used both clinically and experimentally to evaluate vascular conditions of the fundus and iris.[38] It detects lesions in the vascular wall of the retinal vessels or in tight junctions between retinal pigmented epithelial cells, both of which constitute the blood-retinal barrier.[166] When vascular disease is present, changes in the angiogram can be evaluated. When given intravenously, 60% to 80% of the fluorescein is protein bound and does not normally cross the tight junctions between retinal pigment epithelial cells.[166] However, unbound fluorescein readily passes into the choroidal interstitium through large fenestrae after passing into the choriocapillaris.[166] So if there is any abnormality of the RPE, progressive subretinal pooling of the dye will be seen. Because of the absence of a real choroidal barrier and a choroid–optic nerve barrier, the optic nerve becomes progressively fluorescent in the late phase.[166]

Sodium fluorescein is a water-soluble, low-molecular-weight, weak, dibasic acid.[38,166] It fluoresces intensely at a blood pH of 7.4.[166] The 10% (100 mg/ml) solution is commonly used to perform the angiogram.[38,166] The dye is excited by light with a wavelength of 465 to 490 nm (i.e., blue light) and emits light from 500 to 600 nm (yellow-green), with a maximum intensity at a wavelength of 520 to 530 nm.[38,166] Appropriate barrier filters are used to accomplish this event during the angiogram. A blue filter (Kodak Wratten 47A) in the light pathway induces maximal fluorescence, and a yellow filter (Kodak Wratten 15) in the optical pathway provides maximal contrast. The appropriate use of these filters also helps reduce much of the background fluorescence and pseudofluorescence that can make the images undiagnostic.[166] Other dyes are available for angiography and include indocyanine green, pyranine, and rhodamine but their use has not been reported in the horse.[38]

Sedation or general anesthesia is usually required to perform an angiogram in the horse. The pupils must be pharmacologically dilated and the ocular media must be clear. Fluorescein angiography can be performed with a direct or indirect ophthalmoscope, but a fundus camera is preferred for documentation.[38] Because of the rapid occurrence of events during the angiogram,

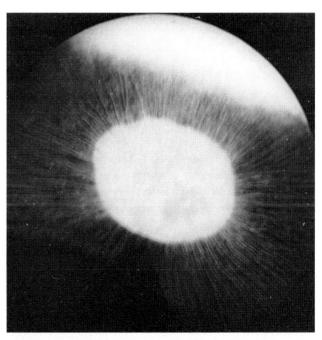

Fig. 1-63 Fluorescein angiography is the recording of dye, after intravenous administration, as it passes through the retinal and choroidal circulation. This is a normal equine example with black and white film. (Fluorescein angiogram image courtesy Dr. Dennis Brooks and Dr. Stacy Andrew.)

some changes may not be seen by the examiner until the serial photographs are evaluated. Models of fundus cameras used to perform fluorescein angiography include Kowa, Topcon, and Zeiss.[38] These models can take pictures as rapidly as three times per second. If the camera is table mounted, however, its use is limited in the horse because of positioning difficulties. Kowa has marketed a handheld fundus camera that could take up to one photograph every 2 seconds.[38] Fluorescein angiography has been reported in the horse with the use of a Kowa Fundus Camera RC-2.[167] Slide film, either black and white or high-speed (400 asa) color film, may be used.

The angiogram consists of six normal phases: the prefilling, choroidal, retinal arteriolar, retinal capillary, retinal venous, and recirculation phases.[166] The prefilling phase occurs before injection. The choroidal phase is rapid and short and is evidenced by a brightening of the background under the RPE, centrally to peripherally, and occurs within 22 seconds in the horse after injection of dye into the jugular vein (i.e., choroidal flush).[167] In small animals, cilioretinal arteries also fill during this phase as fluorescein leaks into the optic nerve from the choroid through the border of Elschnig and the optic nerve begins to fluoresce, although this occurrence has not been documented in the horse.[38,168] The pure choroidal phase is difficult to capture. With incomplete pigmentation of the nontapetal fundus or absence of the tapetal zone, the choroidal phase may be visualized.[38] The retinal arteriolar and retinal capillary phases (i.e., transition to venous) occur next. The retinal venous phase is characterized by a laminar flow pattern.[168] Finally, a recirculation phase (i.e., a second retinal arteriolar phase) can be seen with optimal fluorescence.[166]

Very little information is available on fluorescein angiography in the horse.[167,169,170] Fluorescein angiography will characterize but not diagnose posterior segment lesions.[166] Indications for fluorescein angiography include inflammatory conditions such as uveitis (posterior, anterior), swelling of the optic nerve (neuritis, edema), retinal lesions (with or without associated blindness), and subretinal edema. Fluorescein angiography is also used to monitor progression of disease and response to therapy.[166] Contraindications to fluorescein angiography include a known hypersensitivity to the dye, severe systemic disease, and persistent miosis.[166] Reported complications in veterinary medicine include transient nausea and vomiting in 5% to 10% of small-animal patients, urine and mucous membrane discoloration for 24 to 48 hours, and anaphylaxis.[171] Complications have not been reported in the horse, but emergency cardiac and respiratory drugs (e.g., epinephrine) should be immediately available and the angiogram should be performed in a relatively safe and open environment. Emesis cannot occur in a horse. Because of the possible catastrophic nature of an anaphylactic reaction in a horse, pretreatment with diphenhydramine hydrochloride may be indicated.

A pre-injection (i.e., control) photograph should be taken with routine film for future comparison.[166] This control can minimize misinterpretations caused by pseudofluorescence and autofluorescence. In small animals, the recommendation is to take a photograph at least once every 2 seconds, starting 5 seconds after injection, and after 20 seconds, to take photographs at 1, 5, and 10 minutes after injection.[38] Dye usually appears in the eye of small animals within 5 seconds of injection; however, the time for dye to appear in the eye after jugular injection in the horse has been reported to take up to 22 seconds.[38,167] Therefore photographs after injection should not begin until 15 to 20 seconds have passed or the dye is visualized. Total retinal circulation time was reported as 20.5 seconds, and the late phase occurred within 3 to 5 minutes.[167] The optimal dose of fluorescein reported in the literature is 8 to 10 mg/kg in 20% solution.[167]

Breakdown of the RPE or retinal vascular barrier (e.g., endothelialitis) allows fluorescein to pass into the retina and escape the vascular system. Morphologic analysis of the angiogram takes into consideration overall patterns.[166] The first question to answer is whether an abnormality in the angiogram exists. Abnormalities in the angiogram are then characterized as either hyperfluorescent or hypofluorescent.[166] Hypofluorescence occurs when normally transmitted fluorescence is decreased or blocked.[166] Vascular attenuation or occlusion and visual obstructions such as pigment, hemorrhage, edema, and exudate can block normal fluorescence.[166] Hyperfluorescence occurs when there is autofluorescence, pseudofluorescence (early phase, late phase), or increased transmitted fluorescence.[166] Causes of increased transmitted fluorescence include RPE window defects, which cause increased choroidal visibility, atrophy, vascular abnormalities, active hemorrhage, leakage into the vitreous or subretinal space (e.g., retinal detachment), staining of tissue from leaky retinal or choroidal vessels, and increased accumulation associated with tumors.[166] Psuedofluorescence can occur with poor matching of excitation and barrier filters.[166] Autofluorescence occurs in the tapetal fundus of the cat, lemur, and many other tapetal species such as the horse.[38] This can limit the value of this procedure for detection of tapetal abnormalities. Drusen formation in the optic nerve, lipofuscin in the retina, and normal sclera can also produce autofluorescence.[166]

Fluorescein angiography has been used to study focal chorioretinal lesions caused by EHV-1 in ponies.[169] The chorioretinal lesions fluoresced but did not leak.[169] This suggested focal loss of overlying RPE after infarction of the choroidal vasculature and was confirmed by histopathologic examination.[169]

Corneal Esthesiometry

The corneal reflex is one of the most sensitive reflexes of the body, and its purpose is to protect the eye. Both eyelid closure and a retraction of the globe should occur simultaneously.[43] Corneal sensitivity can be tested empirically by using either a Dacron-tipped applicator or an esthesiometer. Corneal esthesiometers evaluate corneal sensitivity by measuring the corneal touch threshold (CTT), which is the threshold of the stimulus that results in a corneal reflex.[45] Estimation of corneal sensitivity may be used to diagnose and monitor corneal diseases, evaluate progression of corneal diseases after surgery, and monitor the effects of surgery and topical medications. The Cochet-Bonnet esthesiometer (Luneau Ophthalmologie, Chartres Cedex, France) is a well-established tool for evaluation of the CTT in veterinary medicine.[172-174] The instrument contains a nylon or platinum filament with an adjustable length and a defined diameter. The filament is applied in different lengths to the cornea until a corneal reflex is elicited with the same pressure or length of filament.[172,173] The length of the nylon filament estimates the applied pressure on the corneal surface and is readable on a millimeter scale. The shorter the filament, the more pressure is applied to the cornea and vice versa.

Corneal sensitivity has been reported in foals and adult horses. The central area of the cornea, similar to that in other species, has been shown to be the most sensitive; and the dorsal region, the least sensitive.[172,175] A decrease in corneal sensitivity was shown in sick neonatal foals compared with normal adults.[172] Corneas in healthy foals were slightly more sensitive than those in healthy adults.[172]

In humans, it has been shown that the CTT is influenced by age, mental status, iris color, hormone cycle, gravidity, time of day, humidity, room temperature, esthesiometric method, and investigator.[176-181] A decrease in sensitivity has been described in cats with herpes keratitis, in dogs with spontaneous chronic corneal epithelial defects, and in dogs after neodymium:yttrium-aluminium-garnet (Nd:YAG) laser photocoagulation.[182-184] Further investigation into the effects of corneal disease, cyclophotocoagulation, and surgeries such as penetrating keratoplasty on CTT needs to be performed in the horse.

Ultrasonic Pachymetry

Ultrasonic pachymetry is the most accurate and reliable in vivo method currently available to measure corneal thickness in animals and humans.[185-187] Previously, corneal thickness was measured from gross postmortem specimens and histologic specimens. These measurements do not correlate with in vivo measurements because the cornea swells after death.[188] Pachymetry is a technique that measures the corneal thickness in vivo. Ultrasonic pachymetry measures the time required for ultrasonic energy to traverse the cornea, with a preset constant for velocity of sound, and converts this to a measure of thickness.[20,189] Other methods of pachymetry include optical, electromechanical, and laser methods.[38,189] Transparent media are required for full-thickness corneal measurements.[38]

A 20-MHz ultrasonic pachymeter (DGH500, DGH Technology Inc., Exton, Pa) has been used to study the horse. It has been used to determine corneal thickness in healthy juvenile and adult horses, Rocky Mountain horses with cornea globosa, horses that have been given an auriculopalpebral nerve block and xylazine, and healthy Miniature horses.[20,36,69,130] Corneal thickness of enucleated globes was approximately 858 μm centrally, 914 to 939 μm dorsally and ventrally, and 861 to 898 μm laterally and medially.[20] Corneal thickness (mean) was reported to be 793 μm centrally, and thicker peripherally at 831 to 924 μm in vivo.[69] Three reports indicate that the dorsal and ventral portions of the cornea are thicker.[20,36,69] Block, sedation, age, and sex did not affect corneal thickness.[69] However, thickness of the central portion of the cornea may increase up to the age of 6 months in a healthy horse.[36] Corneal thickness in the normal Miniature horse is 785 μm centrally.[130]

Specular Microscopy

Specular microscopy was developed to evaluate the corneal endothelium and lens. Specular microscopy is one of the oldest methods of measuring corneal thickness in vivo. Contact and noncontact scanning specular microscopes, which allow the recording of a larger field of view, can be used. In specular microscopy, differential focusing is used on the corneal epithelial and endothelial cell surfaces at a 45-degree angle. Noncontact specular microscopy has been used to determine corneal endothelial cell counts and corneal thickness in healthy horses (Topcon SP-2000P, Topcon America, Paramus, NJ).[20] The average endothelial cell count was 3155 ± 765 cell/mm². There was not a great difference between eyes of the same horse or various quadrants of the cornea. As in dogs and humans, in the horse the endothelial cell count decreases with age.[20,190]

Corneal edema occurs when a minimal critical cell density is reached. This number has not yet been established in horses. The determination of corneal endothelial cell counts would be useful in evaluation of horses with unexplained corneal edema or penetrating injury and horses that have undergone penetrating keratoplasty or phacoemulsification, and in examination of donor tissue to be used in corneal transplantation.[191,192]

Gonioscopy

Gonioscopy is the examination of the filtration (iridocorneal) angle. The filtration angle is visible through the cornea at the nasal and temporal limbi in the adult horse and 360 degrees in the foal (see Fig. 1-12). Therefore a goniolens is not needed to examine it. Transillumination and biomicroscopy are adequate. The portion of the filtration angle visualized can be assumed to be representative of the rest of the filtration angle. The angle should be examined for width; the character of the pectinate ligaments; goniodysgenesis; and the presence of peripheral anterior synechia, neoplasia, or injury. However, abnormalities in the iridocorneal angle are extremely rare in the horse.

Electroretinography

Electroretinography is used to determine function in the outer layers of the retina by recording the summation of electrical response when the retina is stimulated by light.[193-196] The electroretinogram (ERG) is the recorded total electrical response of the retina to that light. The ERG is not a measure of vision but only a measure of functional integrity of the outer portion of the retina and RPE. A blind animal (e.g., with disease of the inner retina, optic nerve, or central nervous system) can have normal ERG findings. The ganglion cells and their axons, as well as the optic nerve, do not contribute to the ERG recording.

An ERG is indicated whenever visual problems are suspected to be present in the outer retina. In the horse, an ERG is indicated to assess for retinal function in cases of equine recurrent uveitis, corneal or lens opacities that preclude visualization of the ocular fundus (e.g., cataracts, diffuse corneal edema), suspected congenital stationary night blindness, non–equine retinal uveitis–related retinitis and chorioretinitis, retinal detachment, ocular trauma, and chronic glaucoma.[197-200]

The primary components of an electroretinograph are a light source (photostimulator), a high-gain amplifier, and a recorder.[196] Three electrodes are needed, a positive (i.e., active) corneal electrode, a negative (i.e., reference) electrode, and a ground (i.e., indifferent) electrode (Fig. 1-64, A).[196] The clinical ERG consists of three basic waveforms (a-wave, b-wave, and c-wave) (Fig. 1-64, B).[196] The a-wave is an initial negative deflection. This is followed by a positive deflection, the b-wave, which has a higher potential (amplitude) and is followed by an afternegativity. In addition to the a-wave and b-wave, there is usually a second positive deflection, the c-wave, which is more prolonged. The origin of each wave component is complex and

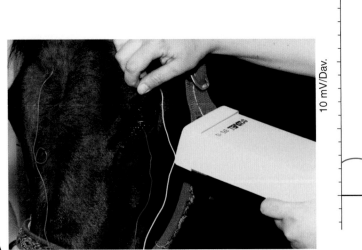

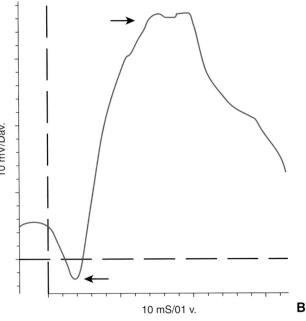

Fig. 1-64 **A,** Three electrodes are in place for performance of an electroretinogram (ERG). **B,** The clinical ERG consists of three basic waveforms (a-wave, b-wave, and c-wave). The a-wave, an initial negative deflection *(bottom arrow),* and the b-wave, positive deflection, which follows the a-wave *(top arrow),* are most prominent in the horse. (ERG image courtesy Dr. Andras Komaromy.)

poorly understood. Latency and implicit times, the time from onset of a stimulus to the peak of a particular response, are also important in evaluating the ERG. In a diseased eye, the amplitudes typically decrease while the implicit times increase.

One of the intrinsic factors that can affect the ERG is the eye's state of light adaptation, classified as scotopic (dark-adapted) and photopic (light-adapted).[196,197] The scotopic state of the eye is primarily a rod response. The photopic state of the eye is primarily a cone response. Rods are more numerous than cones in the horse, so the ERG is primarily a rod response in this species.[197] The rod and cone responses can be separated by repetitive stimuli or flickers of varying frequency, light adaptation state of the retina, and variation in the intensity of the stimulus.[196] Other intrinsic factors that may affect the ERG include age, transparency of the ocular media, retinal integrity, and retinal circulatory disturbances.[196,197] Amplitudes can vary according to species, state of adaptation to light, ocular movements, pupillary dilation, and pathologic state of the eye.[196,197]

Extrinsic factors that affect the ERG include the light stimulus used, electrodes used, and recording equipment.[196,197] The light stimulus may have variations in duration of flash, light intensity, frequency, and color. The positioning and type of electrode affect the level of background noise and amplitude of the ERG. Both extrinsic and intrinsic factors can be minimized and must be monitored by establishing a protocol for evaluating the ERG in the horse.[197]

Three main techniques used in clinical veterinary ophthalmology are the flash ERG, pattern ERG, and visual evoked potentials.[196] In contrast to the flash ERG, the pattern ERG originates in the inner retina and therefore is helpful in the diagnosis of diseases such as glaucoma.[196] Limits to visual resolution can also be established by pattern ERG.[196] Visual evoked potentials, although not ERGs, can be recorded with the same equipment and can record activity from the visual cortex. This activity has been mapped in some breeds of dogs and cats, but not in the horse.[153,201]

Flash electroretinography is the method of choice for assessment of retinal function in veterinary ophthalmology.[196,197] The proper recording of ERGs requires general anesthesia in animals to prevent recording of artifacts from muscle activity and to allow ideal positioning of the eyes. General anesthesia is inherently risky, expensive, and more labor intensive in the horse. Also, the inhalant anesthetics, halothane and isoflurane, have been shown to have a negative effect on the ERG amplitude and inner retinal function in other species.[197,202,203] Electroretinography in the standing horse can be frustrating because the commonly used corneal contact electrodes drop out of the eye easily, especially with head movement.[197] Sedation will not eliminate the almost constant head movement.

Sedated or unsedated, the horse may still shy from the closeness of the stimulator, and even small head movements can easily dislodge the other electrodes and require their replacement.[197] As a result, studies in which electroretinography is used in the horse are rare.

Findings from flash ERGs in horses have been reported, and the implicit times and amplitudes were similar in the various reports.[197,199,204-206] Unfortunately, a lack of detailed description of recording parameters and lack of descriptive statistics of results have made comparisons between studies difficult.[197,199,204] The rod and cone components of the equine flash ERG have been studied.[204,205] Mean reported latencies and amplitudes of the photopic a- and b-waves are 5.19 ± 1.56 and 26.63 ± 2.26 ms and 40.89 ± 20.50 and 184.75 ± 63.26 µV, respectively.[66] Mean latencies and amplitudes of low-intensity flash (0.33 CD/m^2 with 5 minutes of dark adaptation) and high-intensity flash (4.62 CD/m^2 with 5 minutes of dark adaptation) scotopic a- and b-waves, with pseudo-Ganzfield stimulation, Dawson, Trick and Litzkow (DTL) microfiber electrodes (Retina Technologies), and detomidine sedation in the standing horse have been reported.[197] Low-intensity flash scotopic a- and b-wave latency and amplitudes are 5.73 ± 1.88 and 36.95 ± 3.89 ms and 103.18 ± 120.72 and 409.30 ± 319.36 µV, respectively.[197] High-intensity flash scotopic a- and b-wave latency and amplitudes are 5.13 ± 1.34 and 34.75 ± 1.87 ms, and 153.68 ± 94.19 and 374.09 ± 161.93 µV, respectively.[197] ERG flicker-photometry has been used to assess the spectral sensitivities of cones in the horse.[207] Oscillatory potentials have not yet been recorded in the horse.[197,199,204,205]

ADVANCED OCULAR IMAGING TECHNIQUES

Diagnostic Ocular Ultrasonography

Ultrasonography is a rapid, safe, and practical method for examination of the intraocular and retrobulbar structures in an awake horse. Ocular ultrasonography allows examination of the globe in conditions in which opacity of the transmitting media of the eye (cornea, aqueous humor, lens, and vitreous humor) or extreme eyelid swelling otherwise prevents a complete ophthalmic examination.[208-210] In addition, evaluation of intraocular mass lesions, differentiation between solid and cystic structures, examination for a foreign body, axial length determination of the globe and intraocular structures, and examination of orbital structures are all indications for performing ocular ultrasonography.[210] The most common clinical indications for ocular ultrasonography in the horse are to evaluate for the presence of a retinal detachment in eyes after trauma, with uveitis, hyphema, cataract, and severe corneal opacities (e.g., edema, fibrosis), and as a preoperative cataract surgery evaluation.[210] Orbital evaluation is also routinely performed in instances of exophthalmos or orbital trauma. Ultrasonography can also be used to verify the stage and location of a cataract before surgical removal, as well as potential complications (e.g., posterior lenticonus) that would make phacoemulsification more challenging.[208,210] Diagnostic ultrasonography of the equine lens and posterior segment has been reported.[208] The ultrasound dimensions of the extirpated equine globe have been reported and are shorter in length than the ocular dimensions previously reported for the equine eye.[211] More thorough descriptions of the physics, equipment, techniques, and results of ultrasonography in various disease states can be found elsewhere.[210-217]

Ocular Ultrasonography: General Features

Ultrasound is an acoustic wave that consists of an oscillation of particles within a medium.[212] The velocity of the longitudinal wave is dependent on the medium through which it is traveling.[212] Water transmits the wave at a slower velocity than a more solid media, so the wave passes more quickly through the lens than through the aqueous or vitreous.[212] Echoes are produced by acoustic interfaces that are created at the junction of two media that have different acoustic impedances.[212] The greater the difference in the acoustic impedance of the two media that produce the interface, the stronger is the reflection of the ultrasound wave (i.e., the echo).[212] So, the anterior lens capsule would produce a stronger echo when bordered by normal aqueous than when bordered by blood (hyphema). The returning echoes are affected by many factors including the angle of sound incidence; the size, shape, and smoothness of the acoustic interface; absorption; scatter; and refraction.[212] If the sound wave strikes an interface at a perpendicular angle, all of the wave is reflected back to the transducer, and a strong echo results. If the beam is angled, some of the reflected energy is diverted away from the probe and results in a weaker echo. The smoother and straighter an interface is (e.g., retinal surface, lens capsule), the more reflected energy returns directly to the probe, resulting in a strong echo. Higher sound velocities (i.e., higher-numbered transducer probes) and greater tissue thickness increase absorption of the sound wave and weaken the echo. Refraction occurs when a sound wave is directed obliquely to an interface that demarcates two media of different sound velocities.[212] Therefore no refraction occurs when a sound wave is directed perpendicular to an interface or when the velocities of the two media are the same.[212]

Deep tissue penetration is not required for ocular ultrasonography, but high resolution is required.[210] The frequency of the ultrasonic waves emitted by the selected oscillating piezoelectric transducer determines the resolution of the image.[210,212] Transducer probes are available in a range of frequencies (e.g., 3.5, 5, 7.5, 10, 12.5, 20, 35, and 50 MHz), and the frequency is inversely proportional to the wavelength of the sound beam.[210,212] Depth of sound beam penetration is directly proportional to wavelength. Therefore a low frequency transducer (5 MHz) provides poor near-field axial resolution but greater tissue penetration and is therefore useful for imaging more posteriorly located structures such as the orbit. A high-frequency transducer (50 MHz) provides lower tissue penetration but high near-field axial resolution and is therefore useful for imaging more anteriorly located structures.[210,212]

An optimal ophthalmic transducer for general use is a 10-MHz transducer with a focal range of 3 to 4 cm and a small scan head.[210] This probe provides adequate depth of penetration to visualize the retrobulbar structures, enhanced resolution, and ability to visualize the anterior intraocular structures such as the iris, ciliary body, anterior and posterior chambers, and cornea (with the use of an off-set device).[210] Alternately, a 5- MHz or 7.5-MHz transducer will also produce good ophthalmic images and have a better depth of penetration for visualization of retrobulbar structures.[210] Near-field reverberation artifacts will obscure the anterior segment of the globe unless an off-set device or increased sterile coupling gel is used or the ultrasound examination is performed through closed eyelids.[210] The use of probes with frequencies of 20 to 100 MHz is referred to as high-frequency ultrasound biomicroscopy.[218,219] Ultrasound biomicroscopy allows for optimal visualization of the cornea, sclera, anterior and posterior chambers, iris, choroid, and lens and is described in the following section.

Both amplitude-mode (A-scan) and brightness-mode (B-scan) ultrasonography are useful for diagnostic purposes in ocular disease.[212] A-scan ultrasonography produces an anterior-posterior image with peaks reflecting tissues of different identities displayed as a linear series of vertical spikes from a baseline (Fig. 1-65).[212] The time between two spikes can be converted into distance and used to measure anterior-posterior axial length of the globe, anterior chamber depth, axial lens thickness, and vitreous anterior-posterior axial length.[212] B-scan ultrasonography provides a two-dimensional real-time image of the eye and orbit and is the most common mode of ultrasound used clinically in veterinary ophthalmology (Fig. 1-66).[208-211,213-217]

Ultrasonographic images are described as hyperechoic, hypoechoic, and anechoic.[210,212] Four major ocular acoustic echoes (hyperechoic) are generated

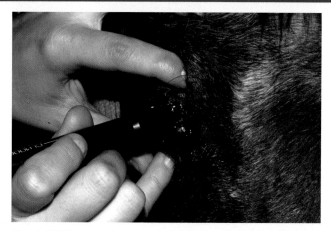

Fig. 1-67 The transducer can be placed directly on the cornea, which provides superior images of the posterior segment or orbit, or the scan may be performed through closed eyelids or with an off-set device.

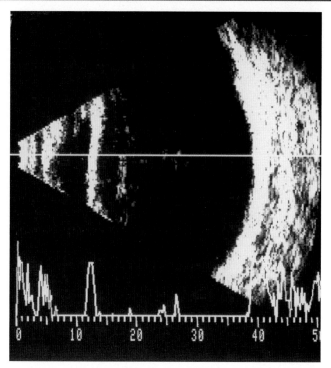

Fig. 1-65 A-scan ultrasonography produces an anterior-posterior image with peaks reflecting tissues of different identities displayed as a linear series of vertical spikes from a baseline. (Ultrasound image courtesy Dr. David Wilkie.)

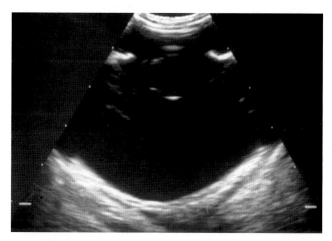

Fig. 1-66 B-scan ultrasonography provides a two-dimensional real-time image of the eye and orbit and is the most common mode of ultrasound used in a clinical setting. Four major ocular acoustic echoes (hyperechoic) are generated within a normal eye. These echoes originate from the anterior cornea, the anterior lens capsule, the posterior lens capsule, and the retina/choroid/sclera. (Ultrasound image courtesy Dr. David Wilkie.)

by the iris, corpora nigra, ciliary body, optic nerve, orbital fat, muscles, and other orbital structures.[210] The optic nerve head/lamina cribrosa appears as a hyperechoic structure with the optic nerve itself seen as a hypoechoic structure extending posteriorly from the optic nerve head.[210,212] The orbital muscle cone appears as an echodensity extending posteriorly from the equatorial region of the globe and converging toward the orbital apex.[210,212] The anterior and posterior chambers, lens cortex and nucleus, and vitreous chamber are normally anechoic.[210,212]

Ocular Ultrasonography Technique

The transducer can be placed directly on the cornea, which provides superior images of the posterior segment or orbit, or the scan may be performed through closed eyelids or with the use of an off-set device (Fig. 1-67). The transducer can be positioned to provide horizontal, vertical, and oblique scanning sections of the eye.[212] The globe should routinely be imaged in the horizontal and vertical planes through the visual axis.[210,212,215] Oblique positioning can then be performed for a complete examination.[210,212,215] The transducer can also be positioned dorsal to the zygomatic arch to scan the orbit.[212,210] The use of a small scan head diameter allows optimal placement on the cornea (Fig. 1-68).[210] When ultrasound biomicroscopy is not being performed, conducting the examination through the eyelids or with the use of an off-set device, which may require an increase in gain setting, will facilitate examination of the anterior portions of the globe.[210] A suitable tissue-equivalent off-set device is available with most transducers, or alternatively, a water-filled balloon or excess coupling gel can be used.[210] A water bath is necessary for ultrasound biomicroscopy.[210]

within a normal eye. These echoes originate from the anterior cornea, the anterior lens capsule, the posterior lens capsule, and the retina/choroid/sclera (see Fig. 1-66).[210,212] The retina, choroid, and sclera cannot be normally differentiated from one another by ultrasonography. Additional echodensities can be generated

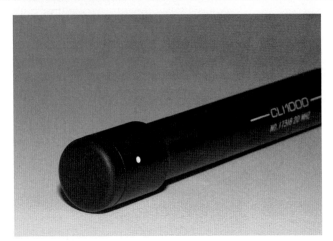

Fig. 1-68 A small transducer head is optimal for transcorneal ultrasound examination.

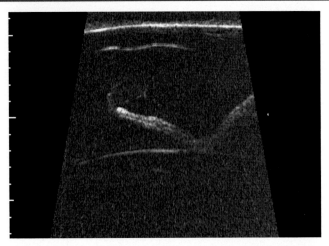

Fig. 1-69 Fibrin appears as a series of disconnected echodensities throughout the anterior chamber, whereas hypopyon is most often seen ventrally and is more uniform in its echodensity. A fibrin clot is shown attached to the tip of the iris (35-MHz probe).

Sedation and/or regional nerve blocks may be required, depending on the temperament and level of discomfort of the horse and globe stability. Topical anesthesia of the cornea (proparacaine 0.5%, Alcaine, Alcon Laboratories) is required for a transcorneal ultrasound examination. Sterile ultrasound coupling gel or K-Y jelly is placed on the transducer tip or on the corneal surface and should be irrigated from the eye on completion of the examination.[210] Cellulose-based coupling gels may cause corneal irritation and should be avoided.[210] Care should also be taken to avoid exposure of the intraocular contents to the coupling gel with full-thickness corneal lacerations and uveal prolapse.[210]

Ultrasonic Evaluation of Ocular Trauma

Ocular ultrasonography is of extreme importance in the evaluation of ocular trauma in the equine patient.[210] The extent and severity of the injury, prognosis, and probable therapy can be determined.[210] In many instances, ultrasonography is the only examination method of value in an eye that is otherwise severely painful or opaque or in an eye in which the eyelids cannot be opened because of swelling.[210] A transpalpebral examination can be performed in the last case. Obviously, if the structural integrity of the globe is compromised, extreme care should be taken when this procedure is performed.[210]

Both blunt and penetrating trauma in the horse can result in significant intraocular changes. Penetrating trauma can result in a shallow anterior chamber; fibrin in the anterior chamber; hyphema; lens capsule rupture; lens luxation, subluxation, or expulsion; vitreous hemorrhage; retinal detachment; and possibly limbal or posterior scleral rupture.[210] In addition, hyphema; vitreous hemorrhage; cataract; lens luxation or subluxation

and rupture; and retinal tear, retinal detachment, and choroidal detachment can all occur with blunt trauma.[210]

In instances of severe trauma, measurements of identifiable structures should be obtained for assessment of the damage.[210] For example, a reduction in the lens-posterior scleral wall axial length may indicate a posterior lens luxation, whereas an increase may indicate an anterior lens luxation or a posterior scleral wall rupture.[210] On ultrasound examination, vitreous and orbital hemorrhage can appear uniform in echodensity, blending together because they are no longer separated by the scleral fibrous tunic.[210] In addition, the normally hyperechoic posterior scleral wall is not identifiable.[210]

Hyphema and inflammatory material (e.g., fibrin, hypopyon) may accumulate in the anterior chamber as a result of trauma or anterior uveitis.[210] Fibrin appears as a series of disconnected echodensities throughout the anterior chamber, whereas hypopyon is most often seen ventrally and is more uniform in echodensity (Fig. 1-69).[210] In addition, the ciliary body and vitreous should be examined for involvement in the inflammatory process, and the lens should be examined for secondary cataract formation.[210]

Ultrasound Examination of Intraocular Masses

Intraocular masses consist of inflammatory, neoplastic, and cystic structures and most commonly arise from the anterior uvea (iris, ciliary body) in the horse (Fig. 1-70), but choroidal mass lesions can occur as well.[210] Because many of these mass lesions arise from the anterior uvea, an off-set device, extra coupling gel, scanning through closed eyelids, or ultrasound biomicroscopy is required to adequately visualize the lesion.[210] Uveal or corpora nigra cysts usually remain attached to the

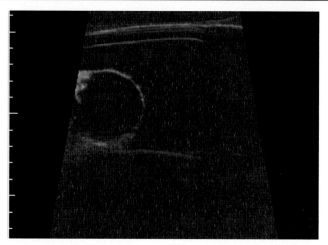

Fig. 1-70 Intraocular masses consist of inflammatory, neoplastic, and cystic structures and most commonly arise from the anterior uvea (iris, ciliary body) in the horse. A corpora nigra cyst is shown with the use of a 35-MHz probe. Air bubbles trapped between the transducer and the cornea result in the hyperechoic structures that look like "snow" throughout the sonogram.

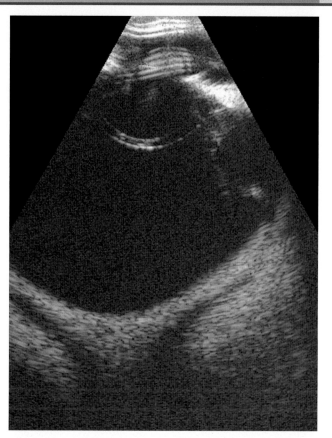

Fig. 1-71 A posterior cortical cataract is apparent as a second line anterior to the posterior lens capsule (12.5-MHz probe).

tissue of origin in the anterior chamber of the horse and can be transilluminated.[210] Mass lesions that are densely pigmented and cannot be transilluminated could be either cysts or melanomas.[210] A cyst will have an echogenic wall but an anechoic, fluid-filled center; whereas a melanoma appears homogeneous in its acoustic density.[210] Other inflammatory and neoplastic intraocular mass lesions could occur in the horse and could appear as hyperechoic, anechoic, or a heterogeneous mix on ultrasonography.[210]

Ultrasound Examination of Lens Abnormalities

When findings of ocular ultrasound examination are normal, the lens appears as two distinct echodensities seen at the anterior and posterior axial lens capsules.[210] The anterior echo is slightly convex, whereas the posterior echo is slightly concave. Internally, the lens is anechoic, and peripherally, the echo is reflected away from the probe. Abnormalities of the lens that can be detected on ultrasonography include abnormalities of lens size, cataract, luxation or subluxation, and lens rupture (Figs. 1-71 and 1-72).[210]

A cataract appears as increased internal echoes within the lens and as increased visualization of the lens periphery other than the anterior and posterior axial portions.[210] The size and intensity of the echoes will depend on the extent and severity of the cataract.[210] Abnormalities of lens size, measured anterior to posterior at the axial position, include both increased and decreased lens dimensions.[210] Enlargement of the lens is typically seen in association with a cataract.[210] A decrease in lens size occurs as a result of resorption of

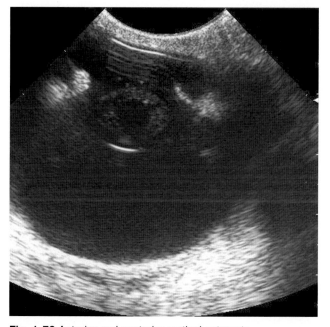

Fig. 1-72 Anterior and posterior cortical cataracts.

liquefied cortical material, as is seen with a hypermature cataract or microphakia (Fig. 1-73).[210]

Ultrasound can be used to evaluate the position of the lens after trauma or during inflammation when the anterior segment is opaque as a result of edema or hemorrhage.[210] Difficulty in obtaining a simultaneous echo of both the anterior and posterior lens capsule and changes in the anterior-posterior axial measurements of the lens or lens-posterior scleral wall may indicate a luxation or subluxation of the lens.[210]

Ultrasound Examination of the Posterior Segment

Ultrasound is used to evaluate the posterior segment for abnormalities of the vitreous or retina in an eye with a cataract, after trauma, or in other conditions in which opacification of the transmitting media may be present (e.g., equine recurrent uveitis).[208,210] The evaluation of the posterior segment in an eye with cataract is probably the second most common indication for ocular ultrasonography in a horse, after trauma.[208]

The vitreous cavity is normally anechoic, appearing dark or black on ultrasonography.[210] Abnormalities

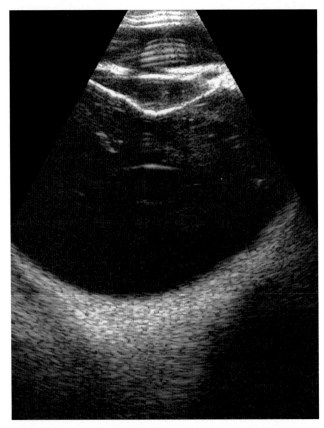

Fig. 1-73 A decrease in lens size occurs as a result of resorption of liquefied cortical material as is seen with a hypermature cataract or microphakia. This hypermature cataract is smaller than normal and the fibrotic lens capsule appears hyperechoic. A reverberation artifact is also present in the vitreous (12.5-MHz probe).

of the vitreous appear as echodensities and include hemorrhage, inflammation, degeneration (syneresis), asteroid hyalosis, and detachment.[210] Vitreal degeneration creates interfaces that result in ultrasonographic echodensities.[210] These appear as multiple, variable echogenic lines within the vitreous cavity and are best visualized by increasing the far-field gain setting on the ultrasound unit.[208,210,213] Clinically, the vitreous degeneration may or may not be visible. Asteroid hyalosis appears as highly reflective, discrete, freely moving echoes that persist even as the gain setting is decreased.[210] Vitreous hemorrhage appears as discrete to diffuse moderate amplitude echoes, which may demonstrate motion.[210] Vitreous inflammation appears as multifocal, disconnected variable echodensities within the vitreous cavity.[210]

The retinal echo is indistinguishable from the underlying choroidal and scleral echo in a normal eye.[210] The retina becomes apparent as a distinct echodensity with a separation of 0.5 to 1.0 mm.[211] When detached, the retina appears as an echo-dense linear structure, most often attached at the optic disc posteriorly and the ora ciliaris retinae anteriorly, resulting in the classic funnel or gull-wing–appearing detachment (Fig. 1-74).[210] A complete or only partial retinal detachment, as well as disinsertion from the ora (usually dorsally), can be present.[210] Initially, retinal detachments will be seen to undulate when viewed in real time, but with chronicity, the retina will become fixed and less mobile.[210] Examination of the subretinal space is important. An anechoic subretinal space indicates fluid such as a transudate, which may resorb, whereas the presence of echo-dense material in the subretinal space may indicate hemorrhage or infiltration of neoplastic or inflammatory cells.[210] Differential diagnoses for a hyperechoic linear structure in the vitreous include choroidal

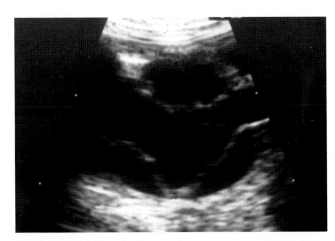

Fig. 1-74 When detached, the retina appears as an echo-dense linear structure, most often attached at the optic disc posteriorly and the ora ciliaris retinae anteriorly, resulting in the classic funnel or gull-wing–appearing detachment. (Ultrasound image courtesy Dr. David Wilkie.)

detachment, vitreous hemorrhage, vitreous detachment, vitreous degeneration, traction bands, and artifacts such as reverberation from the lens. (Fig. 1-75).[210]

Ultrasound Examination of the Orbit

Orbital contents include the extraocular muscles, fat, vascular tissues, glands, and the optic nerve. Exophthalmos and orbital trauma are the two most common indications for orbital ultrasound examination in the horse. Differential diagnoses for exophthalmos in the horse include orbital mass lesions (e.g., neoplasia) or hemorrhage (e.g., after trauma). An orbital mass lesion should be characterized as cystic or solid, and its location within the orbit should be determined.[210] Ultrasound-guided fine-needle aspiration or biopsy of orbital masses is useful.[210] After trauma to the orbit and associated structures, ultrasound may be used to evaluate the retrobulbar space for displaced fractures, hemorrhage, swelling, or compression of the optic nerve, and integrity of the posterior wall of the globe.[210]

Interpretation of Ocular Ultrasound Artifacts

Artifacts may be caused by inaccurate technique (e.g., insufficient amount of coupling gel or air bubbles in the water bath). Types of artifacts that can occur during the examination in the horse include Baum's bumps, absorption artifacts, and reverberation echoes

(i.e., reduplication or multiple-signal echoes).[210] Entrapment of air between the transducer and the eye, resulting in the display of bright echoes across the echogram, can be avoided by ensuring that a sufficient amount of coupling gel is used (see Fig. 1-70).[210,212] Air can also be entrapped by the hair coat when a transpalpebral ultrasound examination is performed, and therefore hair should probably be clipped.[210] Air bubbles in a water bath should be removed. Baum's bumps (Fig. 1-76) are B-scan artifacts that appear as elevations of the fundus.[210] They occur as the sound beam is refracted more quickly through the peripheral versus the central lens.[210-212] As a result, the posterior eye wall appears to be closer to the probe and can be seen as two discrete retinal elevations at the retinal surface.[210] The size of the elevations varies with the scan angle.[210]

An absorption artifact (shadowing, attenuation) occurs when a dense structure causes sound attenuation or complete reflection of sound and produces an absence of echoes posterior to the hyperechoic structure.[210,212] This appears as an anechoic area that can be confused with a mass lesion.[210-212] Structures that can cause this "acoustic shadow" include dense cataracts and intraocular foreign bodies.[210,212] Refraction around

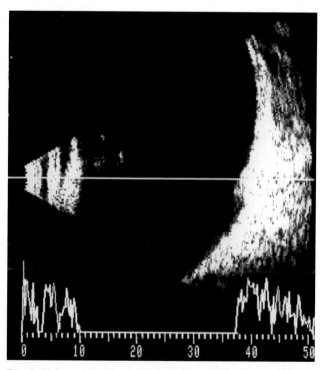

Fig. 1-76 Baum's bumps occur because the normal lens refracts the sound waves from the transducer, resulting in a faster passage of sound through the peripheral lens as compared with the central lens. This may result in the posterior eye wall appearing to be closer to the probe and will be seen as one or two discrete retinal elevations at the retinal surface, the size of which will vary with the scan angle. Only one bump is visible on this scan. (Ultrasound image courtesy Dr. David Wilkie.)

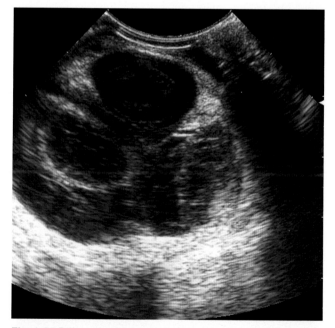

Fig. 1-75 Differential diagnoses for a hyperechoic linear structure in the vitreous include choroidal detachment, vitreous hemorrhage, vitreous detachment, vitreous degeneration, traction bands, and artifacts such as reverberation from the lens.

the edge of an artifact can also occur. This most commonly occurs around the edges of the globe.[212]

Reduplication echoes (reverberation artifacts) occur either between the probe and a highly reflective interface or between two highly reflective interfaces.[212] Because it will take longer for these echoes to reach the probe and return into the eye to be imaged, the artifacts always appear deeper in the globe than the tissue of origin.[212] Multiple signals can occur from the lens capsule, a foreign body, an air bubble, the sclera, or the orbital bone.[210,212] The typical reduplication echo occurs from the lens capsule to the transducer and back again and appears as linear hyperechodensities in the mid to posterior axial vitreous and can be confused with vitreous hemorrhage, inflammatory debris, or degeneration (see Fig. 1-73).[210-212] The true echo and the subsequent artifacts are equidistant and decrease in strength, and the artifact may "move" with movement of the transducer.[212] Reverberation artifacts in the anterior chamber, lens, and posterior segment have been reported as a common finding in a recent study.[208]

High-Frequency Ultrasound Examination and Ultrasound Biomicroscopy

Ultrasound probes with frequencies ranging from 20 to 35 MHz (high-resolution ultrasound) to 50 to 100 MHz (ultrasound biomicroscopy) have been developed and allow imaging at resolutions that are comparable to those achieved with low-power microscopic views.[218,219] Routine ultrasound examination of the eye with 5- to 12.5-MHz probes effectively bypasses the anterior segment of the eye. High-frequency ultrasound biomicroscopy (UBM) allows imaging of the anterior ocular segment at near-microscopic resolution in living patients and provides exceptionally detailed two-dimensional gray-scale images of the conjunctiva, cornea and anterior sclera, aqueous chambers, anterior chamber angle structures, uveal and ectodermal components of the ciliary body, the layers of the lens, zonules, and anterior vitreal face (Figs. 1-77, 1-78, and 1-79).[218,219] The important differences between UBM and conventional ultrasound examination are that the UBM transducer has a much higher frequency (20-100 MHz) and provides much higher image resolution.[218,219] However, UBM requires the use of a water bath that, until recently, necessitated the use of heavy sedation or general anesthesia in most veterinary patients. Self-contained water bath systems that can be used in an upright position have recently become available and will revolutionize this technology for easy clinical use in veterinary patients, especially large-animal patients such as the horse (E-Technologies). General anesthesia is not required—only topical anesthesia or light sedation.

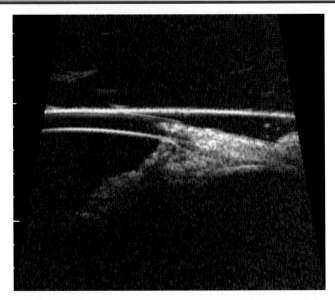

Fig. 1-77 Ultrasound biomicroscopy (UBM) allows imaging of the anterior ocular segment at near-microscopic resolution in living patients. The cornea, iridocorneal angle, iris, and anterior lens capsule can be visualized (35-MHz probe).

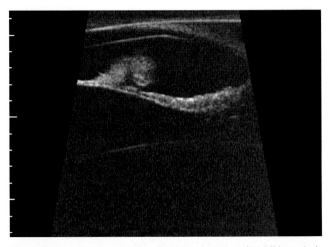

Fig. 1-78 Normal appearance of the corpora nigra (35-MHz probe).

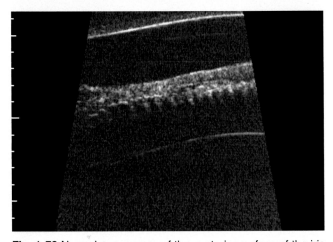

Fig. 1-79 Normal appearance of the posterior surface of the iris and ciliary body (35-MHz probe).

UBM has been used extensively in human medicine to define the dynamic mechanism of angle closure glaucoma, to evaluate the functional status of glaucoma-filtering implants, to evaluate tumors of the iris and ciliary body, to assess intraocular trauma, and to evaluate the position of intraocular lens implants.[220-222] It has been suggested that, in quantitative studies in which high-resolution ultrasound is used, one experienced observer should be employed to minimize variability.[223]

In the horse, UBM can be used to evaluate depth of stromal abscesses, corneal thickness, ocular squamous cell carcinoma, uveal cysts, changes in anterior uveitis, and other anterior segment and lens change, including trauma and cataracts (see Fig. 1-70).[224,225] Scleral thickness has been measured in both fresh and formalin-fixed equine globes.[28] Caliper and UBM measurements on fresh equine tissue revealed that at all sites measured, the thickness of the sclera in fresh tissue was significantly greater than that of tissue fixed in formalin. Thickness ranged from 1.02 ± 0.19 mm at the limbus (inferior), to 0.44 ± 0.06 mm at the equator (superior), to 0.79 ± 0.12 mm at the optic nerve (nasal). There were no significant differences between measurements obtained by caliper and measurements obtained by UBM.

Radiography

The anatomic structures in the equine head are complex and make radiographic evaluation difficult.[10-17,25,34] Radiographic techniques and exposures also vary with the area of the head being examined. Accurate radiographic interpretation becomes possible when knowledge of radiographic anatomy, radiographic signs of disease, and a basic understanding of disease processes involving the skull have been acquired.[25,34,226-231]

Skull Radiography

Skull radiographs in the horse may be most informative if there is involvement of bone in the disease process. Radiography is a valuable diagnostic tool for diseases of the nasal cavity, paranasal sinuses, and surrounding orbital bones (Fig. 1-80).[25,34,227]

Indications for skull radiography for the evaluation of ocular disease in horses include orbital and facial trauma, exophthalmos, and suspected disease of the nasolacrimal duct (e.g., chronic epiphora, dacryohemorrhea).[25,232] Trauma to the skull overlying sinuses or the nasal chambers—primarily the frontal, lacrimal, nasal and maxillary bones—usually results in depressed fractures that can impinge on the orbit or nasolacrimal duct.[232] Radiographic examination can evaluate the extent of displacement and can be used to predict posthealing contour.[232] It will also aid in establishing fracture size and suitability for repair.[232]

Contrast Radiography

Radiographic examination of enucleated globes fixed in Zenker's solution has been described.[233] Resultant radiographs demonstrate normal and abnormal anatomy, providing a new method of studying intact globes. Contrast radiograph techniques include dacryocystorhinography, orbital angiography, orbitography, and thecography, of which, only dacryocystorhinography has been described in the horse.[25,27,234-236]

Dacryocystorhinography

The entire nasolacrimal system can be outlined through contrast radiography (e.g., with barium or iodine) and is termed dacryocystorhinography.[25,27,234-236] This technique has been used to characterize the anatomy and to identify obstructive lesions of the nasolacrimal duct in horses and donkeys.[25,27,236] Dacryocystorhinography outlines the nasolacrimal system, thereby revealing obstructions, dilations, deviations, atresia, and other abnormalities. Indications for dacryocystorhinography include chronic epiphora, orbital trauma, and chronic conjunctivitis.[25,233-236]

Dacryocystorhinography can be performed in a standing, tranquilized patient after successful or unsuccessful irrigation of the duct.[25,234] The upper punctum, which is usually larger and more accessible, or the ventral punctum is cannulated and radiopaque contrast material (3 to 5 ml) is injected into the catheter.[234] If the nasolacrimal system is patent, viscid solutions such as 37% iodized poppy seed oil (Ethiodol; Savage Laboratories, Melville, NY) are preferred, because these slowly traverse the nasolacrimal duct during radiography.[234] Use of 60% barium sulfate (Mallinckrodt Inc., St Louis, Mo) and iodinated contrast medium (iohexol, [Omnipaque]; Amersham Health, Princeton, NJ) has also been described. Contrast is injected until it emerges from the lower punctum, external nares (unless obstruction of the duct is present), or both. After contrast injections, lateral, dorsal ventral, and oblique radiographs (Fig. 1-81) are recommended.[25,234,235] The lateral view provides a more detailed representation of the canaliculi and distal nasolacrimal duct.[25]

Computed tomography dacryocystography (CT-DCG) and magnetic resonance DCG have been used in humans for the evaluation of chronic epiphora, nasolacrimal duct masses, and facial trauma.[237,238] CT-DCG has recently been described in a horse with multiple facial bone fractures for evaluation of the patency of the nasolacrimal duct.[235] The advantages of CT over

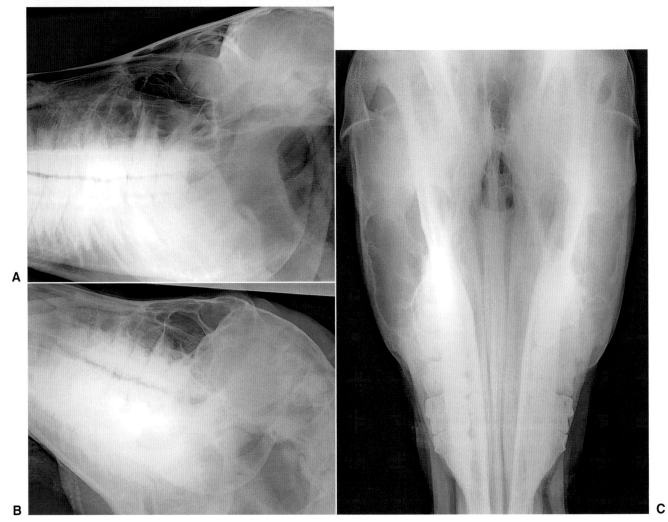

Fig. 1-80 **A,** Lateral radiographic view of the equine orbit and sinuses. **B,** Oblique radiographic view of the equine orbit and nasal sinuses. **C,** Dorsal ventral radiographic view of the equine head.

skull radiography in evaluation of the nasolacrimal duct include the lack of superimposition of bones and the ability to reconstruct three-dimensional images.[235] The disadvantage is the significant increase in cost and the requirement for general anesthesia and general anesthesia's inherent risks in the horse. CT-DCG may be reserved for animals already undergoing CT for evaluation of facial and orbital bone fractures or for those cases in which routine dacryocystorhinography proves nondiagnostic.

Computed Tomography

Computed tomography is the acquisition of cross-sectional, two-dimensional slices (i.e., tomograms) of a tissue.[234] These tomograms are created by a rotating radiation source that transmits x-rays, and the degree of attenuation of the x-rays within the intervening tissue is measured by a synchronous radiation detector array.[234] Gray-scale image reconstruction from the attenuation coefficients can then be digitally performed.[234] The lighter the image, the greater is the absorption of x-rays through that tissue.[234] Fat is black (i.e., low density) and bone, muscle and nerve are various shades of white (i.e., high density).[234] This provides relatively good contrast within the orbit.[234]

The use of cross-sectional CT in the equine head has been proposed to overcome the superimposition of the complex anatomic features of the equine skull that make conventional radiographic interpretation difficult.[239] References for normal transverse CT anatomy of the adult horse and the foal have recently been published, and the reader is referred to these articles for details.[240,241] The requirement for general anesthesia is a risk that must be calculated to gain diagnostic information. The adult equine head can only be scanned in

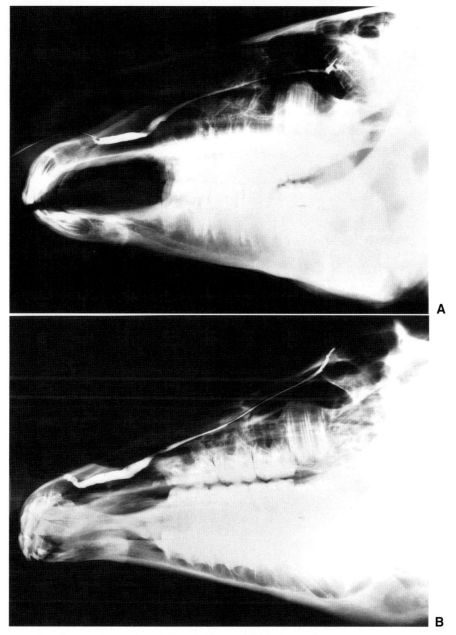

Fig. 1-81 The entire nasolacrimal system can be outlined through contrast radiography (e.g., barium or iodine) and is termed dacrycystorhinography. **A,** Left lateral dacryocystorhinography. **B,** Right lateral, dorsal ventral, and oblique views. (Photographs courtesy Dr. Claire Latimer.)

the transverse plane by CT, at this time, because of the limited diameter of the gantry and weight limitations of the imaging table (Fig. 1-82).[239-242] These images can later be reconstructed into other useful imaging planes.

The large amount of low-density fat in the equine orbit provides good natural contrast for the differentiation of the various soft-tissue structures by CT, although the primary advantage of CT over magnetic resonance imaging (MRI) is its ability to detect osseous changes (Fig. 1-83).[234,243] Disadvantages of CT over skull radiography in the horse include the need for general

anesthesia and the risks associated with recovery from anesthesia, increased cost, and limited accessibility.[243] Disadvantages of CT over MRI in the horse, in addition to the gantry limitations, include greater duration of anesthesia and the risk of irradiation of the lens.[243]

There have been few reports of CT examination of the equine orbit and nasolacrimal duct in disease. Most cases in the literature involving CT of the equine head involve evaluation of the sinuses, brain abscess, pituitary tumors, and skull fractures.[243-254] Very little has directly concerned the orbit (Fig. 1-84).[244,248,254]

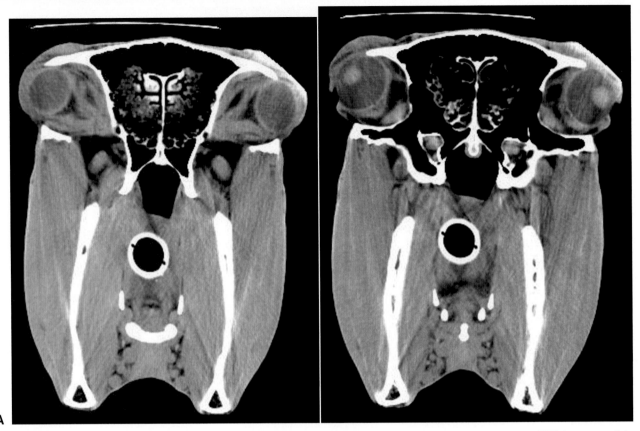

A   B

Fig. 1-82 A, The adult equine head can only be scanned in the transverse plane by computed tomography (CT) because of the limited diameter of the gantry and weight limitations of the imaging table. These images can later be reconstructed into other useful imaging planes. The extraocular muscles can be seen on this scan. **B,** The lens is visible on this scan.

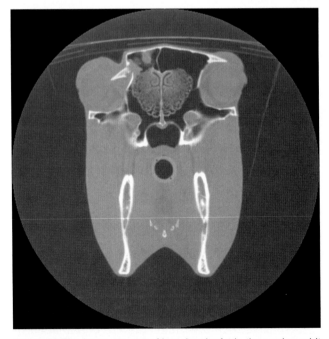

Fig. 1-83 The large amount of low-density fat in the equine orbit provides good natural contrast for the differentiation of the various soft-tissue structures by computed tomography (CT), although the primary advantage of CT over magnetic resonance imaging (MRI) is its ability to detect osseous changes. A supraorbital fracture is present on this CT scan.

Magnetic Resonance Imaging

MRI involves the localization, quantitation, and transformation of emitted resonant energy of protons that have been magnetized.[234,243,255] Standard MRI studies of the head are typically acquired in at least three orthogonal image planes (i.e., sagittal, transverse, and dorsal) relative to the central axis of the head.[244,255] The multiplanar capacity of MRI to acquire images in any desired slice plane without repositioning the patient is an important advantage of MRI over CT.[243,255] Conventional MRI examinations of the head include three types of pulse-echo sequences: the T_1-weighted sequence (performed before and after contrast administration); proton density; and the T_2-weighted sequence.[243] Alternate imaging sequences are available but are not discussed here.[234,243] Contrast enhancement (gadolinium diethylenetriaminepentaacetic acid, Magnevist; Berlex Laboratories, Cedar Knolls, NJ) will result in a hyperintense signal in which the contrast has extravasated (e.g., as a result of breakdown of the blood-brain barrier caused by inflammation or neoplasia).[243] An intravenous dose of 20 ml has been reported to be adequate in the horse.[243] The longitudinal magnetic relaxation time (T_1, spin lattice relaxation

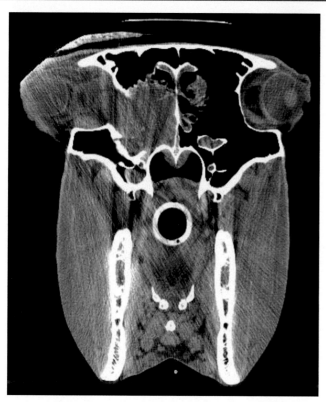

Fig. 1-84 The large amount of low-density fat in the equine orbit provides good natural contrast for the differentiation of the various soft-tissue structures by computed tomography, although the primary advantage of computed tomography (CT) over magnetic resonance imaging (MRI) is its ability to detect osseous changes. A nasal mass that has infiltrated the orbit is seen on this CT scan.

time) and the transverse magnetic relaxation time (T_2, spin-spin relaxation time) are the time needed for energized protons to return from the higher energy state to reestablish alignment with the magnetic field and the rate of decrease in the signal of the excited nuclei of the protons as energy is transferred to adjacent unexcited nuclei, respectively.[234] Proton density weighted images are taken when the protons are relaxed and do not depend on time constants.[234] T_2-weighted images can be differentiated from a T_1-weighted image as a result of the high intensity signal from the vitreous in a T_2-weighted image.[234]

Clinical evaluation of the equine orbit by MRI suffers from the same technical difficulties as CT, including the need for general anesthesia and the risks associated with recovery from anesthesia, weight limitations, and limited accessibility.[243,255] Normal anatomic atlases for the equine orbital structures and sinuses have been published for both T_1-weighted and T_2-weighted magnetic resonance images.[243,255-259]

The order of signal intensity for T_1-weighted images from white to black was as follows: fat > cornea, lens capsule, iris, retina, choroid > brain > extraocular muscles, optic nerve, skin, eyelids > aqueous, vitreous humor > lens, sclera > bone, air.[255] The order of signal intensity for T_2-weighted images from white to black was as follows: vitreous, aqueous humor > brain > extraocular muscles, optic nerve, iris, eyelids, skin > fat, bone, sclera > lens, air.[255] The oblique dorsal and oblique sagittal planes have been reported to be the most valuable for evaluating the orbit and optic pathways.[255] Equine patients <300 lb can be imaged by many of the existent superconductive magnets. Modification of current equipment allows for imaging the adult head. Newer magnets, which are open along the side, may allow imaging of larger horses.[255]

MRI advantages over CT include better resolution of retrobulbar structures, absence of ionizing radiation, direct multiplanar imaging that does not require changes in the position of the patient or gantry, enhanced anatomic detail and tissue characterization, and better assessment of both the intraorbital and extraorbital optic nerves.[234,255] Disadvantages include the requirement for general anesthesia, long data acquisition time, increased tissue slice thickness, poorer spatial resolution, failure to detect defects in cortical bone or soft-tissue mineralization, certain image artifacts, and the need for nonmetallic ventilation during inhalant anesthesia.[234,255] As in humans, T_1-weighted images provide the greatest spatial resolution and the best definition of normal anatomic detail of both the eye and orbit. Pathologic processes are known to predominantly affect T_2-weighted images.[255] Additional magnetic resonance studies on diseased eyes and orbits are needed to determine the value of this imaging tool in equine ophthalmology.

REFERENCES

1. Davidson MG: Equine ophthalmology. In Gelatt KN, editor: *Veterinary ophthalmology,* ed 2, Philadelphia, 1991, Lea & Febiger, pp 576-610.
2. Brooks DE: Equine ophthalmology. In Gelatt KN, editor: *Veterinary ophthalmology,* ed 3, Philadelphia, 1999, Lippincott Williams & Wilkins, pp 1053-1116.
3. Bistner S: Fundus examination of the horse, *Vet Clin North Am Large Anim Pract* 6:541-551, 1984.
4. Cooley PL: Normal equine ocular anatomy and eye examination, *Vet Clin North Am Equine Pract* 8:427-449, 1992.
5. Meredith R, Wolf ED: Ophthalmic examination and therapeutic techniques in the horse. *Comp Contin Ed Pract Vet* 3:s426-s433, 1981.
6. Lavach JD: *Large animal ophthalmology,* St Louis, 1990, Mosby.
7. Riis RC: Equine ophthalmology. In Gelatt KN, editor: *Veterinary ophthalmology,* Philadelphia, 1981, Lea & Febiger, pp 569-605.
8. Lavach JD: *Handbook of equine ophthalmology,* Fort Collins, Colo, 1987, Giddings Studio Publishing.
9. Davis JL et al: The effect of topical administration of atropine sulfate on the normal equine pupil: influence of age, breed, and gender, *Vet Ophthalmol* 6:329-332, 2003.

10. Samuelson D: Ophthalmic anatomy. In Gelatt KN, editor: *Veterinary ophthalmology,* ed 3, Philadelphia, 1999, Lippincott Williams & Wilkins, pp 31-150.

11. Budras KD: *Anatomy of the horse: an illustrated text,* ed 3, Hannover, Germany, 2001, Schlutersche.

12. Dyce KM, Sack WO, Wensing CJG: *Textbook of veterinary anatomy,* ed 3, Philadelphia, 2002, Saunders.

13. Prince JH et al: *Anatomy and histology of the eye and orbit in domestic animals,* Springfield, Ill, 1960, Charles C. Thomas, pp 128-153.

14. Martin CL, Anderson BG: Ocular anatomy. In Gelatt KN, editor: *Veterinary ophthalmology,* Philadelphia, 1981, Lea & Febiger, pp 18-22.

15. Kainer RA: Clinical anatomy of the equine head, *Vet Clin North Am Equine Pract* 9:1-23, 1993.

16. Diesem C: Organs of vision. In Getty R, editor: *Sisson and Grossman's the anatomy of the domestic animal,* ed 5, Philadelphia, 1975, WB Saunders, p 703.

17. Diesem C: Gross anatomic structures of equine and bovine orbit and its contents, *Am J Vet Res* 29:1769-1781, 1968.

18. Miller TL et al: Description of ciliary body anatomy and identification of sites for transscleral cyclophotocoagulation in the equine eye, *Vet Ophthalmol* 4:183-190, 2001.

19. Severin GA: *Veterinary ophthalmology notes,* ed 3, Fort Collins, Colo, 1995, College of Veterinary Medicine and Biomedical Sciences, Colorado State University.

20. Andrew SE et al: Density of corneal endothelial cells and corneal thickness in eyes of euthanitized horses, *Am J Vet Res* 62:479-482, 2001.

21. Simoens P, Muylle S, Lauwers H: Anatomy of the ocular arteries in the horse, *Equine Vet J* 28(Suppl):360-367, 1996.

22. Anderson BG, Anderson W: Vasculature of the equine and canine iris, *Am J Vet Res* 38:1791-1799, 1977.

23. Anderson BG, Wyman M: Anatomy of the equine eye and orbit: histologic structure and blood supply of the eyelids, *J Equine Med Surg* 3:4-9, 1979.

24. Crispin SM: Tear-deficient and evaporative dry eye syndromes of the horse, *Vet Ophthalmol* 3:87-92, 2000.

25. Latimer CA et al: Radiographic and gross anatomy of the nasolacrimal duct of the horse, *Am J Vet Res* 45:451-458, 1984.

26. O'Brien RT, Biller DS: Dental imaging: dentistry, *Vet Clin North Am Equine Pract* 14:259-271, 1998.

27. Said AH et al: Contribution to the nasolacrimal duct of donkeys in Egypt, *Zentralbl Veterinarmed* [C] 6:347-350, 1977.

28. Gilger BC et al: Ocular parameters related to drug delivery in the canine and equine eye: aqueous and vitreous humor volume and scleral surface area and thickness. In Progress.

29. Rubin L: *Atlas of veterinary ophthalmoscopy,* Philadelphia, 1974, Lea & Febiger.

30. Crispin S, Mathews A, Parker J: The equine fundus: examination, embryology, structure, and function, *Equine Vet J* 10(Suppl): 42-49, 1990.

31. Gelatt KN: Ophthalmoscopic studies in the normal and diseases ocular fundi of horses, *J Am Anim Hosp Assoc* 7:158-162, 1971.

32. Matthews A, Crispin S, Parker J: The equine fundus. II. Normal anatomical variants and colobomata, *Equine Vet J* 10(Suppl): 50-54, 1990.

33. De Schaepdrijver L et al: Retinal vascular patterns in domestic animals, *Res Vet Sci* 47:34-42, 1989.

34. Bertone JJ, Biller DS, Ruggles A: Diagnostic techniques for evaluation of the paranasal sinuses, *Vet Clin North Am Equine Pract* 9:75-91, 1993.

35. Scott EA, Duncan JR, McCormack JE: Cryptococcus involving the postorbital area and frontal sinus of the horse, *J Am Vet Med Assoc* 165:626-627, 1974.

36. Ramsey DT, Hauptmann JG, Peterson-Jones SM: Corneal thickness, intraocular pressure, and optical corneal diameter in Rocky Mountain horses with cornea globosa or clinically normal corneas, *Am J Vet Res* 60:1317-1320, 1999.

37. Gelatt KN, Gum GG, Mackay EO: Evaluation of mydriatics in horses, *Vet Comp Ophthalmol* 5:104-107, 1995.

38. Gelatt KN: Ophthalmic examination and diagnostic procedures. In Gelatt KN, editor: *Veterinary ophthalmology,* ed 3, Philadelphia, 1999, Lippincott Williams & Wilkins, pp 427-466.

39. Gelatt KN: Ophthalmic examination and diagnostic procedures. In Gelatt KN, editor: *Veterinary ophthalmology,* ed 2, Philadelphia, 1991, Lea & Febiger, pp 195-235.

40. Williams MM et al: Systemic effects of topical and subconjunctival ophthalmic atropine in the horse, *Vet Ophthalmol* 3:193-199, 2000.

41. George LW: Localization and differentiation of neurologic diseases. In Smith BP, editor: *Large animal internal medicine,* St Louis, 1990, Mosby, pp 145-170.

42. Mayhew IG: *Large animal neurology: a handbook for veterinary clinicians,* Philadelphia, 1989, Lea & Febiger.

43. Scagliotti RH: Comparative neuro-ophthalmology. In Gelatt KN, editor: *Veterinary ophthalmology,* ed 3, Philadelphia, 1999, Lippincott Williams & Wilkins, pp 1307-1400.

44. Crispin SM: Developmental anomalies and abnormalities of the equine iris, *Vet Ophthalmol* 3:93-98, 2000.

45. Gum GG, Gelatt KN, Ofri R: Physiology of the eye. In Gelatt KN, editor: *Veterinary ophthalmology,* ed 3, Philadelphia, 1999, Lippincott Williams & Wilkins, pp 151-181.

46. Neer TM: Horner's syndrome: anatomy, diagnosis, and causes, *Comp Contin Educ Pract Vet* 6:740-746, 1984.

47. Smith JS, Mayhew IG: Horner's syndrome in large animals, *Cornell Vet* 67:529-542, 1977.

48. Purohit RC, McCoy MD, Bergfield WA: Thermographic diagnosis of Horner's syndrome in the horse, *Am J Vet Res* 41:1180-1182, 1980.

49. Bacon CL et al: Bilateral Horner's syndrome secondary to metastatic squamous cell carcinoma in a horse, *Equine Vet J* 28:500-503, 1996.

50. Sweeney RW, Sweeney CR: Transient Horner's syndrome following routine intravenous injection in two horses, *J Am Vet Med Assoc* 185:802-803, 1984.

51. Geiser DR, Henton JR, Held JP: Tympanic bulla, petrous temporal bone, and hyoid apparatus disease in horses, *Comp Contin Educ Pract Vet* 10:740-754, 1988.

52. Adams R, Mayhew IG: Neurological examination of newborn foals, *Equine Vet J* 16:306-312 1984.

53. Gelatt KN: Congenital and acquired ophthalmic lesions in the foal, *Anim Eye Res* 1-2:15-27, 1993.

54. Mayhew IG: Neuro-ophthalmology. In Barnett KC et al, editors: *Color atlas and text of equine ophthalmology,* London, 1995, Mosby-Wolfe, pp 215-222.

55. Latimer CA, Wyman M, Hamilton J: An ophthalmic survey of the neonatal horse, *Equine Vet J* 2(Suppl):9-14, 1983.

56. Enzerink E: The menace response and pupillary light reflex in neonatal foals, *Equine Vet J* 30:546-548, 1998.

57. Brooks DE, Clark CK, Lester GD: Cochet-Bonnet aesthesiometer-determined corneal sensitivity in neonatal foals and adult horses, *Vet Ophthalmol* 3:133-138, 2000.

58. Clark CK, Brooks DE, Lester GD: Corneal sensitivity and tear production in hospitalized neonatal foals. *Proc Am Coll Vet Ophthalmol* 23:134-136, 1996.

59. Latimer CA, Wyman M: Neonatal ophthalmology, *Vet Clin North Am Equine Pract* 1:235-259, 1985.

60. Koch SA et al: Ocular disease in the newborn horse: a preliminary report, *J Equine Med Surg* 2:167-170, 1978.

61. Peiffer RL: Foundations of equine ophthalmology: clinical anatomy and physiology, *Equine Pract* 1:39-46, 1979.

62. Roberts SM: Ocular disorders. In McKinnon AI, Voss JL, editors: *Equine reproduction,* Philadelphia, 1993, Lea & Febiger, pp 1076-1087.

63. Roberts SM: Congenital ocular anomalies, *Vet Clin North Am Equine Pract* 8:459-487, 1992.

64. Munroe G: Survey of retinal haemorrhages in neonatal thoroughbred foals, *Vet Rec* 146:95-101, 2000.

65. Cutler TJ: Ophthalmic findings in the geriatric horse, *Vet Clin North Am Equine Pract* 18:545-574, 2002.

66. Brooks DB: *Ophthalmology for the equine practitioner,* In Brooks DB, editor: *Equine ophthalmology for the equine practitine,* Jackson, Wyo, 2002, Teton NewMedia.

67. Rubin LF: Auriculopalpebral nerve block as an adjunct to the diagnosis and treatment of ocular inflammation in the horse, *J Am Vet Med Assoc* 144:1387-1388, 1964.

68. Manning JP, St. Clair LE: Palpebral, frontal, and zygomatic nerve blocks for examination of the equine eye, *Vet Med Small Anim Clin* 32:187-189, 1976.

69. Van der Woerdt A et al: Effect of auricle-palpebral nerve block and intravenous administration of xylazine on intraocular pressure and corneal thickness in horses. *Am J Vet Res* 56:155-158, 1995.

70. Raffe MR et al: Retrobulbar block in combination with general anesthesia for equine ophthalmic surgery, *Vet Surg* 15:139-141, 1986.

71. Short CE, Rebhun WC: Complications caused by the oculocardiac reflex during anesthesia in a foal, *J Am Vet Med Assoc* 176:630-631, 1980.

72. Brooks DE: Orbit. In Auer JA, editor: *Equine surgery,* Philadelphia, 1992, WB Saunders, pp 654-666.

73. Moore CP: Eyelids and nasolacrimal disease, *Vet Clin North Am* 8:499-519, 1992.

74. Joyce JR, Bratton GR: Keratoconjunctivitis sicca associated with fracture of the mandible, *Vet Med Small Anim Clin* 6:619-620, 1973.

75. Spurlock SL, Spurlock GH, Wise M: Keratoconjunctivitis sicca associated with fracture of the stylohyoid bone in a horse, *J Am Vet Med Assoc* 194:258-259, 1989.

76. Van Kempen KR, James LF: Ophthalmic lesions in locoweed poisoning in cattle, sheep, and horses, *Am J Vet Res* 32:1293-1295, 1971.

77. Spiess BM, Wilcock BP, Physick-Sheard PW: Eosinophilic granulomatous dacryoadenitis causing bilateral keratoconjunctivitis sicca in a horse, *Equine Vet J* 21:226-228, 1989.

78. Collins BK et al: Immune mediated keratoconjunctivitis sicca in a horse, *Vet Comp Ophthalmol* 4:61-65, 1994.

79. Wolf ED, Meredith R: Parotid duct transposition in the horse, *J Equine Vet Sci* 12:143-145, 1981.

80. Reilly L, Beech J: Bilateral keratoconjunctivitis sicca in a horse, *Equine Vet J* 26:171-172, 1994.

81. Firth EC: Vestibular disease and its relationship to facial paralysis in the horse: a clinical study of 7 cases, *Aust Vet J* 53:560-565, 1977.

82. Marts BS, Bryan GM, Prieur DJ: Schirmer tear test measurement and lysozyme concentration of equine tears, *J Equine Med Surg* 1:427-430, 1977.

83. Williams RD, Manning JP, Peiffer RL: The Schirmer tear test in the equine: normal values and the contribution of the gland of the nictitating membrane, *J Equine Med Surg* 3:117-119, 1979.

84. Brightmann AH et al: Decreased tear production associated with general anesthesia in the horse, *J Am Vet Med Assoc* 182:243-244, 1983.

85. Clark CK, Brooks DE, Lester GD. Corneal sensitivity and tear production in hospitalized neonatal foals, *Proc Am Coll Vet Ophthalmol* 23:134-136, 1996.

86. Beech J et al: Schirmer tear test results in normal horses and ponies: effect of age, season, environment, sex, time of day and placement of strips, *Vet Ophthalmol* 6:251-254, 2003.

87. Hamor RE et al: Evaluation of results for Schirmer tear tests conducted with and without application of a topical anesthetic in clinically normal dogs of 5 breeds, *Am J Vet Res* 61:1422-1425, 2000.

88. Massa KL et al. Usefulness of aerobic microbial culture and cytologic evaluation of corneal specimens in the diagnosis of infectious ulcerative keratitis in animals, *J Am Vet Assoc* 215:1671-1674, 1999.

89. Da Silva Curiel JM, et al: Nutritionally variant streptococci associated with corneal ulcers in horses, *J Am Vet Med Assoc* 107:624-626, 1990.

90. Kleinfeld J, Ellis PP: Effects of topical anesthetics on growth of microorganisms, *Arch Ophthalmol* 76:712-715, 1966.

91. Champagne ES, Pickett JP: The effect of topical 0.5% proparacaine HCL on corneal and conjunctival culture results, *Proc Am Coll Vet Ophthalmol* 26:144-145, 1995.

92. Miller TR et al: Herpetic keratitis in the horse, *Equine Vet J* 10(Suppl):15-17, 1990.

93. Collinson PN et al: Isolation of herpesvirus type 2 (equine gamma herpesvirus 2) from foals with keratoconjunctivitis, *J Am Vet Med Assoc* 205:329-331, 1994.

94. Lavach JD et al: Cytology of normal and inflamed conjunctivas in dogs and cats, *J Am Vet Med Assoc* 170:722-727, 1977.

95. Bauer GA, Spiess BM, Lutz H: Exfoliative cytology of conjunctiva and cornea in domestic animals: a comparison of four collecting techniques, *Vet Comp Ophthalmol* 6:181-186, 1996.

96. Wills M et al. Conjunctival brush cytology: evaluation of a new cytological collection technique in dogs and cats with a comparison to conjunctival scraping, *Vet Comp Ophthalmol* 7:74-81, 1997.

97. Richter M et al: Keratitis due to Histoplasma in a horse, *Vet Ophthalmol* 6:99-103, 2003.

98. Forster RK et al. Methenamine-silver stained corneal scrapings in keratomycosis, *Am J Ophthalmol* 82:261-265, 1976.

99. Galle LE et al: Prevalence of equine herpesvirus DNA from conjunctival swabs in Missouri, *Vet Ophthalmol* 6:360-361, 2003 (abstract).

100. Neary A et al: Diagnosis of equine fungal keratitis using polymerase chain reaction, *Vet Ophthalmol* 6 (6):363, 2003 (abstract).

101. Kuonen VJ et al: A PCR-based assay for the diagnosis of equine fungal keratitis, *Vet Ophthalmol* 6:364, 2003 (abstract).

102. Da Silva Curiel JMA et al: Topical fluorescein dye: effects on immunofluorescent antibody test for feline herpesvirus keratoconjunctivitis, *Prog Vet Comp Ophthalmol* 1:99-104, 1991.

103. Feenstra RPG, Tseng SCG: What is actually stained by rose Bengal? *Arch Ophthalmol* 10:984-993, 1992.

104. Kim J: The use of vital dyes in corneal disease, *Curr Opin Ophthalmol* 11:241-247, 2000.

105. Feenstra RPG, Tseng SCG: Comparison of fluorescein and rose Bengal staining, *Ophthalmology* 99:605-617, 1992.

106. Gelatt KN: Vital staining of the canine cornea and conjunctiva with rose Bengal, *J Am Anim Hosp Assoc* 8:17-22, 1972.

107. Slatter DH: Differential staining of the canine cornea and conjunctiva with fluorescein-rose Bengal and Alcian blue, *J Small Anim Pract* 14:291-296, 1972.

108. Laroche RR, Campbell RC: Quantitative rose Bengal staining technique for external ocular diseases, *Ann Ophthalmol* 20:274-276, 1988.

109. Coster DJ: Superficial keratopathy. In Tasman W, Jaeger EA, editors: *Duane's clinical ophthalmology on CD-ROM, vol 4 (17),* Hagerstown, Md, 1999, Lippincott, Williams & Wilkins.

110. Lemp MA, Chacko B: Diagnosis and treatment of tear deficiencies. In Tasman W, Jaeger EA, editors: *Duane's clinical ophthalmology on CD-ROM, vol 4 (14),* Hagerstown, Md, 1999, Lippincott, Williams & Wilkins.

111. Kimura SJ: Fluorescein paper: simple means of insuring use of sterile fluorescein, *Am J Ophthalmol* 34:446-447, 1951.

112. Cello RM, Lasmanis J: Pseudomonas infection of the eye of the dog resulting from the use of contaminated fluorescein solution, *J Am Vet Med Assoc* 132:297-299, 1958.

113. Kim J, Foulks GN: Evaluation of the effect of lissamine green and rose bengal on human corneal epithelial cells, *Cornea* 18:328-332, 1999.

114. Brooks DE et al: Rose Bengal positive epithelial microerosions as a manifestation of equine keratomycosis, *Vet Ophthalmol* 3:83-86, 2000.

115. Dziezyc J: Nasolacrimal system. In Auer JA, editor: *Equine surgery*, Philadelphia, 1992, WB Saunders, pp 630-634.

116. Schumacher J, Dean P, Welch B: Epistaxis in two horses with dacryohemorrhea, *J Am Vet Med Assoc* 200:366-367, 1992.

117. Berliner ML: *Biomicroscopy of the eye*, Vol I, New York, 1949 Paul B. Hoeber.

118. Martin CL: Slit lamp examination of the normal canine anterior ocular segment. I. Introduction and technique, *J Small Anim Pract* 10:143-149, 1969.

119. Martin CL: Slit lamp examination of the normal canine anterior ocular segment. II. Description, *J Small Anim Pract* 10:151-162, 1969.

120. Martin CL: Slit lamp examination of the normal canine anterior ocular segment. III. Discussion and summary, *J Small Anim Pract* 10:1163-169, 1969.

121. Trim CM, Colbern GT, Martin CL: Effect of xylazine and ketamine on intraocular pressure in horses, *Vet Rec* 117:442-443, 1985.

122. Miller PE, Pickett JP, Majors LJ: Evaluation of two applanation tonometers in horses, *Am J Vet Res* 51:935-937, 1990.

123. Cohen CM, Reinke DA: Equine tonometry, *J Am Vet Med Assoc* 156:1884, 1970.

124. McClure JR, Gelatt KN, Manning JP: The effect of parenteral acepromazine and xylazine on intraocular pressure in the horse, *Vet Med Small Anim Clin* 32:1727-1730, 1976.

125. Benson GJ et al: Intraocular tension of the horse: effects of succinylcholine and halothane anesthesia, *Am J Vet Res* 42:1831-1832, 1981.

126. Smith P et al: Tonometric and tonographic studies in the normal pony eye, *Equine Vet J* 10(Suppl):360-368, 1990.

127. Gelatt KN et al: Evaluation of applanation tonometers for the dog eye, *Invest Ophthalmol Vis Sci* 16:963-968, 1977.

128. Gelatt KN, Gum GG: Evaluation of electronic tonometers in the rabbit eye, *Am J Vet Res* 42:1778-1781, 1981.

129. Dziezyc J, Millichamp NJ, Smith WB: Comparison of applanation tonometers in dogs and horses, *J Am Vet Med Assoc* 201:430-433, 1992.

130. Plummer CE, Ramsey DT, Hauptmann JG: Assessment of corneal thickness, intraocular pressure, optical corneal diameter, and axial globe dimensions in Miniature horses, *Am J Vet Res* 64:661-665, 2003.

131. Kotani T et al: Which are the optimal tonometers for different animal species? *Anim Eye Res* 12:55-61, 1993.

132. Gelatt KN, Gum GG, Mackay EO: Estimation of aqueous humor outflow facility by pneumatonography in normal, genetic carrier, and glaucomatous Beagles, *Vet Comp Ophthalmol* 6:148-151, 1996.

133. Smith P et al: Unconventional aqueous humor outflow of microspheres perfused into the equine eye, *Am J Vet Res* 47:2445-2453, 1986.

134. Toris CB et al: Prostaglandin A2 increases uveoscleral outflow and trabecular outflow facility in the cat, *Exp Eye Res* 61:649-657, 1995.

135. Murphy CJ, Howland HC: The optics of comparative ophthalmoscopy, *Vision Res* 27:599-607, 1987.

136. Bunce DF: The use of the ophthalmoscope in veterinary practice, *Vet Med* 50:599-604, 1955.

137. Barnett KC: Principles of ophthalmoscopy, *Vet Med* 62:56-57, 1967.

138. Bistner SI: Techniques and advances in ophthalmology, *Vet Med Small Anim Clin* 78:489-491, 1983.

139. Olin DD: Examination of the aqueous humor as a diagnostic aid in anterior uveitis, *J Am Vet Med Assoc* 171:557-559, 1977.

140. Hazel SJ et al: Laboratory evaluation of aqueous humor in the healthy dog, cat, horse, and cow, *Am J Vet Res* 46:657-659, 1985.

141. May DR, Noll FG: An improved approach to aqueous paracentesis, *Ophthalmol Surg* 22:821-822, 1991.

142. Wurster U, Riese K, Hoffman K: Enzyme activities and protein concentration in the intraocular fluids of ten mammals, *Acta Ophthalmol (Copenh)* 60:729-741, 1982.

143. Glaze MB et al: Immunoglobulin levels in tears and aqueous humor of horses before and after diethylcarbamazine (DEC) therapy, *Vet Immunol Immunopathol* 7:185-198, 1984.

144. Halliwell RE et al: Studies on recurrent equine uveitis. II. The role of Leptospira interrogans serovar pomona, *Curr Eye Res* 4:1033-1040, 1985.

145. Halliwell RE, Hines MT: Studies on recurrent equine uveitis. I. Levels of immunoglobulin and albumin in the aqueous humor of horses with and without intraocular disease, *Curr Eye Res* 4:1023-1031, 1985.

146. Cook CS, McGahan MC: Copper concentrations in cornea, iris, normal, and cataractous lenses and intraocular fluids of vertebrates, *Curr Eye Res* 5:69-76, 1986.

147. Matthews AG, Poulter T: Albumin and immunoglobulins G, A, and M in aqueous humor from clinically normal equine eyes, *Equine Vet J* 18:117-120, 1986.

148. Cantor GH, Palmer GH, Fenwick BW: Analysis of post mortem aqueous humor chemistry in the horse with particular reference to urea nitrogen and creatinine, *Equine Vet J* 21:288-291, 1989.

149. Parma AE et al: Tears and aqueous humor from horses inoculated with Leptospira contain antibodies which bind to cornea, *Vet Immunol Immunopathol* 14:181-185, 1987.

150. Faber NA et al: Detection of *Leptospira* spp. in the aqueous humor of horses with naturally acquired recurrent uveitis, *J Clin Microbiol* 38:2731-2733, 2000.

151. Wollanke B, Rohrbach BW, Gerhards H: Serum and vitreous humor antibody titers in and isolation of *Leptospira interrogans* from horses with recurrent uveitis, *J Am Vet Med Assoc* 219:795-800, 2001.

152. McLaughlin BG, McLaughlin PS: Equine vitreous humor chemical concentrations: correlation with serum concentrations, and postmortem changes with time and temperature, *Can J Vet Res* 52:476-480, 1988.

153. Ofri R. Optics and physiology of vision. In Gelatt KN, editor: *Veterinary ophthalmology*, ed 3, Philadelphia, 1999, Lippincott Williams & Wilkins, pp 183-216.

154. Roberts SM: Equine vision and optics, *Vet Clin North Am Equine Pract* 8:451-457, 1992.

155. Stuhr CM et al: The normal refractive state of the equine, *Vet Ophthalmol* 2:265, 1999 (abstract).

156. Sivak JG, Allen DB: An evaluation of the ramp retina in the horse eye, *Vision Res* 15:1353-1356, 1975.

157. Matthews AG, Handscombe MC: Bilateral cataract formation and subluxation of the lenses in a foal: a case report, *Equine Vet J* 2(Suppl):23-24, 1979.

158. Millichamp NJ, Dziezyc J: Cataract surgery in horses, *Invest Ophthalmol Vis Sci* 37:S763, 1996 (abstract).

159. Ramsey DT et al: Refractive error in Rocky Mountain horses with cornea globosa and with normal corneas, *Invest Ophthalmol Vis Sci* 41:S135, 2000 (abstract).

160. Hamori D: Notes on hereditary myopia in horses, *Vet Bull* 13:136, 1941 (abstract).

161. Miller PE: A limited review of feline and equine vision, *Proc Am Coll Vet Ophthalmol* 26:94-102, 1996.

162. Woimant Z: *Contribution à l'étude du globe oculaire chez le cheval par la skiascopy et l'echographie.* Thesis, École Nationale Vétérinaire d'Alfort, 1976. Referenced from Lavach JD, Large animal ophthalmology.

163. Wouters L, De Moor A: Retinocopische refraktiebepaling bij het paard, *Vlaams Diergeneeskd Tijdschr* 1978;47:445-454. Referenced from Lavach JD, Large animal ophthalmology.

164. Davidson MG: Clinical retinoscopy for the veterinary ophthalmologist, *Vet Comp Ophthalmol* 7:128-137, 1997.

165. Murphy CJ, Zadnik K, Mannis MJ: Myopia and refractive error in dogs, *Invest Ophthalmol Vis Sci* 33:2459-2463, 1992.

166. Berkow JW, Orth DH, Kelley JS: *Fluorescein angiography: technique and interpretation,* San Francisco, 1991, American Academy of Ophthalmology.

167. Walde I: [The fluorescence angiogram of the normal ocular fundus in the dog and horse], *Tierarztl Prax* 5:343-347, 1977.

168. Gelatt KN, Henderson JD, Steffen GR: Fluorescein angiography of the normal and diseased ocular fundi of the laboratory dog, *J Am Vet Med Assoc* 169:980-984, 1976.

169. Slater JD et al: Fluorescein angiographic appearance of the normal fundus and of focal chorioretinal lesions in the horse, *Invest Ophthalmol Vis Sci* 36:S779, 1995.

170. Walde I, Punzet G: Intravital staining of the ocular fundus with fluorescein sodium in the dog and horse, *Weiner Tierärztliche Monatsschrift* 63:216-224, 1976.

171. Davidson MG, Baty KT: Anaphylaxis associated with intravenous sodium fluorescein administration in a cat, *Prog Vet Comp Ophthalmol* 1:127-128, 1991.

172. Brooks DE, Clark CK, Lester GD: Cochet-Bonnet aesthesiometer-determined corneal sensitivity in neonatal foals and adult horses, *Vet Ophthalmol* 3:133-137, 2000.

173. Barrett PM et al: Absolute corneal sensitivity and corneal trigeminal nerve anatomy in normal dogs, *Prog Vet Comp Ophthalmol* 1:245-254, 1991.

174. Blocker T, Van Der Woerdt A: A comparison of corneal sensitivity between brachycephalic and domestic short-haired cats, *Vet Ophthalmol* 4:127-130, 2001.

175. Kaps S, Richter M, Spiess BM: Corneal esthesiometry in the healthy horse, *Vet Ophthalmol* 6:151-155, 2003.

176. Boberg-Ans J: Experience in clinical examination of corneal sensitivity, *Br J Ophthalmol* 39:705-726, 1955.

177. Bonnet R, Millodot M: Corneal aesthesiometry: its measurement in the dark, *Am J Optom Arch Am Acad Optom* 43:238-243, 1966.

178. Millodot M: The influence of age on the sensitivity of the cornea, *Invest Ophthalmol Vis Sci* 16:240-242, 1977.

179. Millodot M: The influence of pregnancy on the sensitivity of the cornea, *Br J Ophthalmol* 61:646-649, 1977.

180. Millodot M: Do blue-eyed people have more sensitive corneas than brown-eyed people? *Nature* 255:151-152, 1975.

181. Kolstad A: Corneal sensitivity by low temperatures, *Acta Ophthalmol* 48:789-793, 1970.

182. Weigt AK, Pickett JP, Herring IP: The effects of cyclophotocoagulation with a neodymium: yttrium-aluminum-garnet laser on sensitivity, intraocular pressure, aqueous tear production, and corneal nerve morphology in eyes of dogs, *Am J Vet Res* 63:906-915, 2002.

183. Murphy CJ et al: Spontaneous chronic corneal epithelial defects (SCCED) in dogs: clinical features, innervation, and effect of topical SP, with or without IGF-1, *Invest Ophthalmol Vis Sci* 42:2252-2261, 2001.

184. Boydell P: Corneal sensitivity in cats with herpetic keratitis, *Proc Am Coll Vet Ophthalmol* 24:98, 1997.

185. Gilger BC et al: Canine corneal thickness measured by ultrasonic pachymetry, *Am J Vet Res* 10:1570-1572, 1991.

186. Moodie KL et al: Postnatal development of corneal curvature and thickness in the cat, *Vet Ophthalmol* 4:267-272, 2001.

187. Gilger BC et al: Corneal thickness measured by ultrasonic pachymetry in cats, *Am J Vet Res* 54:228-230, 1993.

188. Ling T: Osmotically induced central and peripheral corneal swelling in the cat, *Am J Optom Physiol Opt* 64:674-677, 1987.

189. Korah S, Thomas R, Muliyil J: Comparison of optical and ultrasound pachymetry, *Indian J Ophthalmol* 48:279-283, 2000.

190. Gwin RM et al: Decrease in canine corneal endothelial cell density and increase in corneal thickness as a function of age, *Invest Ophthalmol Vis Sci* 22:267-271, 1982.

191. Gwin RM et al: Effects of phacoemulsification and extracapsular lens removal on corneal thickness and endothelial cell density in the dog, *Invest Ophthalmol Vis Sci* 24:227-236, 1983.

192. Bell KD, Campbell RJ, Bourne WM: Late endothelial failure of penetrating keratoplasty: study with light and electron microscopy, *Cornea* 19:40-46, 2000.

193. Gum GG: Electrophysiology in veterinary ophthalmology, *Vet Clin North Am Small Anim Pract* 10:437-453, 1980.

194. Komaromy AM, Smith PJ, Brooks DE: Electroretinography in dogs and cat. Part I. Retinal morphology and physiology, *Comp Contin Educ Pract Vet* 20:343-350, 1998.

195. Komaromy AM, Smith PJ, Brooks DE: Electroretinography in dogs and cat. II. Technique, interpretation, and indications, *Comp Contin Educ Vet Pract* 20:355- 366, 1998.

196. Sims MH: Electrodiagnostic evaluation of vision. In Gelatt KN, editor: *Veterinary ophthalmology,* ed 3, Philadelphia, 1999, Lippincott Williams & Wilkins, pp 483-507.

197. Komaromy AM et al: Flash electroretinography in standing horses using the DTL microfiber electrode, *Vet Ophthalmol* 6: 27-33, 2003.

198. Brooks DE: Equine glaucoma. In Robinson ER, editor: *Current therapy in equine medicine 4,* Philadelphia, 1997, WB Saunders, pp 360-362.

199. Witzel DA et al: Congenital stationary night blindness: an animal model, *Invest Ophthalmol Vis Sci* 17:788-795, 1978.

200. Rebhun WC: Retinal and optic nerve diseases, *Vet Clin North Am Equine Pract* 8:587-608, 1992.

201. Bilge M et al: A map of the visual cortex in the cat, *J Physiol* 191:116P-118P, 1967.

202. Yanase J, Ogawa H: Effects of halothane and sevoflurane on the electroretinogram of dogs, *Am J Vet Res* 58:904-909, 1997.

203. Lalonde MR, Chauhan BC, Tremblay F: Retinal ganglion cell contribution to the multi-focal electroretinogram (MF-ERG): axotomy vs. TTX injections in a porcine model, *Invest Ophthalmol Vis Sci* 42:S147, 2001 (abstract).

204. Wouters L, de Moor A, Moens Y: Rod and cone components in the electroretinogram of the horse, *Zentralbl Veterinarmed A* 27:330-338, 1980.

205. Francois J et al: Morphometric and electrophysiologic study of the photoreceptors in the horse, *Ophthalmologica* 181:340-349, 1980.

206. Gilger BC et al: Long term effect on the equine eye of an intravitreal device used for sustained release of cyclosporine A, *Vet Ophthalmol* 3:105-110, 2000.

207. Carroll J et al: Photopigment basis for dichromatic color vision in the horse, *J Vis* 1:80-87, 2001.

208. Scotty NC et al: Diagnostic ultrasonography of equine lens and posterior segment abnormalities, *Vet Ophthalmol* 7:127-139, 2004.

209. Wilkie DA: Ophthalmic procedures and surgery in the standing horse, *Vet Clin North Am Equine Pract* 7:535-547, 1991.

210. Williams J, Wilkie DA: Ultrasonography of the eye, *Comp Contin Educ Pract Vet* 18:667-677, 1996.

211. Rogers M et al: Evaluation of the extirpated equine eye using B-mode ultrasonography, *Vet Radiol* 27:24-29, 1986.

212. Byrne SF, Green RL: *Ultrasound of the eye and orbit,* ed 2, St Louis, Mo, 2002, Mosby.

213. van der Woerdt A, Wilkie DA, Myers W: Ultrasonographic abnormalities in the eyes of dogs with cataracts: 147 cases (1986-1992), *J Am Vet Med Assoc* 203:838-841, 1993.

214. Dziezyc J, Hagar DA: Ocular ultrasonography in veterinary medicine, *Semin Vet Med Surg* 3:1-9, 1988.

215. Eisenberg HM: Ultrasonography of the eye and orbit, *Vet Clin North Am Small Anim Pract* 15:1263-1274, 1985.

216. Mettenleiter EM: [Sonographic diagnosis (B-mode technique) for the eyes in horses. I. Methods and normal findings], *Tierarztl Prax* 23:481-488, 1995.

217. Mettenleiter EM: [Sonographic diagnosis (B-mode technique) for the eyes in horses. II. Pathological cases], *Tierarztl Prax* 23:588-595, 1995.

218. Liebmann JM, Ritch R, Esaki K: Ultrasound biomicroscopy, *Ophthalmol Clin North Am* 11:421-433, 1998.

219. Pavlin CJ, Foster FS: *Ultrasound biomicroscopy of the eye*, New York, 1995, Springer-Verlag.

220. Pavlin CJ et al: Ultrasound biomicroscopy of anterior segment structures in normal and glaucomatous eyes, *Am J Ophthalmol* 113:381-389, 1992.

221. Trope GE et al: Malignant glaucoma. Clinical and ultrasound biomicroscopic features, *Ophthalmology* 101:1030-1035, 1994.

222. Berinstein DM et al: Ultrasound biomicroscopy in anterior ocular trauma, *Ophthalmic Surg Lasers* 28:201-207, 1997.

223. Bentley E, Diehl KA, Miller PE: Measurement of high resolution ultrasound images: intraobserver and interobserver reliability, *Vet Ophthalmol* 5:286, 2002 (abstract).

224. Bentley E, Miller PE, Diehl K: Use of high-resolution ultrasound as a diagnostic tool in veterinary ophthalmology, *J Am Vet Med Assoc* 223:1617-1622, 2003.

225. Dietrich U, Moore PA: Clinical application of ultrasound biomicroscopy in veterinary ophthalmology, *Vet Ophthalmol* 5:292, 1999 (abstract).

226. Schebitz H, Wilkens H: *Atlas of radiographic anatomy of the horse*, ed 3, Philadelphia, 1978, WB Saunders, pp 10-15.

227. Park RD: Radiographic examination of the equine head, *Vet Clin North Am Equine Pract* 9:49-74, 1993.

228. Wyn-Jones G: Interpreting radiographs 6: radiology of the equine head. II. *Equine Vet J* 17:417-425, 1985.

229. Stickle R: The equine skull. In Thrall DE, editor: *Textbook of veterinary diagnostic radiology*, ed 2, Philadelphia, 1994, WB Saunders, pp 66-72.

230. Latimer JC: Equine nasal passages and sinuses. In Thrall DE, editor: *Textbook of veterinary diagnostic radiology*, ed 2, Philadelphia, 1994, WB Saunders, pp 73-86.

231. Smallwood JE, Spaulding KA: Radiographic anatomy of the dog and horse. In Thrall DE, editor: *Textbook of veterinary diagnostic radiology*, ed 2, Philadelphia, 1994, WB Saunders, pp 556-603.

232. Caron JP et al: Periorbital skull fractures in five horses, *J Am Vet Med Assoc* 188:280-284, 1986.

233. Davidson HJ et al: Radiographic examination of eyes fixed in Zenker's solution, *Vet Pathol* 26:83-85, 1989.

234. Brooks DE: Ocular imaging. In Gelatt KN, editor: *Veterinary ophthalmology*, ed 3, Philadelphia, 1999, Lippincott Williams & Wilkins, pp 467-482.

235. Nykamp SG, Scrivani PV, Pease AP: Computed tomography dacryocystography evaluation of the nasolacrimal apparatus, *Vet Radiol Ultrasound* 45:23-28, 2004.

236. Latimer CA, Wyman M: Atresia of the nasolacrimal duct in three horses, *J Am Vet Med Assoc* 184:989-992, 1984.

237. Ashenhurst M et al: Combined computed tomography and dacryocystography for complex lacrimal problems, *Can J Ophthalmol* 26:27-31, 1991.

238. Takehara Y et al: Dynamic MR dacryocystography: a new method for evaluating nasolacrimal duct obstructions, *Am J Radiol* 175:469-473, 2000.

239. Barbee DD et al: Computed tomography in horses, *Vet Radiol Ultrasound* 28:144-151, 1987.

240. Morrow KL et al: Computed tomographic imaging of the equine head, *Vet Radiol Ultrasound* 41:491-497, 2000.

241. Smallwood JE et al: Anatomic reference for computed tomography of the head of the foal, *Vet Radiol Ultrasound* 43:99-117, 2002.

242. Dik KJ: Computed tomography of the equine head. Abstracts of oral presentations, 10th IVRA meeting, *Vet Radiol Ultrasound* 35:231-251, 1994.

243. Tucker RL, Farrell E: Computed tomography and magnetic resonance imaging of the equine head, *Vet Clin North Am Equine Pract* 17:131-144, 2001.

244. Boroffka SAEB, Van Den Belt AJA: CT/Ultrasound diagnosis: retrobulbar hematoma n a horse, *Vet Radiol* 37:441-443, 1996.

245. Allen JR et al: Brain abscess in a horse: diagnosis by computed tomography and successful surgical treatment, *Equine Vet J* 19:552-555, 1987.

246. Colbourne CM et al: Surgical treatment of progressive ethmoidal hematoma aided by computed tomography in a foal, *J Am Vet Med Assoc* 211:335-338, 1997.

247. Forrest LJ: The head: excluding the brain and orbit, *Clin Tech Small Anim Pract* 14:170-176, 1999.

248. Ragle CA et al: Computed tomographic valuation of head trauma in a foal, *Vet Radiol* 39:206-208, 1988.

249. Sasaki M et al: CT examination of the guttural pouch (auditory tube diverticulum) in Przewalskis's horse (Equus przewalski), *J Vet Med Sci* 61:1019-1022, 1999.

250. Tietje S, Becker M, Bockenhoff G: Computed tomographic evaluation of head diseases in the horse: 15 cases, *Equine Vet J* 28:98-105, 1996.

251. Wallace MA et al: Central blindness associated with a pituitary adenoma in a horse, *Equine Pract* 18:8-13, 1996.

252. Warmerdam EPL, Klein WR, van Herpen BPJM: Infectious temporomandibular joint disease in the horse: computed tomographic diagnosis of two cases, *Vet Rec* 141:172-174, 1997.

253. Baptiste KE et al. Paranasal sinus osteoma in an American Miniature horse: computed tomographic evaluation and surgical management, *Equine Pract* 18:14-19, 1996.

254. Davis JL et al: Nasal adenocarcinoma with diffuse metastases involving the orbit, cerebrum, and multiple cranial nerves in a horse, *J Am Vet Med Assoc* 221:1460-1463, 2002.

255. Morgan R, Daniel GB, Donnell RL: Magnetic resonance imaging of the normal eye and orbit of the horse, *Prog Vet Comp Ophthalmol* 3:127-133.

256. Vazquez JM et al: Magnetic resonance imaging of two normal equine brains and their associated structures, *Vet Rec* 148:229-232, 2001.

257. Arencibia A et al: Magnetic resonance imaging and cross sectional anatomy of the normal equine sinuses and nasal passages. *Vet Radiol Ultrasound* 41:313-319, 2000.

258. Chaffin MK et al: Magnetic resonance imaging of the brain of normal neonatal foals, *Vet Radiol Ultrasound* 38:102-111, 1997.

259. Freestone JF et al: Ultrasonic identification of an orbital tumor in a horse, *Equine Vet J* 21:135-136, 1989.

2 Diseases and Surgery of the Globe and Orbit

Tim J. Cutler

The equine orbit is a complete bony cavity surrounding the globe and other structures. Several disease types are expressed through a few pathologic processes. The globe is subject to trauma, inflammation, neoplasia, congenital disease, and extension of disease into the orbit from adjacent cranial cavities, particularly the sinuses. Advances in imaging hold promise for more elaborate medical and surgical therapy in the near future. More medical conditions of the orbit are now recognized, and improved diagnostic testing is likely to identify additional conditions. The desire for more cosmetic outcomes after serious ocular injury and trauma has resulted in a greater variety of surgical prostheses. Options now permit retention or replacement of the globe with a painted prosthesis or a solid ocular prosthesis placed over a phthisical globe, with normal function of the eyelids. Orbital and globe surgery procedures are described, together with diagnosis and medical management of other conditions.

CLINICAL ANATOMY AND PHYSIOLOGY

The horse is unusual in having a complete bony orbital rim (Fig. 2-1). The globes are positioned laterally on the head and are ideally situated for a wide and panoramic visual field, exceeding 340 degrees.[1] This seems appropriate for the horse's ecologic niche as a grazer, and consequently, a prey animal, but perhaps is less perfect for the activities that it commonly performs in today's society. The horse has a binocular visual field, permitting stereoscopy, and the wide separation of the two globes provides greater depth perception than most other domestic species can attain. The main visual axis is approximately parallel with the long axis of the skull.[2] Equine vision is explored more thoroughly in Chapter 10.

The equine globe is among the largest in the mammalian kingdom, perhaps eclipsed only by that of the giraffe. The axis of the globe in the horse is nearly perpendicular to that of the skull and is angled with respect to the long axis of the orbit. In the adult horse, the average globe dimensions are 43.68 mm anterior-posterior, 47.63 mm vertically, and 48.45 mm horizontally.[1] The globe of the mule is almost identical in size, measuring 43.0 mm, 47.5 mm, and 48.5 mm in the same orientation. The globe is not a sphere but rather is compressed from anterior to posterior, with the ratios of the dimensions previously given being 1:1.09:1.10 for the horse and 1:1.10:1.12 for the mule.[1] The globe is located at the anterior border of the rather large orbit, which averages $62 \times 59 \times 98$ mm. The orbits are separated by 172 mm across the anterior surface of the frontal bone.[1] The remainder of the orbital cavity is filled largely by fat and muscle and is divided into pockets by layers of connective tissue that coordinate ocular mobility.

The orbital bones are the frontal, lacrimal, zygomatic, and temporal bones, traveling clockwise for the right orbit, with the sphenoid and palatine bones forming the deeper internal wall of the orbit that separates it from the calvaria (see Fig. 2-1). The complete bony rim, temporally and dorsally, is composed of the frontal process of the zygomatic bone and zygomatic processes of the frontal and temporal bones. The supraorbital foramen features prominently in the anterior aspect of the frontal bone, forming the dorsal orbital rim. The lacrimal gland proper is closely adhered to the internal orbit near the dorso-temporal orbital rim, a location of minor surgical interest because it is seldom removed during enucleation in the horse. Inferiorly, the zygomatic bone forms the lower rim, and nasally, it is fused to the lacrimal bone, wherein embedded canals provide refuge to the nasolacrimal duct canaliculi (see Fig. 2-1). Beneath the globe, substantial cushioning is provided by fat that separates the globe from the palatine bone. Caudally, the orbital floor is angled inferiorly until it is comprised of soft tissues only, including the substantial pterygoid muscles that exert closing motion for the lower jaw. The boney floor of the orbit ends directly beneath the caudal aspect of the dorsal rim.

Various foramina provide conduits between the orbit and other compartments of the head, particularly

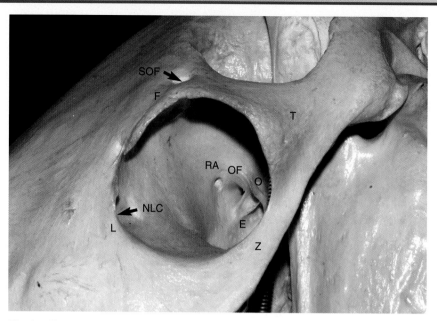

Fig. 2-1 The horse has a complete bony orbital rim. The orbital bones include the frontal *(F)*, lacrimal *(L)*, zygomatic *(Z)*, and temporal *(T)* bones. The sphenoid and palatine bone form the medial wall of the orbit, separating the orbit from the calvaria. The nasolacrimal duct canaliculi *(NLC)* course through the lacrimal bone. The orbital foramina through the sphenoid bone includes—from anterior to posterior—the rostral alar *(RA)*, orbital fissure *(OF)*, optic *(O)*, and ethmoidal *(E)* (see also Table 2-1). The supraorbital foramen *(SOF)* exits through the frontal bone.

Table 2-1	Structures Perforating the Orbit and Their Contents
Structure	**Ostium**
Maxillary artery and nerve	Rostral alar foramen
Ethmoidal artery, vein, and nerve	Ethmoidal foramen
Optic nerve (CN II)	Optic foramen
Oculomotor nerve (CN III)	Orbital foramen
Trochlear nerve (CN IV)	Orbital foramen
Abducens nerve (CN VI)	Orbital foramen
Supraorbital artery, vein, and nerve	Supraorbital foramen
Major palatine artery, vein, and nerve	Caudal palatine foramen
Infraorbital vein, artery, and nerve	Maxillary foramen
Sphenopalatine artery and vein and pterygopalatine nerve	Sphenopalatine foramen

through the calvaria to the brain. The efferent foramina are arranged in a curvilinear fashion along the sphenoid bone that forms the medial orbital wall. From anterior to posterior, they are the rostral alar, orbital fissure, optic, and ethmoidal foramina (Table 2-1) and are evident in Fig. 2-1. The clinical significance of the location of the foramina lies in avoiding their contents during biopsy and exploratory procedures and in closely approaching them to deposit local anesthetic in the performance of the retrobulbar block (Chapter 1). The foramina appear to provide relatively minimal risk for extension of orbital infection or neoplasia, but they may be severely damaged during trauma to the calvaria, with serious consequences for continued ocular function. Fracture of the basisphenoid and basioccipital bones frequently occurs in blunt trauma to the poll. Afferent foramina are located in the extreme anteromedial portion of the orbit and are the caudal palatine (major palatine artery and nerve), the maxillary (infraorbital artery, vein, and nerve), and sphenopalatine (sphenopalatine artery and vein and pterygopalatine nerve).

The infraorbital foramen is the point of egress of the infraorbital nerve, artery, and vein from the orbit, which can be palpated 1 cm rostral and 3 cm dorsal to the rostral edge of the facial crest, one third of the distance to the nostrils (Fig. 2-2). It may be partially obscured by the overlying muscular belly of the levator nasolabialis.[3] The infraorbital nerve arises from the maxillary branch of the trigeminal nerve to provide sensory innervation to the upper lip, nostril, and cheek. Its major significance is in desensitization for laceration repair of those tissues, and infrequently, for nerve blockade to evaluate the contribution of trigeminal summation in clinical head shakers.[4] The infraorbital canal bisects the maxillary sinus.

The orbit is completely lined with a multilayered tenacious periosteum/periorbita. This dense fibrous connective tissue has tremendous surgical importance, because it provides a formidable barrier to the extension of orbital disease beyond the soft tissue contents into the bone architecture. Even moderately extensive stages of squamous cell carcinoma (SCC) may be sufficiently contained by the periosteum, allowing successful and complete surgical removal of the neoplastic expansion. The periorbita is retained in enucleation, and its anterior portion is preferably completely reapposed in closure. In the exenteration procedure the majority of the periorbita is removed. If the periosteal surface overlying orbital bone has lost its thin glossy appearance, suggesting disease, it should be elevated and removed, and deeper lesions should be explored and treated appropriately.

The equine globe resides anteriorly within the orbit, supported by loosely packed retrobulbar tissues. The globe is a fluid-filled cavity divided into anterior and posterior segments by the lens. Reflections of the periorbita together with smooth muscle attach the globe to the orbital rim. The external wall of the globe is a trilayer with the sclera and cornea forming the outer predominantly fibrous tunic, the highly vascular uvea forming the middle layer, and the neural layers of the retina being most internal. The thickness of the sclera is 1.5 to 2.2 mm (average, 1.9 mm) at its thickest, 1.35 mm where the optic nerve penetrates the posterior pole, 1.1 mm where the cornea and sclera meet at the limbus, but a mere 0.5 to 0.3 mm at the equator of the globe.[1] Consequently, during traumatic events, the sclera most frequently ruptures at the equator or more anteriorly at the limbus. The adult cornea measures 29.7 to 34.0 mm horizontally and 23.0 to 26.5 mm vertically.[5] When measured by ultrasonic pachymetry, the corneal thickness averages 0.793 to 0.893 mm with no effect of gender or age but a tendency to be thicker in the dorsal and ventral quadrants.[6,7] Recently, these values have also been reported for Miniature horses, in which average corneal thickness was 0.785 mm, horizontal diameter was 25.8 mm, and vertical diameter was 19.4 mm.[8] Mean intraocular pressure (IOP) was 26.0 mm Hg.[8] The internal volume of the equine globe is capacious. In one study, the mean aqueous humor volume measured in six adult equine eyes was 3.04 ± 1.27 ml, and the mean vitreous humor volume was 26.15 ± 4.87 ml (Gilger BC, Unpublished data, 2004). Total internal volume of the globe has been reported as up to 45 to 50 ml with a weight of 100 mg. The horse is unusual in having a predominantly uveoscleral outflow tract for aqueous humor egress, which is an important feature in equine glaucoma (see Chapter 8). Laterally and medially the entrance to the iridocorneal angle is apparent with the anterior trabeculae visible as an orchestrated fibrillar network. This is an important site for clinical evaluation with the slit lamp because it is often distorted after blunt trauma or severe protracted uveitis. The drainage angle continues superiorly and inferiorly but is not visible because of the architecture of the limbus.

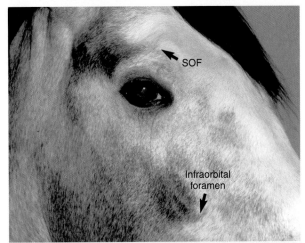

A

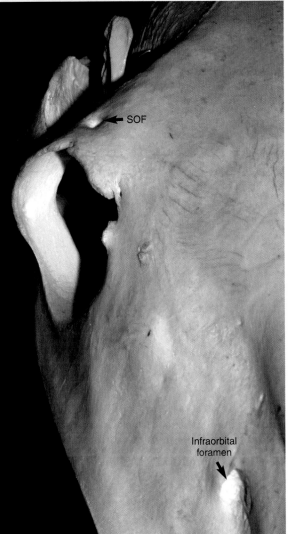

B

Fig. 2-2 A, The infraorbital foramen is the point of egress of the infraorbital nerve, artery, and vein from the orbit. It can be palpated 1 cm rostral and 3 cm dorsal to the rostral edge of the facial crest, one third of the distance to the nostrils *(arrows). SOF,* Supraorbital foramen. **B,** An equine skull viewed from the front, showing the right orbit and infraorbital foramen *(arrow).*

Table 2-2   Orbital and Ocular Muscles: Function and Innervation

Muscle	Function	Innervation
Globe		
Dorsal rectus	Upward motion of globe	Oculomotor (CN III)
Ventral rectus	Downward motion	Oculomotor (CN III)
Medial rectus	Medial motion	Oculomotor (CN III)
Lateral rectus	Lateral motion	Abducens (CN VI)
Dorsal oblique	Rotation nasally and inferiorly	Trochlear (CN IV)
Ventral oblique	Rotation laterally and superiorly	Oculomotor (CN III)
Retractor bulbi	Posterior motion of globe	Abducens (CN VI)
Eyelid		
Levator palpebrae superioris	Elevates upper eyelid	Facial (CN VII)
Levator angularis oculi	Elevates nasal eyelid/eyebrow	Oculomotor (CN III)
Malaris	Opens lower eyelid	Facial (CN VII)
Orbicularis oculi	Forceful closure of eyelids	Facial (CN VII)
Retractor angularis oculi	Retracts lateral canthus	Facial (CN VII)
Arrectores ciliorum	Elevates eyelashes	Sympathetic
Orbitalis (Muller's): superior and inferior tarsus and circular fibers	Retracts eyelid (smooth)	Sympathetic
Corrugator supercilii	Elevates upper eyelid	Facial (CN VII)

CN, Cranial nerve.

The multiple bellies of the retractor bulbi, which attach extensively around the posterior half of the sclera and are innervated by cranial nerve (CN) VI, dominate the extraocular muscles. The eyeball retraction reflex provides one of the major methods of evaluating this nerve's function. The other six muscles have typical attachments (Table 2-2) but have more extensive bulk and insertion than is the case in many other species. Muscular attachments are seldom avulsed in orbital trauma (in contrast to the dog) but may become entrapped and be unable to function after orbital fractures (Fig. 2-3).

The vascular system of the equine orbit has been described in detail, and the interested reader is referred to the excellent work of Simoens, Muylle, and Lauwers.[9] Most vessels cross through the orbit inferiorly and nasally and may be avoided by aspiration and biopsy of the orbit only from a dorsal, lateral, or dorsomedial approach. The orbital branches of the external ophthalmic artery are variably derived from the internal maxillary artery deep within the orbit. Two functional groups, the ciliary arteries rostrally and the chorioretinal arteries caudally, perfuse the globe. Posterior ciliary arteries enter the sclera behind the equator in the cardinal positions to perfuse the choroid and continue forward toward the anterior segment within the sclera. Anterior ciliary arteries enter superiorly and inferiorly caudal to the limbus. Multiple chorioretinal arteries (10 to 20) surround the optic nerve at its entry through the sclera, supplying retinal arteries and contributing to local choroidal perfusion.[9] The primary venous drainage of the eye is through the ophthalmic, orbital, supraorbital, and reflex veins.[1] The superior vortex vein and the palpebral and lacrimal veins course into the dorsal ophthalmic vein, before more caudal contributions from the anterior ciliary, supraorbital, muscularis, and infratrochlear veins and ultimately from the ophthalmic vein at the apex of the orbit. The orbital and internal maxillary veins then provide venous drainage. The inferior vortex vein anteriorly drains into the reflex vein, which also receives venous return from the muscular and palpebral veins and the great palatine, sphenopalatine, and infraorbital veins in the anterior orbit before it enters the facial vein.

The buccal cavity is separated from the orbit in horses because of skull bulk and elongation and the complete bone demarcation of the orbit. Dental disease may still affect the orbit, via the sinuses, but must be substantial to do so. The last premolar and first three molars arise in the maxillary sinus, and the last molar abuts the sphenopalatine sinus. If oral disease is present or suspected, the buccal cavity should be opened and examined, and the individual's ability to prehend food should be further evaluated. Manipulation of the mandible on the maxilla will often elicit information about functional quality of apposition of the dental arcades. Use of an oral speculum is necessary for more detailed analysis, and oral examination should be performed if malodorous breath, evidence of food retention or packing, chronic rhinorrhea, or purulent discharge is present.

The guttural pouch is a diverticulum of the eustachian tube that occupies the area posterior to the mandible and is the site of multiple fragile structures. It extends anteriorly to closely approximate the orbit and enters the pharynx through a slit-like opening, and disease may affect the orbit directly. More commonly, ocular

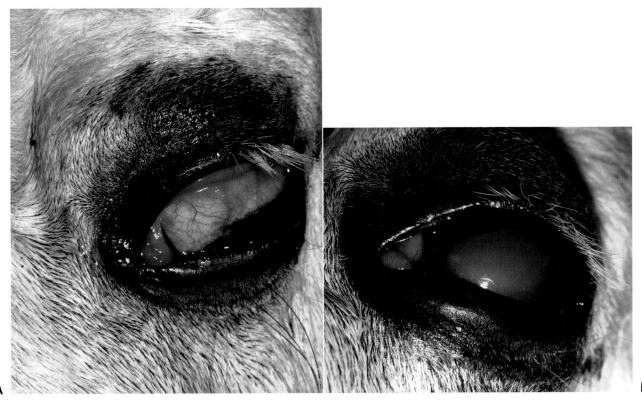

Fig. 2-3 A, Severe ventral strabismus caused by (inferior) orbital fracture in a horse. A displaced fragment of bone impinged on the ventral rectus muscle causes the strabismus. **B,** Three days after orbital exploratory surgery and removal of the bone fragment, the strabismus was resolved, but there remained orbital swelling, corneal ulceration, and corneal edema, which eventually resolved. (Photograph **B** courtesy Dr. Brian Gilger.)

disease may result from damage to the internal carotid artery that passes through the guttural pouch or to the cranial cervical ganglion of the autonomic nervous system. The major conditions are bacterial or fungal infection, empyema, and some of the surgical and medical treatments for empyema. Rupture of the internal carotid artery is a life-threatening condition.

The nasolacrimal duct system originates at moderately large puncta in the upper and lower eyelids and is joined by canaliculi to the lacrimal sac, which is embedded in the lacrimal bone. Damage by fracture, direct blunt trauma, or infectious or inflammatory disease at this site may cause epiphora and chronic irritation. Surgical procedures to rectify this condition are described in Chapter 3. The nasolacrimal duct traverses the maxillary sinus, and sinusitis that causes increased sinus pressure may functionally obstruct the duct, resulting in epiphora.

The periorbital sinuses—the frontal (conchofrontal), maxillary (caudal and rostral), and sphenopalatine sinuses—are close to the orbital bones (Fig. 2-4). Primary sinus diseases may secondarily affect one or both orbits.[10-14] The *frontal sinus* is a shallow, wide sinus, parallel with the frontal bone, which extends anteriorly from a line joining each temporomandibular joint forward almost to the dorsal turbinate bone that represents the conchofrontal sinus. The sinus system is lined with epithelium and filled with air; therefore an open fracture of any sinus is clinically relevant because it is considered a contaminated wound. The *maxillary sinus* extends ventrally from an imaginary line joining the medial canthus and the nasomaxillary notch, to just below the facial crest. The rostral border is the rostral extent of the facial crest, and the caudal border is the midline of the orbit. Diminutive *ethmoidal* and *sphenopalatine sinuses* are present medial to the internal wall of the orbit and are more difficult to identify from external landmarks. Drainage is into the frontal and caudal maxillary sinuses. Ultimately, drainage occurs from these sinuses into the nasal cavity. When surgical drainage is indicated for treatment of sinus disease, trephination dorsal to a line between the infraorbital foramen and the medial canthus can result in nasolacrimal duct damage and must be avoided.[15] Additional sinuses are present in the nasal cavity and communicate with the maxillary sinus but are of minimal clinical interest.

The ethmoid turbinates are located axially and inferiorly to the orbit at the caudal end of the nasal cavity within the skull. This area receives a very rich vascular supply and may be the site of origin of ethmoidal hematomas (which cause chronic nasal disease), as

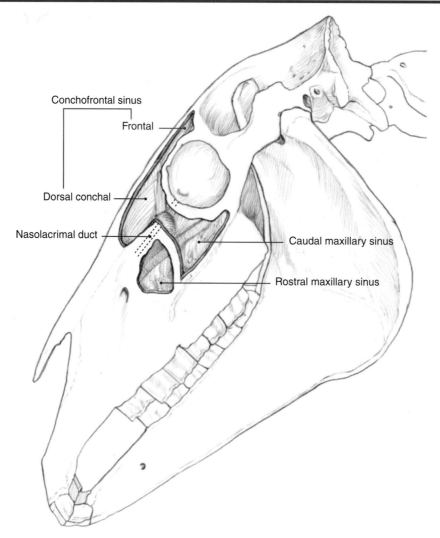

Conchofrontal sinus

Frontal

Dorsal conchal

Nasolacrimal duct

Caudal maxillary sinus

Rostral maxillary sinus

Fig. 2-4 Periorbital sinuses are close to the orbit and include the frontal (conchofrontal), maxillary (caudal and rostral), and sphenopalatine sinuses.

well as aggressive carcinoma. Direct extension of this mass may precipitate exophthalmos.

DIAGNOSTICS

Although the horse typically does not display much independent globe motion, entrapment or compression of the globe within the orbit may be evaluated by taking advantage of the oculokinetic reflexes of the vestibular system. While standing at one side of the horse, the examiner grasps the skull near the distal extremity and makes gentle sweeping motions while observing for primary and secondary adjustments in globe position. A spiraling motion may be used to attempt to determine whether tertiary motions are normal, although this maneuver may be more challenging for the examiner than for the subject.

Passive forced duction testing requires desensitization (e.g., use of topical 0.5% proparacaine) and gentle retraction of the globe in the direction of interest (the motion is passive for the horse). Failure to achieve globe motion is regarded as a positive test result and indicates entrapment or disease of the muscle. Active forced duction testing requires the participation of the patient, and the operator observes and feels for attempted motion of the globe by muscle contraction in the direction of interest.

Fine needle aspiration for cytology and biopsy (Trucut) for histopathologic examination is highly desirable when a mass is present. Imaging studies should be performed to define the location more specifically after a thorough physical examination. Real-time ultrasonography and sampling permit observation of needle placement and reduce the risk of iatrogenic trauma. Strabismus or globe displacement suggests the location of an intraorbital mass, which must be extensive to compress or decenter the globe. Intraconal masses displace the entire globe forward, whereas extraconal masses cause strabismus and possibly exophthalmos. Biopsy of orbital contents may be performed from the supraorbital fossa, from 1 cm lateral to the lateral canthus, and from the medial canthus paralleling the orbital wall and avoiding the inferior quadrant. Needle advancement should be guided by ultrasonography from a different window into the orbit. Avoiding the major vessels and structures of the orbit is critical. Several samples may be acquired if the mass is firm, but hemorrhage may impede later sample acquisition.

Bacterial culture is indicated for samples acquired from any paranasal sinus, and potentially from orbital masses in younger animals in which an abscess or septic cellulitis is suspected. When generalized orbital cellulitis is present, microbial culture is desirable, but an appropriate sample is difficult to acquire, and the entire contents of the orbit appear homogenously expanded on ultrasonography; in such cases, a small biopsy specimen may be preferable to an aspirate for culture purposes. Even when systemic leukocytosis is demonstrated, blood cultures are highly unlikely to be useful unless a severe fever is present concurrently (>105° F).

Orbital Imaging and Diagnostics

Orbital disease may be more challenging to diagnose because many of the structures are hidden from direct examination. In addition to appearance, displacement of adjacent structures permits deduction of involved structures and suggests the tissue of interest. Imaging systems provide confirmation of suspected diagnoses and are frequently an essential part of the diagnostic process. Imaging is described in greater detail in Chapter 1.

Ultrasonography is convenient, efficient, performed in real time, inexpensive, and readily available to most practitioners. Samples may be obtained concurrently with a biopsy instrument, if no vital structures intercede. Although a 10- or 7.5-MHz probe is necessary for adequate imaging of the globe, the deeper aspects of the orbit require a 5- or 7.5-MHz probe (Fig. 2-5). Lesions that are suggestive of disease should be imaged in different axes (vertical, horizontal, and transverse) to localize them spatially, permit mental reconstruction in three dimensions, and confirm that they are not artifacts. The window dorsal to the globe should be used to supplement anterior views. It is salient to recall that even moderately large orbital lesions may not be apparent on some sonograms. In such cases, further imaging should be pursued.

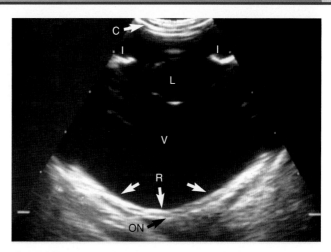

Fig. 2-5 Transcorneal ocular ultrasonography of a normal equine eye obtained with a 7.5-MHz transducer. The deeper aspects of the orbit may require a 5- or 7.5-MHz transducer. *C,* Cornea; *I,* iris; *L,* lens; *V,* vitreous; *R,* location of retina; *ON,* location of optic nerve.

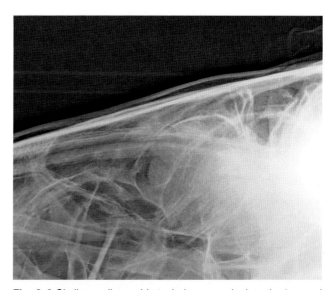

Fig. 2-6 Skyline radiographic technique may isolate the bone of interest against an air-filled background (e.g., frontal sinus). This radiograph is of a frontal sinus fracture caused by blunt trauma, demonstrating subcutaneous emphysema. The globe ruptured at the limbus in the same injury.

Radiography is indicated primarily to identify bone fractures in the individual with an acute trauma injury or bone deformation in the patient with invasive neoplasia or sepsis and to localize cellulitis if gas production is evident. Precise radiographs require general anesthesia to prevent motion, although screening images may be obtained in the standing sedated patient, particularly with the advent of digital radiography. Specific skyline techniques to highlight the bones of interest (Fig. 2-6) may reveal a lesion against an air-filled background (e.g., frontal sinus). Contrast orbitography may be performed by artificially introducing air into the orbit, although the indications for this procedure are decreasing with the advent of computed tomography (CT) and magnetic resonance imaging (MRI). Other contrast materials are seldom indicated and carry a risk of complications. Fluid-air interfaces within the sinus indicate disease that is directly relevant to the orbit.

Radiography is also important in planning resection of orbital neoplasms, particularly SCC that is locally invasive into the orbit. Preemptive knowledge of orbital involvement allows planning for the necessary adjunctive surgery to control the neoplasia. Although infrequently necessary, radiography is also useful for localizing metallic foreign bodies such as gunshot within the orbit. In general, such foreign bodies are preferably left in place, unless direct damage to a blood vessel results in substantial hemorrhage or the object is migrating.

Advanced imaging such as MRI and CT scans provide the best reconstructive images and localize the lesion precisely (Fig. 2-7). Reconstruction is easier to perform with MRI than with CT because it can be more easily reformatted. Certain lesions that are not readily detected by other methods may be readily apparent, and lesions that are nonresectable may be identified without exploratory surgery, and with far less trauma. Images of the soft tissue structures of the orbit may be realigned to sequentially image the optic nerve perpendicularly, permitting a more accurate diagnosis. MRI and CT are not yet routinely performed in the horse, but this will likely change in the near future. Irradiation of cranial and extracranial neoplasms is now commonly performed in companion animals, and in due course, highly targeted tumor irradiation may become feasible in horses. Precise imaging allows computer-guided irradiation of neoplastic tissue with a linear accelerator with minimal dose delivery to adjacent structures.

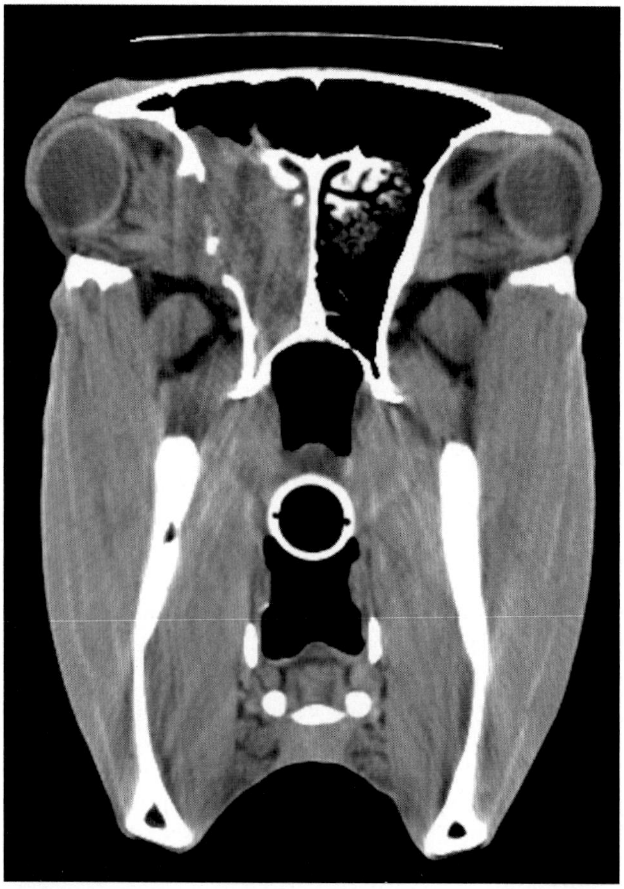

CT-monitored dacryocystography has recently been used to evaluate the integrity of the nasolacrimal duct and may be performed concurrently with evaluation of the skull in cases of complex or severe trauma to the orbit and surrounding tissues.[16]

Vascular diseases of the orbit may be investigated with a CT-monitored contrast venogram or arteriogram, but findings are difficult to interpret, and access to appropriate imaging systems is required. Published protocols for contrast media and doses are not readily available for the horse.

Fig. 2-7 Computed tomography of a horse with right-sided exophthalmos caused by a nasal mass invading the orbit. (Photograph courtesy Dr. Brian Gilger.)

IMPACT OF ORBITAL DISEASE ON THE EQUINE INDUSTRY

Orbital disease is uncommon and of relatively low financial impact in general, although it does have a very substantial and potentially life-threatening impact on the individual. Minor variations in globe size may be discerned relatively commonly, but dramatically abnormal globes are uncommon. The majority of treatable orbital diseases occur in juvenile and young horses and are predominantly traumatic or congenital, whereas the debilitating progressive orbital diseases that occur in older adult horses may be difficult to contain and are often impossible to cure. No epidemiologic studies are available to record the potential annual economic impact of orbital disease, but the major costs are likely related to total loss of use because of loss of vision or loss of life. Precautions to minimize these losses include preventive management strategies in the stall and during handling to reduce trauma; cautious introduction of new individuals into group confinement; and early diagnosis, referral, and imaging of orbital disease in older horses. Earlier surgical intervention may improve the outlook after surgery in older individuals in the future. There are no significant contagious or infectious diseases of the orbit that pose a threat to livestock in the United States. Among exotic diseases, African horse sickness, equine infectious anemia, and infectious diseases causing vasculitis may cause retrobulbar and supraorbital swelling and distension in multiple individuals (see Chapter 12). Quarantine, importation restrictions, and routine serologic testing are the major means of protection against these diseases in the United States, Australia, and nonendemic areas of Europe.

CLINICAL SIGNS OF ORBITAL DISEASE

Abnormalities of Globe Position

Strabismus describes the deviation of the visual axis from the expected orientation, which approaches straight ahead in the horse. When both globes are focused ahead, the conjugate gaze has an overlap of the visual fields, which allows for binocular vision and permits good depth perception as a result of the wide globe separation. The deviation induced by strabismus presumably disturbs the collation and overlap of visual field information from each eye when it is interpreted in the midbrain and visual centers. In humans, misdirection of visual axes results in diplopia or double vision. Strabismus may reflect alteration of orbital contents, distorting the globe from its resting position; or more likely, it may result from disturbance of the ocular muscle innervation or activity caused by stricture, contraction, or mechanical entrapment. Strabismus in young individuals is uncommon and likely to be congenital or breed related.

Neonatal foals most frequently have a physiologic *rotational strabismus* that resolves to the adult orientation within the first 2 to 4 weeks of life. The horizontal pupil is rotated so that the nasal portion is ventral to the temporal portion, and the globe may also be rotated medially. The strabismus is considered physiologic and requires no therapy. Certain breed lines of mules have been reported to have convergent (bilateral) strabismus, or esotropia, and some were described as having visual deficiencies including stumbling. The cause is unknown and no therapy is possible. Appaloosa foals with congenital stationary night blindness may also exhibit a dorsal strabismus (Fig. 2-8).[17,18] The relationship of the strabismus to the congenital stationary night blindness is unclear.

Acquired strabismus is typically traumatic in origin, caused by muscle entrapment after fracture, or less likely, by avulsion of a rectus muscle attachment. The most anterior rectus muscle attachments are for the ventral (8 mm behind limbus) and dorsal (9 mm) rectus muscles, whereas a portion of the lateral rectus attaches within 5 mm of the limbus.[19] Occasionally, central

nervous system (CNS) infections may result in strabismus, most commonly with equine protozoal myeloencephalitis (see Chapter 12).[20-22] Midbrain (oculomotor) lesions most commonly result in a lateral strabismus.[23] Peripheral vestibular disease may result in strabismus, rather than nystagmus, and is often accentuated by elevation of the horse's head. Strabismus may be the only residual sign after recovery from vestibular disease.[23]

Stricture of an ocular muscle after inflammation may result in moderate or severe strabismus but is not commonly identified. In duction tests, the globe cannot be moved in the direction opposite the strabismus. In contrast, muscle avulsion will permit a freely mobile globe, at least until the partner muscle atrophies and fixes the globe position. This strabismus is occasionally identified in horses after severe blunt trauma to the head from the side or front.

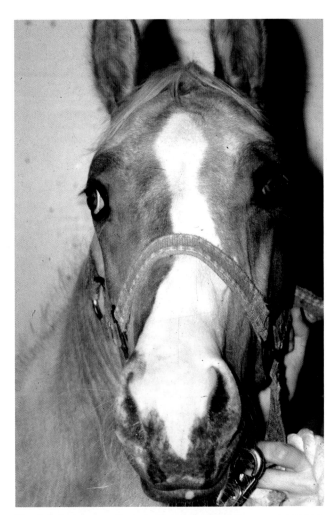

Fig. 2-8 Appaloosa affected with congenital stationary night blindness (CSNB) demonstrating dorsomedial strabismus and an unusual gaze associated with head elevation, termed *star gazing*. The relationship of the strabismus to the CSNB is unclear. (Photograph courtesy Dr. David Wilkie.)

Nystagmus

Nystagmus is an oscillatory movement of the globe, which may be horizontal, vertical, or rotational. Physiologic nystagmus is a normal compensatory reaction that occurs when the head turns and is a direct response to differential stimuli within the inner ear and the vestibular system. This involuntary motion of the globe permits a more stable visual horizon and enhances stability of the visual field. Pathologic forms of nystagmus reflect damage to the vestibulocochlear apparatus (horizontal, rotatory) or CNS disease (vertical). Nystagmus most frequently accompanies CNS disease in the horse, which most often has an infectious cause. Potential causes include equine protozoal myeloencephalitis, the viral encephalitides (Eastern Equine Encephalitis, Western Equine Encephalitis, Venezuelan Equine Encephalitis, West Nile virus), aberrant parasite migration, and bacterial sepsis. Peripheral causes include equine protozoal myeloencephalitis; trauma fracturing the petrous temporal, basisphenoid or basioccipital bones; conditions affecting the guttural pouch diverticulum (empyema, mycosis, chondroids; temporohyoid osteopathy; and osteomyelitis adjacent to the inner ear orbit). Concurrent depression substantially worsens the prognosis. Refer to Chapter 12 (Systemic Disease) for more details on the specific diseases and their treatment.

Abnormalities of Globe Location, Size, and Function

Exophthalmos

Exophthalmos describes the anterior displacement of a normal-sized globe within the orbit. The most common causes are retrobulbar mass, orbital cellulitis, and trauma that reduces the orbital space (Fig. 2-9). Exophthalmos is most easily identified by viewing the head from the front and comparing the angle of the eyelashes, the relative prominence of the globe, and the size of the palpebral fissure (Fig. 2-10). Minimal additional benefit is obtained from observation from above the skull, as compared with observation in other domestic species. An exophthalmometer is a device used to measure relative globe prominence within the orbit, but it is seldom of clinical relevance. Palpation of the globe relative to the orbital rim may provide results similar to those obtained with an exophthalmometer.

Retropulsion reflects the tissue pressure within the orbit and should be attempted in every individual exhibiting exophthalmos. Each globe should be repelled in the same position and direction for the comparison to be valid. It is easier to move the globe directly posterior than inferiorly. Painful exophthalmos typically suggests cellulitis or inflammatory disease, whereas nonpainful exophthalmos is more commonly observed when slowly expanding neoplastic or cystic masses are present. Exophthalmos may induce lagophthalmos, which requires therapy to protect the cornea.

Enophthalmos

Enophthalmos of the globe is typically caused by the loss of orbital contents. It is most commonly found in older horses that are reabsorbing orbital fat but should be differentiated from phthisis occurring in a chronically inflamed eye. Neonatal foals are enophthalmic if they are dehydrated (Fig. 2-11), and this rapidly reverses with return to normal homeostasis. Enophthalmic globes should be comfortable and visual, but vision may be reduced by the prominence of the nictitans, which is no longer held in position by the globe. The supraorbital fossa is more prominent and deep. Secondary complications from enophthalmos relate to inappropriate contact between the eyelid and the globe, typically caused by entropion (see Fig. 2-11). It has been suggested that fat mobilization occurs preferentially from sites with the greatest variation in individual fat cell size. The orbital fat and supraorbital fossa fat cells are the smallest in the body, suggesting that fat resorption in this area occurs as a late outcome.[24]

Trichiasis and chronic ocular discharge from misalignment of the eyelid and puncta are management problems in enophthalmic globes. Entropion of the lower eyelid may be addressed to prevent direct abrasion of the hair on the cornea (see Chapter 3 for more information on management of entropion and trichiasis). Strategies include primary entropion repair, which may result in inappropriate gapping between the globe and the eyelid and accumulation of mucoid debris. Alternatives are cryosurgery of irritating hairs, injection of collagen intradermally to increase eyelid rigidity, or placement of retrobulbar silicone devices to propel the globe forward. The latter procedure is subject to later displacement of the silicone prostheses and recurrence of entropion. Addressing the sequelae in this manner is likely to be successful only temporarily. An alternative strategy to enhance eyelid rigidity and prevent entropion is the injection of autogenous fat into the dermal layers to improve alignment. Pars intermedia dysfunction in horses may accentuate reabsorption of fat and worsen enophthalmos. Orbital fracture may result in enophthalmos if the ventral floor of the orbit is displaced. Finally, enophthalmos may be associated with sympathetic denervation to the smooth muscle between the globe and orbital rim, which is typically somewhat subtle in appearance, but may be associated with nictitans prominence (see Chapters 3 and 12 for more information on Horner's syndrome).

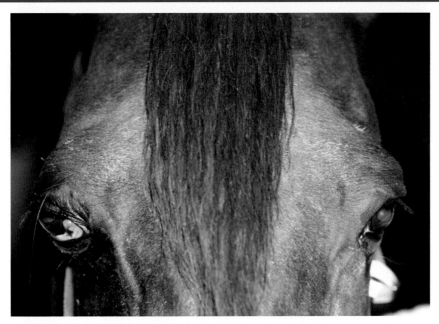

Fig. 2-9 Exophthalmos of the right eye caused by an orbital mass. Note the prominence of the nictitans and mild dorsomedial strabismus, which suggests that the mass is extraconal and nasal within the orbit. (Photograph courtesy Dr. Brian Gilger.)

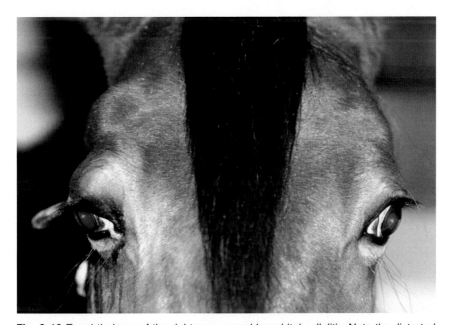

Fig. 2-10 Exophthalmos of the right eye caused by orbital cellulitis. Note the distorted contour of the eyelids, mydriasis, supraorbital fossa swelling, and eyelash angle asymmetry of the right eye compared with the left. (Photograph courtesy Dr. Brian Gilger.)

Spastic enophthalmos may be a prominent sign of pain in horses and is due to the powerful contraction of the retractor bulbi. Resolution of the ocular pain results in return to normal position of the globe.

Phthisis Bulbi

Gradual shrinkage of the globe is due to chronic inflammation and hypotony of the globe, resulting from severe damage to the ciliary body epithelial cells that are responsible for fluid production (Fig. 2-12). When desirable, such globes may have an intrascleral prosthesis inserted to replace the intraocular contents. It is not possible to expand the size of the globe, but further shrinkage may be prevented. See the chapters on uveal diseases (Chapter 5) and equine recurrent uveitis (Chapter 7) for more information and a description of treatments of intraocular inflammatory diseases.

Atrophia Bulbi

Atrophia bulbi is a term that implies the gradual decline in globe size caused by chronic inflammation. In contrast, phthisis bulbi refers to an end-stage, blind eye. See the chapters on uveal diseases (Chapter 5) and equine recurrent uveitis (Chapter 7) for more information and a description of treatments of intraocular inflammatory diseases.

Hydrophthalmos (Buphthalmos)

Hydrophthalmos refers to an unusually enlarged globe, which is universally associated with ocular hypertension secondary to glaucoma. Technically, the term *buphthalmos* indicates a globe typical of a bovine, which purists would observe is generally smaller than that of the horse. The term *hydrophthalmos* indicates that the

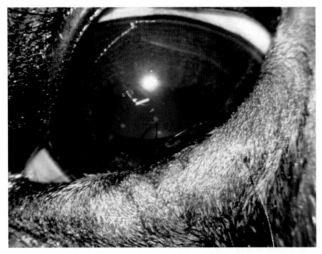

Fig. 2-11 Dehydrated neonatal foal with enophthalmos and lower eyelid entropion. Tacking sutures to roll out the lower eyelid and systemic support will allow the globes to return to their normal position rapidly. (Photograph courtesy Dr. Riccardo Stoppini.)

globe is larger than it was previously, and consequently, may be preferred for describing the horse. In adult horses, globe enlargement occurs slowly and is associated with other clinical signs of glaucoma including corneal edema and endothelial striae (Fig. 2-13). Vision may be present, reduced, or absent at the time of diagnosis. It is not uncommon in horses for vision to return when IOP is subsequently controlled, even if the condition is chronic and mild globe enlargement has occurred. Glaucoma may also be congenital, in which instance, hydrophthalmos may occur rather rapidly with only a temporary retention of ocular function. Congenital glaucoma is usually severe and blinding in the early stages. Hydrophthalmos should be differentiated from exophthalmos of a normal-sized globe. See Chapter 8 for more information on the diagnosis and treatment of glaucoma in horses.

Megalophthalmos

Megalophthalmos refers to a distortion of the globe and has been used to describe the grouping of abnormalities found in Rocky Mountain horses with anterior segment dysgenesis. These clinical signs include increased corneal curvature, iris hypoplasia, congenital miosis, uveal cysts, cataracts, and retinal dysplasia. Persistent pupillary membranes may also be present.[25]

Other Signs of Orbital Disease

In addition to the various displacements of the globe described previously, the following signs suggest orbital disease beyond ocular disease:

- *Prominent nictitans:* The nictitans in the horse is passively displaced by controlled motion of the globe. This temporary physiologic displacement may become chronic and persistent if orbital

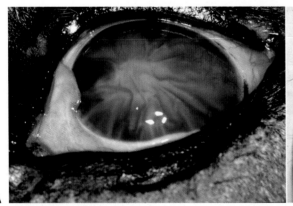
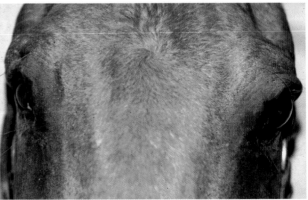

Fig. 2-12 A, Phthisis bulbi, or shrunken globe, from chronic ocular inflammation associated with equine recurrent uveitis. **B,** Phthisis bulbi of the horse's right eye, front view. (Photographs courtesy Dr. Stacy Andrew **[A]** and Dr. David Wilkie **[B].)**

contents are altered in position because of the presence of a mass or absence of adequate globe support, resulting in enophthalmos. The prominence of the nictitans in Horner's syndrome is associated with enophthalmos and may not always be obvious in the horse. Horses with clinical cases of tetanus often exhibit spasm of the nictitans, particularly in response to sudden stimulation. Retropulsion should always be performed when nictitans prominence is observed.

• *Epiphora:* Epiphora is commonly associated with orbital disease but should be differentiated from eyelid swelling and distortion caused by dacryocystitis (Chapter 3) and habronemiasis. In orbital and extraorbital disease, the nasolacrimal duct may be obstructed functionally or anatomically (sinusitis, fracture, neoplasia); or the eyelid puncta may become misaligned as a result of blepharedema, blepharoconjunctivitis, or exophthalmos. Normal tear flow through the nasolacrimal duct depends in part on vacuum development in the duct created by the orbicularis oculi during eyelid closure. Functional obstruction may be differentiated from occlusion by flushing the nasolacrimal duct.

• *Emphysema:* Accumulation of subcutaneous air is due to unidirectional aspiration of air and entrapment between the skin and skull (Fig. 2-14). The most common cause is a sinus fracture, which should be considered an open contaminated wound. A depression or displaced fracture is almost always palpable, but radiography with skyline views is performed if the fracture is not identified clinically. Infrequently, anaerobic bacterial sepsis may result

in gas production, although this is uncommon in skull fractures.

• *Reduced airflow from the ipsilateral nostril:* Reduced airflow from the ipsilateral nostril may be subtle but may be detected by holding a piece of cotton in front of the nostril, or a cool glass slide may be used to detect condensation of warm exhaled air. Partial occlusion of the nasal cavity by a large expanding mass should be suspected if airflow is altered.

• *Sinus percussion:* The mandible should be opened to reduce the mass of tissue being percussed, which improves the sonic qualities, and the bones overlying the sinus should be rapidly percussed to determine whether a fluid pocket, or solid density, can be localized by a more bass tone to the echoing sound. Each side is percussed in sequence for comparative purposes.

• *Episcleral vessel engorgement:* If direct compression of the optic cone results in venous stasis, episcleral

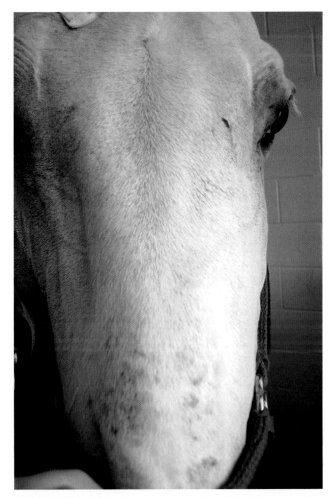

Fig. 2-14 Subcutaneous emphysema from blunt trauma to the left frontal sinus. The accumulation of subcutaneous air is due to unidirectional aspiration of air and entrapment between the skin and skull.

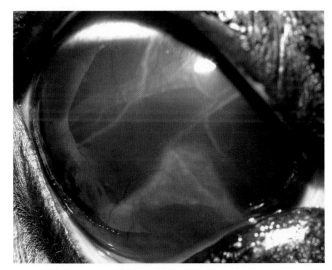

Fig. 2-13 Hydrophthalmos (buphthalmos) in an adult horse with chronic glaucoma. Note additional typical signs of chronic glaucoma such as corneal edema and endothelial striae. (Photograph courtesy Dr. Brian Gilger.)

vessels may become quite prominent. Secondary effects are glaucoma that is typically poorly responsive or unresponsive to hypotensives, despite the importance of uveoscleral outflow in the horse. Exophthalmos may not result, but increased tissue turgor is common. Findings on retropulsion may not be abnormal because the functional obstruction surrounds the cone in the caudal orbit. Blindness may result from concurrent optic nerve compression, even if retropulsion is still possible.

- *Bone deformation:* Sinus neoplasia may result in deformation of adjacent bone, which is typically uncomfortable during firm or deep palpation. Radiographic confirmation of the localized area is usually diagnostic and permits further sample acquisition. Periosteal reaction is less smooth and uniform than that of the normal bone margin and bone sutures.

- *Keratoconjunctivitis sicca.* Keratoconjunctivitis sicca together with ipsilateral facial nerve paralysis suggest trauma to the facial nerve proximal to the geniculate ganglion. Neuroparalytic keratitis results from more distal lesions. The vestibulocochlear nerve (CN VIII) should be evaluated critically if facial (CN VII) nerve disease is identified, because these nerves are commonly injured together in proximity to the petrous temporal bone[19] or the ramus of the mandible.[26] Parasitic migration through the orbit may also result in keratoconjunctivitis sicca.

- *Supraorbital fossa distension:* Supraorbital fossa distension may accompany exophthalmos and space-occupying masses of the orbit. It is a particularly prominent feature of the exotic disease African horse sickness in which hemorrhagic edema causes great distension. Equine viral arteritis results in a panvasculitis and secondary edema that may also cause supraorbital fossa distension and exophthalmos (see Chapter 12 for further details).

CONGENITAL DISEASES

Microphthalmos

Microphthalmos is a congenital or developmental anomaly in which the globes are abnormally small.[27-33] Microphthalmos may be simple or complicated, depending on whether compound abnormalities are present. In the embryo, microphthalmos may result from incomplete closure of the optic fissure, preventing normal sealing and inflation of the globe; or it may be the consequence of a mistimed union of the migrating embryologic tissues. Microphthalmia occurred in 14.7% of foals in one study[28] and in 7% in another.[34]

A case of microphthalmia with brachygnathia has been reported in the foal of an older Friesian mare that received griseofulvin in the second month of gestation; this case was similar to microphthalmia caused by intoxication in other breeds.[31] Multiple ocular colobomas may accompany microphthalmia and result in severely debilitated and blind globes. Staphyloma refers to a diverticulum of uveal tissue prominently displaced through a scleral defect. Cyclopia refers to a single orbit centered in the skull with or without a rudimentary globe. Cyclopia is a very rare condition and is even more rarely associated with an apparently normal globe.

Clinical Appearance and Diagnosis

Microphthalmic eyes appear variably smaller than normal (Fig. 2-15) and commonly have additional abnormalities including cataract and other congenital abnormalities such as retinal coloboma. Nanophthalmos refers to a globe that is functional but smaller than normal. Anophthalmos is the furthest degree of microphthalmos and is extremely uncommon; rather more commonly it is an excessively small globe that is barely recognizable and usually is present as a very diminutive and heavily pigmented spherical mass. In such cases the predominant tissues identified are conjunctivae and nictitans. In the adult animal, differentiating mild microphthalmos from phthisis bulbi as the cause of the small globe may be difficult; however, a poorly developed and small orbit and historical reports of a small or absent globe are most common with microphthalmos. Phthisical globes typically exhibit intraocular changes suggestive of prior substantial uveitis (see Chapters 5 and 7).

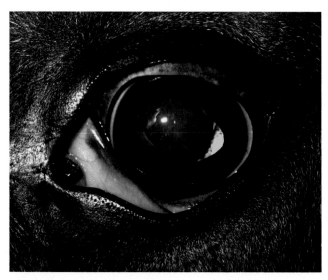

Fig. 2-15 Congenital microphthalmos, a developmental anomaly in which the eyeball is abnormally small, is seen in this foal. Temporally, there is a lens coloboma. (Photograph courtesy Dr. David Wilkie).

Treatment

If the lenses are cataractous but the globes approach normal size, have appropriate light responses, and show no abnormalities on electroretinogram, it is often possible to restore useful vision with the removal of the cataract if surgery is performed early (see Chapter 6). If practical management is a substantial issue and the condition is unilateral, the globe may be removed and replaced with a prosthetic device. More elaborate techniques are being developed in humans to stimulate more normal development of the orbit and involve stepwise inflation of an expandable prosthetic device. Such techniques are unlikely to become practical in horses, given the interventions necessary for a blind globe/orbit.

Long-Term Prognosis and Inheritability Information

Prognosis for vision depends on severity and the presence of other ocular defects. Microphthalmos is more common in Thoroughbreds, and in this breed it is frequently associated with cataract. Inheritance is suspected, but the mode is unknown. Conventional wisdom is to avoid repeating the same sire–dam combination.

Congenital Glaucoma

Congenital glaucoma is uncommon but often quite dramatic in foals. The globe may rapidly enlarge and become a management problem before it becomes blind. Therapy usually carries a poor prognosis for maintaining vision. (For more information, see Chapter 8.)

Orbital Dermoids

Orbital dermoids are particularly rare in the horse but may cause congenital or juvenile unilateral exophthalmos. Skin with or without hair embedded within the orbit may result in a fluid-filled cystic mass that expands.[35] More commonly, noncystic dermoids are located in the dorso-temporal conjunctiva or limbus and are frequently pigmented but not always haired.

Clinical Appearance and Diagnosis

Clinical presentation is the same as for any other space-occupying mass in the orbit. Progressive enlargement and increasing exophthalmos may occur if the dermoid is not removed. The specific diagnosis is likely to be determined at surgery with biopsy confirmation, but may be suggested by findings on presurgical ultrasonography in a juvenile with appropriate history.

Treatment

A space-occupying mass in the orbit requires surgical excision or orbital exenteration.

Long-Term Prognosis

The long-term prognosis depends on the size of the mass, extent of exophthalmos, and damage to the ocular surface. In general, the prognosis for saving the globe is good for small to moderately sized masses. There is no known genetic component in horses. Dermoids of the globe have an excellent prognosis if the dermoids are excised and are not full-thickness. Deeper excisions should be repaired with a conjunctival flap.

Vascular Abnormalities of the Orbit and Globe

Pulsatile exophthalmos has been described to cause prominent exophthalmos after strenuous activity in several nonequine species. Venous dilatations cause more equivocal and stable exophthalmos. Orbital vascular anomalies occur uncommonly as a component of intracranial and extracranial congenital disease in humans. A variety of neuroectodermal dysplasias have been reported in humans, but Sturge-Weber syndrome has been specifically reported in a young horse.[36] In that individual, prominent arterioles affected the choroid plexus of the ventricles intracranially, together with milder vascular abnormalities in the orbit. That horse presented with intermittent seizures and was euthanized. At the University of Florida, the author treated a juvenile Quarter horse filly with unilateral vascular anomalies of the left lower eyelid, orbit, nasal cavity, and anterior buccal cavity; this filly did not exhibit neurologic signs but had progressive dilation of prominent venous sinuses. Orbital varices are often ascribed to traumatic origins.

Clinical Appearance and Diagnosis

Exophthalmos with a palpable or auscultable bruit indicates arterial abnormalities. External orbital vascular abnormalities are very obvious (Fig. 2-16), but orbital

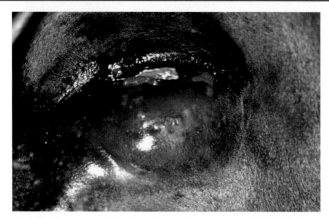

Fig. 2-16 Juvenile Quarter horse filly with unilateral vascular anomalies of the left eyelids, orbit, and anterior buccal cavity.

and intracranial arteriovenous anastomoses are harder to identify, unless seizures or neurologic abnormalities are prominent and imaging studies are performed. Contrast venogram or arteriogram of the orbit may be performed with CT to recreate a three-dimensional image.

Treatment

If nonessential arteriovenous anastomoses can be identified, an intravascular coil may be placed to precipitate embolization. Venous sinus dilatations may be reduced surgically, but access is often limited. In the case of the Quarter horse filly, orbital vessels were demonstrated to be abnormal and asymmetric on CT scan, but a specific site amenable to surgical intervention was not identified.

Prognosis

The prognosis is good for life if no neurologic abnormalities are present. Prognoses for vision and the globe depend on the extent of the anomaly, and surgical intervention may be necessary.

Other Cysts

Maxillary sinus cysts may exhibit behavior clinically similar to that of neoplastic masses but are readily differentiated on imaging studies and are more amenable to surgical control and removal. Cysts in the caudal maxillary sinus may result in exophthalmia.[37] Dentigerous cysts occur uncommonly but may result in exophthalmos or deformation of the orbit. They are typically found close to the petrous temporal bone,

near the base of the external ear. Surgical resection is indicated and should be curative. Radiographs have a pathognomonic appearance.[38]

ACQUIRED DISEASES

Clinical signs of nontraumatic orbital disease are gradual exophthalmos with local orbital distention or deformation, which may extend to deviate and involve the frontal or maxillary sinus, adjacent tooth roots (of the caudal upper cheek teeth), nasal cavity, ethmoid turbinate bones, or guttural pouch. Processes beginning in these structures that impinge on the orbit may be detected primarily because of exophthalmos, strabismus, or blindness. Extension of guttural pouch disease is more commonly due to secondary effects rather than direct mechanical extension.

Traumatic Orbital Disease

Traumatic damage to the orbit occurs more commonly in younger animals, males, and those with fractious personalities or subjected to group confinement. Athletic performance and transportation increase the risk of injury. In particular, rearing and panic-stricken behavior increase the likelihood of sudden blunt trauma, especially to the poll. The dorsal orbital rim and zygomatic arch are at greatest risk of fracture (Fig. 2-17), together with the poll of the skull, which may transmit displacing forces to the sphenoid bones that form the internal orbital wall. Fracture of the frontal or maxillary bones may be further complicated by exposure of the extensive sinuses of the equine head and by laceration of the profuse vasculature at the turbinate bones close to the orbit. Traumatic injury to the ethmoid turbinates or sinus results in epistaxis, entrapped hemorrhagic clots that may become septic, and possibly facial swelling. Palpation and potentially percussion to compare both sides may be supplemented with radiography to localize fractures, hematomas, and fluid. Lavage with large volumes of saline solution has been recommended every 12 hours to prevent prolonged sinusitis and possible development of fistulae. The dental arcade should be specifically evaluated on radiographs to identify periapical tooth root abscesses, fractures of the roots or surrounding maxilla, or other lesions that may greatly affect the outcome. The thin periapical bone may be incomplete overlying the molars, which predisposes that area to formation of abscesses. The constant eruption of equine molar and premolar teeth contributes to the increasing size of the maxillary sinus and likely reduces the impact of dental disease inducing orbital disease.

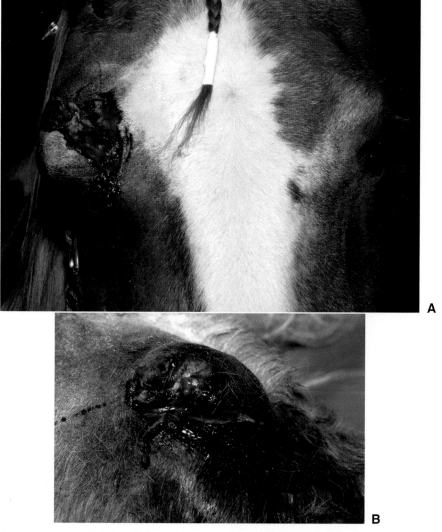

Fig. 2-17 A, Traumatic laceration with fracture of the dorsomedial orbital rim and frontal bone from high-speed blunt trauma. **B,** Traumatic fracture of the dorsal orbital rim in a pony as a result of blunt trauma. (Photograph **A** courtesy Dr. Brian Gilger.)

Globe Perforation

Introduction and Clinical Appearance

A soft fluctuant ocular surface may indicate corneal or scleral perforation if the area is hemorrhagic or if a focal protrusion of tissue is present. Iris prolapse is typically darkly colored, but frequently fibrin and hyphema are also present, resulting in a tan-red surface (Fig. 2-18). A dense red appearance to the entire anterior chamber indicates total hyphema or hemorrhage into the globe as a result of perforation or severe blunt trauma (Fig. 2-19). Hyphema without perforation invariably results in glaucoma and has a grim prognosis. A perforation may initially reseal but remains mechanically unstable and may leak intermittently. Fluid leakage may be confirmed by the Seidel test

(see Chapter 1). Rupture of the globe from blunt trauma most frequently occurs at or near the limbus, and the scleral rupture site may be completely covered with conjunctiva. This should be suspected if the globe is very soft despite complete hyphema and no corneal defect is visible. Scleral perforation posterior to the equator is uncommon. Extrusion of vitreous or the lens extraocularly indicates that severe trauma has occurred, vision will not return, and the perforation is likely too large to repair. Surgical intervention should occur promptly to prevent sepsis and continued severe pain. Keratomalacia, or melting ulcer, presents with a very soft gelatinous appearance; but the corneal surface bulges forwards and is blue, gray, or tan with an undulant but intact surface. Rupture of such an ulcer is recognized by a central brown-tan protrusion of iris, fibrin, and hyphema through the corneal perforation site.

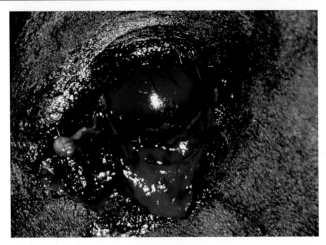

Fig. 2-18 Globe after sudden blunt impact (polo mallet). The limbus is perforated with incarcerated uveal tissue. The globe has mild hypotony and hyphema.

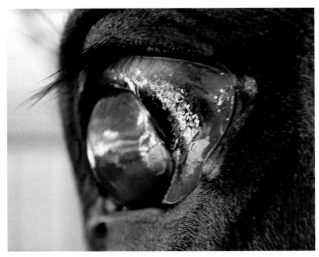

Fig. 2-19 Front view of globe with severe blunt trauma, demonstrating complete hyphema.

Globe rupture during examination occurs if the area is fragile and the horse is resistant. Corneal disease is considered more extensively in Chapter 4.

Diagnosis

The globe's ability to transmit a pupillary light response to the other eye implies that retinal function persists and is a positive indication that vision may be saved. An absent pupillary light response may reflect severe intraocular disease or the intense miosis of the pupil and opacity of the intraocular fluids. Vision return remains possible, but other criteria should be evaluated critically to determine whether surgical intervention should be aimed at preserving vision, placement of a cosmetic globe, or enucleation. With appropriate

restraint, and if not contraindicated by lack of globe integrity, cautious transpalpebral ultrasonography permits evaluation of lens and retinal position (detachment), vitreal or subretinal hemorrhage, posterior globe rupture, and possibly, intraocular foreign bodies. Caution is necessary to avoid complicating the injuries present, and ultrasonography may be better avoided if surgery is certain to be performed. The probe position may be altered (e.g., placed laterally) to prevent complications, and even ultrasonography through the supraorbital fossa may be contributory. Radiography is more useful to determine the extent of fractures and whether bone displacement is present. CT is not routinely available but would be indicated for evaluation of the basisphenoid and basioccipital bones, in cases of complex poll fractures, or to improve the accuracy of diagnosing deep orbital disease. If the patient is ataxic, depressed, or somnolent, a neurologic examination and radiographic examination of the head should be performed to confirm or refute fracture of the calvaria, which greatly affects outcome.

Treatment

Treatment for globe perforations depends on the severity and prognosis for vision. Globes in which vision may be regained (e.g., normal posterior segment and pupillary light response) should have the perforation(s) repaired, usually by suturing of the defect and covering it with a conjunctival flap. If corneal closure is excellent and the laceration is not excessive, a conjunctival flap may be bypassed to reduce long-term fibrosis. Vascularization will still occur and generate a leukoma. It is more difficult to close the surgical margins when they are induced by rupture rather than by a surgical incision because of irregular directional changes (see Chapter 4). The globe should be thoroughly evaluated for other areas of rupture, including the area beneath the conjunctiva. It is not uncommon for multiple independent scleral tears to be present. A peritomy should be performed, and the sclera should be examined in the vicinity of lacerations. If an ulcer perforates, a corneal transplant is the procedure of choice to prevent tissue distortion and is usually supplemented by a conjunctival flap. Eyes with retinal detachments, with large corneal or scleral ruptures, or severe endophthalmitis have very poor visual prognosis and are painful. Horses with these conditions should have an intraocular or hydroxyapatite prosthesis placed or have the globe enucleated with or without the use of an orbital prosthesis. Unfortunately, globe removal is usually associated with the fewest complications and lowest cost. Nonetheless, the degree of trauma that the globe may sustain and yet retain or regain vision and comfort after meticulous surgical repair is remarkable if the repair is performed early.

Long-Term Prognosis

The prognosis for regaining sight after corneal perforation is affected by the length of the prolapse (<10 mm), whether it arose from blunt trauma or ulcer perforation, the presence of a consensual pupillary light reflex, and whether the limbus is involved.[39] Unrepaired globe lacerations have poor prognosis for comfort.

Ocular Injury Associated With Facial Trauma

Facial trauma commonly involves ocular injury because of the prominent orbital location. However, the complete bony orbit does provide substantial protection to the globe. The greatest risk is from lateral blunt impact. The globe itself should be evaluated for normal motion and inflation, any possible mechanical entrapment, vision, and discharge. Concurrent clinical signs to be evaluated include presence of lagophthalmos, emphysema, displacement of skull sutures/bones resulting in an open fracture, appearance of facial asymmetry or deformity, presence or absence of airflow through the nostrils, and the ability to masticate and swallow. The appearance of viscous yellow fluid in the external ear in tandem with a head tilt should be regarded as a particularly serious sign.

Clinical Appearance and Diagnosis

Facial and ocular diseases associated with trauma are quite variable, depending on the type of object (e.g., blunt vs sharp) that the horse has encountered (see Figs, 2-17, 2-18, and 2-19). Globe examination should be sufficiently thorough to ensure that no serious injury is hidden by eyelid, nictitans, or surface swelling. An auriculopalpebral nerve block and sedation will likely be necessary. Initial therapy may allow a better examination within 1 to 2 hours. Diagnostic techniques of value in determining the extent of facial trauma include palpation, oral examination, radiography with air as an inherent contrast agent, and more elaborate imaging techniques as required. Ocular ultrasonography is the alternative approach to determine whether the globe is inflated or whether a perforating injury has been sustained. Measurement of IOP may be of indirect value, but normal IOP does not rule out a perforating injury because temporary closure may occur if intraocular contents are dislodged into the

void, and it is possible to sustain an IOP approaching normal despite slow leakage of aqueous humor, particularly if hemorrhage is extensive.

The proximity of the orbit to the frontal, maxillary, sphenopalatine, and ethmoidal sinuses—together with the nasal cavity and tooth roots—provides ample opportunity for extension of trauma to adjacent cavities. Air may be introduced into the orbit and result in pneumophthalmos and subcutaneous emphysema (see Fig. 2-14). Air aspiration occurs in a valved manner and is entrapped beneath the skin. Differentiation of anaerobic sepsis from air may be difficult, but if clinical signs are suggestive (febrile, leukocytosis, change in mentation, rapid progression), aspiration of fluid for cytologic examination and culture may be most useful. Metronidazole should be administered while test results are pending (Table 2-3).

Treatment

Therapy includes the need to prevent further globe injury, ensuring adequate corneal protection and lubrication, and verification of vision or identifying the need to perform decompression. If eyelid lacerations or other open skin wounds are present, they should be cleaned, clipped, and apposed if appropriate. Eyelid margin defects should be realigned cautiously to ensure that no step defect is introduced and to prevent any sutures from abrading the corneal surface. Specific examination of the tongue is worthwhile, because even extensive lacerations may pass unnoticed in the horse. Deep lacerations may require suturing, and the results may be very rewarding because of the degree of vascular perfusion.

Initial medical therapy should include aggressive administration of systemic antiinflammatory agents (flunixin meglumine, 1.1 mg/kg, given intravenously [IV] or orally [PO]) and broad-spectrum systemic antibiotics if a skin break or sinus fracture is present (see Table 2-3). Surgical interventions to repair bony and soft-tissue trauma of the orbit are discussed later in this chapter.

Penetrating Orbital Foreign Bodies

Introduction and Clinical Appearance

Penetrating orbital foreign bodies, such as gunshot, that become lodged in the orbit may be identified by radiography, and possibly, ultrasonography. Organic foreign bodies are more difficult to detect but may be identified on ultrasonographic evaluation by casting an acoustic shadow. A penetrating tract may

Table 2-3   Parenteral Medications for Orbital disease

Drug	Dose	Notes
IV Antibiotic		
K-penicillin	22,000-44,000 IU/kg IV q6h	
Gentamicin	6.6 mg/kg IV, IM q24h, or 3.3 mg/kg IV, IM q12h	
Ampicillin sodium (trihydrate for IM use only)	20-50 mg/kg tid	Useful if K-penicillin is unavailable
Tetracycline	5-7.5 mg/kg IV q12h	Risk of anaphylaxis; recommend dilution
Oral Antibiotic		
Trimethoprim-sulfa	15-30 mg/kg PO q12h	Broad-spectrum, well tolerated
Doxycycline	10 mg/kg PO q12h	
Enrofloxacin	7.5 mg/kg PO q24h	Off-label use; if indicated on sensitivity
Metronidazole	15 mg/kg PO initial dose 7.5 mg/kg PO q6h	Occasionally indicated for anaerobic infection
Antiinflammatory		
Flunixin meglumine–Banamine	1.1 mg/kg PO, IM, IV q12h 0.5 mg/kg q8h	
Phenylbutazone	2.2-4.4 mg/kg PO q12h	
Aspirin	15-30 mg/kg PO q24h	Least antiinflammatory effect
Gastric Protectant		
Omeprazole	4 mg/kg PO qd 2 mg/kg PO qd (low dose)	For individuals receiving NSAIDs on long-term basis; low dose may be effective
Anthelmintics		
Ivermectin	0.3 mg/kg PO	Habronemiasis
Ivermectin	1.2 mg/kg PO	May repeat at 2- to 3-week intervals for halicephalobiasis or resistant habronemiasis
Fenbendazole	10 mg/kg PO ×5 days, or 50 mg/kg PO every third day	For aberrant strongyles and other nematodes

be apparent. Orbital cellulitis may occur as a delayed complication.

Treatment

Metal fragments that are embedded in the globe may be surgically excised after general anesthesia has been induced if they are readily accessible. Masses embedded within orbital bones should be monitored and not excised unless they result in an unstable fracture, threaten vessels or other structures, or are found in conjunction with orbital cellulitis. Metal fragments within the orbital soft tissue should also be treated with benign neglect, unless they are clinically unstable, which could result in a risk of further damage. Gunshot is typically sterilized by the high firing temperature, whereas metal shards or organic materials that are lodged in the orbit should be treated with broad-spectrum systemic antibiotics, as well as systemic antiinflammatory agents. Organic material should be removed as expeditiously as possible, and aggressive antimicrobial administration is warranted. MRI should not be performed when an intraocular foreign body may be magnetic.

Long-Term Prognosis

The prognosis for vision is usually good unless the foreign bodies have penetrated the globe. Certain metal types may oxidize and discolor, inducing an inflammatory reaction.

Orbital Fat Prolapse

Orbital fat may herniate through weakened episcleral fascia or as a result of trauma to form a fluctuant subconjunctival mass (Fig. 2-20).[40-42] Aspiration or biopsy is recommended if the diagnosis is uncertain. Therapy includes resection of the mass in toto and closure of the conjunctival surface over the exposed area. Future herniation of fat may be prevented by closure of a fascial layer beneath the conjunctiva if sufficient tissue is available (see Chapter 3 for more information).[40-42] Iatrogenic fat prolapse may follow removal of the nictitans if the resulting conjunctival and fascial wounds are not sutured, but it is easily repaired by resecting and closing the herniation site.

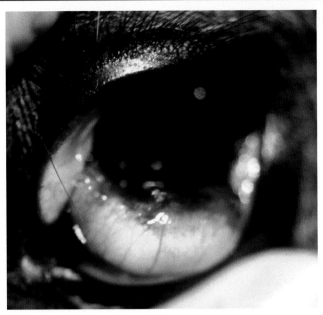

Fig 2-20 Orbital and conjunctival swelling associated with fat prolapse. (Photograph courtesy Dr. Mike Davidson.)

Orbital Proptosis

Introduction and Clinical Appearance

Proptosis is the physical displacement of the globe from the orbit. Fortunately, proptosis is an uncommon condition in horses because it is a devastating injury. If the eyelid margins become entrapped posterior to the equator of the globe, the prognosis for vision substantially worsens. Arterial flow and venous drainage are restricted, and the globe is completely exposed to mechanical trauma and corneal abrasion. Traumatic optic neuropathy results in blindness when the optic nerve is overstretched or sustains a severe whiplash or contrecoup injury, even if proptosis does not occur. The diagnosis is made on the basis of the appearance of extrusions around the optic disc on funduscopic examination, and subsequently, by optic nerve head atrophy (see Chapter 9).

Treatment

The earliest possible decompression (by means of a canthotomy if necessary) and return of the globe to the confines and protection of the orbit should be attempted. If the globe has been expelled from the orbit, sedation and extensive local anesthesia are given immediately, and a brief surgical preparation is performed. General anesthesia may be necessary for repair, but decompression of the proptosis should be performed urgently. Lidocaine 20% mixed with sodium bicarbonate 8.4% (5 to 10 ml, 4:1 vol/vol) is administered at the lateral

canthus and infiltrated along the eyelid margins. The globe should be vigorously cleansed and lubricated. A canthotomy may be performed by briefly crushing the lateral canthus for 10 mm and cutting the marked tissue with large Mayo scissors. With adequate exposure, the fornices are examined for foreign bodies and other lacerations that require intervention. The orbital margin should be evaluated (see discussion of orbital fracture). A subpalpebral lavage system may be placed to permit medication delivery and complete tarsorrhaphy. If no other injuries are present, the globe is gradually retropulsed into the orbit by means of broadly applied pressure. Multiple broad tarsorrhaphy sutures are placed with stents and closed in steps to ensure complete apposition of the eyelids (see discussion of tarsorrhaphy). The canthotomy is closed routinely. Control of ocular and orbital inflammation by systemic antiinflammatory medication is essential if vision is to be preserved (see Table 2-3). Oral corticosteroids have been advocated by some authors and may be more effective if no microbial contamination can be identified (dexamethasone 5 to 20 mg PO every day). Oral antibiotics are commonly administered. Use of topical therapy should be determined on the basis of concurrent cornea ulceration (Table 2-4).

Long-Term Prognosis

Prognosis for vision is poor if the globe is displaced from the orbit and very guarded if the eyelids are entrapped behind the globe. Enucleation or use of a cosmetic implant may be necessary if the globe is severely traumatized or ruptured.

INFECTIOUS ORBITAL DISEASE

Orbital Cellulitis

Orbital cellulitis is not necessarily septic, although that is the most dramatic form. Perforation by a foreign body, direct trauma, and seeding by septic emboli are among the more common causes. The globe is at risk only in the more severe cases, in which therapy has been delayed or additional complications (such as fracture) have occurred. An initial innocuous superficial wound adjacent to the orbital rim may be the only external indicator and may heal rapidly. Deeper extension of the penetrating tract and sepsis subsequently result in more dramatic clinical signs. Extension of inflammatory and infectious conditions from adjacent cavities also occurs commonly. If septic endophthalmitis is untreated or poorly responsive to therapy, it may progress to panuveitis and orbital cellulitis, in which

Table 2-4   Topical Medications for Globe or Orbital Disease

Lubrication	Frequency	Notes
Artificial tears ointment	q1h-tid as needed	If excessive exposure, may become desiccated
Genteal gel severe	q1h-tid	More frequent administration necessary than ointment;
Refresh PM		aids prevention of desiccation
Serum, autologous, homologous	q1h-tid	Refrigerate; viscous lubricant with antienzymatic properties
Adequan in artificial tears solution	q2h-tid	Good viscosity but expensive
Hypertonic saline ointment 3% or 5%	bid-tid	If concurrent corneal edema or bullae are present, at risk for ulceration
Antimicrobial		
Neomycin-polymyxin B-bacitracin ointment	tid-qid	Broad-spectrum; rare drug-induced reaction to neomycin
Neomycin-polymyxin B-gramicidin solution		
Gentamicin or tobramycin 0.3% solution or ointment	tid-qid	Moderate spectrum with minimal epithelial toxicity
Erythromycin ointment	tid-qid	Occasionally irritating, bacteriostatic
Chloramphenicol ointment or solution	tid-qid	Moderate spectrum; bacteriostatic

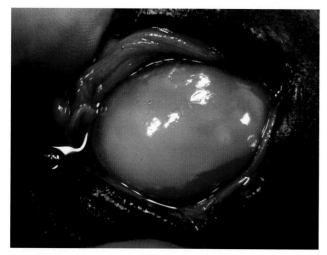

Fig. 2-21 Septic panophthalmitis may extend to the orbit, resulting in exophthalmos.

case the cause will be apparent. In particular, septic panophthalmitis (Fig. 2-21) may lead to devastating spread of bacterial or fungal agents, which would require exenteration to control the process and prevent devastating microbial colonization of deeper tissues. In contrast, orbital cellulitis does not readily induce uveitis within the globe. A more localized and chronic process will result in the formation of a true abscess, rather than generalized cellulitis, and a systemic response (leukocytosis, hyperfibrinogenemia, and fever) is less likely to manifest. Granulomas caused by *Actinomyces* and *Habronema* species may also occur deep in the orbit. *Cryptococcus* infection is reported uncommonly in the orbit and elsewhere in the skull in horses but should be considered as a differential diagnosis for nonresponsive cellulitis.[11] Protracted therapy without attempt at removal of a granuloma allowed

survival for 26 months in one case until the granuloma expanded through the nasal cavity and paranasal sinus and abutted the orbit.[43] *Cryptococcus* infection is initiated in the respiratory or gastrointestinal tract and is spread via lymph nodes until it subsequently localizes. Phycomycosis occurs uncommonly in the orbit but may spread from the guttural pouches or nasopharynx, where it may result in substantial obstruction to respiration and cause secondary clinical signs by local expansion. Organisms include *Conidiobolus* and *Basidiobolus* species. Granulomas are very persistent, locally expansive, and ultimately may be difficult to control.

Clinical Appearance and Diagnosis

The entire contents of the orbit are distorted and enlarged, being forced forward through the palpebral fissure and being restrained only by the eyelids. Blepharedema or blepharitis may be severe, and venous drainage may be obstructed; epiphora may be serous or mucoid, depending on the underlying condition, and is often profuse. The nictitans is displaced anteriorly. The conjunctivae are engorged and may be displaced above the eyelid margin. If the fundus is visible on ophthalmoscopic examination, small white exudates may be present overlying the optic nerve where orbital cellulitis intimately involves the orbital cone. Severe exophthalmos may result in lagophthalmos. IOP is normal until vascular compromise begins and retrobulbar tissue pressure begins to rise, which indicates an unusually severe condition. The only other aperture of the orbit is the supraorbital fossa, which may become turgidly distended. Diagnostic tests of value include a complete blood count to evaluate the degree of systemic inflammatory response (leukocytosis, hyperfibrinogenemia, hypergammaglobulinemia) and imaging to determine whether a section of foreign body is still embedded within the orbit. Fever and general malaise may result from orbital cellulitis or even endophthalmitis; nonetheless, a thorough physical examination including thoracic rebreathing examination should be performed to identify primary or secondary disease elsewhere. Nasopharyngeal obstruction is likely to be a prominent sign with phycomycosis, and diagnosis is made by endoscopy of the nasopharynx, guttural pouches, or both.

Treatment

Antimicrobial agents should be administered systemically at the highest tolerable doses according to diagnostic findings. Aggressive initial nonsteroidal antiinflammatory drug (NSAID) use should attenuate the high intraorbital tissue pressure and preserve globe health. Cold compresses may improve comfort and reduce local inflammation. Abscesses that are truly lined by a capsule are uncommon in the horse, but if one is identified, external surgical drainage may be established after general anesthesia has been induced, and the abscess may be lavaged with broad-spectrum antibiotics such as K-penicillin. When possible, the area should be débrided of malacic material. Considerable caution is necessary to prevent iatrogenic damage, and drainage is more difficult to establish in horses than in other domestic species. Systemic therapy is as for other cases of cellulitis.[44] Therapies proposed for pythiosis include direct intralesional injection of antifungal agents (such as amphotericin B),[45] IV administration of sodium iodide and oral administration of potassium iodide, and laser ablation. Prolonged therapy should be anticipated.

Long-Term Prognosis

Prognosis depends on severity of disease, response to therapy, and the degree and duration of orbital vascular compromise that arises before initiation of therapy. Enucleation may be necessary to control pain from persistent endophthalmitis.

Parasitic Orbital Disease

Parasitic disease of the orbit presents as a space-occupying mass and exophthalmos. Hydatid cysts have been reported in Europe in the United Kingdom and Germany and have been associated with optic nerve atrophy and blindness.[46] Aberrant migration of other nematodes including *Strongylus vulgaris*, *Halicephalobus gingivalis*, and *Draschia megastoma* is more common in the CNS, but these parasites may be found in the orbit. *Strongylus edentatus* has been found in the orbit.[47] *Halicephalobus gingivalis* (syn. *H. deletrix*, syn. *Micronema deletrix*) is a ubiquitous saprophytic soil nematode, which appears to enter the body through damaged mucosal barriers and sporadically causes orbital, neurologic, and diffuse disease in horses and other species.[48] Invasion of the CNS is a common and grave complication. An expanding granuloma present subcutaneously at the orbital rim was successfully removed surgically and medically in one report.[49] Renal involvement is also common with halicephalobiasis. Nematodes are surrounded by macrophages, some eosinophils, a fibrous lining, and localized calcification that may be visible on radiographs. *Echinococcus granulosus equinus* is not of public health significance and cycles between horses and dogs/foxes. Habronemiasis (summer sores) may cause very severe blepharoconjunctivitis, predominantly nasally, but rarely involves the orbit more deeply (see Chapter 3).

Clinical Appearance and Diagnosis

Clinical appearance is typical of a retrobulbar mass. History of inadequate or infrequent deworming is noteworthy. Neurologic abnormalities, hematuria, and other renal abnormalities are poor signs associated with migrating nematode infestation. Uveitis and chorioretinitis have been reported with *H. deletrix*,[50] with diagnosis occurring after histopathologic evaluation. Urine sediment should be examined for rhabditiform nematodes.[51] Ultrasounds or CT scans that reveal a cystic structure are highly suggestive of a hydatid cyst of *Echinococcus* species, and aspiration should typically be avoided to prevent dispersal of the organism.

Treatment

Administration of higher doses of ivermectin (see Table 2-3) is appropriate for many parasitic orbital conditions. For migrating strongyles, or in cases in which ivermectin has already been administered, very high doses of fenbendazole may be administered orally but may not be effective. Orbital hydatid cysts are ideally excised surgically with very cautious dissection to avoid inadvertent puncture and dispersal of the contents. Percutaneous aspiration has been reported as an alternative to removal[52] and should be combined with anthelmintic therapy. *Halicephalobus gingivalis* may be treated by ivermectin (1.2 mg/kg PO every 2 weeks for 3 to 4 treatments).[48] Surgical debulking is indicated if the mass is large or easily accessible.

Long-Term Prognosis

Hydatid cysts are well tolerated unless exophthalmos is present, and cysts are frequently found in other organs at necropsy. Recurrence may accompany cyst rupture. Prognosis for halicephalobiasis depends on severity of disease and response to therapy. Large granulomas may cause blindness, especially if the optic nerve or retina is infiltrated. If signs of CNS involvement are apparent, the prognosis is very poor. Intraocular infection also carries a poor prognosis.[50]

INFLAMMATORY DISEASES OF THE EQUINE ORBIT

Inflammatory orbital disease is less common in horses than in other domestic animals, in part because of the greater separation from the buccal cavity and the greater bony demarcation of the orbit. Penetrating foreign bodies from the oral cavity are considerably less likely to enter into the orbit because of the length of the oral cavity. Sinusitis extending from the maxillary or frontal sinus perhaps poses the greatest threat. Ethmoidal masses may also secondarily induce an inflammatory orbital condition. Control of the primary disease process together with symptomatic orbital therapy is usually sufficient. When the orbit is invaded directly, the condition is managed as a primary orbital cellulitis (see discussion of orbital cellulitis).

Nutritional Myopathy

Uncommonly, nutritional myopathy associated with inadequate dietary intake of selenium, vitamin E, or both may result in severe myonecrosis. Cases localized to the muscles of mastication (particularly the bulky masseter) have been reported. The condition is very painful, especially on deep palpation. A history of inadequate fresh forage and limited pasture access is typical. It has been suggested that stall confinement may protect other muscle groups and predispose the masticatory muscles.[23,53] The condition is less common than, but just as severe as, masticatory myositis in canines.

Clinical Appearance

In one reported case, a horse was presented with acutely swollen masseter and temporalis muscles, exophthalmos, passive displacement of the nictitans, and severe chemosis resulting in herniation of the conjunctiva into the palpebral fissure. Supraorbital fossae were distended. The mouth could only be opened 3 to 4 cm.[53] In general, trismus, an inability to prehend, and a distressed facial expression were apparent.

Diagnosis

Clinical appearance is strongly suggestive of masticatory myositis. Other muscle groups should be evaluated, and the possibility of cardiac myositis should be given consideration. Evaluation of diet, including feed analysis, together with determination of blood selenium and vitamin E levels of the affected individual will confirm the diagnosis. Serum chemistry reflects the severity of the myositis, and urine may be discolored from myoglobinuria.

Treatment

Treatment consists of supplementation with selenium/vitamin E (25 mg/50 mg) and subsequent daily supplementation with selenium to reach a daily intake of 0.3 μg/g. Horses with nutritional myopathy should also be given access to high-quality forage. Daily oral supplementation of vitamin E (5000 to 10,000 IU) would also be reasonable. Supportive care to manage the myonecrosis includes administration of NSAIDs, diuresis (possibly with IV fluid administration), and application of warm compresses to the affected muscles. Nutritional supplementation may be necessary until normal feeding behavior is possible. In the reported case, administration of oral dexamethasone and IV dimethyl sulfoxide was necessary to control the inflammation. Prognosis is poor if debilitation is present, and muscle atrophy may become profound if the patient survives.

Periostitis

Introduction and Clinical Appearance

Periostitis of the nasofrontal bone anastomoses/suture line may result in secondary periocular swelling and severe chemosis. Although predominantly of cosmetic interest,[54] periostitis in the region of the nasolacrimal duct may result in partial or total obstruction and secondary overflow epiphora.[55] Clinical signs may be asymmetric or unilateral. The cause has been suggested to be instability of the junctions of the frontal, nasal, and maxillary bones, although specific traumatic history is often not identifiable.[54]

Diagnosis

Radiography may be indicated to rule out a depression fracture and to determine the extent of the periostitis. Age and history of the patient are important.

Therapy

Therapy involves the use of systemic NSAIDs to control clinical signs as necessary.

Prognosis

A permanent raised distortion of the suture line, akin to a callus, is likely. The significance of this disorder depends on the location of the lesion and its severity but is usually cosmetic only.

Other Inflammatory Orbital Diseases

Other orbital diseases reported in other species may occur uncommonly in the horse, although they have yet to be reported in the literature, such as immune-mediated/eosinophilic myositis and pseudotumor. Pseudotumor is the term used to describe a particularly aggressive inflammatory condition of humans and cats, which is poorly responsive or unresponsive to antiinflammatory therapy.[56-58] The pathogenesis

suggests neoplasia because of its inexorable progression. Reduced retropulsion and dramatic exophthalmos may result, and enucleation may be necessary for control.

NEOPLASIA OF THE ORBIT

Neoplasia of the equine orbit is much less common in the horse than in other domestic species. The most common neoplasms of the orbit are lymphosarcoma (Fig. 2-22) and SCC. SCC of the orbit arises as an extension of neoplasia from another part of the globe. The index of suspicion is raised substantially by identification of a tumor on the globe or eyelids. Belgian and other draft breeds are at increased risk of developing SCC. Lymphosarcoma is a secondary neoplasia that is frequently more insidious and less obviously neoplastic because it frequently presents as gross blepharedema and a reduced palpebral fissure aperture. In one study, ocular lymphosarcoma represented 21 of 79 cases.[59] Eyelid involvement was recorded in 11, nonspecific uveitis in 4, corneoscleral masses in 2, and diffuse retrobulbar infiltration in 2 cases. As is the case in other species, the implication is that early suspicion and confirmation of lymphosarcoma will make early therapy possible and result in an improved short- to medium-term survival for these animals with lymphosarcoma. Biopsy for histopathologic evaluation should be performed early when there is clinical evidence of lymphosarcoma. Lymphosarcoma may also

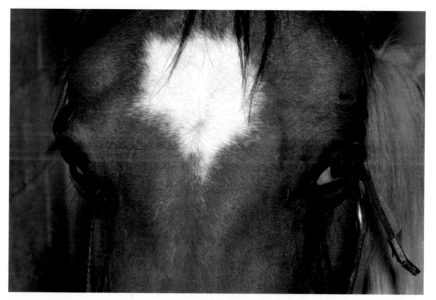

Fig. 2-22 Bilateral exophthalmos in a yearling horse. Note the prominence of the nictitans, epiphora caused by punctal misalignment, bulging of the supraorbital fossa, and distortion of the normal eyelid contour. Generalized lymphosarcoma was diagnosed at necropsy. (Photograph courtesy Dr. Brian Gilger.)

occur as a solitary orbital mass and proceed to rapidly enlarge and result in orbital proptosis.[60]

Other less commonly reported neoplasms of the orbit include melanoma, meningioma, neurofibroma, granulocytic sarcoma, hemangiosarcoma, osteoma, lipoma, ethmoid carcinoma, neuroendocrine tumor, equine sarcoid, multilobular osteoma, medulloepithelioma, and schwannoma. In other species, an age grouping exists, which separates adenocarcinomas (middle-aged individuals) from sarcomas (older individuals).

Clinical Appearance and Diagnosis

Clinical signs of orbital neoplasia are exophthalmos; prominent displacement of the nictitans; orbital swelling; bone surface distortion (possibly with pain on palpation); strabismus if the mass is extraconal; anisocoria, blindness, or both (if the neoplasm is directly compressing the optic nerve); displacement of chemotic conjunctiva through the fissure—and less commonly—epistaxis and signs referable to the involvement of adjacent cavities (see Figs. 2-10, 2-22, and 2-23). Blindness may result from intracranial compression of the optic nerve by pars intermedia masses. The tissue infiltrate may be diffuse and severe; it may be restricted to the orbit or also be present in other locations. Clinical examination should include palpation of the orbital rim to identify evidence of periosteal reaction and bone infiltration. Local lymph nodes should be evaluated by palpation and by cytology if abnormalities are suspected. Lymphosarcoma commonly presents as a diffuse infiltrate of the eyelids, the nictitans, or the orbit. Exophthalmos may be pronounced, and distortion of the eyelids and palpebral conjunctivae may be profound (see Chapter 3 for more information on primary ocular adnexal neoplasia). Exophthalmos may be the

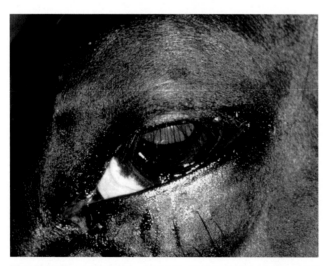

Fig. 2-23 Exophthalmos, elevation of the nictitans, periorbital swelling, and dorsal strabismus with a ventral orbital mass.

presenting complaint for neoplasia that secondarily affects the orbit but arises elsewhere. In such cases, respiratory stridor, epistaxis, purulent discharge, or a fetid odor may be present concurrently and raise clinical suspicion.

Treatment

Treatment consists of surgical removal with or without adjunctive therapies (see later sections in chapter for information on specific neoplasms and Chapter 3 for information on treatment of adnexal neoplasia). If therapy to preserve the globe and eyelids may be of interest to the client, early referral for imaging and surgery is strongly encouraged, and histopathologic samples should be obtained before therapy is initiated. Current medical control of lymphoma is relatively poor but improving, and some individuals will respond well for weeks to months with aggressive use of corticosteroids and other anticancer treatment protocols. Consultation with an oncologist is warranted if therapy may be attempted.

Prognosis

Progress of the disease may be relatively rapid from the point at which the tumor is first recognized as a clinical problem, because the tumor may become quite advanced within the extensive capacity of the equine orbit before clinical signs are apparent. Similarly, masses within the sinus and nasal cavities have considerable space for local expansion before gross deviation of the skull surface or exophthalmos occurs. Consequently, when the tumor becomes overt, much of the normal physiologic function has already been compromised. This is an issue when palliative care and nursing might be an option to allow a short extension of a breeding career or to allow a mare to reach and survive the exertions of foaling. Rapidly enlarging tumors typically do not permit such an approach for more than a short time, and such a management plan is fraught with frustration.

Specific Orbital Neoplasia

A recent case report[22] described a nasal and orbital adenocarcinoma that caused exophthalmos, strabismus, loss of physiologic nystagmus, and specific neurologic signs. A grave prognosis should be attached to secondary metastases to the orbit that also induce neurologic signs or any paraneoplastic syndrome. The mass was identified by means of CT and arose from the maxillary, sphenoid, and frontal sinuses to occupy the orbit and subsequently invade the calvaria. Imaging confirmed parenchymal brain involvement and prevented subjecting the patient to an impossible surgery. Of significance, metastasis was identified in the parotid gland and in fascial planes to the thorax, although no evidence of such involvement was present at clinical examination. The cranial cervical lymph nodes were infiltrated. This case underscores the importance of imaging and consideration of distant metastases, as well as local extension. Thorough palpation may not reveal even sizeable masses, but aspiration and cytology should be performed if even subtle asymmetries are identified on palpation. Thoracic radiography may be of value for identification of masses, but negative findings do not rule out metastasis.[22] Adenocarcinoma of the frontal sinus in a 15-year-old horse expanded through the cribriform plate to enter the orbit and result in exophthalmos.[14] Adenocarcinomas of respiratory epithelium are typically very aggressive in horses, and the delay in making the diagnosis that occurs while the tumor expands to completely occupy the sinus permits substantial destruction before the tumor is manifest. Prognosis is particularly poor when multiple structures are involved.

Osteosarcoma is more readily identified, although it occurs uncommonly because of its early distortion of the bone surface. It has been reported with dramatic distortion of the frontal bone, and radiographic studies are confirmatory.[60]

Melanoma of ocular tissues is frequently benign, and primary excision is curative. However, a subset of these tumors is aggressively recurrent and may invade the orbit. In one case a conjunctival melanoma recurred twice, necessitating orbital exenteration, which was curative for at least 5 years.[61] Specific typing of cell surface receptors may permit identification of more aggressive melanoma types, indicating which individuals require close postoperative scrutiny. In another report, melanoma invading the extraocular muscles appeared to arise from the globe.[62]

Neuroendocrine tumors occur uncommonly in horses but are worthy of consideration because, at exenteration in two horses, hypotension was a potentially serious complication during anesthesia. This was ascribed to the manipulation of the tumor at surgery. After exenteration, the horses were alive at 19 and 24 months before being lost to follow-up.[63] The site of origin may be hard to define because the tumors often involve the orbit, nasal cavity, and paranasal sinus by the time of diagnosis.[10]

A case of medial canthal *hemangiosarcoma* progressed to invade the orbit and maxillary sinus in one individual.[64] Hemangiosarcoma more frequently arises from the globe surface temporally but may rapidly progress caudally and perforate the fascial tunics to invade the orbit.

A *malignant rhabdoid tumor* was treated with exenteration in a 2-year-old filly.[65] The tumor arose from many foci within the globe and the orbit and had spread to the lymph nodes and salivary glands and within the local subcutaneous tissues of the head.

Medulloepithelioma may involve the orbit in young horses, resulting in exophthalmos and intraocular distortion. Medulloepitheliomas may also arise from the uveal tract and optic nerve and require exenteration.[66-68]

Meningioma is rare, but it may cause bilateral blindness in horses because the neoplasm often arises close to the optic chiasm. In one report, a tumor obliterated the maxillary, frontal, and sphenopalatine sinuses but did not invade the calvaria.[69] The diagnosis in that horse was made by histologic examination. Nervous tissue tumors in horses are predominantly peripheral, and the risk reaches a peak at just 4 to 6 years of age and remains stable thereafter.[70]

In rare cases, *odontoma* of normal dentition of young horses may expand to cause maxillary sinus distortion and exophthalmos secondarily.

IATROGENIC ORBITAL DISEASE

Guttural pouch disease in the horse may be remarkably difficult to contain and resolve. Guttural pouch empyema continues to be a challenging condition, and therapy often involves both mechanical and antimicrobial therapies. The use of formalin injection has been advocated for many years and undoubtedly has resulted in control of clinical cases. However, it is important to advise the client that thrombosis of the ophthalmic artery is a possible complication, which is quite likely to result in blindness. Specific cases of severe endophthalmitis have resulted from the occlusion of the internal carotid artery, requiring enucleation to achieve control of severe pain (Fig. 2-24). Surgical occlusion of the external and internal carotid and greater palatine arteries for the treatment of guttural pouch mycosis may cause ischemic optic neuropathy and blindness.[71] However, no ocular complications were observed in patients or experimental animals treated with transarterial coil embolization of the internal and external carotid arteries to prevent hemorrhage associated with guttural pouch infection.[72]

Direct extension of guttural pouch disease is less common, but a case of guttural pouch mycosis resulted in blindness caused by expansion of the plaque to involve the optic nerve and optic chiasm within the calvaria, as well as the retina and orbit.[73]

Complications of oral surgery—specifically dental extraction, wiring of mandibular fractures, and surgical interventions to realign mandibular-maxillary mismatch (parrot-mouth)—may result in moderate or

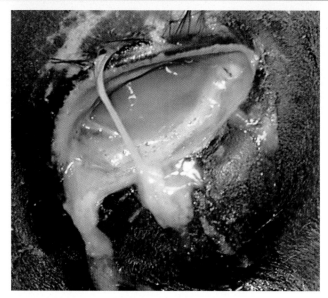

Fig. 2-24 Severe endophthalmitis after formalin injection for treatment of guttural pouch empyema.

severe exophthalmos unilaterally or bilaterally. In addition to symptomatic therapy of the globe(s), diagnostic effort should be invested in locating and identifying an infectious cause for the orbital cellulitis and determining whether removal of any implanted materials is necessary. A thorough systemic physical examination and screening blood work may be extremely useful in identifying further evidence of sepsis such as fever, leukocytosis, and hyperfibrinogenemia. Orbital cellulitis may develop as a result of perforation of the orbital cavity posterior to the conjunctival fornices with a foreign body such as a wood splinter or piece of contaminated metal. The possibility of ingested foreign bodies aberrantly migrating into the orbit is minor in the horse because of the nature of the orientation of the mouth and the soft tissue masses interposed. However, complications of oral surgery intended to repair unstable maxillary fractures or restore symmetry to the maxillary and mandibular occlusion may result in orbital cellulitis, exophthalmos, and lagophthalmos. Therapy is directed toward resolving the underlying cause, removing infected implants, systemic antibiosis and administration of antiinflammatory agents, and treating secondary complications (see discussion of orbital cellulitis for more details).

GENERAL THERAPY OF ORBITAL DISEASE

Topical Medications

Corneal complications of orbital disease are relatively common and may be addressed by frequent use of topical ophthalmic ointment or solutions (see Table 2-4).

If the epithelial surface is intact, protecting the ocular surface tissues with ointment formulations prevents complications from exophthalmos and possibly lagophthalmos and becomes of substantial importance. Failure to adequately lubricate the cornea results in desiccation, trauma, and ulceration that may progress to stromal loss and even globe perforation. Topical ointments are preferred to solutions because of their increased coating ability. Petroleum-based lubricants are ideal if exposure is the primary indication. However, if exposure is sufficient to result in desiccation of the ointment base between applications, a gel-based lubricant should be used in addition. If lagophthalmos is significant, support beyond medical therapy is likely to be necessary, unless the lagophthalmos will resolve rapidly.

Systemic Medications

The parenteral antibiotic of choice in horses with suspected or confirmed sepsis is injectable K-penicillin (22,000 to 44,000 IU/kg IV four times a day) in combination with gentamicin (3.3 mg/kg IV twice a day [bid] or 6.6 mg/kg IV every day) (see Table 2-3). This combination results in very broad-spectrum antimicrobial coverage with excellent distribution to the orbit and globe. The combination is also excellent when emergency anesthesia and surgery are required, although K-penicillin is preferentially given as far in advance of anesthesia induction as possible, to prevent complications from hypotension. When K-penicillin is unavailable, ampicillin sodium may be used in horses (20 to 50 mg/kg IV three to four times a day). The trihydrate form of ampicillin should not be used intravenously. Procaine penicillin requires less frequent administration, but the typical volume of injection (30 to 35 ml) requires distribution over at least two sites and is generally a poor choice for long-term use. Gentamicin has broad effects against gram-negative, and some gram-positive, bacteria. Dosing may be varied, with the high peaks and low troughs of once-daily dosing being preferred in individuals that do not have any contraindications (e.g., renal disease).

For prophylactic antimicrobial therapy, less intensive therapy is usually adequate. Oral antibiotics that achieve good tissue concentrations include trimethoprim-sulfonamide (15 to 20 mg/kg PO bid), which is moderately broad-spectrum and readily tolerated, particularly for intermediate and long-term use. Oral doxycycline (dose 10 mg/kg PO bid) is also well tolerated, but use for orbital disease is not indicated unless sensitivity is confirmed. Doxycycline should not be administered intravenously in horses. Tetracycline is more broad-spectrum and may be preferred in cases of orbital cellulitis. Caution should be used during IV administration of tetracycline to horses to prevent anaphylaxis, and dilution in a moderate volume (100 to 500 ml) of saline solution has been recommended. All orally administered antibiotics in horses may result in diarrhea and bacterial overgrowth that require veterinary attention. Clients should be advised to report any complications that arise with their use.

Antibiotics against anaerobic bacteria are rather limited in horses, but metronidazole (15 mg/kg PO initial dose, then 7.5 mg/kg PO four times a day) is generally very well tolerated. Use is reserved for confirmed or likely cases of cellulitis and when evidence of gas production is present. It may be administered rectally to individuals with gastrointestinal intolerance.

SURGERY OF THE ORBIT

Tarsorrhaphy

Indications for tarsorrhaphy are facial nerve trauma (temporary or permanent), neuroparalytic keratitis, exophthalmos, lagophthalmos, keratoconjunctivitis sicca, and following surgical intervention. A variety of methods have been recommended, but multiple simple interrupted sutures without the use of a stent is recommended. The tarsorrhaphy suture enters the eyelid 3 to 5 mm from the margin, exiting through the gray line of the meibomian gland orifices, and traverses the opposite eyelid in a symmetric manner. Horizontal mattress sutures are better placed with a stent to prevent crushing injury of the eyelid, with adjacent bites being 4 to 6 mm apart. Suture material of choice is a nonabsorbable, 5-0 or 6-0 size, such as surgical silk. However, after surgery, a temporary tarsorrhaphy may be placed with polyglactin 910 7/0 simple interrupted sutures, which may last 7 to 10 days if necessary. A variety of stents may be used on either side of the eyelid, including rubber bands, sections of IV tubing, and a section of surgical drain material. If the stent falls off before the suture is tied, a small-gauge hypodermic needle may be passed through the stent to carry the suture through without repeating the procedure. Tarsorrhaphy may be placed in the standing sedated horse after administration of local anesthetic combined 80:20 vol/vol with sodium bicarbonate 8.4% to increase the pH and promote sensory blockade. An alternative in certain situations may be to use a small amount of tissue glue on the meibomian gland orifice after it has been cleaned and dried. However, caution is warranted to prevent iatrogenic damage caused by inadvertent involvement of the corneal surface.

Retrobulbar blockade is highly recommended in any case of orbital surgery, especially when removal of the globe or evisceration is being performed. Combining epinephrine at 1 to 2:100,000 minimizes any hemorrhage during orbital surgery. The procedure is outlined in detail in Chapter 1.

Orbital Exploration

Orbital exploration is indicated to identify, sample, or remove masses of the equine orbit; to reduce fractures and reverse globe entrapment; to extract foreign bodies; and to investigate nonspecific causes of general orbital disease such as exophthalmos, nictitans prolapse, and generalized tissue displacement. The decision to perform an orbital exploration should not be undertaken lightly, and it behooves the surgeon to consider the potential lesions to be encountered and the surgical manipulations and skills that may be required and to assimilate as many diagnostic results as are available before anesthesia induction. Surgery of the orbit for exploratory purposes may be challenging and requires advance planning and a surgical text for reference. Also of value are an anatomy atlas and a skull model to aid in three-dimensional mental reconstruction of the lesion, its access routes, and its removal. Minor procedures to remove an apparent anterior mass are seldom challenging, but resection and repositioning bone segments, restoring distorted anatomy, and extraction of embedded neoplastic masses while preserving a functional globe are challenging for any surgeon. Specific orthopedic instruments may be necessary to elevate the periosteum, to perform an orbitectomy, and to remove affected areas of bone. Ancillary equipment will frequently be needed to control the disease; for example, cryosurgery may be required to limit the expansion or persistence of neoplastic cells. The layered construction of the orbital contents lends itself to containment of cellulitis or neoplastic disease by remaining outside the affected sheath during surgery where possible. The most aggressive surgical resection is elevation of the periosteum in an attempt to remove the lesion in toto. This requires a meticulous surgical approach, careful dissection, and attention to preventing contamination of the surgical field. If the disease has already breached the surgical containment, the risks of tumor recurrence and persisting infection are increased substantially. Ancillary therapy may still be of value.

Orbital Exploration and Exenteration

Exploration of the equine orbit is rarely performed because of the complex nature of the anatomic structures, together with its infrequent indication. Typically, when exophthalmos is present in an older horse, suggesting an intraorbital mass, imaging reveals the mass to be sufficiently large that surgical debulking is either not reasonable or would also require concurrent removal of the globe. This procedure is described as exenteration and is considered a radical reduction of the orbital bulk in an effort to extend a comfortable life temporarily.

Orbital exploration would be indicated in a younger individual to identify, locate, and remove a mass. Examples of suitable lesions would be parasitic cysts or granulomas; encapsulated orbital abscesses; foreign bodies; circumscribed neoplasia; cystic dilation of the nasolacrimal or salivary apparatus such as the zygomatic gland; or a restrictive mass encircling the optic cone and resulting in secondary ocular disease, glaucoma, and possibly blindness.

The approach to the orbit for exploration depends on the expected location of the mass. Extraconal masses displace the globe and assist in localization. This area should then be subjected to advanced imaging techniques such as CT, MRI, or even contrast radiography with air or a radiopaque fluid. Ultrasonography should be used to supplement these examinations. Diagnostic orbitotomy is uncommon and risks extensive anesthesia and surgical time and dissection but may be necessary if more advanced imaging is not available, if ultrasonography does not yield a specific diagnosis, or if tissue damage is too extensive to obtain satisfactory images. All tissues removed should undergo histopathologic examination, tissue imprints (cytology), and culture as appropriate.

Procedure

Access to the deeper orbit is problematic because of the complete bony orbit. A dorsal orbitotomy approach[63] was used to remove retrobulbar neuroendocrine tumors in three horses. When a dorsal orbitotomy approach is used, a curvilinear skin incision is made just lateral to the sagittal crest of the frontal and parietal bones traveling laterally beyond the zygomatic process of the frontal bone. Retraction of the temporalis muscle attachments exposes the extraocular muscle cone ventrally deep within the orbit. As an alternative, the zygomatic process of the frontal bone may be resected in section by an oscillating bone saw (or osteotome) with appropriate caution to prevent severing the neurovascular bundle within the supraorbital foramen.[74] This step exposes the dorsolateral globe and orbital contents, and the operating window may be further extended by performing a lateral canthotomy. The skin incision is made parallel to the zygomatic process of the frontal bone, with care taken to avoid sectioning nerve fibers that enter the orbicularis oculi laterally. The periosteum is incised anteriorly and reflected off, preserving it to

permit its closure at the conclusion of the procedure. The zygomatic process is removed in an elongated section sufficient to expose the area of interest, after predrilling 20-gauge holes for its subsequent reattachment. Stay sutures may be placed around ocular muscles to permit gentle retraction and dissection of the globe and cone from the mass. Culture and biopsy specimens for histopathologic examination may be obtained. If the mass is to be removed in its entirety, cautious dissection should be performed to prevent inadvertent transection of the myriad vessels, nerves, and muscle attachments. Multiple layers of connective tissue present in the orbit maintain its precise alignment and function. Thus before surgical intervention, it is worthwhile to precisely locate the mass within the orbit and determine whether it is intraconal, extraconal, or subperiosteal. At the conclusion of the surgical procedure, the zygomatic process is repositioned and fixated with stainless steel surgical wire (20 gauge). Periosteal closure may be achieved with simple interrupted absorbable sutures in size 4/0 to 5/0. A subcutaneous closure is performed in a like manner. The skin is reapposed with simple interrupted or cruciate nonabsorbable sutures. If a canthotomy has been performed, it is closed, starting at the eyelid margin, with a buried deep layer and a skin layer that incorporates a figure-8 suture at the canthus. These sutures should be retained for 2 to 3 weeks to prevent subsequent dehiscence because the site is mobile.

Orbital Fracture

Fracture of the orbital rim is a potentially globe-threatening condition, which may result in displacement, impingement, functional restriction, or laceration of the globe. Hemorrhage and increased tissue volume may compress the globe or its vascular channels. Most commonly, the dorsal orbital rim is fractured, and diagnosis is often made by observation and palpation (see Fig. 2-17). The zygomatic arch of the frontal bone may be fractured in a single piece, and it may be manipulated into reduction without further fixation. A bone hook is used to manipulate the arch into reduction without a surgical incision. Comminuted bone chips that are too small to be returned and fixed into position are preferably removed to prevent sequestration and osteomyelitis and a slow protracted healing.[12] The fractured area may be quite painful, and care is indicated to prevent complicating the injury. If multiple bone pieces require reduction, cancellous bone may be used to provide a more cosmetic and mechanically stable healing. Inferior orbital rim fractures may occur from blunt trauma caused by polo balls or mallets; excessive disciplining; and injuries sustained in stalls or during transportation or pasture turnout. Fracture of the lacrimal bone threatens the integrity of the nasolacrimal duct. Fractures that are more extensive result from vehicular accidents and excess struggling of a panicked individual. If the injury involved rearing or falling over backward, damage to the poll may result in fractures to the basioccipital bone, and consequently, to the basisphenoid bone in the inner orbit, resulting in blindness if fractures involve the sphenoid foramina, and probably epistaxis, if the cranial fractures continue rostrally. This dissecting fracture is most likely to occur in individuals younger than 5 years, because the occipitosphenoidal suture line remains incomplete until that time,[38] and concussive force separates preferentially along that line. This area is particularly difficult to visualize with radiographs but is readily apparent on CT. A complete neurologic examination may assist in determining the location of damage. When internal fractures are present, the demeanor and alertness of the patient are often reduced if the calvaria has been traumatized and CNS damage has occurred, which concurrently worsens the prognosis.

When the ultimate cosmetic outcome is desired, closed reduction is highly desirable. After general anesthesia has been induced, zygomatic process fractures may be reduced by manipulation of the bone piece into position with a bone hook.[75] More complex fractures of the dorsal orbital rim may be reduced with a malleable plate or bone plate.[76] If the fracture is repaired by open technique or if an implant is used, parenteral antibiotics are administered. Alignment of the orbital rim is attained more accurately if local tissue inflammation has been attenuated by systemic medications and local compression. Surgical intervention should be initiated early before callus formation becomes significant. Callus formation initiates very rapidly and may be well established at 7 to 10 days. Early stages of second-intention healing are typically advanced by 1 to 2 weeks.[75,77] Fractures of the orbital margin may immediately result in sequelae that require surgical intervention to prevent blinding and painful damage to the globe itself. Entrapment of the ocular muscles, venous stasis, unstable fragment edges, and laceration of blood vessels may necessitate surgical intervention to stabilize the orbit and globe by decompressing the orbit and removal or repositioning of the displaced bones (Figs. 2-25 and 2-26). Hematomas of the orbit are typically stable soon after they form and do not require decompression. If the outflow tract of the globe is not compromised and the optic cone is not encircled, IOP will typically remain normal despite focal soft tissue swelling. However, circumferential compression, or retrobulbar compression, may require urgent reduction in tissue volume to prevent venous stasis and ocular compromise.

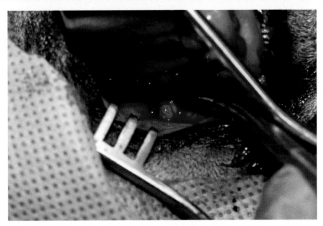

Fig. 2-25 Ventral, transconjunctival approach to the orbit for removal of bone fragments that are impinging on the extraocular muscles, causing ventral strabismus (see clinical appearance in Fig. 2-3). (Photograph courtesy Dr. Brian Gilger.)

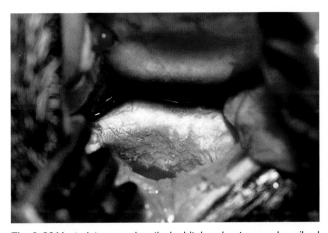

Fig. 2-26 Ventral, transconjunctival orbital exploratory as described in Fig. 2-25. The bone fragment has been isolated and is ready to be removed. (Photograph courtesy Dr. Brian Gilger.)

Fractures of the skull's flat bones may be categorized as displaced or nondisplaced and either open or closed. Closed nondisplaced fractures, together with some closed displaced fractures, are frequently permitted to heal by second intention. Depressed fractures may be realigned by drilling a 2- to 3-mm hole in the bone fragment and inserting angled surgical wire or an instrument to elevate the bone fragment into position. Frequently, it is unnecessary to provide fixation when the bone fragment is repositioned, but fixation with 20-gauge wire is appropriate if necessary. In most such situations, cosmetic outcome is near perfect. Flat bones are likely to heal rapidly and pose little risk of complication if they are not exposed to further stress and extension of the fracture. Stall rest and limited athletic exercise are indicated, together with control of inflammation. Emphysema commonly occurs; it may be monitored for stabilization and treated with parenteral antibiotics because of the open sinus. Fracture pieces may alter position from day to day despite the large bulk of the equine skull. Such motion does not necessarily imply an unstable fracture but should be monitored to ensure that the fragment lines are not progressing. Fractures of the flat bones adjacent to the orbital rim seldom jeopardize the globe. However, if the zygomatic or palatine bone is fractured, the orbital floor may capsize at the time of fracture, and the globe will become ventrally displaced.

Imaging by radiography, and possibly ultrasonography, should be performed before surgical intervention is initiated. Skyline views are helpful for the orbital rim but may be challenging to attain over the sinus (see Fig. 2-6). Despite this, the extent of the fracture may be greater than anticipated from the imaged margins, and a complete evaluation of the injury is necessary before the ideal method of fixation can be determined. When surgical repair is indicated, or the fracture is open, it should be approached with a curvilinear skin incision to provide adequate exposure adjacent to the site, with careful dissection to the location of the fracture. Acute open fractures should be clipped and surgically prepared, and any necrotic or poorly viable skin and subcutaneous tissue should be removed. The exposed surfaces are flushed copiously with sterile saline solution or dilute povidone iodine, which may be administered through a pressure bag, if desired, if appropriate measures to prevent further spread of contaminants are taken. Exposed bone should be débrided aggressively to a healthy vascular supply.

Wiring of fractures may be performed with small-gauge monofilament stainless steel wire (20- to 22-gauge). Alternatively, 2.7-mm or 3.5-mm orthopedic bone plates may be preferred for the repair of certain flat bone fractures. Where comminution occurs or débridement of poorly viable bone results in incomplete fracture reduction, cancellous bone grafts may be incorporated to stabilize bone fragments and reduce mobility within more complicated fractures. If the orbital fracture is extensive, multiple methods of fixation may be required. If fibrous union has already begun or displaced fragments are entrapped, trephine holes may be made near the margin to permit the placement of instruments to elevate and manipulate the fragments into better alignment. However, perfect alignment is much more complex when second-intention healing is advanced and may not be warranted.

Fractures that expose the periorbital sinuses may result in emphysema and epistaxis. Sinus fractures are considered open wounds and should be treated aggressively. If hemorrhage is substantial, prophylactic irrigation with saline solution (possibly through a pressure bag), followed by antibiotic solution is appropriate. A drain may be placed if there is any evidence of infection (purulent exudate, cytologic evidence of bacteria or fungus). Alternatively, comprehensive parenteral antimicrobials and healing by second intention may be elected if displacement is minimal because healing is typically rapid. Tetanus vaccination status should be evaluated, and tetanus antitoxin or toxoid should be administered as appropriate. The sinus egress should be verified, and if drainage is inadequate, the opening into the nasal cavity should be enhanced or an indwelling drain should be established. Microbial colonization of clotted blood within the sinus may lead to severe sinusitis.

Soft Tissue Damage

Initial soft tissue injuries should be treated aggressively with antiinflammatory agents systemically, together with antibiotics if an open wound is present (see Table 2-3). Cold compresses and compression bandages limit tissue volume expansion immediately after injury, which permits more accurate evaluation and reconstruction. Thorough cleansing and minor débridement are important components of first aid care, but if the orbit itself is open, caution is warranted to prevent the introduction of noxious fluids, cleansing agents, or petroleum-based products that may incite an aggressive inflammatory response.

Avulsion of ocular muscles may be repaired in the acute stages if local inflammation is adequately controlled. Alternatively, repair may be delayed for 1 to 2 weeks, during which antiinflammatory agents are administered. The muscle may be avulsed completely or may be strained and lose its mechanical leverage. If the injury is very chronic, an avulsed muscle becomes fibrotic and is too short and mechanically ineffective to reattach. Reattachment of the muscle should be performed with a suture pattern designed to resist tearing or shearing. Sutures are placed adjacent to the original insertion with absorbable material such as 5/0 polyglactin 910. If the muscle and tendon are still inserted but are strained, it may only be necessary to imbricate the weakened tendinous attachment to achieve more normal globe position and restore function. It is often necessary to overcorrect the positional defect at surgery because of the tendency for the suture to loosen during resolution of the inflammation. Exposure of orbit contents, which are predominantly fat, may be resected; and the fascial layers, reapposed over the surface before closure of the conjunctival layer.

Eyelid repair may also be necessary to restore a functional margin without a step defect and to minimize cicatricial sequelae in the conjunctiva. Minor damage to the free margins of the nicitans is common in extensive trauma, and options are either repair with buried sutures or resection. Exposed cartilage poses a minor threat of corneal abrasion. Nasolacrimal duct laceration may be the most challenging to repair functionally. If stricture results, a new drainage conduit into the adjacent sinus may be created. Surgical intervention in the eyelid is reviewed in detail in Chapter 3.

Preoperative Pain Management

If an individual's condition requires stabilization before surgery or if a substantial time interval will elapse before anesthesia induction, there are viable options for preoperative analgesia that will greatly reduce the patient's discomfort (Table 2-5). This makes awaiting major ocular surgery (such as enucleation) the following morning a much more acceptable option for the patient and may permit better overall quality of care than urgent induction of anesthesia to an unstable patient. If the patient is hospitalized and under observation, several options are available. Systemic lidocaine continuous rate infusion reduces the necessary minimum alveolar concentration (MAC) under general anesthesia and may also be administered to awake individuals for pain management. A loading dose of 2.5 to 5 mg/kg is slowly administered as a bolus over a 10-minute period, and a constant rate infusion of 50 to 100 µg/kg/min is continued thereafter. The patient should be generally monitored for signs of muscle fasciculation, recumbency, extensor rigidity, and potentially spontaneous muscular activity that indicate early stages of drug overdose or toxicity. Immediate discontinuation of the drug and bolus administration of IV fluids are typically sufficient to reverse this phenomenon. These signs can typically be avoided by gradual titration of the dose until the patient becomes soporific. Use of a failsafe on the continuous rate infusion is recommended to prevent inadvertent increase

in flow rate. Repeated administration of butorphanol tartrate has more potent analgesic effects and is more suitable for unobserved patients but is more costly. It may also be administered as a continuous rate infusion. If the patient will not be observed, an aseptically administered retrobulbar anesthesia with bupivacaine or mepivacaine (Carbocaine), and possibly epinephrine, would be reasonable (see Chapter 1), together with systemic NSAIDs, but only if the globe is to be removed. Anesthesia to the globe may permit self-trauma that would otherwise not occur.

Enucleation

Enucleation is indicated for the removal of a painful, blind, deformed, or traumatized eye or when extensive neoplasia or infection has rendered survival of the globe unlikely or would require unreasonable duress for the patient. In some situations in which only a single anesthesia induction is tolerable and the ipsilateral globe is visual, enucleation may be preferable to treatment of advanced disease. In individuals considered to be at high risk for complications from anesthesia or who will not tolerate frequent medications and for those cases in which greater economic expenditure is not possible, removal of the globe is a rapid method to restore comfort and prevent further adverse sequelae. Enucleation may be the only humane intervention, but it is important to ensure that the anesthesia and post-operative recovery are not of greater risk than the discomfort of the presenting condition. Removal of an equine globe is a major undertaking, and it should rarely, if ever, be considered in a nonanesthetized individual,[78] and even then, only with appropriate preoperative planning; aggressive analgesia, sedation, and

Table 2-5	Preoperative Pain Management in Surgical Orbital Disease	
Drug	**Dose, route**	**Interval**
Butorphanol tartrate	0.22 mg/kg IM 0.01-0.04 mg/kg IV	Repeat as needed; administer with sedative
Butorphanol tartrate	15-20 µg/kg IV loading dose	Continuous rate infusion of 20-25 µg/kg/h
Retrobulbar block mixture (see Chapter 1)	Retrobulbar (under sedation) Lidocaine/bupivacaine mixture	Repeat every 6-8 h
Lidocaine (requires monitoring for toxicity)	IV loading dose 2.5-5 mg/kg over 10 min	Follow with 50-100 µg/kg/min continuous rate infusion
Lidocaine/mepivacaine (Carbocaine)	Local infiltration at frontal nerve if surface pain is severe	q6-8 h
Xylazine (sedation, minimal analgesia)	0.3-0.6 mg/kg IV or IM	q1-2 h
Detomidine (sedation, minimal analgesia)	10-20 µg/kg IV	q1-4 h
Flunixin meglumine	1.1 mg/kg IV, IM, or PO	q8-12 h

restraint; and appropriate counseling of the client and assisting staff.

A brief candid discussion with the client about alternatives to enucleation is warranted before surgery. All alternatives to enucleation require ongoing maintenance care and have a greater incidence and spectrum of complications, as well as a larger initial and recurring financial investment. For the majority of horses, enucleation remains the most appropriate selection. However, although the client may not initially contemplate

cosmetic alternatives, such alternatives should be offered to prevent the uncomfortable discovery that another procedure would have been preferred if it had been made available. The only postoperative cosmetic alteration that can be performed is implantation of an orbital prosthesis beneath a closed palpebral fissure. Cosmetic alternatives to enucleation are detailed later.

The techniques for enucleation have varied little in recent years, and the major approaches reflect the reason for removing the globe. If neoplasia or severe infection

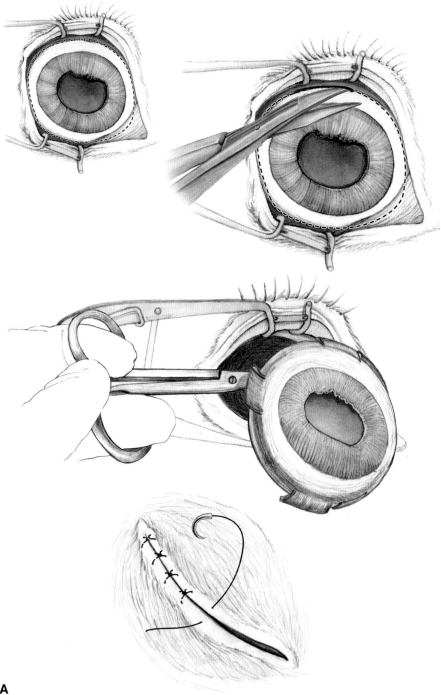

A

Fig. 2-27 A, Transpalpebral and subconjunctival enucleation.

is present, the preferred technique is a closed transpalpebral method (Fig. 2-27). If the ocular disease is contained within the globe or does not threaten the orbit, then a transconjunctival approach is simpler and more easily performed and results in less surgical trauma. Postoperative pain and inflammation are also reduced because fewer tissue planes are interrupted. Routine preparation includes general cleansing of the face; surgical clipping of a 1- to 2-inch margin around the eyelids (in preference to shaving); removal of the eyelashes and possibly the vibrissae; and a surgical scrub of the skin with baby shampoo, chlorhexidine, or Betadine scrub. Detergent is normally avoided on the globe because of its epitheliotoxic effects, but this is not of concern in this procedure. The ocular surfaces may be cleansed with dilute povidone iodine and flushed with sterile saline solution. The head is typically positioned laterally, and the nose is elevated to level the orbit, with the surgeon seated on the dorsal side.

Routine draping is performed to establish a sterile field. A retrobulbar block is recommended (see Chapter 1) to improve anesthetic stability and reduce postoperative discomfort and intraoperative hemorrhage. A portion of the retrobulbar anesthetic mixture can be injected subconjunctivally at the dorsal and ventral limbi. Local auriculopalpebral and sensory nerve blocks may also be performed, together with topical application of proparacaine and phenylephrine. Local anesthesia greatly reduces reliance on general anesthesia and has a more profound effect on pain awareness, thus permitting a generally lighter anesthesia plane. Local anesthetics act to inhibit the action potential by preventing the influx of sodium ions across the axonal membrane. Systemic administration of lidocaine under general anesthesia reduces the MAC, enhancing surgical safety, as well as providing additional analgesia (see the discussion of preoperative pain management).[79]

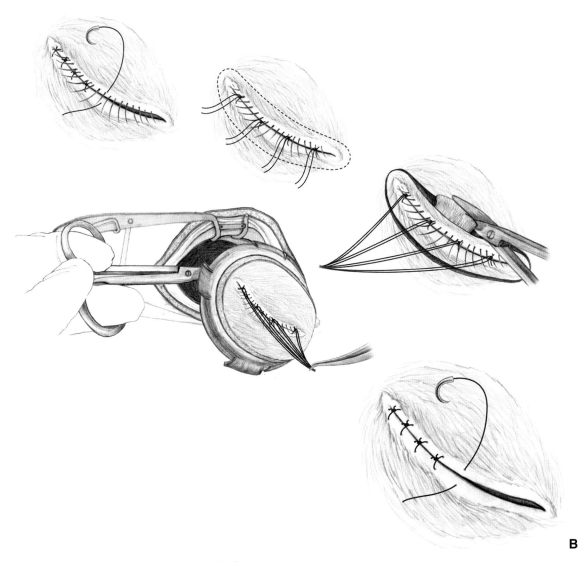

B

Fig. 2-27 cont'd. B, Subconjunctival enucleation.

The transconjunctival enucleation is initiated with placement of an eyelid speculum, and a short lateral canthotomy is performed. A complete peritomy is completed adjacent to the limbus. This is facilitated if a subconjunctival anesthetic has been injected. The extraocular muscles are identified and resected at the globe, permitting its free rotation. The retrobulbar attachments of the recti muscles are very extensive and are resected blindly. A curved clamp may be placed to ligate the optic nerve and vessels. The globe is removed, and if necessary, the orbit may be temporarily packed with gauze. The nictitans may be removed concurrently with the globe or subsequently. It is imperative not to retain the nictitans within the orbit to prevent subsequent dehiscence caused by lacrimal secretions. In contrast, the lacrimal gland is rarely removed and is typically somewhat difficult to identify. The orbital contents should always be inspected to ensure that no disease remains. Capillary seepage is ubiquitous but should not preclude inspection of the orbit. Normal contents include moderate amounts of fat interspersed between fascial layers, the ocular muscles, and the periorbita. The orbit may be flushed with dilute povidone-iodine and may be temporarily packed with sterile gauze. Antibiotic solutions should also be used if the orbit becomes contaminated during surgery, and consideration should be given to establishing a Penrose drain through a stab wound from the ventral orbit (see Table 2-3). The conjunctiva is separated from the eyelid and Tenon's capsule, and the eyelid margin is resected from lateral to medial. Care is exercised to ensure that the medial canthus is completely excised, while avoiding the angularis oculi vein just below it.

An intraorbital prosthesis may be placed to limit the appearance of a hollow orbit visible through the eyelids. Particular attention should be paid to the removal of any surgical powder on the prosthesis by rinsing or wiping with saline or povidone-iodine solution. The prosthesis is aseptically introduced into the orbit. The prosthesis size should be selected to occupy the orbit and approximate the size of the globe removed, typically ranging from 40 to 50 mm in diameter. The contralateral globe may be measured before induction of anesthesia for size comparison. The prosthesis may be fixed in position, if desired, with 2/0 to 3/0 nylon attaching it to the periosteum; or it may be incorporated into a surgical meshwork in an interlocking pattern, with shallow suture bites taken in the prosthesis to maximize stabilization. In some previous surgical descriptions, cutting the anterior face to a flat surface was recommended to prevent a prominent anterior curvature under the eyelid, although this would seem to be a desirable characteristic of the prosthesis. Closure of surgical margins should include complete apposition of a layer between the prosthesis and the eyelid skin to prevent later migration of the prosthesis or

nonabsorbable knots, dehiscence of the wound, and expulsion of the prosthesis.

Closure is performed in several layers. If no orbital prosthesis is placed, the periorbita may be partially approximated with an interlocking layer of 0 to 2/0 nylon in a continuous pattern. The surgical incision may need to be retracted to identify the incised margin of periorbita if it has recoiled, to ensure maximal apposition and closure. It is important to avoid combining the periorbital and subcutaneous layers, which should be closed separately. The knot should be tied by taking adjacent suture bites rather than by tying the knot across the orbital cavity. The subcutaneous layers are closed with an absorbable suture of the surgeon's preference. Either polydioxanone or polyglactin 910 (in sizes of 2/0 to 4/0) is suitable. The pattern may be interrupted, continuous, interlocking, or cruciate as desired, with the former two being most commonly used. Continuous sutures have a greater risk of dehiscence, although this is rarely a practical problem. The skin layer is closed with nonabsorbable sutures in a cruciate or interrupted pattern by using 2/0 to 3/0 nylon or silk. As an alternative, if the patient is difficult to handle, or to avoid suture removal, intradermal skin closure in a continuous pattern of 4/0 polyglactin 910 may be performed. Tetanus vaccination should be verified, or vaccine should be administered if the history is unknown. Tissue swelling is typically minimal at surgical conclusion but increases with recovery from anesthesia and increasing blood pressure. Pressure bandages may be applied or compresses may be used, if the patient tolerates them, although the majority of cases do not require either.

The transpalpebral approach focuses on globe removal with constant separation of exposed surfaces from the orbital cavity. It is preferred for removal of septic globes and malignant neoplasms. The eyelid margins are temporarily tightly apposed with sutures (2-0 nylon) in a continuous or interlocking pattern. Allis tissue forceps may be placed on each knot end for identification and manipulation. An incision is made full thickness through the skin, 5 to 7 mm from the eyelid margin, to expose the subcutaneous tissues, which are bluntly dissected to divide the eyelid into dermal (retained) and tarsal (excised) layers. This is a potential space of embryologic derivation and readily separates. The division is extended to the periorbital margin, with care taken to avoid perforating the inner eyelid and contaminating the orbit with contents of the conjunctival fornix. The medial and lateral orbital ligaments are sharply severed with a surgical blade. Dissection through the reflections of the periorbita/periosteum opens the orbital cavity deeper to the fornix, and minor blunt dissection will rapidly free the globe from its surrounding tissue envelopes. The ocular muscles are resected close to the globe with limited visibility.

The optic nerve may be clamped with curved forceps. A ligature may be applied to the optic cone if desired; otherwise, the clamp is left in position until it must be removed to close tissue layers. The optic nerve is resected immediately anterior to the clamp, 1 to 2 cm posterior to the globe.

Enucleation has a low incidence of complications (<5%). It is imperative to remove the nictitans, the eyelid margins, and the majority (if not all) of the conjunctiva; otherwise, dehiscence is likely to occur, or distension of the orbit with mucoid or mucoserous debris will occur over the long term. Removal of the lacrimal gland from the dorsolateral orbit appears to be unnecessary, and it is rarely entirely removed even when intended because of its protected location. Complete resection of the medial canthus ensures that dehiscence and drainage do not occur at the site of a persistent mucocutaneous junction after suture removal or absorption. When this complication is observed, the surgical correction depends on differentiation of a persistent eyelid margin that may be removed and closed from a draining, possibly septic, tract into the orbit that requires orbital exploration, débridement, flushing, and closure. If the orbit may be septic, it should be débrided and extensively flushed with antibiotic solution, and a drain should be created through a stab wound ventral to the incision closure. The drain tubing is left in position until no further drainage occurs for 24 hours. Alternatively, gauze may be soaked in povidone iodine, rolled up, and placed in the orbit, passing through a stab incision and through a holding suture tied loosely in the skin. A section of gauze is removed (with the patient sedated if necessary) on a daily basis for 3 to 5 days, or until the drainage becomes clear. The stab incision heals by second intention.

Evisceration and Intrascleral Prosthesis

The most common indications for evisceration are a cosmetic alternative to enucleation for blind, painful eyes or globes that are beginning the process of phthisis bulbi. In general, intraocular neoplasia and septic processes should be considered contraindications to retaining the scleral/corneal shell with implant placement. However, intrascleral prostheses (ISPs) have been placed in such cases, and with appropriate informed consent from the client, may not be an absolute contraindication.[80] Cosmetic alternatives that feature an artificial globe are available with the complete removal of the globe but require additional procedures to be performed at the time of first surgery. All prostheses require routine maintenance and greater attention to cleanliness than enucleation. An ISP requires a single surgical procedure but has a less cosmetic outcome

and the potentially more serious complication of future corneal ulcers.

A veterinary ophthalmologist should be consulted before surgery for potential candidates for cosmetic globes. Most owners find an ISP to be preferable to enucleation or retention of a phthisical globe, but it is important to discuss the fact that postoperative corneal ulceration may occur and will require therapy. If stromal loss occurs and is progressive, a conjunctival flap or intensive medication will be required. If perforation occurs and fails to granulate rapidly, enucleation is required, but a prosthetic hydroxyapatite implant remains as a final alternative.

It is pertinent to consider that the cornea will still be at risk of ulceration unless vascularization occurs. Preexisting corneal disease (traumatic or otherwise) increases the risk of complications after surgery, and an advancement conjunctival flap may be placed concurrently if the injury is near the limbus, such as a corneoscleral laceration.[81] If anticipated management or lifestyle changes make daily observation unlikely, then evisceration is not an appropriate surgical choice. Corneal health is somewhat compromised with the removal of aqueous humor, and adequate tear film and eyelid coverage are important for the prevention of future disease. Globes with preexisting keratitis may also be regarded as being at high risk for ulceration. Attempts to quantify tear production are warranted, but findings may not be representative in light of concurrent trauma and pain.

Evisceration is the removal of the ocular contents with preservation of the ocular shell, comprising the cornea, sclera, and its connective tissues and conjunctiva. Surgical preparation is as for other intraocular surgery with removal of eyelashes and fastidious surgical preparation of the skin. The cornea and conjunctival fornices are surgically prepared with dilute povidone iodine, which is adequately flushed with sterile saline solution. A brief sweep of the fornix may be performed with a sterile cotton-tipped applicator to remove loose hairs, particularly from under the nictitans. Topical proparacaine and phenylephrine are applied several times. A self-adhesive drape is preferred to avoid any possible contamination of the intraocular space from the eyelid and skin hair. The conjunctiva and Tenon's capsule are deeply incised over 160 to 180 degrees parallel and 6 to 8 mm posterior to the limbus to completely expose sclera.[82] If the eye has had chronic uveitis, Tenon's capsule may be remarkably thickened, requiring deep incision and blunt dissection to expose sclera. The sclera is incised full thickness in a position to permit easy closure. A shorter perpendicular incision traveling caudally (to complete a T shape) may be made for improved exposure. Dexterity permits the scleral incision to be entirely completed without perforation of the uveal tract. The uveal tract and ocular contents may then be removed by rocking motions alternating between two pairs of nontoothed holding forceps. Alternatively, or if the tract ruptures, a lens loupe or probe may be used to undermine and remove the ocular contents. Caution is used to prevent damaging the corneal endothelium when possible. When the intraocular contents are removed and placed in formalin for histopathologic evaluation, the cavity is examined and débrided of remaining uvea. An intrascleral prosthesis is selected on the basis of corneal diameter, typically 1 to 2 mm larger than the corneal diameter of the ipsilateral or contralateral globe, approximately 36 to 40 mm for most adult horses. The prosthesis is cleaned of residual powder by rubbing it with gauze moistened with dilute povidone iodine or sterile saline solution. The prosthesis is introduced with caution to avoid touching the eyelids and is seated within the ocular tunics. Ability to appose the scleral margins is assessed, allowing accumulated blood to be expelled. The anterior surface of the prosthesis may be cut flat to reduce contact with the corneal endothelium, although this increases the likelihood of blood accumulating in this area and its subsequent imbibition by the corneal stroma. Later, the heme breakdown products may result in a yellow-green corneal discoloration (Fig. 2-28). Closure of the sclera is achieved with interrupted sutures of absorbable material, such as polyglactin 910 (4/0 to 6/0). The margins are apposed without excess tightness because the globe is no longer filled with fluid. The conjunctiva and Tenon's capsule are closed in one layer with absorbable sutures in a continuous or interrupted pattern, ensuring that complete coverage of the scleral incision and suture is achieved with Tenon's capsule to prevent later dehiscence.

A partial temporary tarsorrhaphy is recommended after surgery to reduce exposure and mechanical abrasion. The globe should be adequately lubricated, and routine postoperative therapy should include administration of both topical and systemic antibiotics and systemic antiinflammatory agents. Increasing discharge or discomfort should prompt reexamination and fluorescein staining. Other than corneal ulceration, complications are uncommon but include endophthalmitis (septic or powder-induced), dehiscence of the surgical site if inadequately apposed or if insufficient Tenon's capsule is incorporated, cellulitis from foreign body response to surgical powder, and excessive periocular swelling if extensive dissection was performed. Histopathologic evidence of intraocular neoplasia or sepsis should prompt a discussion with the client about enucleation of the globe in toto with its prosthetic implant. Persistence of small amounts of uveal tissue does not appear to result in complications, but removal of the entire lens should be verified.

Most equine corneas vascularize and fibrose after surgery and may not be very cosmetic initially (Fig. 2-29). If pigmentation occurs, the cornea appears very cosmetic. Corneal tattooing has been described, although it is not universally satisfactory.[83]

Exenteration

The most aggressive orbital diseases are preferably treated by exenteration, which is the removal of all the orbital contents together with the periosteal lining. The intent with this procedure is to encapsulate the pathologic process within multiple natural tissue layers and

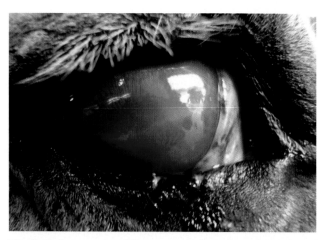

Fig. 2-28 Appearance of the cornea 5 days after evisceration of ocular contents and placement of an intraocular silicone prosthesis. There is corneal edema and ocular discoloration caused by inflammation and resorbing blood products.

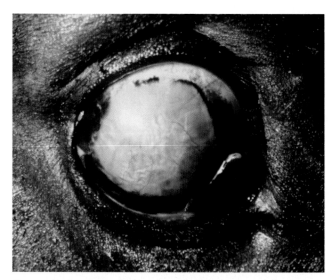

Fig. 2-29 One year after evisceration of ocular contents and placement of an intraocular silicone prosthesis for treatment of chronic glaucoma. The cornea is extensively fibrotic and may become more cosmetic as the cornea pigments. (Photograph courtesy Dr. Brian Gilger.)

remove them without contaminating the orbital cavity itself. Indications for exenteration are control of aggressive neoplasia, severe endophthalmitis, or orbital cellulitis and as a palliative measure in cases of rapidly expanding neoplasia without an attempt to cure. Exenteration may be performed after the failure of enucleation or other local surgical intervention or as the first procedure for aggressive disease. Enucleation procedures may be expanded into exenteration if unexpected orbital contamination is identified, but the advantage of closed tissue layers is usually lost in a converted procedure. A thorough preoperative evaluation will permit the most appropriate procedure to be selected before commencement.

Routine surgical preparation is performed, with a larger area of clipping and prepping. The procedure is performed in a manner similar to transpalpebral enucleation, ensuring preservation of the tissue layers intact. Dissection is performed along the orbital margin to remove as many concentric tissue layers as possible. Neoplastic involvement of the eyelid should be incorporated in the surgical plan as wider surgical margins. When the incision is beyond the level of the conjunctival fornix, dissection is continued close to the orbital margin to remove the tissue layers intact. The periosteum is preferably removed with this procedure if the pathologic process has reached that tissue boundary. A periosteal elevator is necessary. If the periosteum itself is penetrated, adjunctive treatment of the bone margin should be considered by removal with a rongeur or osteotome, followed by either cryotherapy or placement of radiotherapy implants such as iridium beads. The orbit should be flushed with dilute povidone iodine to decontaminate it. If septic endophthalmitis is present, and the tissue layers are compromised, the orbit may be flushed with broad-spectrum antibiotics (see Table 2-3). Orbital evaluation is greatly facilitated if a preoperative retrobulbar block is placed with 1:100,000 epinephrine included. Ligation, hemostats, or cautery should be used as needed to permit a thorough evaluation.

A prosthetic implant is typically contraindicated by disease requiring exenteration. However, if the globe and its shrouds are resected without contamination of the orbit, a meshwork of nonabsorbable suture material (2/0 to 3/0 nylon) may be placed across the orbit in an interlocking or continuous pattern to provide a flat surface on which the dermis can rest, minimizing the tendency to exhibit a gaunt, hollow orbit after recovery. Often, there is minimal periorbita remaining, and the space is spanned with suture material only, which ultimately is likely to break down. The incision knot is tied after a single suture bite at the beginning and end of the pattern. Subcutaneous and skin closure is routine. Alternatively, a preformed mesh may be created to bridge the orbit with a shallow convexity to resemble a globe behind closed eyelids. The prefabricated mesh is attached to the orbital margins.

After final closure of the skin layer, 10 to 20 ml of 0.5% bupivacaine may be aseptically injected transcutaneously to provide inexpensive short-term analgesia for up to 6 hours after recovery. This is particularly useful when a retrobulbar block was not performed before surgical exenteration.

If the orbit was contaminated during or before surgery, in addition to local lavage and antibiotics, a drain site should be created inferiorly; or less optimally, the incision should be maintained open after surgery, to permit drainage of exudate. The wound is managed to ensure drainage and granulation. The patient should be hospitalized, and broad-spectrum systemic antibiotics should be administered. Granulation is typically well advanced by 7 days.

Complications of this procedure are predominantly incomplete removal of the neoplastic mass or infected tissue, allowing persistence of the pathologic process. Excessive swelling is common after exenteration because of the profound disturbance to the tissue layers and destruction of vascular beds. Every effort should be expended to ensure that inadvertent orbital contamination is avoided. More aggressive removal of blood clots and control of hemorrhage are necessary to identify the exact tissue boundaries.

Radical Resection of Eyelid Skin and Globe

A variation of these procedures has been described to permit closure of the orbit when large skin defects remain after neoplasm resection and globe removal.[84] In this procedure, the globe procedure is performed routinely, and any neoplastic mass is excised with a 5- to 10-mm margin. If the skin margins are too widely separated to be apposed, a 10-mm osteotome is used to remove up to 75% of the dorsal and lateral bony orbital rim (the zygomatic process) to reduce the prominence of this landmark and permit more close approximation of the skin wounds. Cruciate sutures are placed in the skin margins, and tension is applied gradually at each site to close the defect. Releasing incisions 10 mm long are then positioned in a staggered pattern parallel and distant to the surgical wound to permit a mesh-like expansion of the surface area. In many situations, this permits a nearly complete closure over the orbit. In the most extreme circumstances, the orbit may remain open. In such cases, the skin is apposed in the most practical and complete method possible, with the use of tension-bearing sutures such as vertical mattress and near-far–far-near sutures, and the remaining area is handled as a granulating open wound. The authors[84] recommend gauze packing of the orbit, protection of the surface, and topical disinfection. Systemic antibiotics are administered until a healthy granulation bed completely covers the internal orbit. Lavage is performed daily with sterile saline solution initially, and after a healthy granulation bed is established in the orbit, lavage is continued with clean water. The authors report excellent outcomes with diligent management and observed no recurrences of the skin tumors that were excised. In circumstances in which options are limited, this procedure may be considered as an in-hospital or referral procedure. Clients should be prepared for prolonged postoperative care and a gradual return to cosmetic appearance. Rotational skin flaps and grafts may be performed but are relatively high risk in the horse. Consultation with a surgeon is recommended to determine the most practical and effective option for each case.

Cosmetic Conformer and Hydroxyapatite Orbital Implantation

More seriously injured globes may be candidates for ocular conformers to be placed over prosthetic globe implants. The process is somewhat involved and requires specialized instruments, but it has been extensively described.[85] The primary candidates for such procedures are individuals in which the utmost cosmetic appearance is required and those with globes that have sustained injuries so substantial that repair is not possible. The cosmetic appearance is superior to that achieved with implantation of an intrascleral prosthesis, and when the initial surgical intervention is healed, the risk of implant expulsion is extremely low. In contrast, the intrascleral prosthesis continues to risk ulceration, infection, and dehiscence via corneal trauma, and the potentially poor cosmetic appearance of an opaque or vascularized cornea.

The surgical procedure for hydroxyapatite-based conformers is performed in a manner similar to transconjunctival enucleation, but only the globe itself is removed. The extraocular muscles, the conjunctival fornices, and other tissues within the orbit are carefully preserved. Cautious microsurgical techniques are necessary. One day before surgery an immediately postmortem globe is acquired, and the sclera are dissected free and submersed in 100% ethanol. Before anesthesia induction, a 40-mm hydroxyapatite sphere prosthesis is soaked in cefazolin for 1 hour and the donor sclera is thoroughly lavaged in sterile saline solution. The sphere is inserted into the sclera by using releasing incisions, which are closed with polyglactin 910 (Fig. 2-30). A stay suture through the eyelid skin and conjunctiva is useful to demarcate the levator muscle

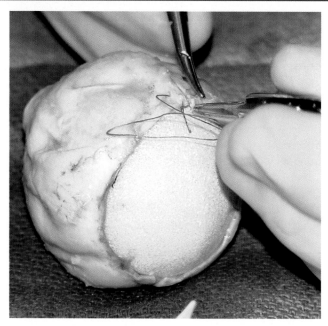

Fig. 2-30 Hydroxyapatite orbital implant and cosmetic corneal-scleral prosthesis. A hydroxyapatite sphere *(white)* is inserted into donor cadaver sclera and placed within the orbit after enucleation. Extraocular muscles are sutured to the donor sclera. (Photograph courtesy Dr. Brian Gilger.)

and the extent of the conjunctival fornix dorsally. A deep peritomy is performed to expose the sclera, and each extraocular muscle is identified and sutured with 5/0 polyglactin 910 and transected at the globe. The retractor bulbi muscles and optic nerve are severed, and the globe is removed. Full-thickness incisions (2 × 4 mm) are made in the donor sclera, 1 cm from the posterior pole. The sclera-clad prosthesis is inserted into the orbit with the exposed coral facing posteriorly (the cornea was removed). Each ocular muscle is inserted through the incision in apposition with the hydroxyapatite and sutured to the interior of the sclera. The oblique muscles are sutured to the sclera directly. Tenon's capsule and fascial layers are apposed across the anterior face of the implant, obscuring it. The peritomy edges are apposed to create a single large conjunctiva-lined fornix (Fig. 2-31). Antibiotic ointment is applied, and a generic plastic extrascleral conformer (prosthesis) is inserted between the eyelids and the conjunctival surface (Fig. 2-32). A tarsorrhaphy is placed temporarily. A compression bandage is placed and changed daily for 3 days. Routine postoperative antibiotics and antiinflammatory agents are administered. After the swelling has subsided, the tarsorrhaphy is removed and the conjunctival fornix is lavaged and treated with topical antibiotics during extended hospitalization for 7 days. With appropriate healing, the patient may be discharged with a prescription for topical antibiotics three times a day for 3 weeks and

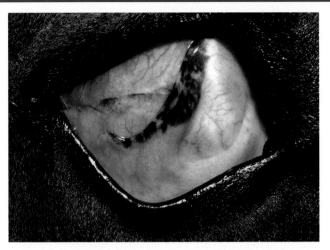

Fig. 2-31 Hydroxyapatite orbital implant and cosmetic corneal-scleral prosthesis. The conjunctiva is apposed over the orbital implant to create a single, large conjunctiva-lined fornix. (Photograph courtesy Dr. Brian Gilger.)

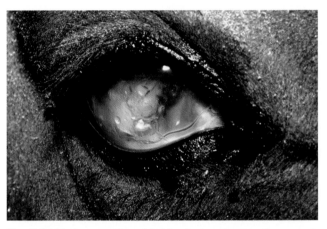

Fig. 2-32 Hydroxyapatite orbital implant and cosmetic corneal-scleral prosthesis. Antibiotic ointment is applied, and a generic plastic extrascleral conformer (prosthesis) is inserted between the eyelids and the conjunctival surface during the healing of the orbit to prevent contracture of the eyelids. (Photograph courtesy Dr. Brian Gilger.)

daily cleaning and repositioning of the conformer. At 4 weeks, the conformer is replaced with a new device to correctly fill the fornix, and measurements are taken for the permanent conformer. Typically, several blank prostheses are used routinely, and one is painted by an ocularist to match the original globe. The individually hand-painted conformers are used only for short periods because of cost (US $3000 to $5000). At the final fitting, any further adjustments in the conformer can be made. Ocular mobility with this procedure may be moderate to excellent, depending on the positioning of the muscles, final prosthesis position, and the amount of tissue between the prosthesis and the conformer. The eyelid position and palpebral fissure size are

determined at the time of surgery by the conformer, which should be placed continuously to ensure that no retraction occurs. If the conformer is cared for appropriately, the final outcome can be excellent (Fig. 2-33). Potential complications of expulsion of the implant or infection are less common with the hydroxyapatite, because its porosity encourages vascular ingrowth and permanent tissue attachment. Owners of potential candidates should be aware that the attempt to increase cosmesis also risks additional complications and that ongoing care of the conformer is necessary.[85]

OTHER SURGICAL PROCEDURES THAT AFFECT THE ORBIT AND GLOBE

Trephination of Sinuses

Trephination may be performed in the standing sedated or recumbent anesthetized horse, depending on the indication and other procedures that must be performed. The maxillary sinus is most commonly involved, because it is the largest and the common exit for the air-filled spaces of the equine skull. Primary indications are exploration, sample acquisition, flushing and drainage of sinusitis and solid masses, and repair of skull fractures. Trephination may be necessary to expose a fracture for repair and is considered an open contaminated site because the sinuses communicate via the maxillary sinus to the nasal cavity. When sinusitis is diagnosed radiographically or clinically, surgery is necessary to obtain samples for culture and cytology, as well as to remove solid material, flush the sinus, and potentially establish drainage. Large volumes of blood should be flushed to prevent bacterial colonization.[75] Draining tracts, although rare, may develop through the orbit and skin. Inferior drainage should be established, and the tract should be treated as a contaminated wound.

The major ocular significance of trephination of the maxillary sinus is the potential puncture and destruction of the nasolacrimal duct or infraorbital nerve. The trephination should be performed dorsal to the facial crest and ventral to the line connecting the medial canthus and the infraorbital foramen. The trephination site should center within this area. Alternatively, if greater access is required, a skin and bone flap may be created after general anesthesia has been induced to flush the sinus and establish drainage.[86] The entire area described is used to create the flap, which opens the caudal maxillary sinus.[37] If the incision is made too dorsal, the nasolacrimal duct may be exposed or perforated, and if it is damaged, it is likely to be difficult to repair. Attempts at repair may be made by cannulating the duct with a flexible retention stylet and

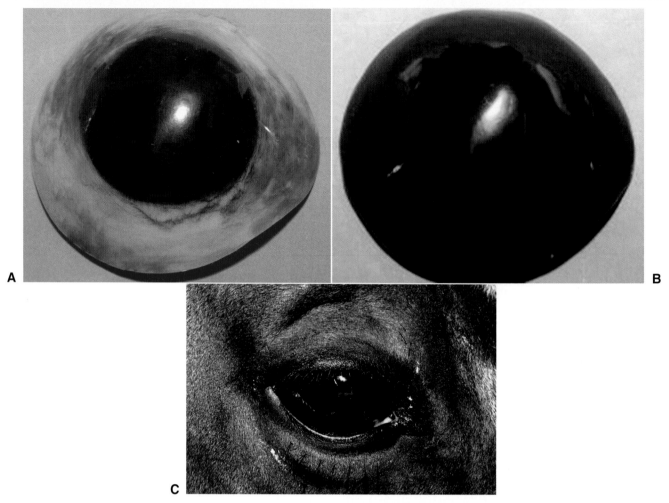

Fig. 2-33 Hydroxyapatite orbital implant and cosmetic corneal-scleral prosthesis. The final corneal-scleral cosmetic prosthesis is made by an ocularist and can be made to appear like a normal eye **(A)** or can be black **(B)**. With either cosmetic shell, the final appearance can be excellent **(C)**. (Photographs courtesy Dr. Brian Gilger.)

realigning the sectioned area across the incision. Sutures should be placed parallel to the long axis of the duct. However, obstruction is likely, and if epiphora results, a canaliculorhinostomy may be required to establish internal drainage. Trephination of the frontal sinus is less commonly performed and is of minor threat to the orbit unless a fracture line extends laterally. A bone flap may be created for greater access, and centers on the midline between the orbits.[37] The sphenopalatine sinus is seldom involved but may be accessed via the maxillary sinus. It is most likely to be damaged by disease that concurrently affects the orbit.

Dental Disease

Dental disease seldom has a direct impact on the equine orbit. The last premolar and first three molars arise in the maxillary sinus, and the last molar is adjacent to the sphenopalatine sinus. Dental disease may result in sinusitis that secondarily affects the orbit, and the caudal cheek teeth may establish tracts from an infected, abscessed tooth root. Spontaneous tracts and fistulas may be identified in the retrobulbar area. Extraction of molars may be challenging, and complications from extraction may ultimately affect the orbit. Complicated surgical treatment of dental misalignment is attempted uncommonly but may place the orbit at risk of sequelae. Surgical correction of prognathism in older individuals has been performed by wiring the maxilla, and the resulting tissue planes may induce cellulitis or sepsis that secondarily involves the orbit. Similarly, implantation of orthopedic plates and screws may result in secondary exophthalmos or lagophthalmos of the globe. Nasolacrimal duct obstruction may also result from the original fracture or from attempts at fixation.[87]

FUTURE RESEARCH

Advancement of imaging modalities will greatly improve the ability to identify, categorize, and diagnose equine orbital disease, and at the same time result in retaining both the globe and vision. Improvements in medical and surgical (irradiation) therapy for orbital neoplasia will ultimately improve the short-term and midterm outcomes of such cases. Improved staging of orbital neoplasia may greatly enhance selection of cases for therapy and the number of visual and comfortable eyes that may be maintained. Further improvements in implant materials will generate new cosmetic procedures for individuals with painful or severely damaged globes. It is to be anticipated that additional pathologic conditions of the equine orbit will be identified in the future with advances in imaging, an increasing population of geriatric horses, and greater expectations of the horse-owning public. Advances in other surgical procedures will limit the consequences of guttural pouch disease and sinus and ethmoid conditions to the globe and orbit. Parasitic diseases will continue to decline in frequency.

REFERENCES

1. Samuelson D: Ophthalmic anatomy. In Gelatt KN, editors: *Veterinary ophthalmology*, ed 3. Baltimore, 1999, Lippincott Williams & Wilkins, pp 31-150.
2. Farrall H, Handscombe M: Equine vision, *Equine Vet J* 31: 354-355, 1999.
3. Wilkins P: Use of an infraorbital nerve block in the diagnosis of headshaking, *Proc Am Assoc Equine Pract* 43:156-157, 1997.
4. Mair TS: Assessment of bilateral infra-orbital nerve blockade and bilateral infra-orbital neurectomy in the investigation and treatment of idiopathic headshaking, *Equine Vet J* 31:262-264, 1999.
5. Ramsey DT, Hauptman JG, Petersen-Jones SM: Corneal thickness, intraocular pressure, and optical corneal diameter in Rocky Mountain horses with cornea globosa or clinically normal corneas, *Am J Vet Res* 60:1317-1321, 1999.
6. van der Woerdt A et al: Effect of auriculopalpebral nerve block and intravenous administration of xylazine on intraocular pressure and corneal thickness in horses, *Am J Vet Res* 56:155-158, 1995.
7. Andrew SE, Willis AM, Anderson DE: Density of corneal endothelial cells, corneal thickness, and corneal diameters in normal eyes of llamas and alpacas, *Am J Vet Res* 63:326-329, 2002.
8. Plummer CE, Ramsey DT, Hauptman JG: Assessment of corneal thickness, intraocular pressure, optical corneal diameter, and axial globe dimensions in Miniature horses, *Am J Vet Res* 64:661-665, 2003.
9. Simoens P, Muylle S, Lauwers H: Anatomy of the ocular arteries in the horse, *Equine Vet J* 28:360-367, 1996.
10. van Maanen C et al: Three cases of carcinoid in the equine nasal cavity and maxillary sinuses: histologic and immunohistochemical features, *Vet Pathol* 33:92-95, 1996.
11. Scott EA, Duncan JR, McCormack JE: Cryptococcosis involving the postorbital area and frontal sinus in a horse, *J Am Vet Med Assoc* 165:626-627, 1974.
12. Modransky P, Welker B, Pickett JP: Management of facial injuries, *Vet Clin North Am Equine Pract* 5:665-682, 1989.
13. Mason BJ: Spindle-cell sarcoma of the equine para-nasal sinuses and nasal chamber, *Vet Rec* 96:287-288, 1975.
14. Hill FW, Moulton JE, Schiff PH: Exophthalmos in a horse resulting from an adenocarcinoma of the frontal sinus, *J S Afr Vet Assoc* 60:104-105, 1989.
15. Latimer CA et al: Radiographic and gross anatomy of the nasolacrimal duct of the horse, *Am J Vet Res* 45:451-458, 1984.
16. Nykamp S, Scrivani P, Pease A: Computed tomography dacryocystography evaluation of the nasolacrimal apparatus, *Vet Radiol Ultrasound* 45:23-28, 2004.
17. Witzel DA et al: Congenital stationary night blindness: an animal model, *Invest Ophthalmol Vis Sci* 17:788-795, 1978.
18. Joyce JR, Witzel DA: Equine night blindness, *J Am Vet Med Assoc* 170:878, 880, 1977.
19. Lavach JD: *Large animal ophthalmology*, St Louis, 1990, Mosby.
20. Green SL et al: Tetanus in the horse: a review of 20 cases (1970 to 1990), *J Vet Intern Med* 8:128-132, 1994.
21. Newton SA: Suspected bacterial meningoencephalitis in two adult horses, *Vet Rec* 142:665-669, 1998.
22. Davis JL et al: Nasal adenocarcinoma with diffuse metastases involving the orbit, cerebrum, and multiple cranial nerves in a horse, *J Am Vet Med Assoc* 221:1460-1463, 1420, 2002.
23. Mayhew I: *Large animal neurology*, Philadelphia, 1989, Lea & Febiger.
24. Bianchi M: Fat cell size in various body regions: a statistical analysis in *Equus caballus*, *Anat Anz* 169:351-366, 1989.
25. Ramsey DT et al: Congenital ocular abnormalities of Rocky Mountain horses, *Vet Ophthalmol* 2:47-59, 1999.
26. Matthews A: Nonulcerative keratopathies in the horse, *Equine Vet Educ* 12:271-278, 2000.
27. Garner A, Griffiths P: Bilateral congenital ocular defects in a foal, *Br J Ophthalmol* 53:513-517, 1969.
28. Priester WA: Congenital ocular defects in cattle, horses, cats, and dogs, *J Am Vet Med Assoc* 160:1504-1511, 1972.
29. Munroe GA, Barnett KC: Congenital ocular disease in the foal, *Vet Clin North Am Large Anim Pract* 6:519-537, 1984.
30. Latimer CA, Wyman M: Neonatal ophthalmology, *Vet Clin North Am Equine Pract* 1:235-259, 1985.
31. Schutte JG, van den Ingh TS: Microphthalmia, brachygnathia superior, and palatocheiloschisis in a foal associated with griseofulvin administration to the mare during early pregnancy, *Vet Q* 19:58-60, 1997.
32. Scotty NC et al: Diagnostic ultrasonography of equine lens and posterior segment abnormalities, *Vet Ophthalmol* 7:127-139, 2004.
33. Williams DL, Barnett KC: Bilateral optic disc colobomas and microphthalmos in a thoroughbred horse, *Vet Rec* 132:101-103, 1993.
34. Roberts SM: Congenital ocular anomalies, *Vet Clin North Am Equine Pract* 8:459-478, 1992.
35. Grant B, Slatter DH, Dunlap JS: *Thelazia* sp. (Nematoda) and dermoid cysts in a horse with torticollis, *Vet Med Small Anim Clin* 68:62-64, 1973.
36. McEntee M et al: Meningocerebral hemangiomatosis resembling Sturge-Weber disease in a horse, *Acta Neuropathol (Berl)* 74: 405-410, 1987.
37. Auer J: *Equine surgery*, Philadelphia, 1992, WB Saunders.
38. Butler J et al: *Clinical radiology of the horse*, Ames, Iowa, 1993, Blackwell Scientific.
39. Chmielewski NT et al: Visual outcome and ocular survival following iris prolapse in the horse: a review of 32 cases, *Equine Vet J* 29:31-39, 1997.

40. Gelatt KN: Herniation of orbital fat in a colt, *Vet Med Small Anim Clin* 65:146-148, 1970.

41. Bedford PGC et al: Partial prolapse of the antero-medial corpus adiposium in the horse, *Equine Vet J* 10:2-4, 1990.

42. Vestre WA, Steckel RR: Episcleral prolapse of orbital fat in the horse, *Equine Pract* 5:135-137, 1983.

43. Roberts MC, Sutton RH, Lovell DK: A protracted case of cryptococcal nasal granuloma in a stallion, *Aust Vet J* 57:287-291, 1981.

44. Hubert J et al: What is your diagnosis? Chronic retrobulbar abscess in a horse, *J Am Vet Med Assoc* 209:1703-1704, 1996.

45. Zamos DT, Schumacher J, Loy JK: Nasopharyngeal conidiobolomycosis in a horse, *J Am Vet Med Assoc* 208:100-101, 1996.

46. Barnett KC, Cottrell BD, Rest JR: Retrobulbar hydatid cyst in the horse, *Equine Vet J* 20:136-138, 1988.

47. Walde I, Prosl H: [Strongylus edentatus as the cause of subconjunctional phlegmon and granuloma formation in the horse], *Tierarztl Prax* 4:493-496, 1976.

48. Pearce SG et al: Treatment of a granuloma caused by *Halicephalobus gingivalis* in a horse, *J Am Vet Med Assoc* 219:1735-1738, 1708, 2001.

49. Isaza R et al: *Halicephalobus gingivalis* (Nematoda) infection in a Grevy's zebra *(Equus grevyi)*, *J Zoo Wildl Med* 31:77-81, 2000.

50. Rames DS et al: Ocular *Halicephalobus* (syn. *Micronema) deletrix* in a horse, *Vet Pathol* 32:540-542, 1995.

51. Kinde H et al: *Halicephalobus gingivalis (H. deletrix)* infection in two horses in southern California, *J Vet Diagn Invest* 12:162-165, 2000.

52. Akhan O et al: Percutaneous treatment of an orbital hydatid cyst: a new therapeutic approach, *Am J Ophthalmol* 125:877-879, 1998.

53. Step DL et al: Severe masseter myonecrosis in a horse, *J Am Vet Med Assoc* 198:117-119, 1991.

54. Trotter G: Paranasal sinuses, *Vet Clin North Am Equine Pract* 1:153-169, 1993.

55. Brooks DE: Equine ophthalmology. In Gelatt KN, editor: *Veterinary ophthalmology*, ed 3, Philadelphia, 1999, Lippincott Williams & Wilkins, pp 1053-1116.

56. Jacobs D, Galetta S: Diagnosis and management of orbital pseudotumor, *Curr Opin Ophthalmol* 13:347-351, 2002.

57. Miller SA, van der Woerdt A, Bartick TE: Retrobulbar pseudotumor of the orbit in a cat, *J Am Vet Med Assoc* 216:356-358, 345, 2000.

58. Weber AL, Romo LV, Sabates NR: Pseudotumor of the orbit. Clinical, pathologic, and radiologic evaluation, *Radiol Clin North Am* 37:151-168, xi, 1999.

59. Rebhun WC, Del Piero F: Ocular lesions in horses with lymphosarcoma: 21 cases (1977-1997), *J Am Vet Med Assoc* 212:852-854, 1998.

60. Rebhun WC: Diseases of the ocular system. In Colahan P, Mayhew I, Merritt A, editors: *Equine medicine and surgery*, ed 4, Goleta, Calif, 1991, American Veterinary Publications, pp 1083-1095.

61. Moore CP et al: Conjunctival malignant melanoma in a horse, *Vet Ophthalmol* 3:201-206, 2000.

62. Ramadan RO: Primary ocular melanoma in a young horse, *Equine Vet J* 7:49-50, 1975.

63. Basher AW et al: Orbital neuroendocrine tumors in three horses, *J Am Vet Med Assoc* 210:668-671, 1997.

64. Bolton JR et al: Ocular neoplasms of vascular origin in the horse, *Equine Vet J* 10:73-75, 1990.

65. Hong C, Van Meter P, Latimer C: Malignant rhabdoid tumour in the orbit of a horse, *J Comp Pathol* 121:197-201, 1999.

66. Ueda Y et al: Ocular medulloepithelioma in a thoroughbred, *Equine Vet J* 25:558-561, 1993.

67. Eagle RC Jr, Font RL, Swerczek TW: Malignant medulloepithelioma of the optic nerve in a horse, *Vet Pathol* 15:488-494, 1978.

68. Bistner S et al: Neuroepithelial tumor of the optic nerve in a horse, *Cornell Vet* 73:30-40, 1983.

69. Kreeger J et al: Paranasal meningioma in a horse, *J Vet Diagn Invest* 14:322-325, 2002.

70. Hayes H, Priester W, Pendergrass T: Occurrence of nervous-tissue tumors in cattle, horses, cats and dogs, *Int J Cancer* 15:39-47, 1975.

71. Hardy J, Robertson JT, Wilkie DA: Ischemic optic neuropathy and blindness after arterial occlusion for treatment of guttural pouch mycosis in two horses, *J Am Vet Med Assoc* 196:1631-1634, 1990.

72. Leveille R et al: Transarterial coil embolization of the internal and external carotid and maxillary arteries for prevention of hemorrhage from guttural pouch mycosis in horses, *Vet Surg* 29:389-397, 2000.

73. Hatziolos BC et al: Ocular changes in a horse with gutturomycosis, *J Am Vet Med Assoc* 167:51-54, 1975.

74. Koch D, Leitch M, Beech L: Orbital surgery in 2 horses, *Vet Surg* 9:61-63, 1980.

75. Caron JP et al: Periorbital skull fractures in five horses, *J Am Vet Med Assoc* 188:280-284, 1986.

76. Brooks DE: Ocular emergencies and trauma. In Auer J, editor: *Equine surgery*, Philadelphia, 1992, WB Saunders, pp 666-667.

77. Blogg JR, Stanley RG, Phillip CJ: Skull and orbital blow-out fractures in a horse, *Equine Vet J Suppl* 2:5-7, 1990.

78. Robertson S: Standing sedation in the horse, *Vet Clin North Am Equine Pract*, 20:485-497, 2004.

79. Doherty TJ, Frazier DL: Effect of intravenous lidocaine on halothane minimum alveolar concentration in ponies, *Equine Vet J* 30:300-303, 1998.

80. McLaughlin SA et al: Intraocular silicone prosthesis implantation in eyes of dogs and a cat with intraocular neoplasia: nine cases (1983-1994), *J Am Vet Med Assoc* 207:1441-1443, 1995.

81. Riggs C, Whitley RD: Intraocular silicone prostheses in a dog and a horse with corneal lacerations, *J Am Vet Med Assoc* 196:617-619, 1990.

82. Meek LA: Intraocular silicone prosthesis in a horse, *J Am Vet Med Assoc* 193:343-345, 1988.

83. Michau T, Gilger BC: Cosmetic globe surgery in the horse, *Vet Clin North Am Equine Pract*, 20:467-484, 2004.

84. Beard WL, Wilkie DA: Partial orbital rim resection, mesh skin expansion, and second intention healing combined with enucleation or exenteration for extensive periocular tumors in horses, *Vet Ophthalmol* 2002;5:23-28.

85. Gilger BC et al: Use of a hydroxyapatite orbital implant in a cosmetic corneoscleral prosthesis after enucleation in a horse, *J Am Vet Med Assoc* 222:343-345, 316 2003.

86. Freeman DE et al: A large frontonasal bone flap for sinus surgery in the horse, *Vet Surg* 19:122-130, 1990.

87. McIlnay TR, Miller SM, Dugan SJ. Use of canaliculorhinostomy for repair of nasolacrimal duct obstruction in a horse, *J Am Vet Med Assoc* 218:1323-1324, 1271, 2001.

3 Diseases of the Eyelids, Conjunctiva, and Nasolacrimal System

Brian C. Gilger and Riccardo Stoppini

Disorders of the eyelids and nasolacrimal system in the horse are among the most common ophthalmic disorders for veterinarians to evaluate and treat. Proper diagnosis and assessment of the disease are especially important in horses with eyelid lesions to ensure proper correction to prevent further ocular damage. Many diseases, such as eyelid trauma and neoplasms, require surgical intervention. Meticulous surgical technique is required to prevent irritation to the underlying sensitive ocular structures. The goal of the chapter is to review the common diseases of the equine eyelids and nasolacrimal system and stress proper diagnostic techniques and surgical therapy.

CLINICAL ANATOMY AND PHYSIOLOGY

Eyelids

The eyelids of the equine eye are composed of thin flexible, mobile skin covering connective tissue, muscle, glandular structures, cilia, and conjunctiva. These structures protect the eye and promote normal ocular physiologic function, such as distribution of tear film and regulation of light.

On the skin surface, the equine eye has three types of hair: vibrissae, cilia, and dermal hair (Fig. 3-1). Two to four vibrissae are typically located 2 to 3 cm dorsal to the medal canthus, and there are 8 to 10 vibrissae located 1 cm ventral and parallel to the lower eyelid. The function of these relatively stiff hairs is to provide tactile stimuli via cranial nerve (CN) V; touching the vibrissae will usually prompt eyelid closure and therefore should be avoided during the ocular examination. Eyelid cilia originate just outside the opening of the tarsal glands on the palpebral margin and may be associated with other modified skin glands (e.g., glands of Zeis and Moll). Eyelid cilia are large and numerous in the upper eyelid but poorly developed or absent in the lower eyelid of the horse (Fig. 3-1).[1] Eyelid cilia also provide tactile input; however, their main function is to protect the cornea and limit the amount of light that enters the eye. Fine, soft dermal hairs cover the eyelid surface in variable degrees of density. The area within 0.5 mm of the eyelid margin generally has few dermal hairs.

The structure and rigidity of the eyelid are provided by the tarsus, which is a narrow dense layer of connective tissue located between the palpebral conjunctiva and the eyelid muscles, such as the orbicularis oculi (Fig. 3-2).[2] The tarsus is larger and firmer in the upper eyelid as compared with the lower eyelid.

The tarsal, or meibomian, glands are a row of sebaceous glands lying along the eyelid at the mucocutaneous junction of the palpebral margin (see Fig. 3-2). The glands open on the upper and lower eyelid margins in a row of evenly spaced orifices ("gray line"). The meibomian glands secrete the lipid layer of the precorneal tear film. Other glandular structures in the equine eyelid include sebaceous glands associated with cilia (i.e., Zeis-like glands) and modified sweat glands (i.e., Moll-like or ciliary glands).[2,3]

The eyelids are very well vascularized by longitudinal vessels that run parallel to the eyelid margins and originate from the malar, superficial temporal, and ventral palpebral arteries.[2,3] The excellent blood supply provides good healing of the eyelids after surgery or traumatic laceration. The eyelids have substantial lymphatic drainage, primarily to ipsilateral parotid and mandibular lymph nodes. This is particularly important with periocular squamous cell carcinoma (SCC) and other neoplasms, because the primary sites of metastasis are these draining lymph nodes.[4]

Motor innervation of the eyelids is from CN III (oculomotor nerve) and CN VII (facial nerve). The blepharospasm often encountered during ophthalmic examination of a horse can be eliminated by blocking the auriculopalpebral nerve (see Chapter 1 for specific locations of these nerve blocks). Sensory innervation of all aspects of the equine eyelid is from CN V (ophthalmic branch of the trigeminal nerve). The upper

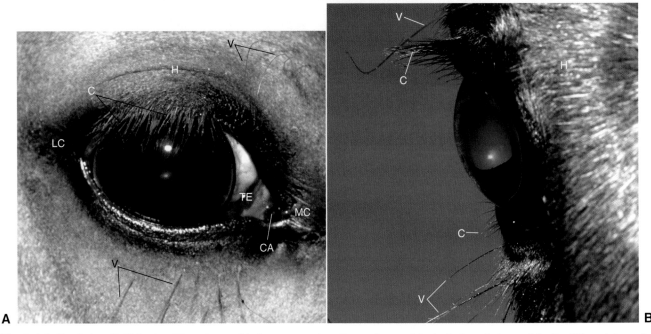

A **B**

Fig. 3-1 A, Front view. **B,** Side view. Three types of hair are present on the equine eyelids, including vibrissae *(V)*, cilia *(C)*, and dermal hair *(H)*. *MC,* Medial canthus; *LC,* lateral canthus; *CA,* lacrimal caruncle; *TE,* third eyelid.

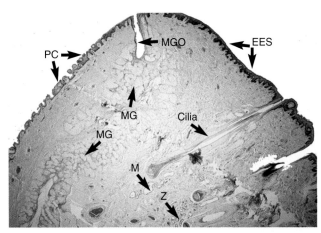

Fig. 3-2 Histologic cross-section of the upper eyelid margin (×40). The meibomian gland orifice *(MGO)* is the location of the muco-cutaneous junction between the palpebral conjunctiva *(PC)* and the external eyelid skin *(EES)*. The meibomian gland *(MG)* is a large sebaceous gland. Sebaceous glands of Zeiss *(Z)* are adjacent to cilia, and apocrine glands of Moll *(M)* are deep to the cilia.

eyelid in the horse can be anesthetized by blocking the frontal (supraorbital) nerve, a branch of CN V. The lower eyelid can be anesthetized by local infiltration near the infratrochlear nerve (Fig. 3-3).

The major muscles of the eyelids consist of the orbicularis oculi muscles, the levator palpebrae superioris, malaris muscle, and Muller's muscle (Table 3-1). The orbicularis oculi muscle surrounds the palpebral fissure to form a sphincter that closes the eyelids. It is innervated by palpebral branch of CN VII (see Fig. 3-3).

The levator palpebrae superioris muscle originates in the posterior orbit, inserts into fibers of the orbicularis oculi muscle of the upper eyelid, and acts to elevate the upper eyelid. It is innervated by CN III, the oculomotor nerve. The malaris muscle attaches to the orbicularis oculi fibers of the lower eyelid and functions to lower the ventral eyelid. It is innervated by a branch of CN VII (facial nerve). Muller's muscle is smooth muscle oriented perpendicular to the eyelid margin that provides the "tone" to the tarsus. It is innervated by sympathetic nerves. Lack of sympathetic tone results in Horner's syndrome. The ptosis portion of Horner's syndrome is a result of the denervation of Muller's muscle.[5,6] Other muscles that control the equine eyelid include the retractor anguli muscle, which retracts and anchors the lateral canthus, and the levator anguli oculi medialis and frontalis muscles, which provide slight elevation of the upper eyelid.

The palpebral fissure has a normal horizontal opening (medial to lateral) of approximately 36 to 51 mm (mean of 43.5 mm) and approximately 25 mm vertically in the adult horse.[7] The lateral canthus is where the upper and lower eyelids adjoin laterally, whereas the medial canthus is where the upper and lower eyelids meet medially (see Fig. 3-1). Structure of the equine eyelids is maintained not only by the palpebral muscles but also by palpebral ligaments. The medial canthal (palpebral) ligament is a firm, ligamentous band anchoring the medial canthus to the dense periorbital fascia and the periosteum of the medial orbital rim. The lacrimal sac lies just deep and ventral to this ligament, and the anguli oculi vein runs just medial to it.

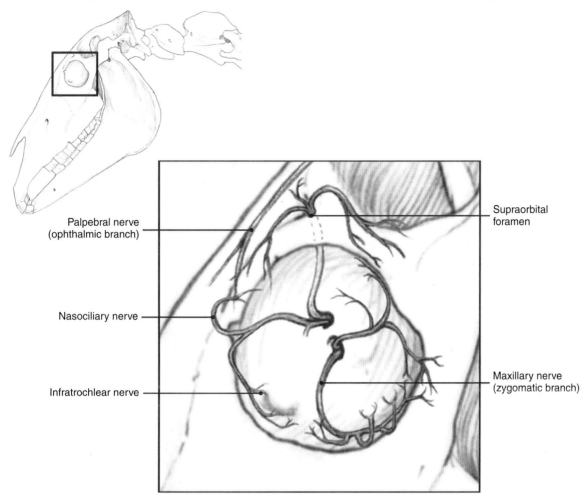

Fig. 3-3 Innervation of the eyelids of the horse. Motor innervation of the eyelids is from cranial nerve (CN) III and CN VII. Sensory innervation of all aspects of the equine eyelid is from CN V. The lower eyelid can be anesthetized by local infiltration near the infratrochlear *(IT)* nerve.

Table 3-1	Muscles and Innervation of the Equine Eyelids	
Muscle	**Innervation**	**Function**
Orbicularis oculi	CN III (oculomotor)	Sphincter that closes the eyelids
Levator palpebrae superioris	CN III (oculomotor)	Elevates the upper eyelid
Malaris	CN VII (facial)	Depresses the lower eyelid
Muller	Sympathetic	Elevates the upper eyelid
Retractor anguli oculi	CN VII (facial)	Lengthens palpebral fissure
Levator anguli oculi medialis	CN VII (facial)	Lengthens and elevates medial canthus
Frontalis	CN VII (facial)	Elevates the upper eyelid

CN, Cranial nerve.

The lateral canthal (palpebral) ligament serves to anchor the lateral canthus.

The lacrimal caruncle lies deep to the medial canthus and external to the third eyelid (see Fig. 3-1). This structure varies in size among horses, and during eyelid closure, it may protrude and prevent the eyelids from conforming as well to the medial aspect of the cornea as compared with the lateral aspect.[1] Conjunctiva, a nonkeratinized squamous epithelium, lines the inner aspect of the upper and lower eyelids (i.e., palpebral conjunctiva) (see Fig. 3-2).

The third eyelid (see Fig. 3-1) in the horse originates in the ventral medial aspect of the orbit and moves passively in the dorsolateral direction with retropulsion of the globe or as the globe is retracted during blinking. The medial and lateral surfaces of the third eyelid are covered with conjunctiva that is richly endowed with goblet cells. A T-shaped cartilaginous structure that conforms to the curvature of the cornea provides structural support along the leading margin of the third eyelid and through the center of the eyelid (Fig. 3-4). The base of third eyelid contains a lacrimal gland (tubuloacinar) that produces portions of the aqueous component of the tear film (Fig. 3-4). A large fat pad is ventral to the gland of the third eyelid.[3]

The function of the eyelids is largely protection of the ocular structures. The blink reflex in response to tactile, chemical, or thermal stimuli of the skin, conjunctiva, or cornea serves to protect the eye. Reflex blinking (and tearing) also helps remove foreign bodies. The eyelids not only produce portions of the tear film (e.g., meibomian glands produce the lipid layer and goblet cells produce the mucin layer of the tear film), they also function to distribute the tear film across the eye during each blink episode.

Conjunctiva

Conjunctiva consists of nonkeratinized stratified columnar cells that are continuous with the corneal epithelium. The conjunctiva consists of three main anatomic regions that are all connected. The anatomic regions include the palpebral conjunctiva, the bulbar conjunctiva, and the fornix. The palpebral conjunctiva is the portion of the conjunctiva that lines the upper and lower eyelids (see Fig. 3-2). The bulbar conjunctiva is attached to the globe. The conjunctival fornix (upper eyelid) and cul-de-sac (lower eyelid) are the junction between the palpebral and bulbar conjunctiva.[3,8] The fornix (dorsally) is located 3 cm from the limbus, whereas the cul-de-sac (ventrally) is 2.5 cm from the limbus.[3] Conjunctiva also covers the anterior and posterior surfaces of the third eyelid (see Fig. 3-4). Conjunctiva is richly vascularized, is pigmented (especially the bulbar conjunctiva), and has many goblet cells that contribute to the tear film. Also, near the limbus, there is an aggregation of lymphoid follicles and lymphatics, termed *conjunctiva-associated lymphatic tissue* that is integral to the ocular immune response and disease.

Nasolacrimal System

The nasolacrimal system of the horse consists of both secretory and drainage portions. The lacrimal gland, a tubuloacinar gland, is located dorsolateral to the globe and has three to five ductules that transport lacrimal fluid from the gland to the dorsal conjunctival fornix. The gland of the third eyelid surrounds the base of the cartilage of the third eyelid and is well anchored compared with the gland of the third eyelid in dogs. The percentage of total lacrimal output produced by the gland of the third eyelid is not known; however, one study demonstrated that horses with the third eyelid removed did not have differences in basal (determined by Schirmer tear test [STT] II) or reflex (determined by STT I) tear production compared with healthy horses.[9] In general, lacrimal function in horses is quite high, and horses produce a large amount of tears in response to stimuli. Furthermore, only a few cases of keratoconjunctivitis sicca (KCS) have been reported in horses.[10-12]

The nasolacrimal drainage apparatus of the horse is a common source of clinical problems, mostly from obstructions.[1,13] Eyelid lacrimal puncta are 2-mm–diameter, slit-like openings located 8 to 9 mm lateral to the medial canthus of the upper and lower eyelids.[14] Through these puncta, lacrimal fluid enters the canaliculi, which are tubes of 3 to 4 mm in diameter that join to form the main nasolacrimal duct (NLD) (Fig. 3-5). Only a slight dilation of the NLD is present where the canaliculi join, and a true "sac" is not observed. The NLD continues distally 7 to 8 cm within the osseous lacrimal canal of the lacrimal and maxillary bones (Fig. 3-6).[14] The duct narrows slightly immediately before its exit from the lacrimal canal of the maxilla bone (see Fig. 3-5). Externally, the course of the NLD through the maxillary bone follows a line from the medial canthus to the infratrochlear foramen (Fig. 3-7).[14] The duct then courses in the submucosa along the nasal wall of the lateral aspect of the middle meatus, then dips ventrally as it courses in the ventral nasal fold. The duct curves laterally over the basal process of the incisive

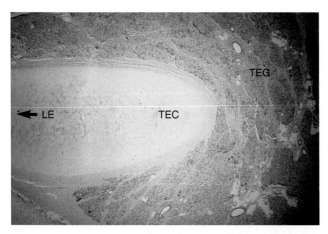

Fig. 3-4 Photograph of the cross-sectional anatomy of the base of the third eyelid (×40). The third eyelid cartilage *(TEC)* runs through the center of the structure with the third eyelid gland *(TEG)* surrounding the base of the third eyelid. The leading edge *(LE)* of the third eyelid is in the direction of the arrow.

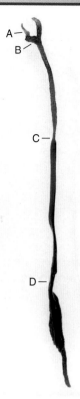

Fig. 3-5 Methyl methacrylate cast of the right nasolacrimal duct. **A,** Lacrimal canaliculus. **B,** Lacrimal sac. **C,** Narrowing of nasolacrimal duct at the exit from the lacrimal canal. **D,** Flattening of the duct by cartilage plate in the sigmoid cartilage. (Photographs courtesy Dr. Clair Latimer, from Latimer CA et al: Radiographic and gross anatomy of the nasolacrimal duct of the horse, *Am J Vet Res* 45:451-458, 1984.)

bone to open at an oval nasolacrimal orifice of 3 to 4 mm in diameter on the ventral floor of the nasal vestibule (Fig. 3-8).[14] Two or more nasolacrimal openings are very common in the nasal vestibule of horses. The total length of the NLD is approximately 24 to 30 cm.[3]

Normal eyelid position is necessary for adequate drainage of the tear film. Closure of the lids occurs from lateral to medial, squeezing the tear film toward and into the nasolacrimal drainage system medially. The vertical component of the eyelid closure distributes the tear film over the surface of the cornea and conjunctiva.

IMPACT OF EYELID DISEASE ON THE EQUINE INDUSTRY

Eyelid and nasolacrimal diseases are among the most common ocular diseases in horses. According to a United States Department of Agriculture 1998 study, the overall prevalence rate for eye diseases was 7.4% in horses older than 6 months.[15] Although this study did not differentiate the ocular problems, eyelid and nasolacrimal diseases likely constitute a large majority of these cases (e.g., eyelid and adnexal diseases are the second most common presenting problem of

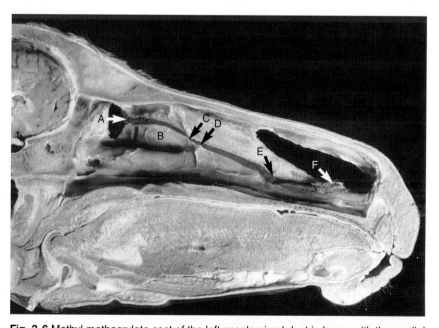

Fig. 3-6 Methyl methacrylate cast of the left nasolacrimal duct in horse with the medial bony orbit and medial wall of the lacrimal canal removed. **A,** Lacrimal sac. **B,** Duct within the lacrimal canal. **C,** Narrowing of nasolacrimal duct at the exit from the lacrimal canal. **D,** Exit of the duct from the lacrimal canal. **E,** Duct pressed laterally by cartilaginous plate in alar fold. **F,** Duct within basal fold. (Photographs courtesy Dr. Clair Latimer from Latimer CA et al: Radiographic and gross anatomy of the nasolacrimal duct of the horse, *Am J Vet Res* 45:451-458, 1984.)

horses, after corneal diseases, admitted to the Equine Ophthalmology Service at North Carolina State University) and therefore would have a high economic impact on the equine industry in general.

CONGENITAL EYELID AND ADNEXAL DISEASES

Entropion in Foals

Entropion, or turning in of the eyelid margins, is the most common ocular abnormality in foals.[16] Usually, the lower eyelid is involved, but both eyelids have been known to be affected. Entropion can be hereditary or acquired. In most foals, the cause of the entropion is loss of orbital fat (cachexia) or dehydration because of systemic illness or maladjustment. The loss of orbital support causes the eye(s) to be retracted into the orbit, allowing the eyelids to roll inward.

Clinical Appearance

Entropion occurs most commonly in neonatal foals and appears as a rolling in, or in-turning, of the eyelid margin. It is usually bilateral and generally involves the lower or lower lateral eyelid (Fig. 3-9). However, unilateral cases and involvement of both upper and lower eyelids do occur. The eyelids roll inward, causing irritation to the cornea because of abrasion by the eyelid cilia and skin hair. The discomfort from this corneal irritation causes severe blepharospasm, further exacerbating the entropion.

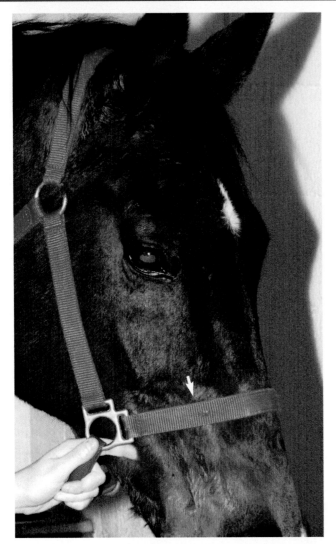

Fig. 3-7 The course of nasolacrimal duct through the maxillary bone follows a line from the medial canthus to the infratrochlear foramen.

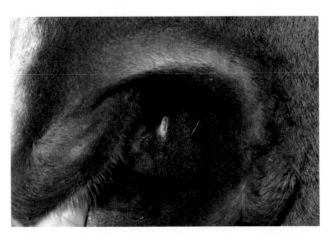

Fig. 3-8 Nasal puncta of the nasolacrimal duct, a 3- to 4-mm, oval orifice on the ventral floor of the nasal vestibule.

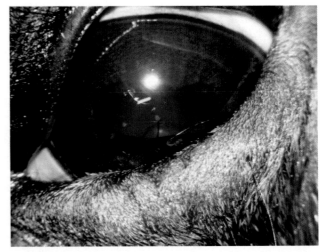

Fig. 3-9 Entropion caused by enophthalmos in a foal with neonatal maladjustment syndrome. (Photograph courtesy Dr. Riccardo Stoppini.)

Differential Diagnosis

The most common cause of the entropion in neonatal foals is systemic disease or maladjustment, as mentioned previously. However, some horses, such as Thoroughbreds[17] and Quarter horses,[1] may be genetically predisposed to entropion. The mode of inheritance and prevalence of the defect are not yet known. Other causes of entropion include microphthalmia, eyelid trauma, scarring (cicatricial entropion), and any disease causing prolonged blepharospasm.[1,18] Entropion in foals must be differentiated from other congenital eyelid abnormalities, such as ankyloblepharon, coloboma, dermoids, and cilia abnormalities (Table 3-2).

Treatment

The goal of treatment for entropion is the temporary eversion of the eyelid margin and protection of the cornea until the foal recovers and orbital structures reestablish eyelid support and return to normal. In rare instances, the entropion persists, and permanent entropion repair is required. In these foals, permanent repair of the eyelid should be delayed as long as possible, without causing permanent damage to the cornea, because the high rate of facial and head growth may result in ectropion or poor cosmetic results.

Medical Therapy

Medical therapy for entropion consists most commonly of corneal protection with frequent (e.g., every 4 to 6 hours) application of topical ophthalmic antibiotic ointment on the affected eyes and medical management and support of the systemic illness. Appropriate management of a corneal ulcer or secondary uveitis, if present, must also be done. However, systemic nonsteroidal medications and topical atropine should be used with caution in these sick foals.

Surgical Therapy

Temporary surgical repair of the entropion is almost always needed to break the chain of discomfort (i.e., entropion, corneal irritation, blepharospasm, and more entropion) to allow the cornea to heal without mechanical irritation, and to provide time for the orbital structures to reestablish support as the foal recovers and grows.

Temporary Entropion Repair Techniques

Everting Sutures (Tacking Sutures)

With the foal heavily tranquilized, usually with xylazine and ketamine, tacking sutures can be placed. These are essentially vertical mattress sutures. Nonabsorbable, 4-0 to 5-0 monofilament suture is recommended, but silk can be used. First, the rolling-in eyelid is everted and placed into its correct anatomic position. Second, a suture is passed in the center of the entropic eyelid, beginning 1 to 2 mm away from the eyelid margin perpendicular to the eyelid. The suture must not go through the eyelid margin because tearing out of the sutures may result in a large eyelid defect. The next step is to take an additional bite of skin distal to the original bite. The distance between the two bites will determine the amount of eversion of the eyelids that will occur after tying the sutures. Therefore if a large eversion is needed, then a distance of 1 to 2 cm between the two bites may be required. Additional sutures are placed in identical fashion adjacent (usually 5 mm between sutures) to the central suture (Fig. 3-10). The number of sutures required depends on the length of the entropic eyelid in the individual foal. After the suture has been tied with multiple knot throws, the end of the suture nearest the cornea should be cut short, and the opposite end should be cut longer to make removal of the suture easier. Application of a drop of cyanoacrylic adhesive to the knots will help ensure

Table 3-2	Congenital Eyelid Abnormalities		
Abnormality	**Appearance**	**Associated defects**	**Breeds**
Ankyloblepharon	Adhesion of the eyelid margins (upper and lower) after birth	Microphthalmos	
Eyelid coloboma	Full-thickness absence of the eyelid margin	Corneal or conjunctival defects or coloboma	
Entropion	Turning in of the eyelid margin	Corneal ulceration, enophthalmos, neonatal maladjustment syndrome	Quarter horse Thoroughbred
Dermoid	Misplaced normal skin	Conjunctival, corneal, or third eyelid dermoids	

Data from references 3, 16, and 18 to 24.

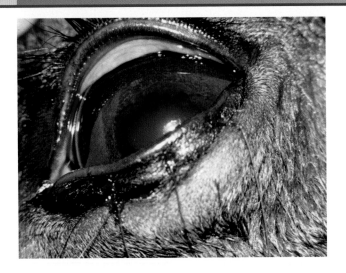

Fig. 3-10 Temporary tacking sutures to roll out the eyelid margin in the foal with entropion in Fig 3-9. (Photograph courtesy Dr. Riccardo Stoppini.)

that they stay in place. After the foal recovers from tranquilization, the surgeon must ensure that the foal can blink adequately to protect the cornea. If the eyelids are held too far open, removal of one or more sutures may be necessary. Sutures remain in place for 2 to 4 weeks in most foals.

Injectable Materials

A large variety of materials have been injected into the eyelid to temporarily evert the margins. Materials used include saline solution, penicillin G, silicone, hyaluronic acid, and liquid paraffin.[3] Although these materials may be effective, the need for repeated injections, the risk of inflammation, and the potential for scarring make this technique undesirable.

Permanent Entropion Correction

Permanent correction of entropion should only be done after several attempts at temporary correction have been made. If the foal regains health and grows normally, but the entropion persists, then permanent fixation is required. If the permanent fixation is done before orbital health is regained, then ectropion, or turning out of the eyelid margin, is possible.

Use of a Jaeger eyelid plate (or other stabilizing device) will help support the eyelid and facilitate an accurate incision. The initial incision is made 2 mm from and parallel to the eyelid margin. A second elliptical incision is made distal to the initial incision.

That portion of skin required to correct the entropion should be excised (Fig. 3-11). Closure is performed with 4-0 to 6-0 monofilament nonabsorbable sutures in a simple interrupted pattern. Sutures are first placed at the central aspect of the incision, and the incision is then closed in either direction. The suture ends should be trimmed so the suture end toward the cornea is short (avoids corneal trauma) and the other end is long (easy to grasp for removal). Sutures should be removed in 10 to 14 days.

Other Congenital Diseases of the Adnexa

Other congenital diseases in foals are much less common than entropion. These abnormalities include ankyloblepharon, eyelid agenesis, coloboma, dermoids (Fig. 3-12), and cilia abnormalities.[3,16,18-21] Features of these conditions are listed in Table 3-2. Congenital ankyloblepharon, or fusion of the eyelids together after birth, is not normal in foals, because horses have fully developed eyes and adnexa at birth.[3] Separation of the eyelids should first be attempted manually, then with blunt dissection, starting at the medial canthus.[19]

CONGENITAL DISEASES OF THE NASOLACRIMAL SYSTEM

Epiphora, or overflow of tears, can occur from excessive lacrimation because of ocular irritation or because of an eyelid abnormality (e.g., entropion) or obstruction of the NLD. Obstructions of the NLD are commonly a result of bacterial infections (e.g., dacryocystitis) and have a profound mucopurulent discharge.

Congenital deficiency in tear production or KCS has not been reported in horses but may occur. In fact, spontaneous development of KCS in horses, in general, is very uncommon and the KCS that has been reported is caused by trauma or other inflammatory disorders.[10-12]

Nasolacrimal Duct Atresia

The most common congenital defect of the NLD is NLD atresia.[3,16,18-21] The most common defect is an imperforate nasal punctum, although eyelid punctal atresia or incomplete formation of the duct can occur anywhere along its course (see Figs. 3-5 and 3-6).

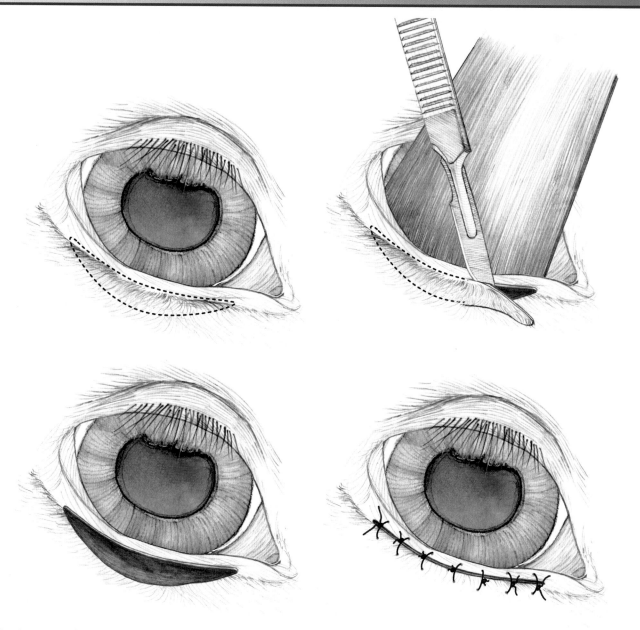

Fig. 3-11 Holtz-Celsus entropion repair.

Clinical Appearance

The most common initial clinical appearance is mild to moderate, unilateral or bilateral epiphora (see Fig. 3-13), but by 4 to 6 months of age the predominate clinical sign is severe mucopurulent ocular discharge, likely caused by the development of secondary bacterial dacryocystitis. Diagnosis is made by direct observation of the nasal vestibule (i.e., lack of punctual openings) and inability to irrigate the nasolacrimal system from the eyelid puncta. Swelling of the nasal epithelium distally, near the area of normal punctal opening, may also suggest atresia.[3,22,23] Rarely, eyelid punctal atresia may occur, resulting in failure of nasolacrimal irrigation (retrograde) and conjunctival swelling.[18]

Differential Diagnosis

Acquired obstructive diseases of the NLD should be differentiated from true atresia. In cases of acquired obstructions, punctal openings are generally visible (see Fig. 3-8) but lack the ability to irrigate the nasolacrimal system. Because nearly all cases of nasolacrimal punctal atresia (either eyelid or nasal) have secondary dacryocystitis, bacterial culture and sensitivity should be performed to help manage the

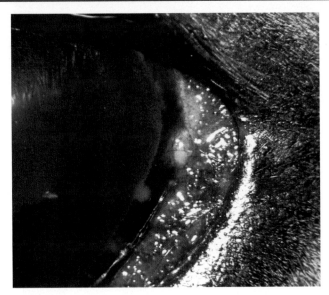

Fig. 3-12 Conjunctival dermoid in a young horse. (Photograph courtesy Dr. Riccardo Stoppini.)

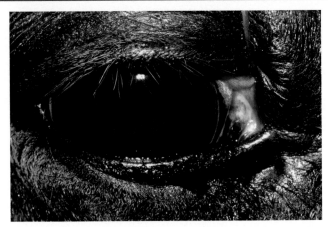

Fig. 3-13 Epiphora in a foal with congenital nasolacrimal duct atresia.

infection after surgery. Furthermore, because of the possibility of concurrent NLD agenesis (or partial agenesis, i.e., narrowing of the NLD) contrast radiography (i.e., dacryocystorhinography) should be performed (see Chapter 1 for description of the technique). This will determine the type of surgery that may be needed (i.e., incision of duct and stent placement vs dacryocystorhinotomy/sinusotomy) and the long-term prognosis.[24]

Treatment

Treatment consists of relieving the obstruction by creating a new opening, whether it be proximally or distally, treating the secondary bacterial infection, and preventing re-obstruction.

Medical Therapy

Topical or systemic antibiotics are only beneficial after surgery to relieve the obstruction, although use of these medications before surgery will decrease epiphora and mucopurulent discharge temporarily. However, the improvement in clinical signs is only observed during the treatment, and unless the obstruction is relieved, the infection and clinical signs will quickly return.

Surgical Therapy

Surgical opening of the obstructed or atretic puncta is always required, unless the NLD is agenic.

Preoperative determination of the location(s) of the obstruction is critical for success. Usually, the obstruction is just at the opening to the nasal puncta, and creation of a new opening at the site is curative. However, preoperative determination of the location of the obstruction(s) can be difficult, and careful physical examination (i.e., careful observation for submucosal swelling), dacryocystorhinography, and possibly advanced radiography (e.g., computed tomography) can allow accurate location of the obstruction. With the horse heavily sedated or anesthetized, an attempt can be made to locate and open a presumed distal atretic puncta manually. A 5 Fr male silicone rubber (Silastic) or plastic urinary catheter (with or without wire stent) is threaded normograde (from proximal to distal) through the dorsal canaliculi into the NLD. The catheter is advanced until resistance is encountered. The catheter should not be forced ventrally if resistance is encountered, because severe hemorrhage may develop.[25] If it is only the nasal puncta that are occluded, the tip of the catheter will be palpable under the nasal mucosa. Occasionally, the duct terminates proximal to the normal puncta site, and careful palpation along the course of the NLD is required to locate the catheter tip. An incision is made over the catheter through the nasal mucosa, and the catheter is pulled through the nares. Profound hemorrhage from the incision through the nasal mucosa is common; therefore only a single bold cut should be made. For the purpose of re-creating a punctal opening, the silicone rubber tubing is sutured in place for 30 days (Fig. 3-14). After surgery, topical and systemic antibiotics should be given according to culture sensitivity results; however, frequently, the choice is topical triple antibiotic solution (every 8 hours) and oral sulfamethoxazole-trimethoprim (10 mg/kg every 12 hours) until the tube is removed.

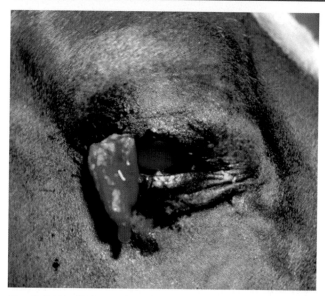

Fig. 3-15 Eyelid laceration of a horse, beginning medially and extending laterally. This hanging eyelid fragment should not be excised, but instead because of the excellent eyelid blood supply, this fragment can be replaced and it usually remains viable. (Photograph courtesy Dr. Mike Davidson.)

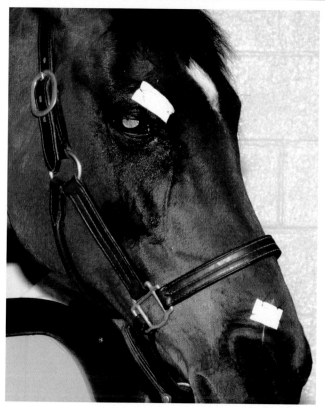

Fig. 3-14 Nasolacrimal stent in place to treat a horse with nasolacrimal duct atresia. The 5 Fr male urinary catheter has been threaded through the nasolacrimal duct and exits the dorsal eyelid puncta and the newly created nasal punctal opening. The ends of the catheter have been sutured to the skin with waterproof tape anchors. The catheter will remain in place for 30 days while the new punctal opening heals.

ACQUIRED EYELID DISEASES

Traumatic Eyelid Diseases

Because of the horse's environment, temperament, and the prominent positioning of the eyes on the side of the head, periocular eyelid trauma is very common. Even in the nicest and cleanest stable, many objects that will traumatize a horse's eye can be found. Many horses tend to react to stimuli by exaggerated and sometimes uncontrolled movements of their heads. These features contribute to the frequent traumatic injuries observed in equine eyelids.

Eyelid Lacerations

Eyelid lacerations are commonly encountered in horses. Generally, lacerations are acute and easily noted by the horse owner. Occasionally, if the horse is not monitored closely, the horse can be presented several days after the injury with a severe mucopurulent ocular discharge.

In most cases, the severity of the appearance of the lesion does not have much bearing on the overall prognosis. Because of the excellent blood supply to the eyelids,[8] most lacerations can be repaired to achieve a relatively well-functioning and cosmetic eyelid, even in the presence of secondary blepharitis. Therefore an attempt should be made to surgically repair all eyelid lacerations, and a hanging eyelid fragment should never be excised (Fig. 3-15). Despite the severity of the eyelid laceration (whether major or minor), a thorough ocular examination is required to identify and treat any associated lesion, such as a corneal ulcer or uveitis.

Common Differential Diagnoses

Some cases of severe and ulcerative eyelid blepharitis and some neoplasms (more information can be found in the following sections) may appear as lacerations or injuries (Fig. 3-16). Most of these lesions are chronic and progressive. If the clinician is unsure of the pathogenesis, then a biopsy, culture, or both should be performed.

Pathogenesis of Disease Process and Progression

Lacerations likely occur in three ways. Blunt trauma from a crushing injury of the upper eyelid against the dorsolateral orbital rim may cause a laceration that is very irregular with substantial eyelid swelling. Sharp objects, such as a nail or metal edge, can cause a laceration that is generally straight. These first two types of eyelid injury commonly have underlying ocular damage in addition to the eyelid trauma. The third type of eyelid laceration is caused by ripping, which occurs when the eyelid is caught on a hook, such as a bucket handle. The typically rapid and uncontrolled retraction of the horse's head from the hook results in a ripping of the eyelid. This wound commonly begins at the lateral canthus and extends parallel to the upper eyelid (Fig. 3-17). These types of eyelid lacerations rarely cause underlying ocular damage.

Treatment

Medical Therapy

No medical therapy exists; surgical correction is needed. However, horses should receive tetanus vaccine or a

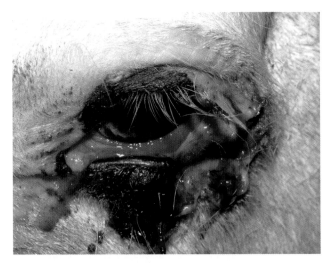

Fig. 3-16 This is a severe ulcerative lower eyelid squamous cell carcinoma. Severe and ulcerative eyelid blepharitis or neoplasms (such as those seen here) must be differentiated from a laceration or trauma injury.

booster dose of tetanus antitoxin after they have sustained an eyelid laceration.

Surgical Therapy

Because of the rich blood supply, even severely lacerated eyelids frequently heal readily. The wound should be minimally débrided, and the tissue should be closed very carefully in two layers. The eyelid margin cannot be re-created surgically, so every attempt must be made to preserve it.[3] The deep, subconjunctival layer is closed initially, and this is required to ensure that the inside of the eyelid does not gape during healing and induce scar formation, which may be irritating to the underlying cornea. Absorbable sutures, such as 5-0 to 6-0 polyglactin 910, are used in a continuous pattern immediately external to the tarsal conjunctiva in the eyelid connective tissue. Extreme care should be taken to ensure that all knots are buried and that no suture material can come in contact with the cornea. The eyelid skin is closed by initially lining up the eyelid margin. A figure-eight suture pattern or a mattress pattern of nonabsorbable 4-0 to 6-0 sutures is useful to perfectly appose the eyelid margins (see Fig. 3-17).[3,26,27] Incorrect closure of this margin or failure to use a two-layer closure may lead to chronic corneal irritation (Figs. 3-18 and 3-19).

Long-Term Prognosis

Prognosis after eyelid laceration repair is generally very good, providing that the surgery was performed accurately, because of the excellent healing capability of the equine eyelid. However, the prognosis generally depends on whether there is any underlying ocular

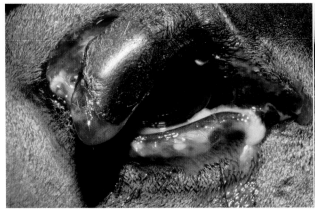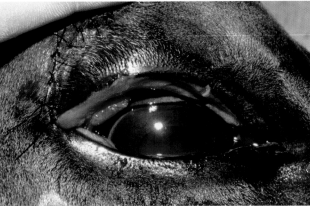

A   **B**

Fig. 3-17 Eyelid laceration in the upper eyelid of a horse. **A,** This laceration is typical of a ripping injury after the hooking of the eyelid on a blunt object such as a bucket handle. **B,** Immediately after repair of the laceration with a 2-layer closure.

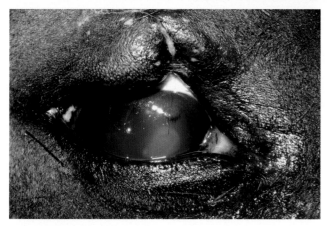

Fig. 3-18 Eyelid scarring 2 months after a skin-only closure of a central upper eyelid laceration. Trichiasis is now present from the upper cilia, resulting in a superficial corneal ulcer.

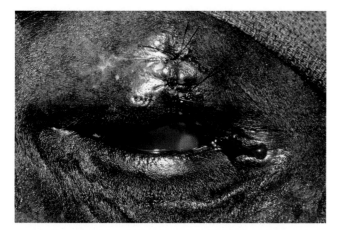

Fig. 3-19 Repair of the cicatricial eyelid lesion in Fig. 3-18. A V-plasty procedure was performed to remove the scarred portion of the eyelid, followed by a standard 2-layer closure.

damage, and therefore a thorough ocular examination is needed.

Blepharoedema

The horse eyelid has a tremendous propensity to swell (Fig. 3-20). This may occur because of the minimal adipose tissue that is present in the equine eyelid.[3,8] A swollen, drooping eyelid is referred to as pseudo-ptosis.[3] Common differential diagnoses for unilateral and bilateral blepharoedema are listed in Box 3-1. Treatment is directed at the underlying cause and protection of the cornea if eyelid function is compromised.

Blepharitis

Inflammation of the eyelids, or blepharitis, is uncommon in the horse as a separate entity or disease. There are numerous causes for blepharitis (Table 3-3), but usually it is result of trauma, bacterial or fungal infection, or parasitic infestation.

Infectious Blepharitis

The most common cause of blepharitis in the horse is bacterial infection after penetrating trauma.[1] Blepharitis has been reported after blunt trauma associated with an orbital bone sequestrum[28] and with primary *Moraxella* sp. infection.[29] Fungal surface infections or granulomas can also cause blepharitis.[1,3] Fungal organisms reported to cause blepharitis include

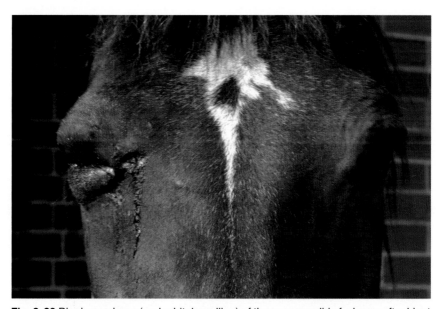

Fig. 3-20 Blepharoedema (and orbital swelling) of the upper eyelid of a horse after blunt trauma. The horse eyelid has the tremendous ability to become edematous and swell. (Photograph courtesy Dr. Mike Davidson.)

Trichophyton spp., *Microsporum* spp., *Histoplasma farcimi-nosus* (i.e., epizootic lymphangitis), *Cryptococcus mirandi*, *Aspergillus* spp., and *Rhinosporidium seeberi*.[1,3,30,31] Parasites may also cause variable degrees of eyelid inflammation and include *Habronema* spp., *Thelazia lacrymalis*, and *Demodex* spp.[1,20,32-39] *Thelazia* and *Demodex* infections are usually asymptomatic; however, a rare blepharitis characterized by meibomian gland inflammation, hair loss, and papulopustular dermatitis has been reported as a result of *Demodex* infestation.[1] With the widespread use of ivermectin in the 1990s, the prevalence of habronemiasis decreased; however, in the past 2 to 3 years, the increasing number of cases being diagnosed suggests the development of resistant strains.

Clinical Appearance and Diagnosis

Blepharitis, in general, appears as swelling and inflammation of the eyelid. Because of its prominence, the upper eyelid is more commonly affected than the lower eyelid. Bacterial infections after trauma injury are associated with swelling surrounding an open wound with or without necrotic draining tracts. Fungal infections may appear as bacterial infections or as an alopecic, scaling of the eyelid skin.[1] Habronemiasis (*Habronema muscae*, *H. microstoma*, and *Draschia megastoma* are potential causative organisms)[3] appears as a raised, granulomatous, ulcerative lesion on the conjunctiva or mucocutaneous junction of the eyelid (Fig. 3-21). This disease is also known as summer sores, swamp cancer, and granular dermatitis,[32,36,39] because the condition

Box 3-1	Causes for Blepharoedema or Swelling of The Equine Eyelid

Unilateral
Blunt trauma
Self-trauma
Insect bite
Snake bite
Foreign body reaction
Abscess formation
Orbital fat prolapse

Bilateral
Self-trauma
Systemic diseases*
   Equine viral arteritis
   Babesiosis
   Lymphosarcoma
   Influenza
Allergy/hypersensitivity
Ocular parasites

Data from references 1 and 3.
*See Chapter 13 for discussion of ocular manifestations of systemic diseases.

Table 3-3	Blepharitis						
	Trauma	**Bacterial**	**Viral**	**Fungal**	**Parasitic**	**Immune/Allergic**	**Actinic**
Clinical signs	Unilateral	Unilateral	Unilateral or bilateral	Unilateral	Unilateral or bilateral	Bilateral	Unilateral or bilateral
	Acute	Subacute Mucopurulent discharge Abscess	Chronic Papillomas Pustular dermatosis	Chronic Alopecia Scales Draining tracts Granuloma Granulation tissue	Chronic Gritty, caseous Pruritus Meibomianitis Alopecia Edema Epiphora	Acute: Pruritic Edema Hyperemic Chronic: Skin induration Hyperpigmentation Decreased palpebral fissure	Hyperemic Ulcerated Scaly Alopecia Discharge Depigmented
Causes	Blunt trauma	*Moraxella* spp. *Streptococcus equi* Other	Papova virus (papillomas) Horse pox	*Trichophyton* spp. *Microsporum* spp Phycomycosis *Histoplasma farciminosum* *Cryptococcus mirandi*	Habronemiasis *Demodex* spp. *Thelazia* spp. Fly bite dermatitis	Atopy: Environmental allergens Sprays ± drugs, etc. Eosinophilic granuloma (nodular necrobiosis) Immune-mediated: Pemphigus foliaceous Bullous pemphigoid	High UV radiation Sun exposure

appears during the hot and humid summer months when the main vectors, house and stable flies, are most prevalent. Infection of the ocular tissue is by *Habronema* larvae. Adult *Habronema* organisms live in the equine stomach; larvae are passed in the feces, are ingested by fly larvae, become infective in the fly pupae, and are deposited near the eye (or other mucocutaneous junctions or wounds).[3,39] Dermal lesions may also develop on other areas of the body (Fig. 3-22). The medial canthus and the caruncle area are the most common areas in the eye, and the lesion typically has discrete nodules or multilobulated masses with occasional mineral- or "sulfur"-appearing nodules. Hypersensitivity to the organisms (especially dead organisms) results in pruritus, periocular alopecia, and occasionally secondary ocular disease such as corneal ulceration and uveitis.

Common Differential Diagnoses

Table 3-3 lists the main causes of blepharitis, including the infectious causes. For bacterial and fungal blepharitis, the definitive diagnosis is based on identification of the organism(s) by cytology and culture. Biopsy and histopathologic examination are recommended if the lesion is chronic and unresponsive to initial therapy. Habronemiasis is diagnosed on the basis of the clinical appearance of the lesion (i.e., gritty, caseous, granulomatous lesion of the medial canthus, occurrence during summer months) and identification of the organisms by cytology or biopsy (Fig. 3-23). Because of the numerous neutrophils, eosinophils, mast cells, and plasma cells in the cytologic samples from habronemiasis lesions, it must be differentiated from mast cell

tumors, *Phycomycetes* spp., eosinophilic granulomas (nodular necrobiosis), and eosinophilic keratoconjunctivitis.[1,3,32,40,41] Therefore biopsy and histopathologic examination are recommended for definitive diagnosis.

Treatment

Medical Therapy

Penetrating eyelid injuries with secondary infectious bacterial or fungal blepharitis usually heal rapidly with appropriate treatment because of the eyelid's excellent blood supply. The wound should be cultured (bacterial and fungal culture and sensitivity); and a cytologic sample should be collected, then shaved, flushed with a copious amount of 1:50 povidone-iodine (Betadine) solution, and probed for foreign material (which should be removed if found). The horse should be given systemic antibiotics (e.g., sulfamethoxazole-trimethoprim, 20 mg/kg by mouth every 12 hours). The antibiotic regimen may be altered once culture and sensitivity results have been obtained. Warm compresses can be applied every 8 to 12 hours for the first 5 days. The cornea should be protected with topical

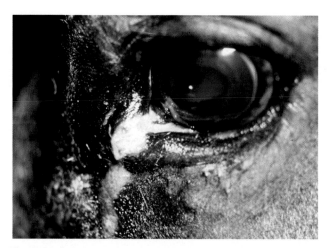

Fig. 3-21 Caseous, granulomatous lesion of the medial canthus typical of habronemiasis ("summer sores") infection in the medial canthus. These infections are raised, granulomatous, ulcerative lesions on the conjunctiva or mucocutaneous junctions. (Photograph courtesy Dr. Mike Davidson.)

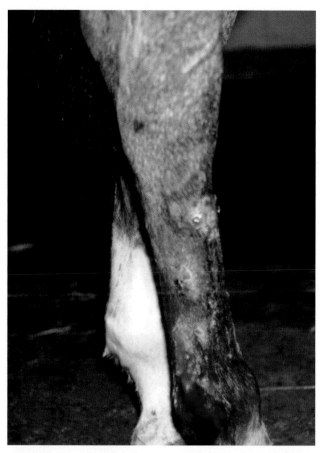

Fig. 3-22 Habronemiasis infectious can occur at mucocutaneous junctions or at sites of injury. Here is habronemiasis on a front leg. (Photograph courtesy Dr. Mike Davidson.)

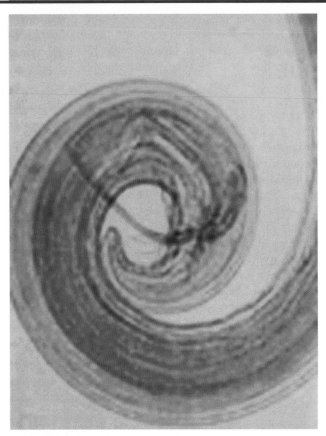

Fig. 3-23 *Habronema muscae* (×100). Note the spinous process on the tail.

ointment every 8 hours. Treatment of habronemiasis is by killing of the parasites, decreasing periocular inflammation, decreasing the size of the lesion, and preventing recurrence. Fly control and regular treatment with ivermectin are recommended to reduce the incidence of habronemiasis.[42] Ivermectin (200 μg/kg by mouth) is given initially and repeated in 30 days. In one study, ivermectin alone caused marked improvement in habronemiasis lesions within 7 days in 87% of horses.[43] A dose of flunixin meglumine (1.1 mg/kg administered intravenously) or other systemic nonsteroidal antiinflammatory medication should be given for 1 to 3 days after administration of ivermectin to decrease inflammation associated with larvae dying in situ. Topical therapies for habronemiasis lesions vary, and recommendations have included preparations of trichlorfon, nitrofurazone, and dimethyl sulfoxide (DMSO)[36]; trichlorfon, nitrofurazone, dexamethasone, and DMSO[33]; and nitrofurantoin, ronnel solution, dexamethasone, and DMSO[32]—each applied every 12 hours to the lesion. Topical 0.03% echothiophate every 12 hours may be helpful as a larvacide,[3] but it is not likely needed in addition to systemic ivermectin. Intralesional injections of triamcinolone or methylprednisolone may decrease inflammation in the lesion.[1,3]

Surgical Therapy

For most cases of blepharitis, appropriate wound management (as described in the preceding section) and use of antibiotics (chosen on the basis of results of culture and sensitivity of the wound) will help the lesion resolve. However, in cases of abscessation, the fluid should be drained, the wound should be flushed copiously, and a drain should be placed for 3 to 7 days. With habronemiasis lesions, debulking or excising granulomatous lesions (to remove a source of chronic immune stimulation[3]), followed by topical, intralesional, or systemic treatment with corticosteroids provided healing within a few weeks in one study.[42]

Long-Term Prognosis

With appropriate diagnosis and treatment, most of these lesions heal readily. Eyelid defects and other ocular damage as a result of the blepharitis depend on the extent and chronicity of the blepharitis.

Allergic, Immune-Mediated, and Actinic Blepharitis

Blepharitis can also be caused by local or systemic allergic diseases (more information on systemic diseases can be found in Chapter 13), immune-mediated diseases, and exposure to sunlight (with or without photosensitization) (Table 3-4). Local or systemic allergic diseases are usually associated with acute onset, bilateral blepharoedema, hyperemia, and pruritus. Over the long term, allergic conditions can cause hyperpigmentation and scarring. Causes include chronic fly-bite irritation and environmental allergens such as molds, dust, sprays, and certain drugs. The eyelids can also be affected with immune-mediated diseases such as pemphigus foliaceous and bullous pemphigoid.[1] Typically, other mucocutaneous junctions on the body are also affected and these lesions are chronic, bilateral, and pruritic. Actinic blepharitis can occur in nonpigmented periocular tissues that have been exposed to sunlight on a long-term basis. The lesions appear hyperemic and ulcerated, typically at the eyelid margin (Fig. 3-24). Actinic blepharitis lesions may be precursors to the development of SCC.[4,44] Use of a high-ultraviolet radiation blocking fly mask is recommended for all horses that lack periocular pigmentation to prevent actinic blepharitis and SCC.

Ciliary Disorders

Ciliary disorders, such as distichiasis, ectopic cilia, and trichiasis, are uncommon in horses, especially compared with other domestic species.[45-47] Usually, these

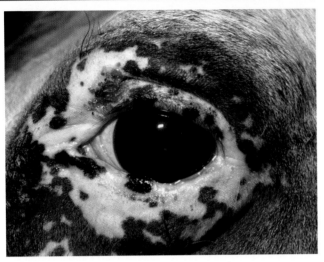

Fig. 3-24 Actinic blepharitis in the eyelids of an Appaloosa horse. Note the hyperemic, ulcerated, and scarred eyelid and third eyelid margins. (Photograph courtesy Dr. Mike Davidson.)

aberrant hairs cause chronic irritation by rubbing on the cornea or conjunctiva. Distichia or ectopic cilia may be congenital, but the clinical manifestations may not be evident for months to years.[1] Trichiasis, which is hair rubbing on the eye from a normal skin location, is the most common cilia abnormality and most frequently occurs after eyelid scarring following laceration or surgery.[46]

Clinical Appearance and Diagnosis

The presenting problem for most horses with ciliary disorders is ocular irritation. Chronic blepharospasm, epiphora, corneal ulceration, or corneal scarring may be the initial concern. Careful evaluation with magnification (usually by biomicroscopy) of the eyelid margin for hairs exiting the meibomian gland openings (i.e., distichiasis) and the palpebral conjunctival surface (i.e., ectopic cilia) is critical in all cases of cornea ulceration and surface corneal irritation. Most commonly, distichia and ectopic cilia involve the upper eyelid in horses. Distichia may consist of dense large hairs, which are very irritating to the ocular surface, or small soft hairs, which may cause no symptoms. Trichiasis is simply misdirected normal cilia that usually develop after eyelid scarring (see Figs. 3-18 and 3-19).

Common Differential Diagnoses

The causes for chronic irritation to the surface of the eye should be considered in addition to cilia abnormalities. Differential diagnoses to be considered include burdock bristle keratitis,[48] other foreign bodies, infectious keratitis,[49-52] KCS,[10-12,53] and other noninfectious keratopathy.[40,41,52,54]

Pathogenesis of Disease Process and Progression

Ectopic cilia and distichiasis are cilia that develop correctly but exit the eyelid at abnormal locations. Cilia may enter a meibomian gland and exit through the ductules, a path of least resistance, resulting in distichiasis. Ectopic cilia exit directly through the conjunctiva instead of the eyelid margin.

Treatment

Removal of the abnormal or misdirected hair or correction of the eyelid scarring is essential in the treatment of the ocular irritation.

Medical Therapy

Medical therapy, without surgical removal of the offending hairs, will not alleviate the irritation. However, topical ointments may help protect the cornea until surgery can be performed.

Surgical Therapy

The underlying cause of trichiasis should be corrected, whether it is eyelid scarring, entropion, or another eyelid abnormality. With eyelid scarring and cilia trichiasis, the scarred area of the palpebral margin should be excised, and the margin should be resutured with perfect anatomic alignment (see Figs. 3-18 and 3-19). Temporary tacking sutures (see previous discussion of everting sutures and Fig. 3-10) can be placed or a permanent Holtz-Celsus entropion repair can be done to correct the entropion.[3,46] The treatment of choice for distichiasis is cryotherapy of the hair follicle at the base of the meibomian gland.[1] A 4-mm cryoprobe is placed on the conjunctival surface of the eyelid, centered over the base of the meibomian gland adjacent to the distichia that is to be removed. The tissue freezing extends from the cryoprobe and is continued until it extends just beyond the distichia. Once the eyelid thaws, epilation of the distichia is attempted. Adequate cryotherapy has been performed if there is no resistance to the epilation of the distichia. Multiple distichia may exit a single meibomian gland orifice. Partial tarsal plate excision or lid splitting has been attempted, but scarring and contracture may occur after surgery.[47] A small entropion repair or V-lid excision of a small portion of eyelid can also be done if there is a focal area

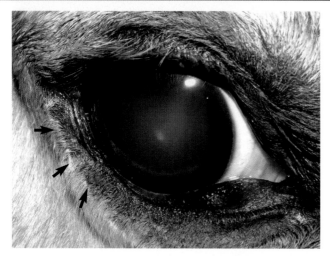

Fig. 3-25 A 29-year-old horse with bilateral lateral eyelid entropion. The horse had mild enophthalmos from muscle atrophy, entropion, and mild blepharospasm and epiphora *(arrows)*.

Common Differential Diagnoses

At times, it is difficult to determine the primary abnormality in entropion. For example, did the corneal ulcer cause blepharospasm and spastic entropion, or did the entropion cause the corneal ulcer? In horses, the entropion is usually secondary. Therefore the primary cause needs to be determined. Causes of blepharospasm, enophthalmos, eyelid scarring, or phthisis bulbi need to determined. If it cannot be determined whether the entropion is the cause or the effect of the ocular irritation, tacking sutures can be used to eliminate the entropion temporarily. Other causes of ocular irritation should also be considered such as burdock bristle keratitis,[48] presence of foreign bodies, infectious keratitis,[49-52] KCS,[10-12,53] and other noninfectious keratopathy.[40,41,52,54]

Pathogenesis of Disease Process and Progression

Turning in of the eyelid margin from a lack of eyelid support causes or contributes to ocular irritation.

Treatment

Adequate treatment of adult-onset entropion and prevention of recurrence in horses requires management of the primary underlying cause. Cicatricial entropion can be repaired surgically by removing the scarred eyelid.[46] Resolution of the cause of ocular irritation, such as corneal ulceration or removal of a foreign body, will help alleviate spastic entropion. However, some conditions cannot be reversed, such as phthisis bulbi or enophthalmos from fat atrophy. Enucleation of a severely phthisical eye is recommended. Entropion repair can be considered for mild phthisis bulbi or enophthalmos.

Medical Therapy

Medical therapy, without repair or resolution of the primary problem, will not reverse the entropion. However, topical ointment application may help protect the cornea until surgery can be performed.

Surgical Therapy

Holtz-Celsus entropion repair is required to permanently roll out the eyelid margin. Again, resolution of the primary problem is essential to prevent recurrence. General anesthesia is recommended for entropion surgery to ensure precise microsurgery. However, minor

of distichia. Ectopic cilia usually consist of a single hair or a focal group of hairs that should be removed by en block excision.

Long-Term Prognosis

If all of the offending hair can be located and removed, or the eyelid abnormality or scarring is minor and repairable, the long-term prognosis is excellent.

Entropion in Adult Horses

Entropion, or turning in of the eyelid margin, is a form of trichiasis that can cause significant ocular irritation and corneal damage in the horse. However, spontaneous entropion is rare in the horse. In the horse, entropion generally occurs after eyelid trauma (i.e., cicatricial entropion) or severe blepharospasm (i.e., spastic entropion).[3,46] Entropion can also occur with a decrease in orbital support of the eyelids, such as in cases of phthisis bulbi formation or enophthalmos. Bilateral entropion can occur in elderly horses with atrophy of orbital fat and development of secondary enophthalmos.

Clinical Appearance and Diagnosis

As in foal entropion, the eyelid margin is turned inward toward the eye with the cilia and eyelid hairs rubbing the surface of the cornea (Fig. 3-25). Associated conditions, such as corneal ulceration, enophthalmos, eyelid scarring, and phthisis bulbi may be present.

entropion repair may be performed with the horse standing after appropriate eyelid blocks have been performed and a tranquilizer has been administered.[55] Use of a Jaeger eyelid plate (if not available, a tongue depressor or Bard-Parker scalpel blade handle can be used) is recommended to help support the eyelid and facilitate an accurate incision. The initial incision is made 2 mm from and parallel to the eyelid margin. A second arching incision is made distal to the initial incision as illustrated in Fig. 3-11. The distance between the two incisions is equal to the amount of entropion repair that is desired and determined before surgery is performed. That portion of skin required to correct the entropion is then excised. Closure is performed with 4-0 to 6-0 monofilament nonabsorbable sutures in a simple interrupted pattern. Sutures are first placed at the central aspect of the incision, and the incision is then closed in either direction. The suture ends should be trimmed so that the suture end toward the cornea is short (avoids corneal trauma) and the other end is long (easy to grasp for removal) (see Fig. 3-11).

Long-Term Prognosis

Prognosis for entropion depends on the underlying cause. For example, if the source of irritation in spastic entropion can be alleviated, then the long-term prognosis is excellent. However, in cases of phthisis bulbi or enophthalmos, the underlying cause of the entropion is generally progressive and severe, and prognosis for elimination of the entropion is poor.

Conjunctivitis

Conjunctival tissue is highly reactive because of its high concentration of blood vessels and lymphoid tissue or follicles. Therefore conjunctiva can demonstrate profound clinical changes, such as hyperemia (redness) and chemosis (swelling) as a result of adjacent inflammatory diseases (i.e., secondary conjunctivitis). Common examples include hyperemic conjunctiva associated with corneal stromal abscesses (Fig. 3-26), glaucoma, or uveitis (Table 3-4). Differentiating primary conjunctivitis from these more serious ocular conditions is essential. Primary conjunctivitis is uncommon in the horse, and many of the causes of primary conjunctivitis also cause systemic disease (see Table 3-4, p. 126).

Clinical Appearance and Diagnosis

Depending on the cause, the appearance of conjunctivitis may vary (see Table 3-4, p. 126). Typically, there is chemosis and hyperemia (Figs. 3-26 and 3-27).

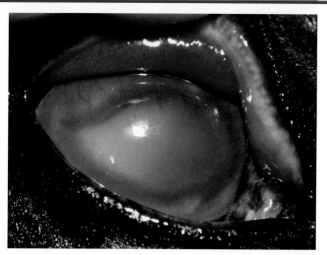

Fig. 3-26 Severe palpebral conjunctival hyperemia and chemosis in a horse with a corneal stromal abscess.

Mucopurulent discharge (Fig. 3-28), follicle formation, and depigmentation (Fig. 3-29) can also develop.

Common Differential Diagnoses

A complete and thorough ophthalmic examination should be done to rule out all ocular causes of secondary conjunctivitis. A bacterial culture and sensitivity, followed by cytologic examination of conjunctival scrapings, should be done on all eyes with chronic conjunctivitis and eyes with mucopurulent discharge. A thorough understanding of the normal bacterial and fungal flora is essential for interpretation of the results of a culture. See Chapter 4 for a review of various studies of the normal corneal and conjunctival bacterial and fungal flora. Viral or fungal isolation, culture, or polymerase chain reaction should be done if any of these organisms are suspected as the cause (see Table 3-4, p. 126). Many systemic diseases have conjunctivitis as a clinical sign (see Fig. 3-5) (see discussion of systemic disease in Chapter 13). Every equine eye with conjunctivitis should have topical fluorescein dye applied to rule out corneal ulceration and NLD obstruction.

Treatment

Treatment of the underlying condition or disease is the primary method for resolution of conjunctivitis.

Medical Therapy

Topical antibiotic therapy based on culture and sensitivity and cytology results is the mainstay of therapy.

Table 3-4 Conjunctivitis

Classification	Etiology	Predominant Clinical Signs
Secondary Conjunctivitis		
	Corneal disease	Corneal ulcer, abscess, blepharospasm, etc.
	Uveitis	Aqueous flare, miosis, hypopyon, etc.
	Glaucoma	High intraocular pressure, corneal edema
	Dacryocystitis	Purulent discharge, blocked nasolacrimal duct
	KCS[10-12,53,86]	Dry cornea, mucoid discharge
Primary Conjunctivitis		
Immune-mediated	Follicular	Follicles on bulbar conjunctiva, epiphora
	Eosinophilic[11,40,41]	Thick, cheesy exudates ± corneal disease
	Allergic	Hyperemia, chemosis, serous discharge
Bacterial	*Moraxella equi*[29,217]	Mucocutaneous erosions, mucopurulent ocular discharge, blepharospasm
	Streptococcus equi[218]	Regional lymphadenitis (strangles), conjunctivitis, and a mucopurulent nasal discharge
	Chlamydia and *Mycoplasma* spp.[219]	Possible respiratory disease or polyarthritis
Fungal	Histoplasmosis[31] and blastomycosis[3]	Conjunctivitis and lymph node involvement
	Aspergillus spp.[3]	Granulomatous conjunctivitis
	Rhinosporidium seeberi[3]	Granulomatous conjunctivitis
Viral	EHV type 2[50,220,221]	Recurrent conjunctivitis ± corneal ulceration
	EHV type 1[222]	
	Equine viral arteritis[223-225]	Conjunctivitis and blepharoedema
	Adenovirus[226]	Keratouveitis, mucopurulent discharge
Parasitic	Onchocerciasis[227]	Lateral limbal depigmentation ± uveitis
	Thelazia lacrimalis[38,228]	Mild conjunctivitis, epiphora
	Ophthalmomyiasis externa[229]	
	Habronemiasis[32]	Granuloma formation, mucopurulent exudate
	Trypanosoma evansi[230]	Fever, anemia, conjunctivitis, edema of the legs and lower parts of the body, progressive weakness, loss of condition, and loss of appetite
Trauma	Blunt trauma	Subconjunctival hemorrhage
	Foreign body	Severe blepharospasm and epiphora
Solar/actinic	UV radiation	Neoplastic precursor

EHV, Equine herpes virus; *KCS,* keratoconjunctivitis sicca.

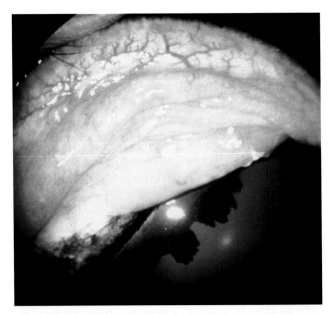

Fig. 3-27 Bulbar and palpebral conjunctival hyperemia and chemosis in a horse with equine herpesvirus keratoconjunctivitis. (Photograph courtesy Dr. Mike Davidson.)

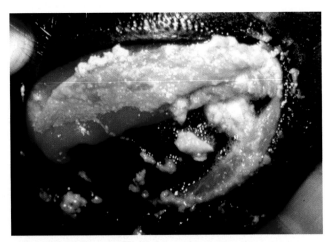

Fig. 3-28 Severe caseous discharge and conjunctivitis in a horse with eosinophilic keratoconjunctivitis. (Photograph courtesy Dr. Mike Davidson.)

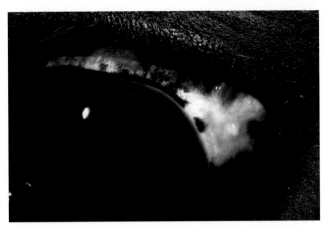

Fig. 3-29 Lateral limbal depigmentation and conjunctivitis associated with chronic *Onchocerca* spp. infection.

Topical application of broad-spectrum antibiotics, such as oxytetracycline or triple antibiotic ointment three to four times a day, is good initial therapy. Antiviral or antifungal therapy (see discussion of corneal diseases in Chapter 4) may be required if these organisms are found.

Surgical Therapy

There are no surgical treatments for conjunctivitis.

Long-Term Prognosis

The prognosis for resolution of conjunctivitis is usually good with primary infections, because most conjunctival infectious respond well to topical therapy, generally within 5 to 7 days. However, viral infections can be recurrent, and many systemic diseases (that have conjunctivitis as a clinical sign) can have serious and life-threatening complications (see Table 3-4, p. 126).

Neurologic Disorders of the Eyelids

Several neurologic conditions may affect the eyelids and periocular structures. Neurologic conditions affecting the orbit and extraocular muscles are covered in Chapter 2. The two most common neurologic diseases of the ocular adnexa in the horse are Horner's syndrome and facial nerve paralysis.

Horner's Syndrome

The autonomic nervous system is also known as the involuntary, visceral, or vegetative nervous system.

The autonomic nervous system is composed of two main divisions: the sympathetic nervous system and the parasympathetic nervous system. Horner's syndrome is a result of the loss of sympathetic innervation to the head. It can be unilateral or bilateral. Knowledge of the sympathetic nerve pathway is essential to understanding the pathogenesis, workup, treatment, and prognosis of a horse with Horner's syndrome. The sympathetic nervous system pathway begins in the hypothalamus and extends down the intermediolateral cell columns of the spinal cord to synapse at C8-T3. The axons from these cells exit the anterior nerve root of the spinal cord though the white ramus. The fibers (preganglionic fibers) course through the brachial plexus, through the thoracic inlet and ascend in the sympathetic trunk (with the jugular vein) and synapse at the cranial cervical ganglion. Postganglionic fibers then pass near the middle ear, through the orbital fissure, and form the sympathetic root of the ciliary ganglion. Short ciliary nerves (along with contributory fibers to the long ciliary nerves) extend to the dilator muscle of the iris. Therefore damage of the pathway from the hypothalamus to the short ciliary nerves may cause denervation and Horner's syndrome. Lesions that occur proximal to the ciliary ganglion are termed preganglionic, whereas those distal to the ciliary ganglion are referred to as postganglionic.

Clinical Appearance and Diagnosis

The predominant clinical signs of Horner's syndrome in horses are ptosis, sweating on the head and neck, and increased cutaneous temperature in the denervated area (Fig. 3-30).[5,6,56-60] Enophthalmos, miosis, elevated third eyelid, and increased lacrimation (common clinical signs in other animals) are variable, inconsistent, or mild in horses.[5,6,56-60] There are no vision deficits with sympathetic denervation, and the diagnosis is based on recognition of clinical signs.

Common Differential Diagnoses

Damage to the sympathetic trunk anywhere along its pathway may result in signs of Horner's syndrome (Box 3-2) (see discussion of systemic diseases in Chapter 13). Trauma to the neck and spinal cord or vagosympathetic trunk (e.g., during jugular venepuncture) can cause Horner's syndrome.[3,59] Horner's syndrome associated with jugular venepuncture was mild and resolved within 14 hours.[59] Other possible causes of Horner's syndrome in horses include idiopathic, guttural pouch infections, obstructive esophageal

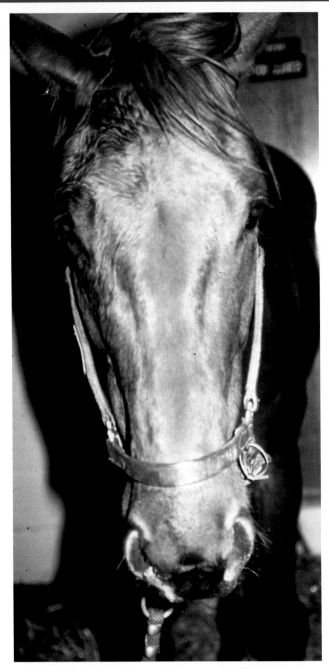

Fig. 3-30 Right-sided Horner's syndrome. Note the predominant clinical signs of ipsilateral sweating above the eye and mild ptosis. Enophthalmos, miosis, and elevated third eyelid (which are common clinical signs in other animals) are not prominent in this horse. (Photograph courtesy Dr. David A. Wilkie.)

Box 3-2	Causes of Horner's Syndrome in The Horse[5,6,56-64]

- Idiopathic
- Trauma to neck or spinal cord
- Jugular venepuncture or other trauma to vagosympathetic
- Guttural pouch infections
- Obstructive esophageal disorders
- Anterior thoracic disorders
- Metastatic neoplasia (melanoma, squamous cell carcinoma)
- Surgical procedures (carotid artery catheterization, cervicothoracic [stellate] ganglion blocks)

Data from references 5, 6, and 56-64.

catheterization.[5] The induced disease appeared nearly identical to naturally occurring clinical cases.[6,60]

Workup for horses with unilateral or bilateral Horner's syndrome should consist of a complete ophthalmic and physical examination. Endoscopic examination of the ipsilateral guttural pouch, laryngeal function, and upper esophagus should be considered. Thoracic ultrasonography or radiography should be considered to detect the presence of anterior thoracic masses or infection.

Pharmacologic testing in Horner's syndrome is the application of topical medications to the eye to help locate the site of sympathetic nervous system damage.[64,65] However, pharmacologic testing is inconsistent in the localization of lesions in horses.[6] The law of denervation hypersensitivity provides the pharmacologic basis for differentiating preganglionic from postganglionic lesions in both the sympathetic and parasympathetic nervous systems. In other words, the receptors in the adjacent neuron (ganglion) or in the neuromuscular junction (effector organ) will be supersensitive to their agonists when the preceding nerve or nerve ending is destroyed. Topical drugs that have been used include cocaine, hydroxyamphetamine, and phenylephrine. Understanding how a specific drug works allows localization of the site of the lesion. Cocaine (6%) blocks the reuptake of norepinephrine at the receptor sites of the iris dilator cells, which results in an accumulation of this neurotransmitter at the receptor site. There is no direct action on the receptor. Therefore a dilated pupil in response to topical cocaine would suggest a preganglionic lesion. Hydroxyamphetamine (1%) stimulates endogenous release of norepinephrine from adrenergic nerve endings. It does not directly stimulate the receptors. As with cocaine, dilatation in response to topical hydroxyamphetamine suggests a preganglionic lesion. Phenylephrine (2.5%) causes direct stimulation of the adrenergic receptors, and dilation after topical application suggests a postganglionic lesion.

disorders,[61] melanoma,[5,56,57] anterior thoracic disorders,[57] metastatic SCC,[58] and surgical procedures such as carotid artery catheterization[5] and cervicothoracic (stellate) ganglion blocks.[62,63] Horner's syndrome may also be associated with concurrent laryngeal hemiplegia.[6] Horner's syndrome has been experimentally induced by transection of the cervical sympathetic and vagosympathetic trunk[6,60] and by carotid artery

Treatment

Treatment is based on eliminating the underlying cause if possible. Horner's syndrome caused by minor trauma to the sympathetic trunk will resolve spontaneously in hours to days. Idiopathic Horner's syndrome will spontaneously resolve in weeks to a month.

Medical Therapy

Topical phenylephrine will temporarily resolve the clinical signs, but this is not a long-term therapy.

Surgical Therapy

Surgery is only performed to manage an underlying cause, such as guttural pouch infection or an esophageal disorder.

Long-Term Prognosis

Prognosis depends on the underlying cause and varies tremendously. Prognosis for resolution of signs is excellent for Horner's syndrome associated with mild trauma.[59] Prognosis for resolution of the syndrome and life is poor for metastatic neoplasia.[56-58]

Facial Nerve Paresis/Paralysis

Facial nerve paralysis is the most common cranial nerve abnormality in horses.[66] In one study, facial nerve paralysis represented the largest number of all neurologic diseases in horses in Australia.[66] The facial nerve in the horse originates posterior to the pons, enters the internal acoustic meatus, travels through the facial canal of the petrous temporal bone, passes through the stylomastoid foramen, extends around the guttural pouch and under the parotid salivary gland, crosses the ramus of the mandible (externally) 4 cm ventral to the temporomandibular joint, then divides into dorsal and ventral buccal branches.[3]

Clinical Appearance and Diagnosis

Clinical features of facial nerve paralysis include ptosis, lagophthalmos, ventral displacement, decreased motility of the ear pinna, decreased nostril function, flaccid lips, and deviation of the nose (either away from the lesion with acute facial nerve paralysis or toward the lesion with chronic paralysis) (Fig. 3-31).[1,3,66-69] Diagnosis is based on clinical signs and lack of facial nerve function

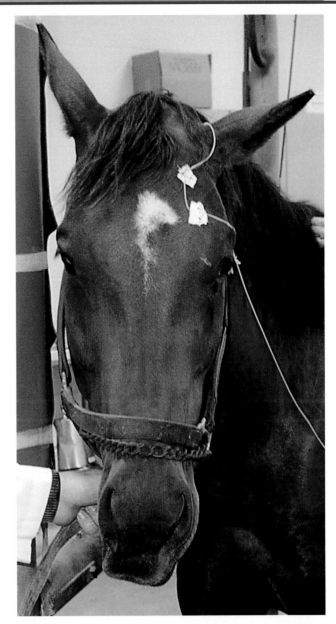

Fig. 3-31 Acute left-sided facial nerve paralysis. A subpalpebral lavage catheter has been placed to assist in the medical management of corneal disease. (Photography courtesy Dr. Stacy Andrew.)

(i.e., lagophthalmos and decreased or absent facial muscle function).

Common Differential Diagnoses

Facial nerve paralysis should be differentiated from other causes of ptosis, such as Horner's syndrome. Because of the proximity of the facial nerve, inflammation of the inner ear, guttural pouch, or salivary glands or fractures to the stylohyoid bone, petrous temporal bone, or ramus of the mandible can damage the facial nerve.[68] Because of the external course of the nerve over the ramus of the mandible, trauma frequently affects this nerve, including prolonged recumbency during illness or anesthesia.[69] A clinical sign of equine protozoal myeloencephalitis (EPM), a disease caused by *Sarcocystis neurona*, is facial nerve paralysis (see discussion of systemic disease in Chapter 13 for more information).[70-72] There was also a report of facial nerve paralysis associated with temporohyoid osteoarthropathy that was diagnosed on the basis of proliferation of the temporohyoid joints and stylohyoid bones on radiographs and results of guttural pouch endoscopy.[67]

Treatment

Treatment for facial nerve paralysis primarily consists of treating the underlying cause, if possible, and providing protection for the cornea.

Medical Therapy

Topical artificial tear ointment should be applied 4 to 6 times a day to keep the cornea moist and to prevent ulceration. If a corneal ulcer is present, it should be treated with topical antibiotics to help prevent infections and to assist in reepithelialization (see discussion of corneal diseases in Chapter 4).

Surgical Therapy

Surgery is only performed to treat a primary abnormality, such as a fracture or guttural pouch abnormality. A partial temporary tarsorrhaphy with a single horizontal mattress suture of 4-0 nylon in the lateral palpebral fissure is recommended. This will help protect the eye until facial nerve function returns.

Long-Term Prognosis

Prognosis depends on the underlying cause. If improvement does not occur in 3 to 4 weeks, the prognosis is poor and the facial nerve deficit is likely to be permanent. In these cases, a permanent partial lateral tarsorrhaphy (i.e., closure of the lateral fourth of the eyelid margins by removals of the eyelids and closure in a two-layer manner) should be considered for increased protection of the cornea. Because most horses with facial nerve paralysis have retractor bulbi function, they can retract the eye and elevate the third eyelid as a form of "blinking." This generally protects the medial two

thirds to three fourths of the cornea, leaving the lateral cornea exposed. The lateral tarsorrhaphy then helps to protect this exposed lateral cornea.

Third Eyelid Disorders

The third eyelid, or nictitating membrane, in the horse originates in the ventral medial aspect of the orbit and moves passively in the dorsolateral direction. The medial and lateral surfaces of the third eyelid are covered with conjunctiva; therefore nearly all diseases discussed in the conjunctivitis section could also involve the third eyelid. The base of third eyelid contains a lacrimal gland (tubuloacinar) that produces portions of the aqueous component of the tear film and can become inflamed. Many of the conditions of the third eyelid are caused by other abnormalities of the globe and orbit. The most common clinical disease of the third eyelid is SCC of the leading edge.[3]

Clinical Appearance and Diagnosis

The leading edge of the third eyelid is visible in the healthy horse, and it may or may not be pigmented (see Fig. 3-1). A nonpigmented third eyelid may appear elevated or more prominent but is not abnormal.[3] An elevated third eyelid can be caused by enophthalmos (i.e., from fat atrophy), retraction of the globe (e.g., with ocular discomfort such as corneal ulceration, uveitis, or photophobia), phthisis bulbi (Fig. 3-32), or an orbital space-occupying mass (e.g., a neoplasm, granuloma, or abscess)[73-76]; or it can result from sympathetic denervation and Horner's syndrome.[5,6,56-59] Bilateral third

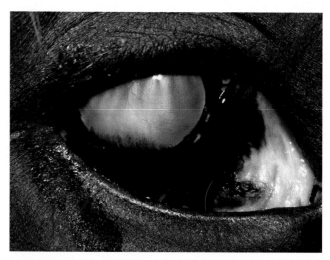

Fig. 3-32 An elevated third eyelid caused by phthisis bulbi. The small size of the eye has allowed the third eyelid to passively extend anteriorly.

eyelid elevation has been associated with tetanus,[77] ear tick (*Otobius megnini*) infestations,[78] and possible other systemic disease in horses (see discussion of systemic diseases in Chapter 13). Conjunctivitis, ulceration, swelling, and eventually erosion of the leading edge of the unpigmented third eyelid are common in horses (see Fig. 3-24), especially those that have pigmented eyelids but nonpigmented third eyelids.[3] Solar or actinic radiation and environmental irritants are usually the causes. These lesions may be precursors to SCC. Inflammation of the third eyelid has been associated with granuloma formation with habronemiasis.[42] Prolapsed gland of the nictitans has not been reported in horses. However, prolapsed orbital fat (specifically the anteromedial corpus adiposum) around the third eyelid can cause protrusion and a clinical appearance similar to that of a gland prolapse (Fig. 3-33).[79,80] Trauma to the third eyelid can result in lacerations of the conjunctiva, cartilage, or both; hemorrhage; and swelling. In general, if the only abnormality is a conjunctival laceration, hemorrhage, or chemosis, then the injury will rapidly heal without surgery. Topical antibiotics may be helpful to prevent injury and to protect the surface of swollen tissue. If substantial chemosis of the third eyelid conjunctiva is present that is not covered when the eyelids close, desiccation and additional swelling may occur. In cases of severe swelling, a partial temporary tarsorrhaphy is recommended to protect the cornea and to prevent desiccation.[3] A single, horizontal mattress suture placed in the medial fourth of the eyelid is generally all that is needed. The lateral palpebral fissure is allowed to remain open so that the horse can still see out of the eye and topical medications can be instilled on the ocular surface. If the cartilage is lacerated, surgical fixation or removal of the third eyelid is recommended.

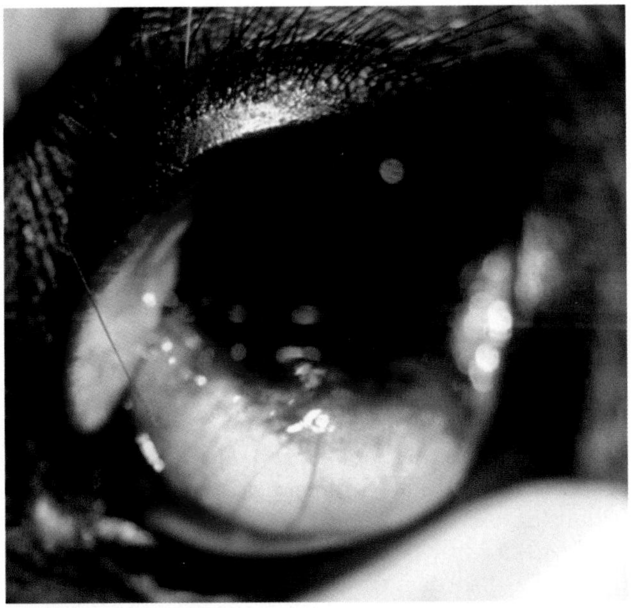

Common Differential Diagnoses

Third eyelid position abnormalities must be differentiated from primary ocular and orbital diseases (see discussion of diseases of the globe and orbit in Chapter 2), such as mass lesions in the orbit, enophthalmos, ocular discomfort, and phthisis bulbi. Third eyelid inflammation should be differentiated from medial canthal habronemiasis and primary conjunctivitis. Lesions can be differentiated by culture, cytology, and biopsy. These tests are especially recommended in any case of chronic or nonreponsive inflammation or swelling. Evidence of primary orbital (i.e., exophthalmos or inability to retropulse the globe) or ocular disease (i.e., small size or phthisis bulbi) suggests the need for further diagnostic procedures to determine the cause of the clinical signs (see discussion of diseases of the globe and orbit in Chapter 2).

Treatment

Treatment should be directed at the underlying cause of the inflammation or swelling.

Medical Therapy

Topical antibiotics are generally used initially; however, if the disease is unresponsive, then treatment should be guided by culture and sensitivity results, cytology results, and findings on histopathologic examination.

Surgical Therapy

Lacerations involving the cartilage of the third eyelid should be surgically repaired, or the third eyelid should be removed entirely. Partial removal of the third eyelid is not recommended because exposed cartilage of the third eye could be irritating to the cornea. In general, the goal of surgical therapy is to eliminate the source of irritation without causing additional irritation. All sutures and suture knots must be either buried under the conjunctiva or placed on the external aspect of the third eyelid. General anesthesia is recommended because the third eyelid and retractor bulbi muscles remain functioning even when the animal is tranquilized. Retrobulbar nerve block is an option for surgery

Fig. 3-33 Prolapsed orbital fat near the base of the third eyelid. The clinical appearance is similar to a prolapse of the gland of the third eyelid, which usually does not occur in horses. (Photograph courtesy Dr. Mike Davidson.)

of the third eyelid[55]; however, it is not recommended for fine microsurgery of the eyelids.

Removal of the third eyelid is a common procedure that is usually performed after diagnosis of a leading edge SCC. With the horse anesthetized or, less ideally, tranquilized and with a retrobulbar nerve block, the third eyelid is grasped and elevated. A full-thickness incision is made on the medial and lateral aspects of the third eyelid, beyond the T-piece of the cartilage. Usually, approximately 2 cm of the third eyelid is removed. The conjunctiva on the medial and lateral aspects of the third eyelid is cut at the base of the cartilage. After the conjunctival incision has been made, the third eyelid is further elevated, and the dense fibrous tissue anchoring the third eyelid is excised. The entire cartilage should be removed, and palpation of the third eyelid before and after excision is recommended. The medial and lateral conjunctiva is sutured together with a continuous pattern of 6-0 polyglactin 910 or similar sutures.

Long-Term Prognosis

Assuming that further damage to the eye does not occur from chronic third eyelid abnormalities or poor placement of sutures during surgery of the third eyelid, prognosis for most third eyelid injuries is good.

Procedure for Retrobulbar Nerve Block

Certain minor ocular surgical procedures, such as biopsies and third eyelid removal, can be done with the horse standing and the use of tranquilization and a retrobulbar nerve block.[55] This block will paralyze the retrobulbar nerves, stop retractor bulbi function, and keep the eye immobile. The orbital fossa above the dorsal orbital rim and zygomatic arch is first clipped and aseptically prepped with povidone-iodine (Betadine) scrub and alcohol. Care must be taken to avoid getting surgical scrub or alcohol on the ocular surface because severe irritation and corneal ulceration may develop. Once prepped, a 22-gauge, 2.5-inch spinal needle is placed through the skin perpendicular to the skull, in the orbital fossa, just posterior to the posterior aspect of the bony dorsal orbital rim. The needle is advanced posterior to the globe until it reaches the retrobulbar orbital cone (Fig. 3-34). When the needle advances to this location, the eye will have a slight dorsal movement as the needle passes through the fascia of the dorsal retrobulbar cone into the retrobulbar space. Once positioned, 10 to 12 ml of 2% lidocaine hydrochloride is injected into the retrobulbar space. During the injection, the globe is pushed

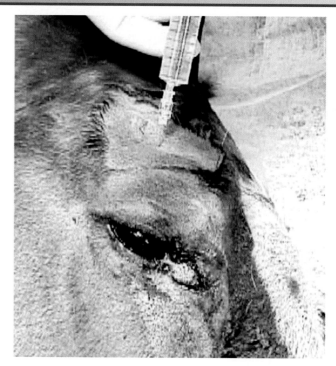

Fig. 3-34 A retrobulbar nerve block with 10 ml of lidocaine can assist in keeping the horse immobile during standing surgery. After surgical preparation of the supraorbital fossa, a 22-gauge 2.5-inch spinal needle is placed through the skin perpendicular to the skull just posterior to the posterior aspect of the bony dorsal orbital rim. The needle is advanced posterior to the globe until it reaches the retrobulbar orbital cone. Once through the retrobulbar cone, the lidocaine is slowly injected into the retrobulbar space (see text for more details).

externally (i.e., slight exophthalmos), indicating an accurate placement of lidocaine. The lidocaine will take effect and anesthetize the eye in 5 to 10 minutes. The duration of effect is approximately 1 to 2 hours. Because the eye is anesthetized, ocular sensation, blink reflex, and vision will be compromised. Therefore stall rest and protection of the eye with lubricants are recommended for 2 to 4 hours after anesthesia.

ACQUIRED NASOLACRIMAL DISORDERS

Nasolacrimal Duct Obstruction

NLD obstruction is a very common problem in horses. Congenital nasolacrimal atresia is one of the most common congenital ocular diseases in horses and usually causes signs of ocular discharge, first noted in foals at 2 to 6 months of age (see discussion of congenital ocular disorders earlier in this chapter). Causes of acquired nasolacrimal disorders include obstructions from inflammation (dacryocystitis), strictures, foreign bodies, and trauma (Fig. 3-35).[1,13,81-84]

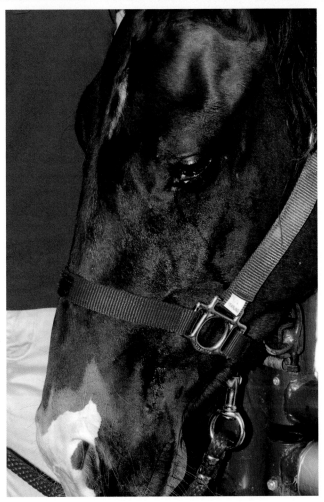

Fig. 3-35 Epiphora and hemorrhagic discharge associated with a blocked nasolacrimal duct caused by dacryocystitis.

Clinical Appearance and Diagnosis

Obstruction of the NLD occurs most commonly as a result of intraluminal foreign material, and clinical signs include epiphora, conjunctivitis, and mucopurulent discharge. Foreign material is often removed by retrograde saline flush (see discussion of atresia earlier in this chapter; see Chapter 1 for technique).[3,83] Initial diagnosis is made by inability of topical fluorescein dye to exit the ventral nasolacrimal puncta. Inflammation or trauma to the NLD may cause hemorrhage from the ventral nasolacrimal meatus, a condition called dacryohemorrhea.[85]

Common Differential Diagnoses

In all cases of epiphora, the clinician needs to differentiate between increased lacrimation (causing overflow of tears) and obstruction of tear outflow (Fig. 3-36). The most common cause of increased lacrimation is ocular pain, caused by conditions such as corneal disease or uveitis. Some horses have seasonal epiphora or dacryocystitis, which is usually bilateral. This may be caused by environmental changes (e.g., increase in dry, dusty environment), allergies, or insects. Diagnostic methods in horses with nasolacrimal obstruction or suspected dacryocystitis include bacterial culture and sensitivity and cytology of the discharge. After these tests have been done, retrograde nasolacrimal irrigation should be attempted with the horse tranquilized (see Chapter 1 for description). If the obstruction can be dislodged, copious irrigation of the duct should be done to clean out all debris. If the obstruction cannot be broken down, overt pressure should not be applied to prevent rupture or other damage to the NLD. If the irrigation is unsuccessful, the horse should be anesthetized and the irrigation should be repeated. Many times, with the animal totally relaxed under general anesthesia, the obstruction can be irrigated. If irrigation is still unsuccessful, or if there are additional NLD obstructions, then a dacryocystorhinography should be performed to determine whether there is an anatomic lesion of the NLD or surrounding bone.[14,25,82,83] Computed tomography[84] or microvideo endoscopy may also be used to visualize the defect in the NLD.

Pathogenesis of Disease Process and Progression

Dacryocystitis, or inflammation of the NLD, is generally a result of a complete or partial obstruction, secondary retention of tears in the duct, and bacterial proliferation in the stagnant tear fluid. Obstructions can be caused by accumulation of environmental debris in the NLD, especially in areas of normal narrowing of the duct, such as immediately before its exit from the lacrimal canal of the maxilla bone.[25] Damage to the lacrimal canal of the maxillary bone from external trauma, sinus infections, or upper arcade dental disease may cause strictures of the NLD.[1,13,81,82]

Treatment

Medical Therapy

After relief of the obstruction in the NLD, topical broad-spectrum antibiotic solution (type determined according to culture and sensitivity results) should be used

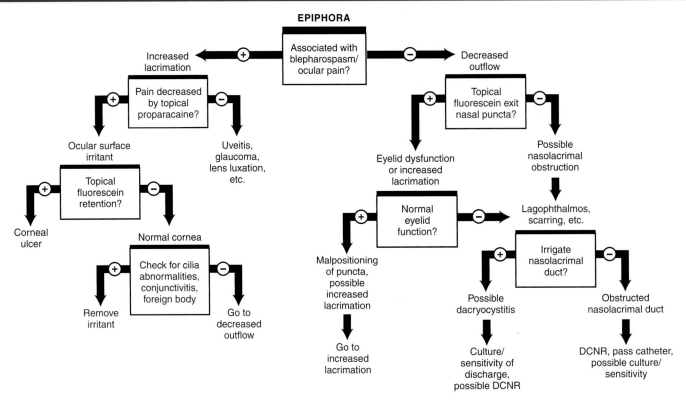

Fig. 3-36 Algorithm for diagnosis and treatment of epiphora.

every 6 hours. Solutions may be better than ointments because they can pass through the NLD more easily. A topical corticosteroid (e.g., 0.1% dexamethasone or 1% prednisolone acetate) is also recommended to decrease swelling in the NLD if there are no ocular surface contraindications (e.g., a corneal ulcer). Treatment should be continued for at least 2 weeks. Topical corticosteroids require a decreasing dosage schedule, or taper, to prevent rebound inflammation. If repeated obstructions were found or dacryocystitis was present, if the obstruction was difficult to resolve, or if there was stricture of the duct visualized by dacryocystorhinography or other imaging modalities, then a surgical stent or catheter should be placed for 4 weeks. A 5 Fr silicone rubber (Silastic) or plastic canine urinary catheter (with or without wire stent) is threaded normograde (from proximal to distal) or retrograde. The catheter is advanced until resistance is encountered. The catheter should not be forced if resistance is encountered, because severe hemorrhage may develop.[25] Once passed, the silicone rubber tubing is sutured in place for 30 days (see Fig. 3-13). After surgery, topical and systemic antibiotics should be given according to culture sensitivity results; however, frequently, the choice is topical triple antibiotic solution (every 6 hours) and oral sulfamethoxazole-trimethoprim (10 mg/kg every 12 hours) until the tube is removed.

Surgical Therapy

Surgery to correct NLD obstruction is uncommon but includes two main categories. The first is a group of procedures designed to remove the surrounding tissue abnormality that is compressing the NLD. This includes surgery to relieve swelling from sinusitis or dental disease or to repair facial fractures or canaliculi lacerations.[1,13,81] If the NLD cannot be opened or is permanently destroyed, a new tear outflow pathway must be created. Creating a pathway from the canaliculi to the nasal cavity (canaliculorhinostomy)[83] or from the ventral medial conjunctival surface to the maxillary sinus (conjunctivosinostomy)[24] can eliminate the epiphora. These procedures involve drilling a hole with a Steinmann pin or drill through the lacrimal bone into the maxillary sinus or nasal cavity, then placing a stent to allow the incisions to heal. Although successful, the procedure can be challenging because of the risk of significant hemorrhage, the density of facial bones in the horse, and the propensity of the new opening to stricture over time.

Long-Term Prognosis

The prognosis for NLD obstructions and dacryocystitis is good, unless the horse has recurrent problems.

It is essential to determine the location, extent, and cause of the obstruction to adequately treat it. Some horses can tolerate mild epiphora if the owners can keep the area ventral to the eye clean and prevent fly infestation. Decreasing environmental debris, dust, and other sources of material that may accumulate in the NLD, allergens, and insects can decrease severity in most horses. Other horses with severe and recurrent NLD obstructions may need a new drainage pathway, such as canaliculorhinostomy or conjunctivosinostomy. The long-term success of these techniques is not yet known.

Keratoconjunctivitis Sicca

KCS, or dry eye, is very uncommon in horses.[10-12,53,86,87] Nearly all cases of KCS in horses have been associated with trauma,[10,12] and there has not been a definitive case of immune-mediated lacrimal gland adenitis, which is the most common cause of KCS in dogs.[88-90] Crispin[87] subdivides KCS into tear-deficient dry eye and evaporative dry eye, which is desiccation of the ocular surface as a result of facial nerve paralysis (or other eyelid dysfunction), loss of corneal sensation, and other primary ocular surface diseases.

Clinical Appearance and Diagnosis

Clinical signs of possible dry eye in horses include blepharospasm; mucopurulent ocular discharge; a dry, lusterless cornea; and keratitis. Definitive diagnosis is made by assessment of clinical signs and STT values. The STT should be performed before manipulation of the eye and orbit during examination to minimize reflex tearing (see discussion of ocular examination in Chapter 1 for the technique for performing an STT in a horse). Healthy horses have been reported to have an STT I (measurement of tears without the use of a topical anesthetic) range of 11 to greater than 30 mm wetting/min and 15 to 20 mm wetting/30 sec.[9,91,92] A study of the STT in the horse revealed no differences between STT I and STT II (i.e., with topical anesthetic) values or an effect of age, season, environment, sex, time of day, or location, or placement of strips.[92] Tranquilization does not effect STT values; however, general inhalant anesthesia with halothane does affect the STT for up to 3 hours.[91] STT measurements of 10 to 15 mm wetting/min or less with clinical signs of dry eye are suggestive of KCS.

Common Differential Diagnoses

An STT is indicated if evidence of CN VII dysfunction (e.g., after trauma, facial paralysis) is observed, if the cornea or conjunctiva appears dry, if tenacious mucoid discharge is present, if persistent corneal vascularization or ulceration is present, or if an underlying cause cannot be identified. KCS is most commonly the result of CN V or CN VII trauma but has also been reported in cases of fractures of the mandible and stylohyoid bone, locoweed poisoning, eosinophilic dacryoadenitis, and in association with corneal stromal sequestration.[1,3,10-12,86] The clinician must differentiate KCS from other much more common diseases, especially primary keratitis and NLD obstruction.

Treatment

Medical Therapy

Medical therapy is the mainstay of treatment of equine KCS. Initial therapy should consist of application of topical broad-spectrum antibiotic ointment to help reduce the secondary bacterial infections that commonly develop. Use of once-daily eye irrigation for the first week of therapy may help with secondary infections also, but the owner must be warned not to overuse the wash because it can dry the cornea. Topical artificial tear ointments, used three to four times daily, will help keep the corneas of most horses healthy. However, the importance of the continued use of the medication must be stressed to the owners. Use of topical 0.25% pilocarpine, vitamin A, and acetylcysteine once a day has been recommended for treatment of horses with KCS[3]; however, their efficacy has not been reported. Topical cyclosporine has also been recommended for equine KCS,[3] and improvement of clinical signs has been reported.[86] However, because horses are not known to have lacrimal adenitis, the value of cyclosporine for equine KCS is questionable. Application of topical corticosteroids may also initially improve clinical signs of KCS, but they should be used with extreme caution because of the risk of corneal ulceration.

Surgical Therapy

Occlusion of the nasolacrimal puncta by cauterization has been recommended for mild cases of equine KCS,[3] but the efficacy of this technique is unknown. In horses with facial nerve deficits, loss of corneal sensation, or chronic unrelenting KCS, a temporary or permanent lateral tarsorrhaphy may help protect the cornea. In severe cases of dry eye that do not respond to medication or other treatment, enucleation of the eye should be considered. A parotid duct transposition (to provide salivary secretion to the corneal surface) has been attempted in a horse, but long-term results were not reported.[93]

Long-Term Prognosis

Acute KCS associated with trauma, anesthesia, or systemic disease will generally resolve as the horse recovers from the primary cause. KCS associated with increased evaporation of the tears caused by lagophthalmos or loss of corneal sensation will resolve if, and when, the neurologic disease resolves. Generally, these lesions resolve in 3 to 4 weeks, and the cornea needs to be meticulously protected until then. The prognosis for primary KCS is good in the short term (i.e., usually medications can improve clinical signs initially); however, long-term therapy is difficult for most owners, and most eyes will develop progressive corneal edema, vascularization, and scarring that decreases vision.

NEOPLASIA

Of all of the diseases that affect the equine eyelids and adnexa, neoplasms are the most common and can be among the most frustrating to treat. Approximately 10% of equine neoplasms are eye-related.[94,95] Identical treatments to similarly appearing tumors may have different clinical outcomes. Why one horse responds well to therapy and another does not requires further study. The most common periocular masses are sarcoids, SCC, papilloma, lymphosarcoma, and melanoma.[1,3,13,73,94-96]

Sarcoids

Sarcoids are the most common tumors or neoplasms in horses.[96-98] These masses can occur in nearly any location on the skin, and their size and location dictate their clinical significance. Although not technically considered to be malignant, sarcoids are commonly invasive and recurrent. Periocular or eyelid sarcoids are common and may cause ocular irritation by disrupting eyelid function or by directly rubbing on the eye.[99-101] In one series, periocular sarcoids represented 14% of total sarcoids.[102] Because of proximity to the sensitive eye, some aggressive treatments used for sarcoids elsewhere on the body cannot be used on the eyelid.[103]

Clinical Appearance and Diagnosis

The clinical appearance of sarcoids varies, and they are most commonly classified into five broad categories: occult, verrucose, nodular (A and B), fibroblastic (A and B), and mixed equine sarcoids.[103,104] An occult sarcoid appears as an alopecic area with fine epidermal nodules. Verrucose sarcoids are thickened and hyperkeratotic with extensive flaking of the skin.

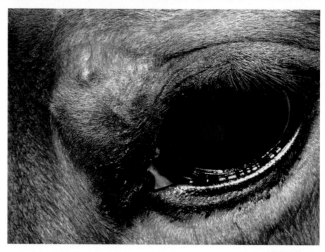

Fig. 3-37 A nodular type A sarcoid in the upper medial eyelid of a horse. Nodular type A sarcoids are well defined, ovoid, and entirely subcutaneous.

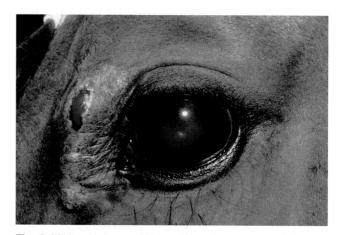

Fig. 3-38 A nodular type B sarcoid in the upper medial eyelid and medial canthus of a horse. Nodular type B sarcoids are well defined and ovoid and involve the epidermis.

Nodular type A sarcoids (Fig. 3-37) are well defined, ovoid, and entirely subcutaneous; whereas type B sarcoids are similar but involve the epidermis (Fig. 3-38). Fibroblastic sarcoids appear fleshy and ulcerated and can have a pedunculated (type A) or broad base (type B) (Fig. 3-39). Mixed sarcoids have one or more of the features of the other types of sarcoids (Fig. 3-40). Periocular sarcoids are most commonly nodular, fibroblastic, or mixed. Sarcoids usually develop in young horses between 3 and 6 years of age; however, sarcoids have developed in horses as young as yearlings.[102] Nearly all breeds have been reported to have sarcoids. However, Quarter horses may be at increased risk, whereas Standardbreds may be at decreased risk.[105]

Common Differential Diagnoses

A surgical biopsy is always required for definitive diagnosis. Exuberant granulation tissue may be present

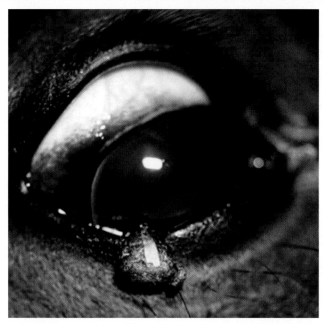

Fig. 3-39 Fibroblastic sarcoids appear fleshy and ulcerated and can have a pedunculated (type A) or a broad base (type B). A type A fibroblastic sarcoid is shown here.

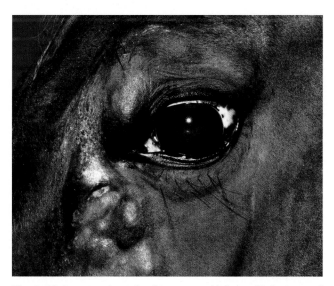

Fig. 3-40 An extensive mixed type sarcoid (i.e., with features of one or more types) of the medial upper eyelid and medial canthus of a horse.

and difficult to distinguish clinically from sarcoids.[102] Histopathologic examination may also be needed to rule out other pathologic conditions of the eyelids such as habronemiasis, melanoma, SCC, papilloma, and orbital fat prolapse. Histologically, all clinical types of sarcoids have increased density of dermal fibroblasts (i.e., fibroblastic proliferation). Epidermal hyperplasia, hyperkeratosis, and rete peg formation were only found consistently in the verrucous and mixed types but not consistently in occult and nodular

sarcoids in one study.[104] Sarcoids commonly invade the subcutis and the deeper muscular structures around the eye.[103,106]

Pathogenesis of Disease Process and Progression

Sarcoids have long been thought to have a viral origin. This infectious origin was supported by the fact that epizootics have occurred in individual herds.[102,107] Numerous studies have associated bovine papilloma virus (BPV) and equine sarcoids.[102,104,108-117] Intradermal inoculation into horses with cell-free extracts from bovine skin tumors caused by BPV caused lesions that resembled equine sarcoids both clinically and histologically.[108,110,118] BPV has not been detected by electron microscopy in natural cases of equine sarcoid,[102] but DNA sequences of BVP (BVP-1 and BVP-2) have been found in equine sarcoid by Southern blotting and polymerase chain reaction studies in most sarcoids.[112-117,119-121] Equine sarcoids appear to contain detectable viral DNA and RNA and are also known to express the BPV types 1 and 2 major transforming protein, E5, but do not appear to produce infectious virions.[102,113-117,120] In one study, no mutations of the tumor suppressor gene *p53* were identified in equine sarcoids, suggesting that these mutations do not have a primary role in equine sarcoid pathogenesis. However, the authors of this study speculated that the high rate of BPV infection associated with equine sarcoid may indicate the functional inactivation of *p53* by BPV-encoded E6 protein.[122] Another study demonstrated that no telomerase activity could be detected in sarcoids, suggesting that telomerase does not play a major role in the development of sarcoids in the horse.[123]

A genetic susceptibility may also exist with equine sarcoid. Sarcoid occurrence was associated with the major histocompatibility complex–encoded class I equine leukocyte antigen (ELA) W3,B1 haplotype in Irish-, Swiss-, and French-bred Warmbloods.[124] An association between sarcoid susceptibility and the major histocompatibility complex–encoded class II allele ELA W13 has also been found in several breeds.[102,125] An association between early-onset sarcoids and A5 ELA, increased recurrence rates after surgery and W13 ELA, and increased prevalence of sarcoid and A3W13 ELA was also found.[126] Another study demonstrated a correlation between the development of sarcoids and heterozygosity for the equine severe combined immunodeficiency allele.[127]

Treatment

Treatments for periocular sarcoids are listed in Table 3-5.

Table 3-5   Treatment for Periocular Sarcoids

Medical Therapy				
Type of Therapy	Drug	Dose	No. of Cases	Nonrecurrence (%)
Topical	AW4-LUDES ointment[103]	Once daily for 5 days	146	35
	5% 5-fluorouracil[103]	Twice a day for 5 days, then once daily for 5 days, then qod for 5 applications	9	67
Immunotherapy	BCG[100]	1 ml/cm² tumor surface every 2-4 wk	26	100
	BCG[103]			
	Occult, verrucose, mixed	1 ml/cm² every 2-4 wk	52	0
	Nodular or fibroblastic	1 ml/cm² every 2-4 wk	300	69
Chemotherapy	Cisplatin[135]	1 mg/cm³ every 2 wk for 4 treatments	19	95
	Cisplatin[103]	1 mg/cm³ every 2 wk for 4 treatments	18	33

Surgical Therapy			
Type of Therapy	Description	No. of Cases	Nonrecurrence (%)
Surgical excision[97]	Excision	—	50
Surgical excision[103]	Excision	28	18
Cryotherapy[143]	Double or triple freeze–thaw to −25° C		9
Cryotherapy[103]	Double or triple freeze–thaw to −25° C	23	9
Hyperthermia[103]	Tissue temperatures between 41° C and 45° C	2	0

Brachytherapy			
Radioisotope	Dose Range	No. of Cases	Nonrecurrence (%)
Radon 222 seeds[150]	6000 cGy	19	92
Gold 198 seeds[152]	7000 cGy	19	90
Iridium 192 seeds[101]	60 Gy	115	87
Iridium 192 pins[103]	7000-9000 cGy	53	98

BCG, Bacille Calmette-Guérin; *qod,* every other day.

Medical Therapy

Topical

Several topical substances (e.g., oil of rosemary, arsenic powder, engine grease, tea tree oil), mostly irritants, have been used for treatment of sarcoids.[3,103] A popular topical product, XXTERRA (Larson Laboratories, Fort Collins, Colo) has bloodroot (*Sanguinaria canadensis*) as the active ingredient. The topical herbal substance irritates the sarcoid, which stimulates the immune system to recognize it and mount an immune response. Anecdotally, there has been a 95% response rate. Because these substances are irritating, they induce severe keratitis and should not be used on or near the eye. AW4 ointment, which consists of 10% 5-fluorouracil and oil of rosemary (applied once daily for 5 days), was used in 146 periocular sarcoids in one study and resulted in a nonrecurrence rate of 35%.

Immunotherapy

The most common immunotherapy[99,100,102,103,128-132] for sarcoids has been the injection of bacille Calmette-Guérin (BCG).[100,103,129-131] The goal is to potentiate the immune system to produce regression of the tumors. The technique is to saturate the tumor with BCG typically at a dose of 1.0 ml/cm² of tumor surface (Figs. 3-41 to 3-43).[100] The injection is repeated at variable intervals (most commonly every 2 to 4 weeks) until complete regression of the tumor occurs. In one study, complete regression was observed in 100% of periocular tumors in 31 horses, with an average of 11.7 ml per treatment, 3.2 treatments per tumor, and a range of 14 to 252 days to achieve remission.[100] Local and systemic anaphylaxis have been noted, especially after the second injection.[130] Pretreatment with flunixin meglumine, antihistamines, and/or corticosteroids may be required. Other substances have been used for immunotherapy

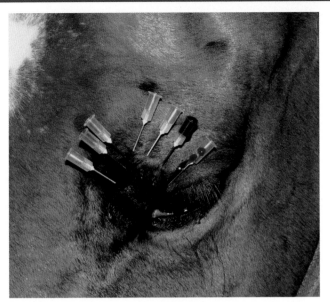

Fig. 3-41 Preplaced needles for infiltration of a nodular sarcoid with bacille Calmette-Guérin or cisplatin.

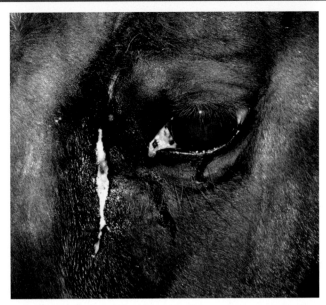

Fig. 3-43 Same horse as shown in Figs. 3-40 and 3-42 after excision of a large mixed sarcoid and three intralesional cisplatin treatments.

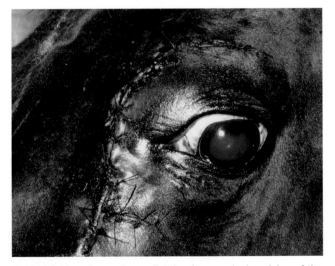

Fig. 3-42 Horse's eye immediately after surgical excision of the large medial canthal mixed sarcoid shown in Fig. 3-40.

in the treatment of sarcoids and include autogenous tumor vaccines, other mycobacterial cell wall fragments, recombinant human tumor necrosis factor-α, and xanthate compounds.[99,130,133] In a review of cases of periocular sarcoids,[103] immunotherapy with intralesional BCG had poor results with verrucose, occult, and mixed sarcoids; whereas BCG immunomodulation therapy for fibroblastic and nodular lesions had a good overall response of 69% (see Table 3-5). Side effects were observed and included development of sinus tracts in 15% and transient swelling after injections.[103]

Chemotherapy

Intralesional cisplatin has been the most common type of chemotherapy for sarcoids.[101,134-136] Use of topical 5-flurouracil has also been reported, with six of nine verrucose or occult sarcoids demonstrating a good response.[137] However, only those sarcoids away from the eye and eyelid margins should be treated with 5-flurouracil because of the irritating qualities of the drug. Treatment with an oily emulsion of cisplatin consisted of four sessions at 2-week intervals at a dose of 1 mg of cisplatin per cubic centimeter of tumor tissue. The oily emulsion is used to infiltrate the tumor with a method similar to that used for BCG injections (see Fig. 3-41). Complete regression was observed in 95% of the sarcoids with a 1-year relapse-free rate of 87%.[135] Adverse effects and toxicity associated with the chemotherapy were minimal.[135] Electrochemical stimulation may enhance the effectiveness of cisplatin chemotherapy of sarcoids.[134] After cisplatin injection, an electropulsator was used to deliver pulses of 0.1 ms at a 1-Hz frequency with a 1.3-kV voltage to the sarcoid. Although an excellent regression of the tumors was noted, the effect on the eye and the tolerance of horses to the electrostimulation of the sensitive periocular tissues was not reported. In a review of 18 cases of periocular sarcoids, use of intralesional chemotherapy resulted in nonrecurrence in 33%.[103]

Surgical Therapy

Surgical Excision

In general, surgical excision of sarcoids without adjunctive therapy (e.g., cryotherapy, interstitial irradiation, immunotherapy, or cryotherapy) has a 1-year recurrence rate of approximately 50%.[97] Split-thickness autogenous skin grafts improved cosmetic results after excision of sarcoids, and there were no recurrences in the three horses in the study.[138] Carbon dioxide (CO_2) laser ablation of sarcoids is associated with a lower recurrence rate than surgical excision alone; however, unless the skin is closed primarily, exuberant granulation may develop.[102,139] In a review of 28 cases of periocular sarcoids treated by surgical excision alone, a recurrence rate of 92% was found.[103] Early onset, long duration, and large size all appeared to increase risk of recurrence,[126] and the likelihood for local recurrence was greater when sarcoids had a surgical margin that was positive for BPV DNA.[120]

Cryotherapy

Cryotherapy is a commonly used surgical treatment for sarcoids, either alone or after surgical debulking of the tumor.[3,103,140-142] The sarcoid is destroyed and the ensuing eschar separates from the underlying granulation bed. Healing after cryotherapy always occurs by second intention. Principles of cryotherapy to ensure proper freezing include a double or triple freeze-thaw cycle with a rapid freeze and slow thaw. Tissues must be frozen to a least −25° C, and a margin of 0.5 cm should be allowed around the periphery of each tumor.[143] Use of thermocouple temperature needles is recommended to ensure that the desired tissue temperature is achieved. Liquid nitrogen provides the fastest freeze, but the surgeon must be very careful around the eye so that liquid run-off does not inadvertently damage the eye. A probe can be used, but more time and overlapping of the sites are needed to compensate for the slow freezing and lack of penetration.[143] Sloughing of tissue will occur 2 to 4 weeks after cryotherapy, and tissue depigmentation may remain for 6 months or more. Repeated treatments may be required for large or recurrent lesions.[144]

Hyperthermia

Neoplastic tissues are more sensitive to elevated temperatures than normal cells, and temperatures between 41° C and 45° C will preferentially destroy neoplastic tissue but not normal cells.[143] Minimal changes were seen in the normal equine eye as a result of hyperthermia.[145] Several studies have been conducted to evaluate hyperthermia in the treatment of equine SCC,[1,3,146,147] but only a few have included treatment of sarcoids. In a review of cases of periocular sarcoids, two were treated by hyperthermia and both of them recurred.[103]

Brachytherapy

In brachytherapy, small gamma radioactive sources are placed on or within neoplasms, allowing a high dose of radiation to be delivered to the tissue and minimal radiation to surrounding tissues.[101,143,148,149] The radioactive sources are usually removed once the desired dose is delivered to the tissue. The length of time that is required depends on the isotope used. Isotopes that have been used include gold 198, iridium 192, radon 222, cesium 137, and tantalum 182.[143,150] Iridium 192 is most commonly used, and the isotope is contained within stainless steel rods at 1-cm intervals in a plastic coating or within needles that are placed in the tumor in parallel rows approximately 1 cm apart (Fig. 3-44).[101,149,151] Iridium 192 has a half-life of 74.2 days, and typical doses of 5000 to 9000 cGy require approximately 7 to 14 days of implantation before removal.[151] A 94% tumor-free incidence at 1 year in 16 cases of sarcoids was found in one study.[151] In a study of periocular sarcoids treated with ^{192}Ir brachytherapy at a dose of 60 Gy (minimum dose), the 1- and 5-year progression-free survival rates for sarcoids were 86.6% and 74.0%, respectively.[101] In another study of periocular sarcoids treated with ^{192}Ir brachytherapy (n = 53), a nonrecurrence rate of 98% was found.[103] Use of other brachytherapy in sarcoids has had similar results (see Table 3-5, p. 138).[101,148-153] Side effects of the radiation therapy are uncommon, but some long-term ocular effects such as palpebral fibrosis, cataract, keratitis, corneal edema, bone sequestrum, and corneal ulceration have been reported.[101,103,154]

Long-Term Prognosis

Failure to induce complete regression of periocular sarcoids will frequently result in regrowth of the tumor, and in many cases, this recurrence may be more aggressive (i.e., extensive local infiltration and faster growth). Therefore potent and aggressive therapy is recommended from the beginning of treatment to more

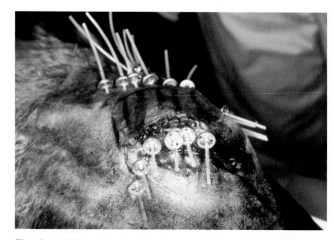

Fig. 3-44 Iridium implants for treatment of an upper eyelid sarcoid. The plastic tubes are preplaced and the iridium is quickly inserted. Total treatment time is typically 7 to 10 days, and then the tubes are removed. (Photograph courtesy Dr. R. David Whitley.)

quickly destroy the tissue and prevent recurrences.[103] However, the clinician must be aware that the periorbital tissues are less tolerant of damage than other tissues, and certain treatment methods, such as surface irritants, should be used with great caution in the vicinity of the eye.[103]

Squamous Cell Carcinoma

SCC and sarcoids are the most common periocular neoplasms. In a study of general neoplasms in horses, sarcoids were most common (43.6% sarcoids vs 24.6% SCC),[94] whereas in another study, SCC was more common (15.3% SCC vs 12.9% sarcoids).[95] At one institution, ocular SCC represented approximately 10% of all equine ocular disease.[4]

Clinical Appearance and Diagnosis

Increased prevalence of SCC is associated with an increase in longitude, decreased latitude, increased altitude, and increased mean annual exposure to solar radiation.[44] An increased prevalence of ocular SCC may occur with increased age and in draft breeds and Appaloosas.[4,44] Mean age at diagnosis of horses with ocular SCC in three studies was 9.8 years,[155] 11.8 years,[4] and 11.1 years,[44] respectively, with an approximate range of 3 to 26 years.[156] Sex predisposition was noted, with a high prevalence of SCC in castrated male horses, double that of mares and five times that of intact male horses, suggesting the possibility that concentrations of circulating androgens, estrogens, or both may be associated with ocular SCC development in the horse.[44] In another study, no sex predisposition was noted.[147] Horses with light hair and skin

have a higher prevalence of ocular SCC.[4,44] Unilateral involvement is most common, but in one study, bilateral ocular SCC was observed in 16% of horses.[157] The most common ocular locations for SCC are the nictitating membrane or medial canthus (approximately 28%) (Fig. 3-45), limbus (approximately 28%) (Fig. 3-46), lower eyelid (approximately 23%) (Fig. 3-47), and other locations (21%) (e.g., cornea, conjunctiva, orbit).[4,73,157,158]

SCC typically starts as a hyperemic area of the eyelid with dark exudates, then progresses to ulceration with hemorrhage to papillomatous masses (Fig. 3-48).[3] The tumors progress to fleshy masses with variable degrees of ulceration, necrosis, and inflammation (see Figs. 3-16 and 3-45 to 3-48).

Common Differential Diagnoses

A diagnosis of SCC should always be suspected in any new growing adnexal mass until it is eliminated by histologic examination. Differential diagnoses include tumors (papilloma, melanoma, mastocytoma, basal cell carcinoma, schwannoma, adenoma and adenocarcinomas, hemangioma and hemangiosarcoma, lymphoma and lymphosarcoma), conjunctivitis (lymphoid hyperplasia and follicular conjunctivitis), inflammatory lesions (abscesses, granulation tissue, foreign body reaction, solar-induced inflammation), and parasites (*Habronema*, *Onchocerca*, and *Thelazia* species).*

Definitive diagnosis of SCC is based on histopathologic findings. There are four basic types of SCC: plaque (i.e., carcinoma in situ), papillomatous, noninvasive SCC, and invasive SCC.[164] Plaque formation primarily involves the proliferation of the stratum

---

*References 3, 32, 73, 74, 79, 80, 103, 159-163.

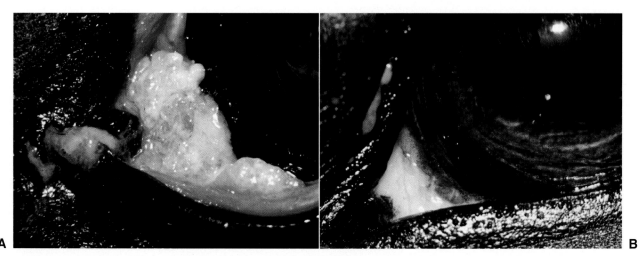

Fig. 3-45 A, An infiltrating third eyelid squamous cell carcinoma. **B,** Two weeks after total excision of the third eyelid and continuous suturing of limbal conjunctiva. (Photographs courtesy Dr. Riccardo Stoppini.)

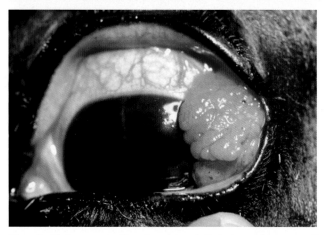

Fig. 3-46 Large proliferative lateral limbal squamous cell carcinoma.

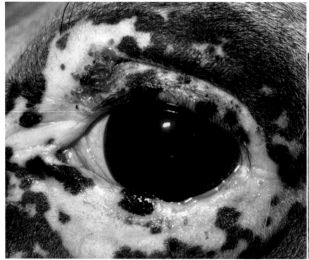

Fig. 3-47 Lower eyelid squamous cell carcinoma in a paint horse. Note how the neoplastic tissue involves only the nonpigmented eyelid margin and stops where the pigmentation begins.

spinosum; however, all layers of the epithelium can be proliferative. When the underlying connective tissue proliferates into the epithelium, which develops hyperkeratosis, a papilloma develops. Noninvasive SCC exhibits malignant transformation of the basilar layer of the epithelium with development of hyperchromatic nuclei, increased mitotic figures, pleomorphism, and loss of polarity. Invasive SCC extends past the basal epithelium into the subepithelial tissue and can have variable degrees of differentiation. Well-differentiated neoplasms are characterized by whorl formation, keratinized foci (i.e., "keratin pearls"), and intercellular bridges (Fig. 3-49). In poorly differentiated SCC, neoplastic cells are frequently arranged in cords or nests but have minimal cellular keratinization.[164]

An inflammatory infiltrate composed mostly of CD3+ T lymphocytes, CD79+ B cells, macrophages, and numerous immunoglobulin G plasma cells is commonly associated with SCCs.[165] In one study, no significant correlation was found between the nature of the inflammatory infiltrate and the SCC histologic grade or degree of invasion.[165] However, expression of major histocompatibility complex II by neoplastic epithelial cells may induce an improved local antitumor immune response.[165]

Pathogenesis of Disease Process and Progression

Any chronic irritation may promote neoplastic change of epithelium to SCC, especially at vulnerable locations, such as mucocutaneous junctions. Unlike sarcoids, equine SCCs have not been shown to exhibit viral antigens.[166] Irritation from actinic and/or ultraviolet radiation has been thought to promote the development of SCC. Clinically, animals exposed to higher elevations and increased sunlight have had a higher incidence of SCC.[44] Ultraviolet radiation may promote

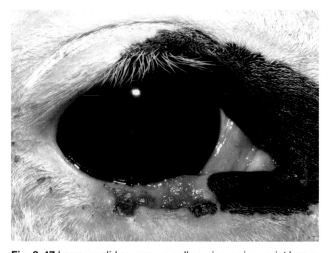

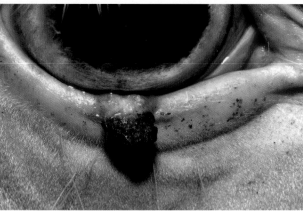

Fig. 3-48 A, Ulcerated lower eyelid typical of early (e.g., plaque, carcinoma in situ) squamous cell carcinoma. **B,** Proliferative, papillomatous lower eyelid SCC. (Photograph **A** courtesy Dr. Mike Davidson.)

mutation in the tumor suppressor protein, p53, and overexpression plays an important role in the development of most SCCs of the animal species studied.[122,167-169] The p53 antigen could be detected immunohistochemically in formalin-fixed tissues of SCCs of domestic animals.[122,168,169] In two separate studies, 100% of equine ocular SCCs overexpressed p53.[167,169]

Treatment

Medical Therapy

Medical treatments for SCC are listed in Table 3-6.

Immunotherapy

Historically, immunotherapy has not been used as commonly for ocular SCC as it has for equine sarcoids.

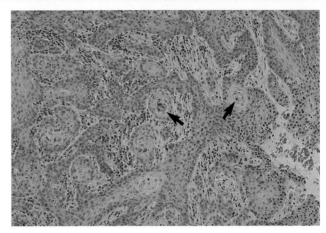

Fig. 3-49 Histologic section of an eyelid squamous cell carcinoma (hematoxylin and eosin stain; ×400). This well-differentiated neoplasm is characterized by whorl formation, keratinized foci (i.e., "keratin pearls" [arrows]), and intercellular bridges.

Table 3-6 — Treatment for Ocular Squamous Cell Carcinoma

Medical Therapy

Type of Therapy	Drug	Dose	No. of Cases	Nonrecurrence (%)
Immunotherapy	BCG[170]	2 ml/cm² of tumor surface every 2-4 wk	1	100
	Noncommercial vaccine[157]	—	2	—
Chemotherapy	Cisplatin[135]	1 mg/cm³ every 2 wk for 4 treatments	7	71

Surgical Therapy

Type of Therapy	Description	No. of Cases	Nonrecurrence (%)
Surgical excision[147]	Excision	18	56
Cryotherapy[147]	Double or triple freeze-thaw to −25° C	6	33
Cryotherapy[178]	Double or triple freeze-thaw to −25° C	5	100
Cryotherapy[176]	Double or triple freeze-thaw to −25° C	3	67
Hyperthermia[147]	Tissue temperatures between 41° C and 45° C	1	100
Hyperthermia[146]	Tissue temperatures between 41° C and 45° C	8	75
CO₂ laser ablation[187]	Ablate tissue	4	100

Brachytherapy

Radioisotope	Dose Range (cGy)	No. of Cases	Nonrecurrence (%)
Cobalt 60 or cesium 137[179]	5000	19	73.6
Gold 198 seeds[152]	7000	3	100
Iridium 192 pins[231]	7000	21	100
Radon 222, iodine 125, iridium 192[156]	5000-10,000	10	80
Iridium 192[147]	—	10	75
Iridium 192[101]	6000	52	81.8
Strontium 90[185]	25,000	27	89
Strontium 90[156]	10,000	8	88
Strontium 90[186]		24	76
Strontium 90[147]	—	7	100

BCG, Bacille Calmette-Guérin.

Immunotherapy can only be used for eyelid SCCs, not third eyelid, limbal, corneal, or orbital SCCs (Box 3-3).[157,158,170] The most common immunotherapy for ocular SCC has been the injection of BCG, although other "vaccines" have been used.[157,158,170] The goal is to potentiate the immune system to produce regression of the tumors. The treatment technique is similar to the treatment of sarcoids: the tumor is saturated with BCG, typically at a dose of 1.0 ml/cm^2 of tumor surface (see Figs. 3-41 to 3-43).[100] The injection is repeated at variable intervals (most commonly every 2 to 4 weeks) until complete regression of the tumor occurs. In one case report, a pony with ocular SCC and regional lymph node metastasis had complete regression after BCG therapy.[170]

Intralesional Cisplatin

Intralesional cisplatin has been the most common type of chemotherapy for ocular SCC.[136,171] Topical 5-flurouracil has also been successfully used on SCC of

---

Box 3-3	Recommended Treatment Modalities According to Site of Ocular Squamous Cell Carcinoma

Eyelid (Upper or Lower Eyelid or Medial Canthus External to Third Eyelid)
Surgical excision (plus any of the following)
- Brachytherapy
- Cryotherapy
- Hyperthermia
- Intralesional chemotherapy

Third Eyelid
Surgical excision (only if small leading edge SCC)
Surgical excision (if extensive) (plus any of the following)
- Brachytherapy
- Cryotherapy
- Hyperthermia

Conjunctival (Palpebral)
Surgical excision and (plus any of the following)
- Cryotherapy
- Hyperthermia
- Beta radiation (strontium-90)
- CO$_2$ laser ablation

Limbal, Bulbar Conjunctival, or Corneal SCC
Surgical excision (e.g., superficial keratectomy) (plus any of the following)
- Beta radiation (strontium-90)
- CO$_2$ laser ablation

Orbital SCC
Surgical excision (exenteration) (plus any of the following)
- Intralesional chemotherapy
- Brachytherapy

---

the external genitalia,[137] but there are no reports of its use on ocular tissues with SCC. Chemotherapy can only be used for eyelid SCC, not third eyelid, limbal, corneal, or orbital SCC (see Box 3-3). Treatment with an oily emulsion of cisplatin consists of four applications at 2-week intervals. The dose is 1 mg of cisplatin/cm^3 of tumor tissue. The oily emulsion is used to infiltrate the tumor with a method similar to that used for BCG injections (see Fig. 3-41). Complete regression was observed in five of seven cases (71%) of SCC with a 1-year relapse-free rate of 65% (see Table 3-6, p. 143).[135] Adverse effects and toxicity associated with the chemotherapy were minimal.[135] Another study showed no difference in outcome between tumors that were injected immediately after cytoreductive surgery and those treated after the skin had healed, except in aggressive tumors that had cellular regrowth within the postoperative period.[136] Therefore it was recommended that treatment be done immediately after surgery when the tumor proliferation index is not known.[136]

Metastatic SCC (i.e., from the primary site at the lip to the submandibular lymph nodes) was successfully treated (i.e., no recurrence 5 years after therapy) with oral piroxicam (80 mg every 24 hours).[172] After 90 days of treatment, the primary and metastatic SCC had resolved. Several bouts of colic occurred, and the piroxicam was reduced to a maintenance dose of 80 mg every 48 hours indefinitely without further gastrointestinal difficulties.[172]

Surgical Therapy

Surgical excision or debulking is almost always indicated to obtain histologic confirmation of disease and to remove the mass and decrease the tumor load. Surgical excision can be curative if the surgeon removes a 2-cm tumor-free margin on all sides of the mass. This is nearly impossible (even with extensive blepharoplastic procedures) on all types of ocular SCC because of the nature of the ocular tissue itself and the need to preserve as much functioning eyelid margin as possible. Because the equine facial skin is firmly attached to the underlying connective tissue and has poor superficial blood supply, blepharoplastic procedures (e.g., advancement flaps, rhomboidal flaps) are rarely successful (Fig. 3-50).[3,173] However, an excellent tumor-free margin can be obtained with an enucleation or complete excision of a third eyelid with a small leading margin SCC. With eyelid, limbal, or corneal SCC, surgical excision (i.e., debulking to visually normal tissue) combined with an adjunctive therapy—such as chemotherapy, cryotherapy, hyperthermia, or radiation therapy—is recommended (see Box 3-3). When SCC has extended into the orbit, an exenteration (i.e., removal of the entire orbital contents—wide surgical excision) is generally the only surgical option (see Box 3-3). With extensive tumors, partial orbital rim resection, mesh skin expansion, and second-intention healing can be used to close the large skin wounds.[174] In one study, surgical excision alone (without additional therapies) of the third eyelid had an SCC recurrence rate of 33% (6 of 14 cases), whereas 66% (2 of 3) of limbal SCCs recurred with surgical excision alone (see Table 3-6, p. 143).[147]

Cryotherapy

Cryotherapy is a commonly used surgical treatment for ocular SCC, usually after debulking of the tumor.[140,144,147,175-177] The technique for use of cryotherapy for SCC is the same as described earlier for sarcoids with a double or triple freeze-thaw cycle with a rapid freeze (−25° C) and slow thaw (Fig. 3-51).[143] Use of thermocouple temperature needles is recommended to ensure that the desired tissue temperature is achieved. Liquid nitrogen provides the fastest freeze, but the surgeon must be very careful around the eye so that liquid run-off does not inadvertently damage the eye. Use of a piece of Styrofoam cup and a liberal amount of sterile lubrication should adequately protect the cornea. A cryoprobe can be used instead of a spray, but more time and overlapping of the sites are required to compensate for the slow freezing and lack of penetration. Sloughing of tissue will occur 2 to 4 weeks after cryotherapy, and tissue depigmentation may remain for 6 months or more. Repeated treatments may be required for large or recurrent lesions.[144] In three small studies of ocular SCC treated with cryotherapy, one of three (33%),[176] one of six (17%),[147] and zero of five [178] cases had recurrence (see Table 3-6, p. 143). However, in another study, recurrence of SCC was 2.5 times more likely after cryosurgery compared with third eyelid removal.[157]

Hyperthermia

Hyperthermia has been used as an adjunctive therapy for equine sarcoids and bovine and equine SCC. It is recommended for eyelid, conjunctival, and limbal SCC, but not for SCC with deep penetration (see Box 3-3).[146] Temperatures between 41° C and 45° C will preferentially destroy neoplastic tissue but not normal cells.[143] Typically, a radiofrequency hyperthermia device is placed against the tissue and heated to 50° C for 30 seconds. Minimal changes from hyperthermia were seen on the normal equine eye.[145] Several studies have evaluated hyperthermia in the treatment of equine SCC.[3,146,147,157] In one study, ocular SCC in eight horses was treated by radiofrequency hyperthermia, resulting in 75% complete regression and 25% partial regression. Complete regression occurred in 66% of tumors given a second hyperthermic treatment (see Table 3-6, p. 143).[146]

Brachytherapy

In brachytherapy, small gamma radioactive sources are placed on or within neoplasms, allowing a high dose of radiation to be delivered to the tissue and minimal radiation to surrounding tissues (see Fig. 3-44).[143] Brachytherapy is recommended for eyelid and conjunctival SCC but not for limbal or orbital SCC (see Box 3-3). The type of radioactive sources, surgical technique, and complications of brachytherapy for use with ocular SCC are identical to those described earlier for sarcoids.[101,148,152,156,179-181] Brachytherapy has a higher nonrecurrence rate than any other therapy (see Table 3-6, p. 143). However, the high cost and human radiation exposure risks make this mode of therapy less desirable in many cases.

Treatment Modalities Based on Anatomic Location

Eyelid SCCs are best managed by a combination of surgical excision and brachytherapy, cryotherapy, hyperthermia, or intralesional chemotherapy (see Box 3-3). The prognosis for eyelid SCC is worse compared with the other sites of the eye.[157]

The third eyelid is reported to be involved in about 30% of cases of ocular SCC[147] and is the primary site with secondary involvement of the nasal canthus conjunctiva, eyelid, and cornea in 50% to 60% of cases.[147,157]

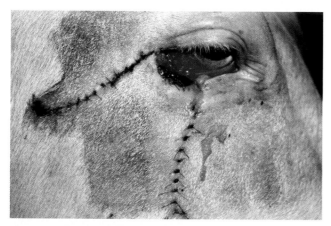

Fig. 3-50 H-plasty or advancement eyelid flap for reconstruction after excision of a lower eyelid squamous cell carcinoma. The leading edge of the flap has become necrotic, which is common after blepharospastic procedures in the horse. (Photograph courtesy Dr. Mike Davidson.)

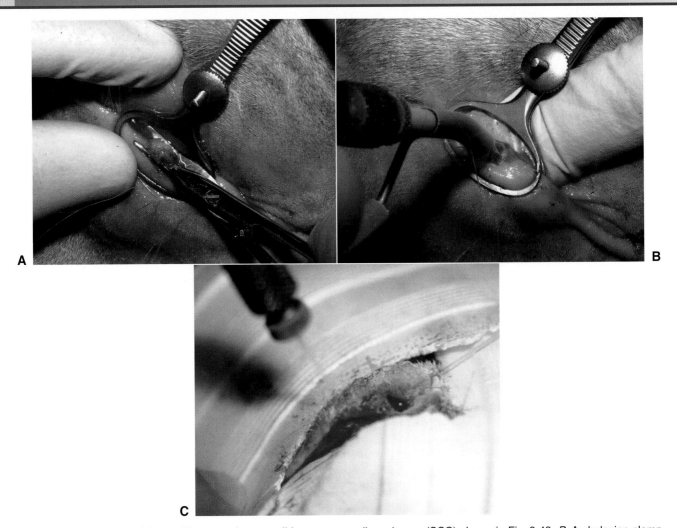

Fig. 3-51 **A,** Debulking of the papillomatous lower eyelid squamous cell carcinoma (SCC) shown in Fig. 3-48, *B.* A chalazion clamp is being used to stabilize the mass and control hemorrhage. **B,** Double freeze-thaw cryotherapy with a liquid nitrogen probe is being performed. **C,** Extensive SCC of the lower eyelid in a horse; cryotherapy is being performed with liquid nitrogen spray (double freeze-thaw). The cornea and adjacent eyelids are protected with lubrication and Styrofoam.

If the mass is at the leading edge of the third eyelid and 1 to 2 cm of normal conjunctiva surrounds the mass, then total excision of the third eyelid is generally all that is required. However, if the mass extends medially or laterally, then adjunctive therapy such as cryotherapy is recommended. Other tumors of the third eyelid, such as basal cell tumors[182] and sebaceous adenocarcinomas,[183] would be treated similarly.[184]

Palpebral conjunctival SCC is best managed by a combination of surgical excision and cryotherapy, hyperthermia, beta radiation, or carbon dioxide (CO_2) laser ablation (see Box 3-3, p. 144).[155] Bulbar conjunctival masses should be managed in the same way as limbal and corneal masses.

Two adjunctive procedures have been used to decrease the recurrence rate of corneal or limbal SCC after a superficial keratectomy: beta-irradiation with a strontium 90 probe and CO_2 laser treatment of the superficial keratectomy site (see Box 3-3, p. 144).[185-187]

Both therapies are thought to be equally effective; however, each has its advantages and disadvantages. Advantages of beta-irradiation include less postoperative inflammation and possibly less eventual fibrosis of the superficial stroma. However, the lack of availability, strict licensing, and human health risks make this mode of therapy less desirable. CO_2 laser units are becoming much more accessible, are easy to operate, and when used properly, pose little health risk.

After a complete superficial keratectomy of no deeper than one fourth of the depth of the cornea (Fig. 3-52), the CO_2 laser is used to ablate the superficial stroma and surrounding normal-appearing corneal and conjunctival epithelium. The laser (LX 20SI; Luxar, Bothell, Wash) has a 0.4-mm tip and is set at 3 J power in continuous mode. With a defocused beam, the laser is used to char the corneal tissue (Fig. 3-52). Laser energy is applied to the entire surface of the keratectomy site (Fig. 3-52). The surgeon must be careful not to allow

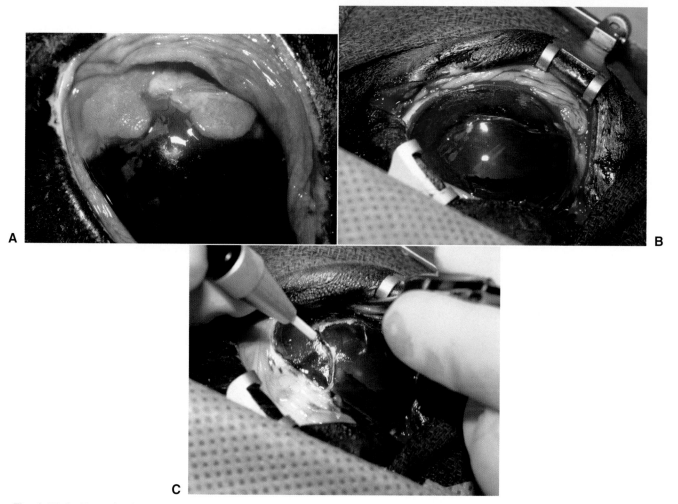

Fig. 3-52 A, Extensive lateral corneal squamous cell carcinoma (SCC) that had extended from the lateral limbus. **B,** Superficial keratectomy has been performed to remove the corneal and limbal SCC. **C,** Carbon dioxide laser ablation is being performed on the surgical bed to destroy remaining SCC cells.

deep penetration of a focused laser beam into the cornea. This could result in significant corneal scarring at best and a corneal perforation at worst. After surgery, the eye is treated for a corneal ulcer and secondary uveitis, which are always present after keratectomy and laser therapy. Topical prophylactic antibiotics (e.g., triple antibiotic ointment every 6 hours), atropine (every 12 to 24 hours), and systemic antiinflammatory medication (e.g., flunixin meglumine 0.5 mg/kg administered orally or intravenously) are typically prescribed. The eye is reevaluated every 3 to 5 days to monitor the healing of the corneal ulcer and to assess the level of uveitis. Once the cornea has re-epithelealized (i.e., no fluorescein dye retention) and if there is no corneal cellular infiltrate (i.e., a yellow-white corneal infiltrate), then topical 0.1% dexamethasone hydrochloride (every 12 hours) can be used to decrease scar formation. Penetrating keratoplasty may be required for persistent or recurrent corneal SCC.[188]

Wide surgical excision (exenteration of the orbit) is required for orbital or invasive SCC (see Box 3-3,

p. 144). See Chapter 2 for description of the surgical technique.

Long-Term Prognosis

Recurrence of ocular SCC, when all tissue sites and treatments were included, was 42.2%[4] and 30.4%[157] of cases. Mean survival after diagnosis in one study was 47 months; however, treatment before referral, multiple versus single tumors at initial examination, and treatment modality used did not influence survival.[157] Tumor location did influence survival; SCC involving the eyelid or orbit was associated with the poorest prognosis, and SCC of the limbus and third eyelid was associated with a better prognosis.[157] Larger masses, orbital extension, and recurrent SCC were associated with shorter survival time.[157] However, in another study, SCC location and treatment modality used had no influence on final outcome.[4] Instead, the willingness of owners to pursue and continue treatment of the SCC correlated with a better outcome.[4]

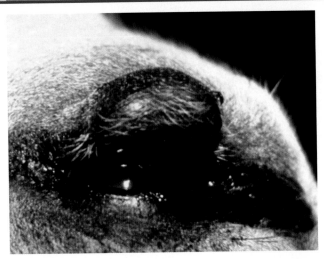

Fig. 3-53 Large upper eyelid melanoma. (Photograph courtesy Dr. Mike Davidson.)

Metastasis of ocular SCC is uncommon and was observed in 6% of cases in one study[4] and 15% in another.[155] Metastasis, when it does occur, most commonly is to the regional (submandibular) lymph nodes, salivary glands, thorax or extends into the orbit, sinus, and calvaria.

Melanoma

Melanoma is a relatively uncommon tumor of the horse involving between 3.8% and 4.8% of total neoplasms.[94-96] In one study in which 84 cases of melanoma in horses were reviewed, the most common sites of occurrence were under the tail (93.9%), the perianal region (43.0%), the lips (33.0%), and the eyelids (24.0%).[189] Melanoma usually involves the eyelids and is most common in horses with gray or white hair and skin.[3,158] A slowly progressive, cutaneous, partially alopecic, pigmented mass of the eyelids is most typical of melanoma (Fig. 3-53). Older horses are predisposed to the development of melanoma, possibly because proliferation of melanocytes is a manifestation of aging.[158,190] Fleury[191] found that melanoma development, size of mass, and number of masses were significantly correlated with older Camargue-type gray-skinned horses (a prevalence of 67% at ages >15 years). Development of melanoma was not associated with sex or sun exposure.[191] In a study of 296 gray Lipizzaner horses, dermal melanomas were found in 148 (50%), with a higher incidence in older horses.[192] Genetic predisposition in the development of dermal melanoma was also suggested.[192]

The size and location of the mass will dictate the clinical signs, varying from no irritation on masses adjacent to the lower eyelid to blepharospasm and corneal irritation on masses of the upper eyelid. A malignant conjunctival melanoma in a horse has been described.[193]

Common Differential Diagnoses

Melanoma of the eyelids needs to be differentiated from other causes of eyelid tumors or swelling such as sarcoids, habronemiasis, SCC, papilloma, lymphosarcoma, and orbital fat prolapse. Biopsy and histopathologic examination are recommended for definitive diagnosis. Four distinct clinical syndromes of dermal melanomas have been described in horses: melanocytic nevus, dermal melanoma, dermal melanomatosis, and anaplastic malignant melanoma.[194]

Equine melanomas have highly variable histologic and cytologic patterns, which can make definitive diagnosis difficult. Epithelioid, round, and spindle cell types occur in equine melanomas with variable and inconsistent tumor pigmentation. The site of the tumor, the depth of invasion, and the number of mitotic figures per high-power field are used histologically to predict biologic behavior. However, in one study, histologic characteristics of dermal melanomas were not predictive of malignancy in most horses.[195] Melanoma cells are usually positive for vimentin, S100, neuron-specific enolase, and Melan-A, and negative for cytokeratin.[196]

Currently, there is no single technique capable of differentiating benign from malignant melanocytic neoplasms or predicting survival time. In one study, most metastatic melanomas showed overexpression of p53 and demonstrated apoptosis, but no differences were observed between malignant and benign dermal melanomas in growth fraction, S-phase index, or DNA configuration.[197] It was concluded that equine melanomas had substantially different phenotypic characteristics in comparison with melanocytic tumors in dogs, cats, and humans.[197]

Treatment

There are few reports of the treatment of equine adnexal melanomas, so success rates of various treatments are not known. Before therapy is initiated, careful evaluation of the entire horse is recommended to rule out metastatic disease. The examination should include a thorough skin evaluation, oral inspection, chest radiography, rectal palpation, and inspection for masses under the tail and in the perianal area.

Medical Therapy

There are no known studies on the effectiveness of intralesional chemotherapy or immunotherapy on melanomas. Oral cimetidine (dose 2.5 mg/kg body weight, every 8 hours) has been used to shrink non-ocular melanomas in horses,[198] but no studies have been done to determine the effect of cimetidine on eyelid masses.

Surgical Therapy

Surgical excision, CO_2 laser ablation, and cryotherapy have been recommended. Success rates have not been published; however, in one study the successful removal of a nonocular dermal melanoma by CO_2 laser ablation in a horse was described.[199] Excision of an eyelid melanoma is usually curative, because most of the masses are benign. However, in a case report of a conjunctival melanoma, recurrence and metastasis were described.[193]

Long-Term Prognosis of Melanoma

Malignant melanoma does occur in horses,[56,57,189,192,193,195-197,200-202] but the overall rate of malignancy is unknown. In one study, the most common sites for metastases were the lymph nodes, liver, spleen, skeletal muscle, lungs, and vascular beds.[195] Horses may have dermal melanomas for years (range, 1 to 6 years) before metastatic disease develops.[195]

Lymphosarcoma

Lymphosarcoma is a relatively uncommon neoplasm in the horse, especially as compared with other domestic animals, such as cows, dogs, and cats.[203,204] Lymphosarcoma represented 1.3% and 4.8% of all tumors in horses in two separate studies.[94,95] Unilateral and bilateral ocular lesions have been reported with equine lymphosarcoma.[161,162,205,206]

Common Differential Diagnoses

Ocular lesions occurred in 27% of horses with systemic lymphosarcoma in one study.[161] Infiltration of the eyelids and conjunctiva is the most common ocular manifestation of lymphosarcoma (Fig. 3-54).[161,205,206] Orbital and third eyelid lesions can also be seen (Fig. 3-55).[161,206] Adnexal lymphosarcoma needs to be differentiated from other causes of eyelid tumors or

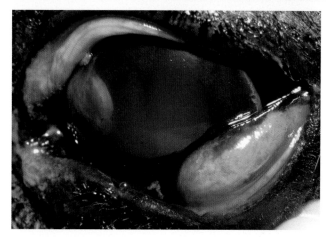

Fig. 3-54 Lower eyelid and conjunctival primary lymphosarcoma.

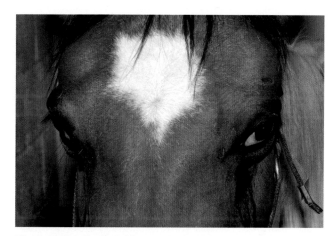

Fig. 3-55 Yearling paint horse with systemic lymphosarcoma with ocular and orbital invasion.

swelling such as sarcoids, habronemiasis, SCC, papilloma, melanoma, and orbital fat prolapse. Biopsy and histopathologic examination are required for definitive diagnosis.

Pathogenesis of Disease Process and Progression

Immunohistologic study of equine malignant lymphomas revealed that they were composed of a heterogeneous cell population with most tumors containing B and T lymphocytes.[207] In this study, 42% of the lymphomas contained primarily neoplastic B lymphocytes, 35% had diffuse large B-cell lymphoma with 40% to 80% nonneoplastic T lymphocytes (called T-cell–rich, large B-cell lymphomas), and 19% had primarily neoplastic T lymphocytes.[207]

Treatment

There are no reports of treatment of local or systemic lymphosarcoma in the horse. However, localized eyelid lesions have been successfully treated with surgical debulking and intralesional corticosteroids (Dr. Dravid Wilkie, personal communication, 2003). Further study is needed.

Long-Term Prognosis

In general, the long-term prognosis for survival is poor for horses with lymphosarcoma.[3]

Conjunctival Pseudotumors or Bilateral Nodular Lymphocytic Conjunctivitis

Conjunctival pseudotumors, or nodular lymphocytic conjunctivitis, appear as unilateral or bilateral, nodular or smooth, pink, nonulcerated conjunctival masses (Fig. 3-56).[208,209] In one study of five horses, the masses were nodular in two cases and relatively flat and more diffuse in three cases.[209] The third eyelid was involved in three cases, and the bulbar conjunctiva and cornea were involved in two cases.[209]

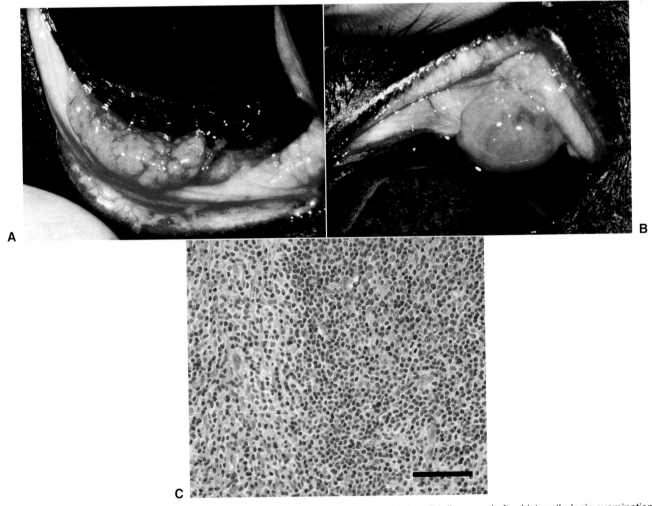

Fig. 3-56 A, Conjunctival proliferative lobulated mass at the basal portion of the third eyelid diagnosed after histopathologic examination as a nodular lymphocytic conjunctivitis or conjunctival pseudotumor. **B,** Another proliferative conjunctival mass located at the dorsal limbus, also confirmed on histopathologic examination as nodular lymphocytic conjunctivitis or conjunctival pseudotumor. **C,** On histologic examination, both masses had similar findings of a heterogeneous population of mononuclear cells with predominantly small mature lymphocytes on the right half of the field and larger histiocytes on the left half (bar = 50 μm). (Photographs courtesy Dr. Riccardo Stoppini.)

Common Differential Diagnoses

Conjunctival pseudotumors need to be differentiated from other causes of eyelid masses or swelling such as sarcoids, habronemiasis, neoplasia (e.g., SCC, papilloma, or melanoma), and orbital fat prolapse. Biopsy and histopathologic examination are required for definitive diagnosis.

On histopathologic examination, characteristic nodular lymphoid components and lymphocytes, plasma cells, and histiocytes were found.[208] The bulbar conjunctiva was infiltrated by small nodular masses composed of dense aggregates of primarily small mature lymphocytes admixed with less mature, usually intermediate-sized, lymphoblasts, histiocytes, and rare neutrophils. The cellular infiltrate often formed follicles of lymphocytic hyperplasia. Etiologic agents were not discernible when hematoxylin and eosin or other more specialized stains were used.[208,209] As determined by immunohistochemistry, scattered infiltrating cells were B lymphocytes, T lymphocytes, and macrophages and other histiocytes.[208]

Pathogenesis of Disease Process and Progression

Equine conjunctival inflammatory pseudotumor is suspected to have an immune-mediated pathogenesis because of the nature of the inflammatory cell infiltrate and the absence of infectious agents, parasites, or foreign bodies.[208,209]

Treatment

Treatment should consist of partial or complete surgical excision and local administration of antiinflammatory agents (i.e., intralesional corticosteroids with or without topical corticosteroids).[208,209]

Long-Term Prognosis

The prognosis for equine conjunctival pseudotumors appears to be good when lesions are treated as described previously.[209] Rapid recurrence of the lesions is possible and would require repeated treatment.[208]

Other Adnexal Neoplasms

Angiomas, angiosarcomas, hemangiosarcoma,[210-213] fibroma, fibrosarcoma,[153,214] adenoma, adenocarcinoma, lacrimal gland carcinoma,[94] basal cell carcinoma,[182]

and mast cell tumors have been reported to involve the eyelids or conjunctiva of horses.

Common Differential Diagnoses

As for other mass lesions of the eyelid or conjunctiva, histopathologic examination is needed to rule out exuberant granulation tissue, habronemiasis, melanoma, SCC, papilloma, and orbital fat prolapse. Immunohistochemical staining with factor VIII–related antigen will help to confirm whether the mass has a vascular endothelial origin (e.g., angiomas, angiosarcomas, hemangiosarcoma).[213,215] Vascular neoplasms must be differentiated from intravascular papillary endothelial hyperplasia, a benign proliferative lesion.[216]

Treatment

Treatment varies, depending on the neoplasm; however, excision with an adjunctive therapy such as cryotherapy is generally recommended.

FUTURE RESEARCH FOR EYELID, CONJUNCTIVAL, AND NASOLACRIMAL DISEASES

Future study is needed for many aspects of eyelid, conjunctival, and nasolacrimal diseases in the horse. The inheritance and diagnosis of the gene defect need to be determined for nearly all equine adnexal diseases, especially entropion and NLD atresia. The pharmacokinetics and ocular distribution of most systemically administered antibiotics are not known in the horse, and this information is needed to treat resistant infectious blepharitis. Enhanced imaging techniques need to be evaluated for diagnosis and monitoring of treatment for nasolacrimal drainage disorders. Earlier diagnosis and more effective treatment protocols are sorely needed for sarcoids and SCC in horses.

ACKNOWLEDGMENTS

We thank Beth Salmon, Elaine Smith, and Melissa Hammon for technical assistance and photography. We also thank Dr. Stacy Andrew for reviewing the manuscript.

REFERENCES

1. Moore CP: Eyelid and nasolacrimal disease, *Vet Clin North Am Equine Pract* 8:499-519, 1992.
2. Samuelson D: Ophthalmic anatomy In Gelatt KN, editor: *Veterinary ophthalmology,* ed 3, Baltimore, 1999, Lippincott Williams & Wilkins, pp 31-150.
3. Lavach JD: *Large animal ophthalmology,* St Louis, 1990, Mosby.
4. Schwink K: Factors influencing morbidity and outcome of equine ocular squamous cell carcinoma, *Equine Vet J* 19:198-200, 1987.
5. Firth EC: Horner's syndrome in the horse: experimental induction and a case report, *Equine Vet J* 10:9-13, 1978.
6. Simoens P et al: Horner's syndrome in the horse: a clinical, experimental and morphological study, *Equine Vet J Suppl* 10: 62-65, 1990.
7. Wyman M, Anderson BG: Anatomy of the equine eye and orbit: gross anatomy of the lids, *J Small Anim Pract* 2:307-311, 1978.
8. Anderson B, Wyman M: Anatomy of the equine eye and orbit: histological structure and blood supply of the eyelids, *J Equine Med Surg* 3:4-14, 1979.
9. Williams RD, Manning JP, Peiffer RL Jr: The Schirmer tear test in the equine: normal values and the contribution of the gland of the nictitating membrane, *J Equine Med Surg* 3:117-119, 1979.
10. Joyce J, Bratton G: Keratoconjunctivitis sicca secondary to fracture of the mandible, *Vet Med* 68:619-620, 1973.
11. Speiss B, Wilcock B, Phyick-Sheard P: Eosinophilic granulomatous dacryadenitis causing bilateral keratoconjunctivitis sicca in a horse, *Equine Vet J* 21:226-228, 1989.
12. Spurlock SL, Spurlock GH, Wise M: Keratoconjunctivitis sicca associated with fracture of the stylohyoid bone in a horse, *J Am Vet Med Assoc* 194:258-259, 1989.
13. Freestone JF, Seahorn TL: Miscellaneous conditions of the equine head, *Vet Clin North Am Equine Pract* 9:235-242, 1993.
14. Latimer CA et al: Radiographic and gross anatomy of the nasolacrimal duct of the horse, *Am J Vet Res* 45:451-458, 1984.
15. United States Department of Agriculture: Equine morbidity and mortality: national health monitoring system, *USDA:APHIS* 1998, pp.
16. Latimer CA, Wyman M: Neonatal ophthalmology, *Vet Clin North Am Equine Pract* 1:235-259, 1985.
17. Barnett K: The eye of the newborn foal, *J Reprod Fertil Suppl* 23:701-703, 1975.
18. Brooks DE: Equine ophthalmology In Gelatt KN, editor: *Veterinary ophthalmology,* ed 3, Philadelphia, 1999, Lippincott Williams & Wilkins, pp 1053-1116.
19. Fox L, Thurmon J: Bilateral ankyloblepharon in a newborn foal, *Vet Med Small Anim Clin* 63:237-238, 1969.
20. Grant B, Slatter DH, Dunlap JS: *Thelazia* sp. (Nematoda) and dermoid cysts in a horse with torticollis, *Vet Med Small Anim Clin* 68:62-64, 1973.
21. Priester WA: Congenital ocular defects in cattle, horses, cats, and dogs, *J Am Vet Med Assoc* 160:1504-1511, 1972.
22. Mason TA: Atresia of the nasolacrimal orifice in two Thoroughbreds, *Equine Vet J* 11:19-20, 1979.
23. Lundvall R, Carter J: Atresia of the nasolacrimal meatus in the horse, *J Am Vet Med Assoc* 159:289-291, 1971.
24. Theoret CL, Grahn BH, Fretz PB: Incomplete nasomaxillary dysplasia in a foal, *Can Vet J* 38:445-447, 1997.
25. Latimer CA, Wyman M: Atresia of the nasolacrimal duct in three horses, *J Am Vet Med Assoc* 184:989-992, 1984.
26. Schoster J: Surgical repair of equine eyelid lacerations, *Vet Med* 83:1042-1049, 1988.
27. Rebhun WC: Repair of eyelid lacerations in horses, *Vet Med Small Anim Clin* 75:1281-1284, 1980.
28. Boulton CB, Campbell K: Equine recurrent blepharitis and ulcerative keratitis, *Vet Med Small Anim Clin* 22:1057-1058, 1982.
29. Hughes DE, Pugh GW Jr: Isolation and description of a Moraxella from horses with conjunctivitis, *Am J Vet Res* 31:457-462, 1970.
30. Connole M: Equine phycomycosis, *Aust Vet J* 49:214-215, 1973.
31. Singh T: Studies on epizootic lymphagitis, *Indian J Vet Sci* 36: 45-59, 1966.
32. Rebhun WC et al: Habronemic blepharoconjunctivitis in horses, *J Am Vet Med Assoc* 179:469-472, 1981.
33. Moore CP, Sarazan R, Whitley RD: Equine ocular parasites: a review, *Equine Vet J (Suppl)* 2:76-85, 1983.
34. Lyons ET et al: Prevalence of selected species of internal parasites in equids at necropsy in central Kentucky (1995-1999), *Vet Parasitol* 92:51-62, 2000.
35. Desch CE Jr, Nutting WB: Redescription of Demodex caballi (= D. folliculorum var. equi Railliet, 1895) from the horse, Equus caballus, *Acarologia* 20:235-240, 1979.
36. Glaze MB: Equine Adnexal habronemiasis. *Equine Vet J Suppl 2* pp. 71-76, 1983.
37. Joyce JR, Hanselka DW, Boyd CL: Treatment of habronemiasis of the adnexa of the equine eye, *Vet Med Small Anim Clin* 22:1008-1009, 1972.
38. Patton S, McCracken MD: The occurrence and effect of Thelazia in horses, *Equine Pract* 3:53-55, 1981.
39. Vasey JR: Equine cutaneous habronemiasis, *Comp Contin Educ Pract Vet* 3:290-298, 1981.
40. Ramsey DT et al: Eosinophilic keratoconjunctivitis in a horse, *J Am Vet Med Assoc* 205:1308-1311, 1994.
41. Yamagata M, Wilkie DA, Gilger BC: Eosinophilic keratoconjunctivitis in seven horses, *J Am Vet Med Assoc* 209:1283-1286, 1996.
42. Pusterla N et al: Cutaneous and ocular habronemiasis in horses: 63 cases (1988-2002), *J Am Vet Med Assoc* 222:978-982, 2003.
43. Herd RP, Donham JC: Efficacy of ivermectin against cutaneous *Draschia* and *Habronema* infection (summer sores) in horses, *Am J Vet Res* 42:1953-1955, 1981.
44. Dugan SJ et al: Epidemiologic study of ocular/adnexal squamous cell carcinoma in horses, *J Am Vet Med Assoc* 198:251-256, 1991.
45. Miller W: Aberrant cilia as an aetiology for recurrent corneal ulcers: a case report, *Equine Vet J* 20:145-146, 1988.
46. Vestre WA, Brightman AH: Correction of cicatricial entropion and trichiasis in the horse, *Equine Pract* 2:13-16, 1980.
47. Wilkinson JD: Distichiasis in the horse treated by partial tarsal plate excision, *Vet Rec* 94:128-129, 1974.
48. Rebhun W, Georgi M, Georgi J: Persistent corneal ulcers in horses caused by embedded burdock pappus bristles, *Vet Med* 86:930-935, 1991.
49. Hamor RE, Whelan NC: Equine infectious keratitis, *Vet Clin North Am Equine Pract* 15:623-646, 1999.
50. Kershaw O et al: Detection of equine herpesvirus type 2 (EHV-2) in horses with keratoconjunctivitis, *Virus Res* 80:93-99, 2001.
51. Andrew SE et al: Equine ulcerative keratomycosis: visual outcome and ocular survival in 39 cases (1987-1996), *Equine Vet J* 30:109-116, 1998.
52. Gratzek AT et al: Ophthalmic cyclosporine in equine keratitis and keratouveitis: 11 cases, *Equine Vet J* 27:327-333, 1995.
53. McLellan GL, Archer FJ: Corneal stromal sequestration and keratoconjunctivitis sicca in a horse, *Vet Ophthalmol* 3:207-212, 2000.
54. Moore CP et al: Post traumatic keratouveitis in horses, *Equine Vet J* 30:366-372, 1998.
55. Gilger B: How to perform standing ocular surgery in the horse. Proceedings of *Am Assoc Equine Practitioners* 48:43-55, 2002.
56. Milne JC: Malignant melanomas causing Horner's syndrome in a horse, *Equine Vet J* 18:74-75, 1984.
57. Murray MJ et al: Signs of sympathetic denervation associated with a thoracic melanoma in a horse, *J Vet Intern Med* 11:199-203, 1997.

58. Bacon CL et al: Bilateral Horner's syndrome secondary to metastatic squamous cell carcinoma in a horse, *Equine Vet J* 28:500-503, 1996.

59. Sweeney RW, Sweeney CR: Transient Horner's syndrome following routine intravenous injections in two horses, *J Am Vet Med Assoc* 185:802-803, 1984.

60. Purohit RC, McCoy MD, Bergfeld WA III: Thermographic diagnosis of Horner's syndrome in the horse, *Am J Vet Res* 41:1180-1182, 1980.

61. Craig DR et al: Esophageal disorders in 61 horses. Results of nonsurgical and surgical management, *Vet Surg* 18:432-438, 1989.

62. Skarda RT, Muir WW, Couri D: Plasma lidocaine concentrations in conscious horses after cervicothoracic (stellate) ganglion block with 1% lidocaine HCl solution, *Am J Vet Res* 48:1092-1097, 1987.

63. Skarda RT et al: Cervicothoracic (stellate) ganglion block in conscious horses, *Am J Vet Res* 47:21-26, 1986.

64. Morgan RV, Zanotti SW: Horner's syndrome in dogs and cats: 49 cases (1980-1986), *J Am Vet Med Assoc* 194:1096-1099, 1989.

65. Bistner S et al: Pharmacologic diagnosis of Horner's syndrome in the dog, *J Am Vet Med Assoc* 157:1220-1224, 1970.

66. Tyler CM et al: A survey of neurological diseases in horses, *Aust Vet J* 70:445-449, 1993.

67. Yadernuk LM: Temporohyoid osteoarthropathy and unilateral facial nerve paralysis in a horse, *Can Vet J* 44:990-992, 2003.

68. Waldridge BM, Holland M, Taintor J: What is your neurologic diagnosis? Stylohyoid bone fracture and possible petrous temporal bone fracture, *J Am Vet Med Assoc* 222:587-589, 2003.

69. Grandy JL et al: Arterial hypotension and the development of postanesthetic myopathy in halothane-anesthetized horses, *Am J Vet Res* 48:192-197, 1987.

70. MacKay RJ et al: Equine protozoal myeloencephalitis, *Vet Clin North Am Equine Pract* 16:405-425, 2000.

71. Gray LC et al: Suspected protozoal myeloencephalitis in a two-month-old colt, *Vet Rec* 149:269-273, 2001.

72. Furr M et al: Clinical diagnosis of equine protozoal myeloencephalitis (EPM), *J Vet Intern Med* 16:618-621, 2002.

73. Lavach JD, Severin GA: Neoplasia of the equine eye, adnexa, and orbit: a review of 68 cases, *J Am Vet Med Assoc* 170:202-203, 1977.

74. Rebhun WC: Tumors of the eye and ocular adnexal tissues, *Vet Clin North Am Equine Pract* 14:579-606, vii, 1998.

75. Barnett KC, Cottrell BC, Rest JR: Retrobulbar hydatid cyst in the horse, *Equine Vet J* 20:136-138, 1988.

76. Freestone JF et al: Ultrasonic identification of an orbital tumor in a horse, *Equine Vet J* 21:135-136, 1989.

77. Green SL et al: Tetanus in the horse: a review of 20 cases (1970 to 1990), *J Vet Intern Med* 8:128-132, 1994.

78. Madigan JE et al: Muscle spasms associated with ear tick (*Otobius megnini*) infestations in five horses, *J Am Vet Med Assoc* 207:74-76, 1995.

79. Vestre WA, Steckel RR: Episcleral prolapse of orbital fat in the horse, *Equine Pract* 5:135-137, 1983.

80. Bedford PGC et al: Partial prolapse of the antero-medial corpus adiposium in the horse, *Equine Vet J* 10:2-4, 1990.

81. Wilson D, Levine SA: Surgical reconstruction of the nasolacrimal system in the horse, *J Equine Vet Sci* 11:232-234, 1991.

82. Cruz AM, Barber SM, Grahn BH: Nasolacrimal duct injury following periorbital trauma with concurrent retinal choroidal detachment in a horse, *Equine Pract* 19:20-23, 1997.

83. McIlnay TR, Miller SM, Dugan SJ: Use of canaliculorhinostomy for repair of nasolacrimal duct obstruction in a horse, *J Am Vet Med Assoc* 218:1323-1324, 1271, 2001.

84. Nykamp SG, Scrivani PV, Pease AP: Computed tomography dacryocystography evaluation of the nasolacrimal apparatus, *Vet Radiol Ultrasound* 45:23-28, 2004.

85. Schumacher J, Dean P, Welch B: Epistaxis in two horses with dacryohemorrhea, *J Am Vet Med Assoc* 200:366-367, 1992.

86. Reilly L, Beech J: Bilateral keratoconjunctivitis sicca in a horse, *Equine Vet J* 26:171-172, 1994.

87. Crispin SM. Tear-deficient and evaporative dry eye syndromes of the horse. *Vet Ophthalmol* 3:87-92, 2000.

88. Kaswan R, Salisbury M, Ward D: Spontaneous canine keratoconjunctivitis sicca. A useful model for human keratoconjunctivitis sicca: treatment with cyclosporine eye drops, *Arch Ophthalmol* 107:1210-1216, 1989.

89. Kaswan RL, Martin CL, Dawe DL: Keratoconjunctivitis sicca: immunological evaluation of 62 canine cases, *Am J Vet Res* 46:376-383, 1985.

90. Kaswan RL, Martin CL, Chapman WL Jr: Keratoconjunctivitis sicca: histopathologic study of nictitating membrane and lacrimal glands from 28 days, *Am J Vet Res* 45:112-118, 1984.

91. Brightman AH et al: Decreased tear production associated with general anesthesia in the horse, *J Am Vet Med Assoc* 182:243-244, 1983.

92. Beech J et al: Schirmer tear test results in normal horses and ponies: effect of age, season, environment, sex, time of day and placement of strips, *Vet Ophthalmol* 6:251-254, 2003.

93. Wolf ED, Merideth R: Parotic duct transposition in the horse, *J Equine Vet Sci* 1:143-145, 1981.

94. Sundberg JP et al: Neoplasms of equidae, *J Am Vet Med Assoc* 170:150-152, 1977.

95. Baker JR, Leyland A: Histological survey of tumours of the horse, with particular reference to those of the skin, *Vet Rec* 96:419-422, 1975.

96. Cotchin E: A general survey of tumours in the horse, *Equine Vet J* 9:16-21, 1977.

97. Ragland WL, Keown GH, Spencer GR: Equine sarcoid, *Equine Vet J* 2:2-11, 1970.

98. Genetzky RM, Biwer RD, Myers RK: Equine sarcoids: causes, diagnosis, and treatment, *Comp Contin Educ Pract Vet* 5:S416-S420, 1983.

99. Murphy JM et al: Immunotherapy in ocular equine sarcoid, *J Am Vet Med Assoc* 174:269-273, 1979.

100. Lavach JD et al: BCG treatment of periocular sarcoid, *Equine Vet J* 17:445-448, 1985.

101. Theon AP, Pascoe JR: Iridium-192 interstitial brachytherapy for equine periocular tumours: treatment results and prognostic factors in 115 horses, *Equine Vet J* 27:117-121, 1995.

102. Marti E et al: Report of the first international workshop on equine sarcoid, *Equine Vet J* 25:397-407, 1993.

103. Knottenbelt DC, Kelly DF: The diagnosis and treatment of periorbital sarcoid in the horse: 445 cases from 1974 to 1999, *Vet Ophthalmol* 3:169-191, 2000.

104. Martens A et al: Histopathological characteristics of five clinical types of equine sarcoid, *Res Vet Sci* 69:295-300, 2000.

105. Angelos J et al: Evaluation of breed as a risk factor for sarcoid and uveitis in horses, *Anim Genet* 19:417-425, 1988.

106. Knottenbelt DC, Matthews JB: A positive step forwards in the diagnosis of equine sarcoid, *Vet J* 161:224-226, 2001.

107. Ragland WL, Keown GH, Gorham JR: An epizootic of equine sarcoid, *Nature* 210:1399, 1966.

108. Ragland WL, Spencer GR: Attempts to relate bovine papilloma virus to the cause of equine sarcoid: immunity to bovine papilloma virus, *Am J Vet Res* 29:1363-1366, 1968.

109. Voss JL: Transmission of equine sarcoid, *Am J Vet Res* 30:183-191, 1969.

110. Ragland WL, McLaughlin CA, Spencer GR: Attempts to relate bovine papilloma virus to the cause of equine sarcoid: horses, donkeys and calves inoculated with equine sarcoid extracts, *Equine Vet J* 2:168-172, 1970.

111. England J, Watson RE Jr, Larson KA: Virus-like particles in an equine sarcoid cell line, *Am J Vet Res* 34:1601-1603, 1973.

112. Nasir L et al: Screening for bovine papillomavirus in peripheral blood cells of donkeys with and without sarcoids, *Res Vet Sci* 63:289-290, 1997.

113. Nasir L, Reid SW: Bovine papillomaviral gene expression in equine sarcoid tumours, *Virus Res* 61:171-175, 1999.

114. Carr EA et al: Expression of a transforming gene (E5) of bovine papillomavirus in sarcoids obtained from horses, *Am J Vet Res* 62:1212-1217, 2001.

115. Martens A, De Moor A, Ducatelle R: PCR detection of bovine papilloma virus DNA in superficial swabs and scrapings from equine sarcoids, *Vet J* 161:280-286, 2001.

116. Chambers G et al: Sequence variants of bovine papillomavirus E5 detected in equine sarcoids, *Virus Res* 96:141-145, 2003.

117. Chambers G et al: Association of bovine papillomavirus with the equine sarcoid, *J Gen Virol* 84:1055-1062, 2003.

118. Olsen C, Cook R: Cutaneous sarcoma-like lesions of the horse caused by the agent of bovine papilloma, *Proc Soc Exp Biol Med* 77:281-284, 1951.

119. Angelos JA et al: Characterization of BPV-like DNA in equine sarcoids, *Arch Virol* 119:95-109, 1991.

120. Martens A et al: Polymerase chain reaction analysis of the surgical margins of equine sarcoids for bovine papilloma virus DNA, *Vet Surg* 30:460-467, 2001.

121. Otten N et al: DNA of bovine papillomavirus type 1 and 2 in equine sarcoids: PCR detection and direct sequencing, *Arch Virol* 132:121-131, 1993.

122. Bucher K et al: Tumour suppressor gene p53 in the horse: identification, cloning, sequencing and a possible role in the pathogenesis of equine sarcoid, *Res Vet Sci* 61:114-119, 1996.

123. Argyle D et al: Equine telomeres and telomerase in cellular immortalisation and ageing, *Mech Ageing Dev* 124:759-764, 2003.

124. Lazary S et al: Equine leucocyte antigens in sarcoid-affected horses, *Equine Vet J* 17:283-286, 1985.

125. Gerber H, Dubath M, Lazary S: Association between predisposition to equine sarcoid and MHC in multiple-case families. In Powell D, editor: *Equine infectious diseases,* Lexington, 1998, The University Press of Kentucky, pp 272-277.

126. Brostrom H: Equine sarcoids: a clinical and epidemiological study in relation to equine leucocyte antigens (ELA), *Acta Vet Scand* 36:223-236, 1995.

127. Ding Q et al: DNA-PKcs mutations in dogs and horses: allele frequency and association with neoplasia, *Gene* 283:263-269, 2002.

128. Wyman M et al: Immunotherapy in equine sarcoid: a report of two cases, *J Am Vet Med Assoc* 171:449-451, 1977.

129. Webster CJ, Webster JM: Treatment of equine sarcoids with BCG, *Vet Rec* 116:131-132, 1985.

130. Owen RA, Jagger DW: Clinical observations on the use of BCG cell wall fraction for treatment of periocular and other equine sarcoids, *Vet Rec* 120:548-552, 1987.

131. Klein WR et al: The present status of BCG treatment in the veterinary practice, *In Vivo* 5:605-608, 1991.

132. Kinnunen RE et al: Equine sarcoid tumour treated by autogenous tumour vaccine, *Anticancer Res* 19:3367-3374, 1999.

133. Otten N et al: Experimental treatment of equine sarcoid using a xanthate compound and recombinant human tumour necrosis factor alpha, *Zentralbl Veterinarmed A* 41:757-765, 1994.

134. Tamzali Y, Teissie J, Rols M: First horse sarcoid treatment by electrochemotherapy: preliminary experimental results. Proceedings of *Am Assoc Equine Practitioners* 49:72-78, 2003.

135. Theon AP et al: Intratumoral chemotherapy with cisplatin in oily emulsion in horses, *J Am Vet Med Assoc* 202:261-267, 1993.

136. Theon AP et al: Comparison of perioperative versus postoperative intratumoral administration of cisplatin for treatment of cutaneous sarcoids and squamous cell carcinomas in horses, *J Am Vet Med Assoc* 215:1655-1660, 1999.

137. Fortier LA, MacHarg MA: Topical use of 5-fluorouracil for treatment of squamous cell carcinoma of the external genitalia of horses: 11 cases (1988-1992), *J Am Vet Med Assoc* 25:1183-1185, 1994.

138. Wilson D, Peyton L, Wolf G: Immediate split-thickness autogenous skin grafts in the horse, *Vet Surg* 16:167-171, 1987.

139. Palmer S: Carbon dioxide laser removal of verrucous sarcoid from the ear of a horse, *J Am Vet Med Assoc* 195:1125-1127, 1989.

140. Farris HE, Fraunfelder FT, Mason CT: Cryotherapy of equine sarcoid and other lesions, *Vet Med Sm Anim Clin* 12:325-329, 1965.

141. Joyce JR: Cryosurgery for removal of equine sarcoids, *Vet Med Small Anim Clin* 70:200-203, 1975.

142. Lane JG: The treatment of equine sarcoids by cryosurgery, *Equine Vet J* 9:127-133, 1977.

143. Houlton JEF: Treatment of periocular equine sarcoids, *Equine Vet J Suppl* 2:117-122, 1983.

144. Harris H, Fraunfelder FT, Mason CT: Cryotherapy of equine sarcoid and other lesions, *Vet Med Small Anim Pract* 71:325-329, 1976.

145. Neumann SM, Kainer RA, Severin GA: Reaction of normal equine eyes to radio-frequency current-induced hyperthermia, *Am J Vet Res* 43:1938-1944, 1982.

146. Grier RL et al: Treatment of bovine and equine ocular squamous cell carcinoma by radiofrequency hyperthermia, *J Am Vet Med Assoc* 177:55-61, 1980.

147. King TC et al: Therapeutic management of ocular squamous cell carcinoma in the horse: 43 cases (1979-1989), *Equine Vet J* 23:449-452, 1991.

148. Lewis RE: Radon implant therapy of squamous cell carcinoma and equine sarcoid, *Proc Am Assoc Equine Pract* 10:217-233, 1964.

149. Walker M et al: Iridium-192 brachytherapy for equine sarcoid, one and two year remission rates, *Vet Radiol* 32:206-208, 1991.

150. Frauenfelder HC, Blevins WE, Page EH: 222Rn for treatment of periocular fibrous connective tissue sarcomas in the horse, *J Am Vet Med Assoc* 180:310-312, 1982.

151. Turrel J, Stover S, Gyorgyfalvy J: Iridium-192 interstitial brachytherapy of equine sarcoid, *Vet Radiol Ultrasound* 26:20-24, 1985.

152. Wyn-Jones G: Treatment of periocular tumours of horses using radioactive gold198 grains, *Equine Vet J* 11:3-10, 1979.

153. Hilmas DE, Gillette EL: Radiotherapy of spontaneous fibrous connective-tissue sarcomas in animals, *J Natl Cancer Inst* 56:365-368, 1976.

154. Slatter DH, Nelson A, Smith G: Ocular sequelae of high-dose periocular gamma irradiation in a horse, *Equine Vet J Suppl* 2:110-111, 1983.

155. Gelatt KN et al: Conjunctival squamous cell carcinoma in the horse, *J Am Vet Med Assoc* 165:617-620, 1974.

156. Walker M, Goble D, Geiser D: Two-year non-recurrence rates for equine ocular and periorbital squamous cell carcinoma following radiotherapy, *Vet Radiol* 27:146-148, 1986.

157. Dugan SJ et al: Prognostic factors and survival of horses with ocular/adnexal squamous cell carcinoma: 147 cases (1978-1988), *J Am Vet Med Assoc* 198:298-303, 1991.

158. Dugan SJ: Ocular neoplasia, *Vet Clin North Am Equine Pract* 8:609-626, 1992.

159. Vestre WA, Turner TA, Carlton WW: Conjunctival hemangioma in a horse, *J Am Vet Med Res* 180:1481-1482, 1982.

160. Turner LM, Whitley RD, Hager D: Management of ocular trauma in horses. II. Orbit, eyelids, uvea, lens, retina and optic nerve. *Mod Vet Pract* 10:341-347, 1986.

161. Rebhun WC, Del Piero F: Ocular lesions in horses with lymphosarcoma: 21 cases (1977-1997), *J Am Vet Med Assoc* 212:852-854, 1998.

162. Rebhun WC, Bertone A: Equine lymphosarcoma, *J Am Vet Med Assoc* 184:720-721, 1984.

163. Goodrich L et al: Equine sarcoids, *Vet Clin North Am Equine Pract* 14:607-623, vii, 1998.

164. Peiffer R et al: Fundamentals of veterinary ophthalmic pathology. In Gelatt KN, editor: *Veterinary ophthalmology,* ed 3, Philadelphia, 1999, Lippincott Williams & Wilkins, pp 355-426.

165. Perez J et al: Immunohistochemical study of the inflammatory infiltrate associated with equine squamous cell carcinoma, *J Comp Pathol* 121:385-397, 1999.

166. Junge RE, Sundberg JP, Lancaster WD: Papillomas and squamous cell carcinomas of horses, *J Am Vet Med Assoc* 185:656-659, 1984.

167. Sironi G et al: p53 Protein expression in conjunctival squamous cell carcinomas of domestic animals, *Vet Ophthalmol* 2:227-231, 1999.

168. Pazzi KA et al: Analysis of the equine tumor suppressor gene p53 in the normal horse and in eight cutaneous squamous cell carcinomas, *Cancer Lett* 107:125-130, 1996.

169. Teifke JP, Lohr CV: Immunohistochemical detection of P53 overexpression in paraffin wax-embedded squamous cell carcinomas of cattle, horses, cats and dogs, *J Comp Pathol* 114:205-210, 1996.

170. McCalla TL, Moore CP, Collier LL: Immunotherapy of periocular squamous cell carcinoma with metastasis in a pony, *J Am Vet Med Assoc* 200:1678-1681, 1992.

171. Theon AP, Pascoe JR, Meagher DM: Perioperative intratumoral administration of cisplatin for treatment of cutaneous tumors in Equidae, *J Am Vet Med Assoc* 205:1170-1176, 1994.

172. Moore AS et al: Long-term control of mucocutaneous squamous cell carcinoma and metastases in a horse using piroxicam, *Equine Vet J* 35:715-718, 2003.

173. Gelatt KN: Blepharoplastic procedures in horses, *J Am Vet Med Assoc* 151:27-44, 1967.

174. Beard WL, Wilkie DA: Partial orbital rim resection, mesh skin expansion, and second intention healing combined with enucleation or exenteration for extensive periocular tumors in horses, *Vet Ophthalmol* 5:23-28, 2002.

175. Joyce JR: Cryosurgical treatment of tumors of horses and cattle, *J Am Vet Med Assoc* 168:226-229, 1976.

176. Hilbert BJ, Farrel RK, Grant BD: Cryotherapy of periocular squamous cell carcinoma in the horse, *J Am Vet Med Assoc* 170:1305-1308, 1977.

177. Schoster J: Using combined excision and cryotherapy to treat limbal squamous cell carcinoma, *Vet Med* 32:357-365, 1992.

178. Harling D, Peiffer RL, Cook C: Excision and cryosurgical treatment of five cases of squamous cell carcinoma in the horse, *Equine Vet J Suppl* 2:105-109, 1983.

179. Gavin P, Gillette E: Interstitial radiation therapy of equine squamous cell carcinomas, *Vet Radiol Ultrasound* 19:138-141, 1978.

180. Chahory S et al: Treatment of a recurrent ocular squamous cell carcinoma in a horse with iridium-192 implantation, *J Equine Vet Sci* 22:503-506, 2002.

181. Wilkie DA, Burt J: Combined treatment of ocular squamous cell carcinoma, using radiofrequency hyperthermia and interstitial 198Au implants, *J Am Vet Med Assoc* 196:1831-1833, 1990.

182. Baril C: Basal cell tumour of third eyelid in a horse, *Can Vet J* 14:66-67, 1973.

183. Kunze DJ, Schmidt GM, Tvedten HW: Sebaceous adenocarcinoma of the third eyelid of a horse, *Am Anim Hosp Assoc* 3:452-455, 1979.

184. van der Linde-Sipman JS, van der Gaag I, van der Velden MA: Solid carcinoma of the glandula superficialis palpebrae tertiae in a horse, *Zentralbl Veterinarmed A* 33:208-211, 1986.

185. Frauenfelder HC, Blevins WE, Page EH: 90Sr for treatment of periocular squamous cell carcinoma in the horse, *J Am Vet Med Assoc* 180:307-309, 1982.

186. Rebhun WC: Treatment of advanced squamous cell carcinomas involving the equine cornea, *Vet Surg* 19:297-302, 1990.

187. English RE, Nasisse MP, Davidson MG: Carbon dioxide laser ablation for treatment of limbal squamous cell, *J Am Vet Med Assoc* 196:439-442, 1990.

188. van der Woerdt A, Gilger BC, Wilkie DA: Penetrating keratoplasty for treatment of recurrent squamous cell carcinoma of the cornea in a horse, *J Am Vet Med Assoc* 208:1692-1694, 1996.

189. Fleury C et al: The study of cutaneous melanomas in Camargue-type gray-skinned horses. I. Clinical-pathological characterization, *Pigment Cell Res* 13:39-46, 2000.

190. Ohmuro K et al: Morphogenesis of compound melanosomes in melanoma cells of a gray horse, *J Vet Med Sci* 55:677-680, 1993.

191. Fleury C et al: The study of cutaneous melanomas in Camargue-type gray-skinned horses. II. Epidemiological survey, *Pigment Cell Res* 13:47-51, 2000.

192. Seltenhammer MH et al: Equine melanoma in a population of 296 grey Lipizzaner horses, *Equine Vet J* 35:153-157, 2003.

193. Moore CP et al: Conjunctival malignant melanoma in a horse, *Vet Ophthalmol* 3:201-206, 2000.

194. Valentine BA: Equine melanocytic tumors: a retrospective study of 53 horses (1988 to 1991), *J Vet Intern Med* 9:291-297, 1995.

195. MacGillivray KC, Sweeney RW, Del Piero F: Metastatic melanoma in horses, *J Vet Intern Med* 16:452-456, 2002.

196. Smith SH, Goldschmidt MH, McManus PM: A comparative review of melanocytic neoplasms, *Vet Pathol* 39:651-678, 2002.

197. Roels S et al: Proliferation, DNA ploidy, p53 overexpression and nuclear DNA fragmentation in six equine melanocytic tumours, *J Vet Med A Physiol Pathol Clin Med* 47:439-448, 2000.

198. Goetz T et al: Cimetidine for treatment of melanomas in three horses, *J Am Vet Med Assoc* 196:449-452, 1990.

199. McCauley CT et al: Use of a carbon dioxide laser for surgical management of cutaneous masses in horses: 32 cases (1993-2000), *J Am Vet Med Assoc* 220:1192-1197, 2002.

200. Rodriguez F et al: Metastatic melanoma causing spinal cord compression in a horse, *Vet Rec* 142:248-249, 1998.

201. Patterson-Kane JC et al: Disseminated metastatic intramedullary melanoma in an aged grey horse, *J Comp Pathol* 125:204-207, 2001.

202. Tarrant J et al: Diagnosis of malignant melanoma in a horse from cytology of body cavity fluid and blood, *Equine Vet J* 33:531-534, 2001.

203. Malatestinic A: Bilateral exophthalmos in a Holstein cow with lymphosarcoma, *Can Vet J* 44:664-666, 2003.

204. Dobson JM et al: Prognostic variables in canine multicentric lymphosarcoma, *J Small Anim Pract* 42:377-384, 2001.

205. Murphy CJ et al: Bilateral eyelid swelling attributable to lymphosarcoma in a horse, *J Am Vet Med Assoc* 194:939-942, 1989.

206. Glaze MB et al: A case of equine adnexal lymphosarcoma, *Equine Vet J Suppl* 10:83-84, 1990.

207. Kelley LC, Mahaffey EA: Equine malignant lymphomas: morphologic and immunohistochemical classification, *Vet Pathol* 35:241-252, 1998.

208. Stoppini R et al: Bilateral nodular lymphocytic conjunctivitis in a horse, *Vet Ophthalmol* 2004;In press.

209. Moore CP et al: Equine conjunctival pseudotumors, *Vet Ophthalmol* 3:57-63, 2000.

210. Bolton JR et al: Ocular neoplasms of vascular origin in the horse, *Equine Vet J Suppl* 10:73-75, 1990.

211. Hacker DV, Moore PF, Buyukmihci NC: Ocular angiosarcoma in four horses, *J Am Vet Med Assoc* 189:200-203, 1986.

212. Hargis AM, McElwain TF: Vascular neoplasia in the skin of horses, *J Am Vet Med Assoc* 184:1121-1124, 1984.

213. Moore PF, Hacker DV, Buyukmihci NC: Ocular angiosarcoma in the horse: morphological and immunohistochemical studies, *Vet Pathol* 23:240-244, 1986.

214. Fatemi-Nainie S, Anderson LW, Cheevers WP: Identification of a transforming retrovirus from cultured equine dermal fibrosarcoma, *Virology* 120:490-494, 1982.

215. Johnson GC et al: Histologic and immunohistochemical characterization of hemangiomas in the skin of seven young horses, *Vet Pathol* 33:142-149, 1996.

216. Herrera HD et al: Intravascular papillary endothelial hyperplasia of the conjunctiva in a horse, *Vet Ophthalmol* 6:269-272, 2003.

217. Huntington PJ et al: Isolation of a *Moraxella* sp from horses with conjunctivitis, *Aust Vet J* 64:118-119, 1987.

218. Dalgleish R et al: An outbreak of strangles in young ponies, *Vet Rec* 132:528-531, 1993.

219. McChesney AE, Becerra V, England JJ: Chlamydial polyarthritis in a foal, *J Am Vet Med Assoc* 165:259-261, 1974.

220. Borchers K et al: Virological and molecular biological investigations into equine herpes virus type 2 (EHV-2) experimental infections, *Virus Res* 55:101-106, 1998.

221. Collinson PN, et al: Isolation of equine herpesvirus type 2 (equine gammaherpesvirus 2) from foals with keratoconjunctivitis, *J Am Vet Med Assoc* 205:329-331, 1994.

222. Studdert MJ: Equine herpesviruses. IV. Concurrent infection in horses with strangles and conjunctivitis, *Aust Vet J* 47:434-436, 1971.

223. Holyoak GR et al: Pathological changes associated with equine arteritis virus infection of the reproductive tract in prepubertal and peripubertal colts, *J Comp Pathol* 109:281-293, 1993.

224. Jones TC: Clinical and pathologic features of equine viral arteritis, *J Am Vet Med Assoc* 155:315-317, 1969.

225. Wood JL et al: First recorded outbreak of equine viral arteritis in the United Kingdom, *Vet Rec* 136:381-385, 1995.

226. McChesney AE, England JJ, Rich LJ: Adenoviral infection in foals, *J Am Vet Med Assoc* 162:545-549, 1973.

227. Cello RM: Ocular onchocerciasis in the horse, *Equine Vet J* 3:148-154, 1971.

228. Giangaspero A et al: Occurrence of *Thelazia lacrymalis* (Nematoda, Spirurida, Thelaziidae) in native horses in Abruzzo region (central eastern Italy), *Parasite* 7:51-53, 2000.

229. Heyde RR, Seiff SR, Mucia J: Ophthalmomyiasis externa in California, *West J Med* 144:80-81, 1986.

230. Silva RA et al: Outbreak of trypanosomosis due to *Trypanosoma evansi* in horses of Pantanal Mato-grossense, Brazil, *Vet Parasitol* 60:167-171, 1995.

231. Wyn-Jones G: Treatment of equine cutaneous neoplasia by radiotherapy using iridium 192 linear sources, *Equine Vet J* 15:361-365, 1983.

4 Diseases of the Cornea and Sclera

Stacy E. Andrew and A. Michelle Willis
With contributions from Franck J. Ollivier and Andy Matthews

Corneal disorders are frequent causes of presentation of horses to veterinarians. They can be rather impressive in appearance and therefore are noticed by horse owners. Corneal disease is most often a primary problem, but it can also signify intraocular disease. This chapter concentrates on various clinical conditions observed and diagnosed in the horse cornea and sclera. Normal anatomy and physiology are described with a focus on corneal wound healing. Prevalence of corneal and scleral diseases is also addressed. Congenital malformations and neonatal diseases are discussed, followed by acquired diseases.

CLINICAL ANATOMY AND PHYSIOLOGY

Anatomy

The normal horse cornea consists of five layers (Fig. 4-1). The outermost stratified squamous epithelium is approximately eight to ten cell layers thick[1] and includes three cell types: nonkeratinized stratified squamous cells, wing cells, and basal cells. A thin epithelial basement membrane anchors the epithelium to the underlying corneal stroma, which comprises approximately 90% of the corneal volume.[2] Corneal stroma is 75% to 80% water, and the remaining 20% to 25% is made up of collagen fibrils, glycoproteins, and glycosaminoglycans.[3] The predominant glycosaminoglycans in the equine corneal stroma are chondroitin sulfate, dermatan sulfate, and keratan sulfate. Sulfation of equine corneal chondroitin sulfate has recently been shown to vary, with more superficial molecules having higher sulfation values.[4] Chondroitin 4-sulfate is more prominent in the deep central and peripheral horse cornea, as well as the middle central layer, compared with chondroitin 6-sulfate.[4] This may be important because chondroitin 6-sulfate tends to hold more water than chondroitin 4-sulfate. Internal to the stroma are Descemet's membrane and the innermost corneal

endothelium. Descemet's membrane is a basement membrane secreted by the corneal endothelium. Because it is produced continuously throughout life, the thickness of Descemet's membrane increases with horse age. The endothelium is a single layer of hexagon-shaped cells, which interdigitate with one another[2] and act as a barrier between the stroma and aqueous humor to limit imbibition of water and solutes from the anterior chamber into the corneal stroma.[5] Corneal nutrition is supplied by the precorneal tear film anteriorly and the aqueous humor posteriorly. The tear film provides glucose and electrolytes to the avascular cornea and also permits transfer of oxygen.[3] Corneas are transparent and have no blood vessels, as is fitting for a tissue with the purpose of transmitting light, but they are richly innervated superficially with sensory endings of the trigeminal nerves. The peripheral temporal and nasal cornea may normally appear white or gray near the limbus because of iridocorneal angle pectinate ligament insertions into the cornea (Fig. 4-2).

Corneal Diameters

The normal horse cornea is oval in shape, with the horizontal diameter being slightly larger than the vertical diameter (Fig. 4-3). Normal adult horse corneal diameters average 29.7 to 34.0 mm horizontally and 23 to 26.5 mm vertically.[6,7] In younger horses, the mean horizontal diameter ranges from 20.5 to 26.6 mm and the vertical diameter ranges from 19.5 to 24.0 mm.[7,8] Mean horizontal corneal diameter in Miniature horses is 25.8 mm and mean vertical corneal diameter is 19.4 mm.[9] In normal Rocky Mountain horses, optical corneal diameter increases with age.[7]

Corneal Thickness

Several recent studies have been performed to measure corneal thickness in horses. When ultrasonic

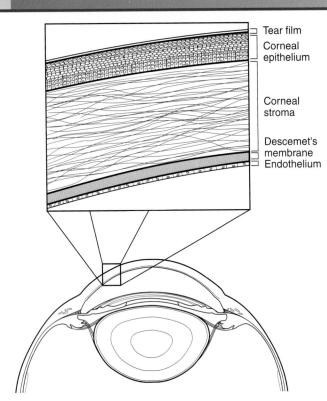

Fig. 4-1 Schematic of equine corneal layers.

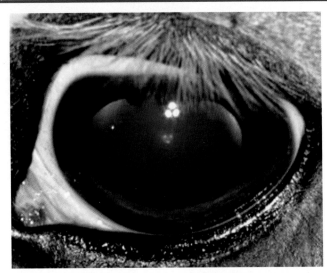

Fig. 4-3 Normal equine cornea demonstrating a horizontal diameter that is larger than the vertical diameter.

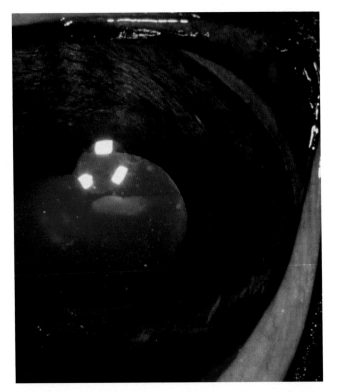

Fig. 4-2 "Grey line" or the insertion of pectinate ligaments into the cornea seen temporally in this 8-year-old American Quarter horse.

pachymetry was used in two studies, the thickness of the central cornea in healthy horses was reported to range between 770 μm [7] and 793 μm,[10] and both studies revealed the peripheral cornea to be thicker than the central cornea. In enucleated eyes of euthanized horses, the central cornea measured 893 μm, with the dorsal and ventral quadrants being significantly thicker than the central cornea and the medial and temporal quadrants.[11] No correlation was found between corneal thickness and sex, age, or endothelial cell density.[11] It has been determined that diagnostic auriculopalpebral nerve block and sedation with xylazine (0.3 mg/kg administered intravenously [IV]) have no effect on corneal thickness measurement in healthy horses.[10] Healthy Miniature horses were found to have a mean corneal thickness of 785.6 μm.[9] Similarly, no correlation was found between corneal thickness and sex or age, meaning that corneal thickness did not increase with increasing animal age.[9] A positive correlation between increasing age and corneal thickness has been noted in healthy Rocky Mountain horses.[7]

Corneal Curvature

The only known report of corneal curvature in healthy horses is from Rocky Mountain horses not affected with cornea globosa, which were found to have a curvature of 20.59 ± 1.72 diopters.[12] The radius of curvature has been reported to be 16.6 mm vertically and 17.9 mm horizontally.[6]

Normal Refractive State

The cornea is the primary refractive structure in the eye because of the large change in refractive index at its

Table 4-1A Gram-Positive Bacterial Isolates From Conjunctival/Corneal Collections in Healthy Horses

Author Country (state) Organism % (number/total)	Lundvall[371] US	Cattabiani[18] Italy	Whitley and Moore[372] US (FL)	Whitley et al.[373] US (WI)	Moore et al.[16] US (MO)	Andrew et al.[17] US (FL)
Actinomyces	33 (82/250)					6 (135/2357)
Aerobacter	<1 (2/250)					
Bacillus	98 (244/250)	12 (7/59)	12	18 (6/33)	11 (11/96)	17 (398/2357)
Corynebacterium		7 (4/59)	14	21 (7/33)	26 (25/96)	29 (689/2357)
Dermatophilus						<1 (3/2357)
Enterococcus					3 (3/96)	
Lactobacillus						<1 (1/2357)
Micrococcus	78 (194/250)	49 (29/59)		2 (1/33)	7 (7/96)	2 (53/2357)
Rhodococcus						<1 (5/2357)
Staphylococcus	6 (15/250)	19 (11/59)	18	26 (9/33)	16 (15/96)	22 (513/2357)
Streptococcus	11 (28/250)	7 (4/59)	2	2 (1/33)		4 (87/2357)
Streptomyces				18 (6/33)	11 (11/96)	<1 (19/2357)
Unidentified					2 (2/96)	<1 (6/2357)

anterior surface.[13] Normal index of refraction is 1.337 with a focal length of −59 mm anterior cornea and +79 mm posterior cornea.[6] In a survey of 82 horses, the normal refractive state was found to be approximately 0.25 diopters horizontally and vertically.[14] Most horses are near emmetropia, but some are myopic or hyperopic by as much as 3 diopters.[13] Astigmatism is uncommon in horses.[15] Astigmatism was detected in 7.3% (6 of 82), myopia in 20.7% (17 of 82), and hyperopia in 24.4% (20 of 82) of healthy horses.[14]

Endothelial Cell Density

Endothelial cell density is important for corneal clarity because a significant decrease in cells results in an inability to pump water out of the cornea.[5] Disturbance of corneal endothelial cell arrangement or density may have a profound effect on corneal transparency. The corneal endothelium may be compromised by a number of inherent disease processes or by surgical manipulations of the cornea or the anterior chamber of the eye. Mean endothelial cell density in healthy horses is 3155 ± 765 cells/mm², and the density decreases with age.[11]

Microflora

Corneal and conjunctival microflora are grouped together as ocular surface microflora because the eyelid conjunctiva is in direct contact with the cornea each time a horse blinks. The conjunctival and corneal microflora of the horse normally consist of mainly gram-positive bacteria and fungi (Tables 4-1A, 4-1B,

and 4-2). In Missouri horses, 96 species of aerobic bacteria and 57 species of fungi were isolated. *Corynebacterium* spp., *Bacillus* spp., *Staphylococcus* spp., and *Streptomyces* spp. were the gram-positive bacteria isolated most frequently, and less than 25% of isolates were gram-negative (*Neisseria* spp., *Moraxella* spp., and *Acinetobacter* spp.).[16] In Florida horses, 24 genera of bacteria and 35 genera of fungi were recovered. *Corynebacterium* spp., *Staphylococcus* spp., *Bacillus* spp., and *Moraxella* spp. were the bacteria most frequently isolated.[17] In Italy, normal equine conjunctival bacterial flora consist of *Bacillus* spp., *Moraxella* spp., *Streptococcus* spp., and *Corynebacterium* spp.[18] Environmental fungi including *Cladosporium* spp. and *Alternaria* spp. accounted for 50% of fungal isolates in Missouri horses[16]; whereas mold and dematiaceous mold, *Chrysosporium* spp., *Cladosporium* spp., and *Aspergillus* spp. were the most frequently recovered fungi in Florida.[17] In New York, 88% (44 of 50) of horses had fungi, and the two most common genera were *Aspergillus* and *Cladosporium*.[19] The common fungal flora isolates from horses in Brazil included *Aspergillus* spp., *Penicillium* spp., *Scopulariopsis* spp., *Trichoderma* spp., and yeast.[20] It appears that inherent weather conditions such as temperature and humidity may play a role in the normal conjunctival and corneal microflora because many of the organisms are considered to be environmental contaminants.[21]

Corneal Sensitivity

The cornea is one of the most sensitive tissues in the body. It is densely innervated by sensory nerve

Table 4-1B Gram-Negative and Anaerobic Bacterial Isolates From Conjunctival/Corneal Collections in Healthy Horses

Author Country (state) Organism % (number/total)	Lundvall[371] US	Cattabiani et al.[18] Italy	Whitley and Moore[372] US (FL)	Whitley et al.[373] US (WI)	Moore et al.[16] US (MO)	Andrew et al.[17] US (FL)
Achromobacter					1 (1/96)	
Acinetobacter		5 (3/59)		2 (1/33)	5 (5/96)	
Alcaligenes						<1 (2/2357)
Escherichia	<1 (2/250)				1 (1/96)	<1 (2/2357)
Enterobacter						<1 (1/2357)
Klebsiella						<1 (5/2357)
Moraxella		12 (7/59)	2	2 (1/33)	5 (5/96)	10 (225/2357)
Neisseria		8 (5/59)	2	2 (1/33)	7 (7/96)	
Pasteurella					1 (1/96)	<1 (4/2357)
Proteus	<1 (1/250)					<1 (1/2357)
Pseudomonas	<1 (1/250)		0			<1 (1/2357)
Sphingomonas						<1 (1/2357)
Stentophomonas						<1 (2/2357)
Unidentified	7 (18/250)					9 (204/2357)

endings of the trigeminal ganglia, namely the ophthalmic branches of cranial nerve V. Ciliary nerve trunks enter the middle stromal layer of the cornea at the limbus; as they travel superficially toward the center of the cornea, collateral branches form anterior stromal and subepithelial plexi.[22] These fibers continue to branch and penetrate the epithelium with terminal enlargements at the wing cell level.[22] Corneal sensitivity in healthy horses has been reported. Mean central corneal touch threshold (CTT) as measured with a Cochet-Bonnet esthesiometer in adult horses and was 5.54 ± 0.57 cm in one study (n = 12 eyes)[23] and 2.12 ± 0.62 cm in another larger (n = 100 eyes) study.[24] The adult horse central cornea was more sensitive than the limbal cornea in both studies, and the dorsal quadrant was the least sensitive area.[23,24] Healthy foals appear to have more sensitive corneas (CTT 5.01 ± 0.61 cm, n = 10 eyes) than do adult horses, but ill or hospitalized foals were found to have the least sensitive corneas (CTT 3.21 ± 0.24 cm, n = 22 eyes).[23]

Opioid Receptors

Opioid growth factor (OGF) and its receptor have been detected by immunocytochemical methods in the corneal epithelium of healthy horses.[25] OGF has been shown to inhibit wound healing in ulcerated corneas,[26] and studies have shown faster corneal epithelialization with blockade of the OGF receptor system.[26,27] Further studies need to be performed to determine whether the OGF-OGF receptor system can be manipulated to facilitate corneal wound healing in horses.

Physiology

Nutrition

Most of the metabolic requirements for glucose, amino acids, vitamins, and other nutrients are supplied to the cornea through the aqueous humor, with lesser amounts available in the tears or through limbal vessels. In addition, glucose can be derived from glycogen stored in the corneal epithelium for energy use under stressful conditions, such as after trauma or the development of surgical wounds. If glycogen stores are depleted, normal healing of the epithelium and cellular locomotion over the surface are inhibited.[28] In the absence of oxygen, as when eyelids are closed, energy is provided through anaerobic glycolysis.

Corneal Wound Healing

Epithelial Maintenance and Healing

The primary functions of the corneal epithelium are to form a barrier to invasion of the eye by pathogens and to prevent uptake of excess fluid by the stroma. The corneal epithelium is maintained by a constant cycle of apoptotic shedding of superficial cells and proliferation of cells in the basal layer.[5] Epithelial cell mitosis is limited to the basal layer. A balance of cell shedding, mitosis of basal cells, and renewal of basal cells by centripetal migration of limbal stem cells maintains the corneal epithelium.

Table 4-2   Fungal Isolates From Conjunctival/Corneal Collections From Healthy Horses

Author Country (state) Percentage of Isolate (No./total)	Rosa et al.[20] Brazil	Samuelson et al.[21] US (FL)	Moore et al.[16] US (MO)	Riis[19] US (NY)	Lundvall[371] US	Andrew et al.[17] US (FL)
Absidia			2 (1/57)		8 (20/250)	
Acremonium						5 (25/541)
Alternaria		7 (6/88)	23 (13/57)	Yes	3 (7/250)	2 (11/541)
Aspergillus	37 (75/204)	26 (23/88)	5 (3/57)	41 (18/44)	24 (60/250)	6 (30/541)
Botrytis		1 (1/88)				
Candida		1 (1/88)	4 (2/57)			<1 (3/541)
Cephalosporium			4 (2/57)			
Cladosporium	6 (13/204)	7 (6/88)	30 (17/57)	39 (17/44)	4 (11/250)	8 (44/541)
Chrysosporium						8 (44/541)
Cunninghamella			4 (2/57)			
Curvularia					<1 (2/250)	<1 (3/541)
Drechslera						1 (7/541)
Epicoccum					2 (6/250)	1 (6/541)
Epidermophyton			2 (1/57)			
Eurotium	2 (4/204)					
Fonsecaea						<1 (1/541)
Fusarium	<1 (1/204)		5 (3/57)	Yes	8 (20/250)	1 (8/541)
Geotrichum	1 (2/204)	2 (2/88)				<1 (2/541)
Gliocladium		6 (5/88)	2 (1/57)			<1 (1/541)
Gliomastix	<1 (1/204)					
Helminthosporium		1 (1/88)				
Memnoniella		1 (1/88)				
Monotospira				Yes		
Mucor	2 (5/204)					
Nigrospora						<1 (2/541)
Paecilomyces				Yes		1 (6/541)
Papulaspora						<1 (1/541)
Penicillium	29 (60/204)	22 (19/88)	5 (3/57)		16 (40/250)	5 (29/541)
Phialophora						<1 (2/541)
Phoma				Yes		
Pseudallescheria						<1 (1/541)
Pullularia				Yes		
Rhizopus	1 (2/204)					5 (25/541)
Saccharomyces			5 (3/57)			
Scedosporium						<1 (2/541)
Scopulariopsis	18 (37/204)			Yes	<1 (1/250)	2 (10/541)
Sordaria					<1 (2/250)	
Sporothrix						<1 (2/541)
Staphylotrichum						
Syncephalastrum	2 (5/204)					
Torula		1 (1/88)				
Torulopsis						<1 (2/541)
Trichcladium						<1 (2/541)
Trichoderma	21 (43/204)	2 (2/88)		Yes	2 (4/250)	
Trichophyton						<1 (2/541)
Trichosporon						<1 (2/541)
Tripospermum						<1 (1/541)
Verticillium	<1 (1/204)	2 (2/88)		Yes		<1 (1/541)
Wallemia						<1 (1/541)
Wangiella						<1 (2/541)
Unidentified		8 (7/88)	7 (4/57)	Yes		
Unidentified dematiaceous mold						16 (84/541)
Unidentified mold					12 (30/250)	30 (161/541)
Unidentified yeast	11 (23/204)	13 (11/88)	4 (2/57)			3 (18/541)

After epithelial abrasion, mitosis ceases and the cells at the wound edge retract, thicken, and lose their hemidesmosomal attachments to the basement membrane. The cells enlarge and the epithelial sheet begins to migrate by ameboid movement to cover the defect. This process is initiated within hours of cellular injury.[5] The leading edge of the migrating cells is only one cell thick, but a multilayered sheet made up of both basal and squamous cells eventually covers the wound. After wound closure, mitosis resumes and restores the epithelium to its normal configuration.[29] The corneal epithelium can be completely replaced in 2 weeks.[30] Migration of corneal epithelial cells during wound repair is accompanied by an increase in protein synthesis, which promotes the adhesion of the epithelial cells to the basement membrane during the healing process. If the basement membrane of the cornea is damaged or removed, weeks to months may be required for regeneration to occur, and the epithelium may be easily removed from the stroma.[29]

The healing rate of experimentally induced corneal ulcers has been evaluated in horses.[1] Corneal ulcers to the depth of the anterior third of the stroma were created surgically in both eyes of 10 ponies. One eye in each pony was treated topically with chloramphenicol and 1% atropine ophthalmic ointments three times per day; the contralateral eye was not treated topically. The median healing time of the treated eyes (11 days) and the median healing time of the untreated eyes (13.5 days) were not found to be significantly different, which calculates to 0.6 mm/day healing time. Clinically, however, more severe complications arose in the untreated eyes.[1] These results suggest that the use of cycloplegics and prophylactic topical antimicrobial agents is warranted even for superficial corneal wounds in horses.

Stromal Healing

Stromal wound healing involves the re-synthesis and cross-linking of collagen, alterations in proteoglycan synthesis, and gradual wound remodeling leading to the restoration of tensile strength.[5] Polymorphonuclear cells appear around areas of cellular necrosis within hours of a penetrating stromal injury, followed thereafter by monocytes. Adjacent cells undergo a process of transformation leading to an accumulation of fibroblasts. In perforated wounds, collagen fibers are first replaced by a fibrin matrix. During the 2 weeks after injury, fibroblasts proliferate and rapidly synthesize collagen and other components of the extracellular matrix. Fibronectin is produced by stromal fibroblasts only during wound healing. It is a multifunctional extracellular matrix glycoprotein that stimulates cell adhesion, cell migration, and protein synthesis.[31]

Fibronectin stimulates fibroblast migration chemotactically, thus promoting stromal wound healing. Stromal keratocytes may begin to lose their interconnections and go through morphologic changes, some undergoing hypertrophy, proliferation, and finally reformation of cellular processes and connecting gap junctions.[32] Collagen fibrils in the regenerating stroma are disorganized, and corneal transparency is decreased.

Endothelial Healing

Although some species and age variation in endothelial regenerative capacities exists, minimal to no mitosis occurs in the adult corneal endothelium of humans,[33] nonhuman primates,[34] cats,[35] and dogs.[36] When endothelial cells are lost as a result of surgical trauma, disease, or the aging process, replacement of endothelial cells occurs primarily by enlargement and migration of adjacent cells, rather than by cell division. This results in an overall reduction in endothelial cell numbers. A summary of the steps involved in three-layer corneal wound healing is presented in Fig. 4-4.

The Role of Growth Factors in Corneal Healing

Peptide growth factors, which are produced both locally and systemically, act to coordinate and regulate the wound healing processes in the cornea.[37] Because the cornea is normally avascular, the stimulation and regulation of healing depend on growth factors that reach a corneal wound through the aqueous, tears, and limbal vessels. Several growth factors are known to affect corneal wound healing in humans and dogs. Epidermal growth factor (EGF) increases RNA, DNA, protein synthesis, and mitosis in corneal epithelium and stromal fibroblasts.[38] Platelet-derived growth factor (PDGF) stimulates the synthesis of fibronectin, hyaluronic acid, collagenase, and other growth factors for corneal wound healing.[31] Transforming growth factor-β (TGF-β) can stimulate chemotaxis of inflammatory cells and synthesis of extracellular matrix.[31,38] Several of these growth factors have recently been evaluated for their potential in aiding corneal healing in the horse. Platelet-derived growth factor and EGF stimulated but TGF-β inhibited the proliferation of equine corneal epithelial cells and keratocytes in cell culture.[39] The ability of EGF to modulate the rate of corneal epithelial healing in horses has also been evaluated in vivo.[40] The healing of corneal epithelial wounds created by mechanical debridement of the limbus was evaluated in conjunction with the use of topical EGF. The beneficial effects of administration of a high dose of EGF (50 μg/ml) for acceleration of healing of corneal defects in eyes of horses were reportedly outweighed by the intensity of the associated inflammatory response. A profound increase in the degree of inflammation, neovascularization, melanosis, and scarring was observed in eyes treated with the high dose of EGF. Healing of corneal ulcers in horses is often associated with profound corneal stromal fibrosis and scar formation, resulting in visual impairment. Connective tissue growth factor (CTGF) is a fibrogenic cytokine involved in wound healing and scarring.

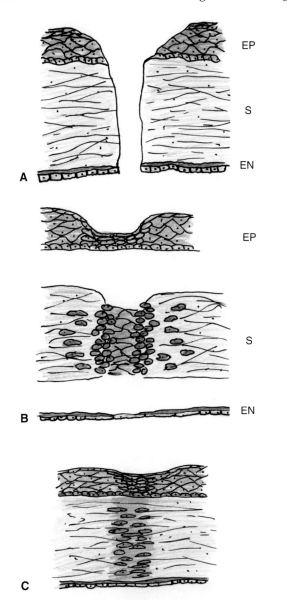

Fig. 4-4 Healing of a full-thickness corneal wound. **A,** Full-thickness corneal wound. **B,** Epithelium *(EP)*. Cells peripheral to wound edge migrate within hours of injury. Mitosis of epithelial cells begins within 24 to 36 hours of injury. Stroma *(S)*. Fibrin matrix is secreted into wound. Leukocytes and fibroblasts proliferate and migrate to wound edge. Fibroblasts undergo mitosis with subsequent collagen secretion. Endothelium *(EN)*. Cells at wound edge enlarge and migrate to cover defect. Migrated cells thin and flatten. **C,** Wound modification. Epithelium differentiates to stratified squamous layer within 2 weeks. Macrophages remove cellular debris in stroma. Stromal fibroblasts synthesize collagen that is disorganized, reducing corneal transparency. Endothelium is incapable of mitosis.

CTGF is present in horse tear fluid and derives, at least in part, from the lacrimal gland. Corneal disease was found to lead to a decrease of CTGF concentrations in equine tears.[41] The reduction in tear CTGF may be due to a reduction in CTGF production or may be associated with increased utilization of this growth factor. Although promising effects may eventually be achieved, further research is required before growth factors can be recommended as a safe and effective adjunctive therapy in corneal disease in horses. A summary of the relationships between growth factors and their effects on corneal wound healing is depicted schematically in Fig. 4-5.

Sequelae to Corneal Wounding

Vascularization

The equine cornea is normally avascular and transparent, but many keratopathies promote superficial or deep corneal vascularization. Corneal neovascularization is a result of vascular cellular sprouting from the perilimbal vessels.[5] The angiogenic process has three basic steps: enzymatic degradation of the basement membrane, endothelial cell movement, and endothelial cell proliferation. Migrating vascular endothelial cells elongate and form a solid sprout, which later develops a lumen. Polymorphonuclear cell infiltrates are important in stimulating corneal angiogenesis,[42] as are the cyclooxygenase and lipoxygenase inflammatory pathways.[43] Various cytokine growth factors, such as acid fibroblast growth factor, basic fibroblast growth factor, EGF, and TGF-α appear to have a direct effect in

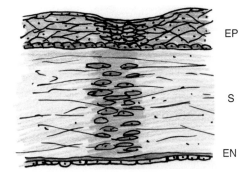

Fig. 4-5 Role of growth factors in corneal wound healing. Epithelium *(EP):* Epidermal growth factor (EGF) increases epithelial cell migration and proliferation and promotes adhesion; stimulates cell differentiation; transforming growth factor–(TGF)-β2 stimulates healing; its specific role is unclear; TGF-β1 decreases epithelial cell proliferation; antagonizes effect of EGF. Stroma *(S):* EGF increases fibroblast numbers; platelet-derived growth factor (PDGF) increases wound strength; TGF-β1 increases fibroblast numbers and increases collagen synthesis. Endothelium *(EN):* EGF increases endothelial cell density and promotes mitosis (in vivo); TGF-β1 increases in concentration; its specific role is unclear.

inducing vascular endothelial cell proliferation into the cornea. Lymphatics follow the blood vessels into the diseased cornea.

Corneal vascularization has both positive and negative effects on the healing of the equine cornea. Some keratopathies are routinely seen to elicit delayed or ineffective vascularization. A stromal abscess, for example, does not completely heal until it becomes vascularized, either directly from a conjunctival graft or from centripetal corneal vascular ingrowth.[44] Corneal vascularization in this condition is desired to promote the influx of plasma, leukocytes, antibodies, and systemically administered antimicrobials into the diseased area. Impairments to vascularization of these lesions can be related to the host, characteristics of the inciting infectious agent, or the presence of topical or systemic pharmacologic inhibitors of angiogenesis. The normally avascular equine cornea appears to vascularize at an extremely slow rate, especially when centrally located stromal abscesses are present.[45] This can lead to deep progression of the abscess with potential rupture into the anterior chamber. It has been proposed that fungal organisms produce metabolites that inhibit angiogenesis.[46] A recent in vitro study suggested that certain fungal organisms produce metabolites that may play a significant role in altering the host vascular response to fungal infections of the horse cornea.[46] Flunixin meglumine, an inhibitor of the cyclooxygenase pathway, is frequently used in cases of equine keratopathies such as ulcers and stromal abscesses to control the associated anterior uveitis. The use of this medication may slow progression of corneal vascularization in horses with stromal abscesses.[44] There appears to be an important balance in the use of flunixin meglumine between reducing the iridocyclitis, which can potentially blind a horse regardless of whether the cornea heals, and achieving resolution of the stromal keratitis by allowing more rapid vascularization.[44] Additionally, patients treated with topical corticosteroids may have delayed vascularization of corneal lesions. Although topical or systemic corticosteroids may temporarily reduce the severity of the uveitis associated with ulcerative keratomycosis and stromal abscesses, therapy is very risky and not advised.[47]

Corneal vascularization and fibrosis can have undesirable results, as a result of a loss of transparency and potential vision compromise. This has particular significance in the performance horse. Corneal grafting procedures (e.g., lamellar keratoplasty and therapeutic penetrating keratoplasty) are frequently indicated in equine keratopathies to remove diseased tissue and provide tectonic support. The incidence of corneal graft rejection after such procedures is apparently common and can be attributed to vascularization and fibrosis of the grafted tissue (Fig. 4-6).[48] Vascularization of grafts begins 5 to 10 days after surgery. The normal

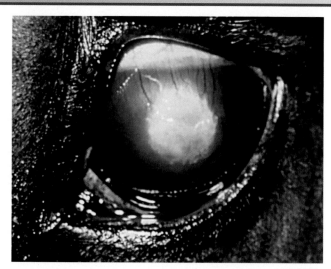

Fig. 4-6 Although disease resolution was achieved, corneal fibrosis, vascularization, and edema represent effective rejection of the corneal allograft used to provide tectonic support after a penetrating keratoplasty for treatment of a corneal stromal abscess in this horse. The photo was taken 6 weeks after surgery.

cornea has a decreased immune response as a result of the lack of a blood supply and a lack of intrinsic immune cells, which is theoretically why a high success rate of corneal transplantation is expected with allografts.[49] Dendritic cells and macrophages extend into the peripheral cornea, but the central cornea is essentially devoid of immune cells, including B and T lymphocytes.[50] In human patients with vascularized or inflamed corneas, however, corneal allografts experience a much lower rate of success, because these tissues no longer function as immune privileged sites.[51,52] Studies have demonstrated that a deficit of antigen-presenting cells in the normal cornea is a critical component in the corneal immune privilege.[53,54] The CD4+ T cell is considered to be a key player in instigating rejection of corneal grafts. Macrophages are typically recruited and activated by CD4+ T cells and can govern the cornea graft rejection process.[54] Because the causes associated with the need for corneal transplantation in horses are typically inflammatory in nature (e.g., stromal abscesses), affected corneas routinely have some level of vascularization at the time of surgery, which alters the corneal immune response. This undoubtedly influences the extent of graft rejection and eventual degree of corneal opacification that occurs after surgery in horses.[48]

Pigmentation

Corneal pigmentation is a common sequela of chronic keratitis (Fig. 4-7). The severity of the pigmentation correlates with the degree of inflammation. Superficial corneal pigmentation is the result of the migration of

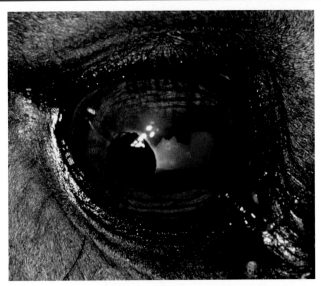

Fig. 4-7 Corneal pigmentation is noted in the center of this 14-year-old Westphalian gelding's cornea. The cause is unknown but presumed to have occurred after surgery.

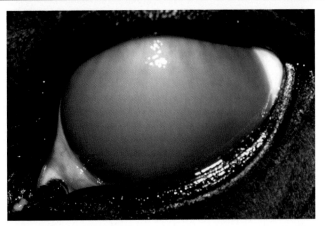

Fig. 4-8 The corneal stroma has an inherent tendency to imbibe water and swell, resulting in severe corneal edema.

melanocytes from the limbal and perilimbal tissues,[55] and it can accompany any condition that produces chronic inflammation, irritation, or exposure of the cornea. Melanocytic pigment becomes deposited in the basal epithelial cells of the epithelium and the anterior stroma. Melanocytes can become deposited within the deeper stroma with deeper wounds that are infiltrated with stromal inflammatory cells and granulation tissue.[55] Pigment can also be introduced into the stroma of the cornea with the transposition of a conjunctival pedicle graft. Deep stromal and endothelial melanosis can be observed in some horses with anterior segment dysgenesis, and iris pigment can become incorporated into the posterior corneal stroma.[56] Endothelial surface pigment can occur as a result of exfoliation from or rupture of anterior uveal cysts and may also be seen in chronic uveitis or with uveal melanoma. Pigment can become incorporated into the endothelial cells, possibly as a result of phagocytosis.[55]

Edema

The state of corneal hydration depends on many factors. The integrity of the corneal epithelium and endothelium provide two-way anatomic barriers against the influx of tears and aqueous humor. Endothelial cell membranes contain transporters for ions, amino acids, and sugars but no active transport mechanism that directly transports water molecules. Instead, water moves osmotically down gradients set up by the active transport of ions. Normal corneal hydration represents a balance between the fluid leak across the corneal endothelium and the extrusion of

fluid via the endothelial metabolic pump. The corneal stroma has an inherent tendency to imbibe water and swell (Fig. 4-8).[5] This is associated with the water-binding capacity of the proteoglycans in the extracellular matrix. Penetrating, blunt and surgical trauma (manual trauma or trauma induced by unbalanced intraocular irrigating solutions) can alter the status of the endothelial cells and render the tissue incapable of maintaining the deturgescence of the stroma in the area affected.

The normal human cornea maintains a constant thickness in the presence of intraocular pressure (IOP) up to 50 mm Hg.[57] This is because the normal stromal swelling pressure is also in a similar range. In eyes with IOP above 50 mm Hg or in those with abnormal endothelial function, there will be resultant epithelial edema and an increase in stromal thickness. Stromal swelling pressure decreases precipitously with increased corneal thickness. Mild corneal edema, combined with slightly elevated IOP, can therefore lead to high imbibition pressure and subsequent microbullous epithelial edema.[5] The sequelae of corneal edema include visual impairment caused by corneal opacification and potentially recurrent corneal ulcers resulting from rupture of epithelial bullae.

Proteases

Franck Ollivier

The normal equine precorneal tear film contains many soluble proteins essential to corneal health. These include matrix metalloproteinases (MMPs) and serine proteinases such as neutrophil elastase, as well as proteinase inhibitors such as tissue inhibitors of MMPs, α_1-proteinase inhibitor, α_2-macroglobulin, growth factors, and cytokines (interleukin-1, interleukin-8).

Important physiologic functions in normal tissues, such as turnover and remodeling of corneal stroma, are performed by proteolytic enzymes. Proteolytic enzyme activity is normally balanced by natural protease inhibitors, which prevent excess degradation of normal healthy tissue. Disproportionate amounts of proteases can create an imbalance. Increased amounts of proteases can cause pathologic degradation of collagen and proteoglycans in the cornea.[58-60] The rapid degradation of corneal stroma in horses with corneal ulcers appears to be caused by various proteolytic enzymes acting on components of the stromal extracellular matrix, including collagen and proteoglycans. Proteolytic enzymes are produced by and released from inflammatory cells, corneal epithelial cells, and fibroblasts.[58] Two important families of enzymes that affect the cornea are the MMPs and serine proteases.[61-64] MMP-2 and MMP-9 are of major importance in terms of remodeling and degradation of the corneal stromal collagen.[62] Higher amounts of MMP-2, MMP-9, and neutrophil elastase have been found in the tear film of ulcerated horse eyes, compared with values for the tear film of eyes of age-matched control horses.[65] Recent work showed that total proteolytic activity in the tear fluid from diseased eyes was significantly higher than that from normal eyes and the normal contralateral eyes of horses with ulcers (Fig. 4-9). Increased total MMP activity in tears has also been shown to prolong corneal ulcer healing time.[66] MMPs have been shown to be produced directly by microorganisms including *Pseudomonas aeruginosa* and *Aspergillus* sp. but not by *Staphylococcus aureus* or β-hemolytic *Streptococcus* spp.[67] Medical and surgical therapy of corneal ulcers results in measurable decreases in MMP activity, and measurement of tear film MMP activity may offer a way to objectively quantify ulcerative keratitis healing.[68] Surprisingly, systemic administration of flunixin meglumine, as well as topical oxytetracycline and topical 1% prednisolone acetate, do not appear to change MMP-2 or MMP-9 activity in the tears of healthy horses.[69] A great deal of research on protease inhibitors and their use in ulcerative keratitis is currently being conducted (see p. 175).

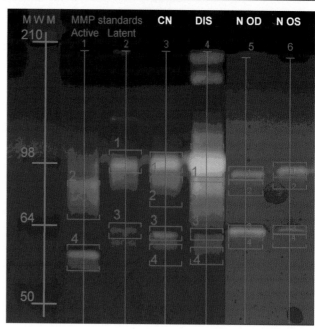

Fig. 4-9 Gelatin zymography and measurement of optical density are used to evaluate the matrix metalloproteinase *(MMP)* activity in tear fluid samples. Human standards of the active forms of MMP-9 *(bracket 2, lane 1)* and MMP-2 *(bracket 4, lane 1)* and the latent forms of MMP-9 *(bracket 1, lane 2)* and MMP-2 *(bracket 3, lane 2)*, as well as the molecular weight markers *(MWM)* were loaded on this gel. Tear fluid samples for the ulcerated *(DIS, lane 4)* and the contralateral normal *(CN, lane 3)* eyes of one horse and the tear fluid samples from the two healthy eyes *(N OD, lane 5 and N OS, lane 6)* of another horse are demonstrated. The red line on the tear fluid samples shows the bracket of the four detected bands. Proteolytic activity for each of the proteases detected is increased in the tear fluid samples from the diseased and the contralateral eyes compared with the level in the healthy eyes.

IMPACT OF CORNEAL AND SCLERAL DISEASE ON THE EQUINE INDUSTRY

Corneal diseases are very common in horses. One report indicated that 57% of equine ophthalmology problems were cornea related.[1] Between the years 1964 and 2003, 599,820 total equine case reports were filed with the Veterinary Medical Data Base (VMDB).[70] Of these, 6122 (1% of total reports) were cornea related (Table 4-3A) and affected 52 breeds of horses. American Quarter horses (1934/6084; 31.8%), Thoroughbreds (1038/6084; 17.1%), and Arabians (560/6084; 9.2%) are the three

breeds most commonly mentioned as having corneal problems in the VMDB (Table 4-3B).[70] American Quarter horse (178,858/518,389; 34.5%), Thoroughbred (90,938/518,389; 17.5%), and American Trotter/Pacer (51,749/518,389; 10%) were the breeds most commonly mentioned for all problems. Equine corneal problems are exceedingly prevalent in many parts of the world and may be exacerbated by season and weather conditions.

CONGENITAL DISEASES

Megalocornea

Prevalence and Literature Review

Megalocornea is a typically bilateral, developmental anomaly of the cornea, which is of abnormally large size at birth. Megalocornea, or corneal globosa, was evident in 43 of 71 Rocky Mountain horses with multiple ocular indolent ulcers, and they should be treated as such. Please refer to the discussion of indolent ulcers, p. 234.

Traumatic Corneal Edema

Prevalence and Literature Review

Corneal edema is probably the most common clinical sign of eye disease in the horse. Corneal edema may be a primary corneal problem and is also seen with virtually any type of corneal and intraocular disease and is therefore extremely prevalent. It can be seen with corneal diseases including ulceration and stromal abscess but is also noted with intraocular problems such as uveitis or glaucoma. In virtually every case report or case series describing a corneal or intraocular problem, corneal edema is listed as a clinical sign. A diagnosis of corneal edema was made in 6.3% (383/6122) of entries related to corneal problems in the VMDB from 1964 to early 2003,[70] although traumatic corneal edema was not entered separately.

Clinical Appearance

The edematous eye appears gray to white, and the condition may be focal or diffuse (Fig. 4-69). The edema may be in the pattern of the object, such as a whip or a branch, that caused the insult. Edematous corneas are usually thickened, and epithelial bullae may be noted. Corneal edema itself is not painful, but vesicles and bullae may rupture, causing painful ulcers. Horses may exhibit signs of pain such as lacrimation, photophobia, and blepharospasm. Depending on the degree of edema, a menace response may be absent.

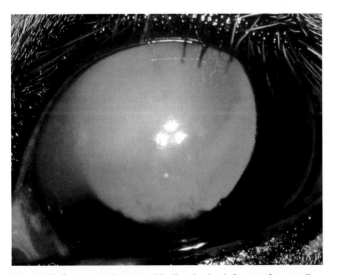

Fig. 4-69 Corneal edema and bullae in the left eye of a yearling Arabian colt that had been struck with a whip during training.

Differential Diagnoses

The list of differential diagnoses for causes of corneal edema is exhaustive. For posttraumatic edema the main differential diagnoses are glaucoma, corneal laceration, endothelial dysfunction, corneal ulcer, chemical keratitis, intraocular disease, intraocular neoplasia, and endotheliitis. Primary corneal edema caused by decreased endothelial cell density is believed to occur in horses but has not been reported.

Pathogenesis

Corneal edema is the result of a disturbance of the lamellar arrangement of corneal collagen caused by hydration of the glycosaminoglycan ground substances.[5] The overhydration and disorder of the collagen lamellae causes scattering of light rays seen clinically.[5] Traumatic corneal edema is usually the result of a separation of the endothelium and Descemet's membrane from the stroma, which allows aqueous humor to enter the stroma.

Medical Treatment

Symptomatic treatment with a topical hyperosmotic agent such as 5% sodium chloride ointment (Muro-128; Bausch & Lomb Pharmaceuticals, Tampa, Fla) every 4 to 6 hours can help to dehydrate the epithelium and stroma. It is especially useful in cases with epithelial vesicles and bullae.

Surgical Treatment

In humans, corneal transplantation is routinely performed for corneal edema caused by endothelial cell loss with Fuchs's dystrophy (23%), as well as for pseudophakic bullous keratopathy (32%).[294] The graft survival rate is much higher in humans than in horses, with 5- and 10-year success rates of 97% and 90% respectively, for Fuchs's dystrophy.[294] Corneal transplantation is not used for corneal edema treatment in horses because of the significant complication and rejection rates reported in horses.[248]

Thermokeratoplasty has been used in horses with corneal edema and bullae that periodically form and rupture, causing additional pain. The goal is to create superficial scarring in the anterior stroma[93] to bind the epithelium to the stroma and prevent recurrent bullae and ulcers. This procedure is usually performed with the horse under general anesthesia, but it can be done in a standing, sedated horse after application of topical anesthetic. Corneal epithelium is débrided to a 2-mm limbal rim with a No. 64 Beaver blade or alcohol-moistened cotton-tipped applicators. Thin-tipped, hand-held cautery is used to make a series of burns through the superficial stroma, with burns being placed 1 to 2 mm apart over the entire corneal surface.[295] The surgeon must use caution to avoid penetrating too deeply with the cautery because burns can occur quickly.[93] After the procedure, horses are treated with a topical broad-spectrum antibiotic, topical atropine, and a systemic NSAID to prevent infection and offer pain relief. Treatment should continue until the cornea re-epithelializes.

Prognosis

The prognosis depends greatly on the underlying cause of the corneal edema and the age of the animal. Younger horses are usually given a better prognosis because their endothelial cells can spread to fill in gaps left after trauma. Many cases will resolve in weeks to months, whereas others may be left with permanent edema.

Chemical Burns

Prevalence and Literature Review

Chemical burns are likely more frequent in horses than other animal species, but they are less common than chemical burns in humans.[19] Only one reported case can be found in the literature in which a mare was presented with presumed organophosphate fly wipe contact.[296] However, as a result of horse handling and environmental and stabling conditions, it is likely that there are far more cases than are reported.

Clinical Appearance

Clinical signs are nonspecific and can include photophobia, blepharospasm, epiphora, chemosis, corneal edema, focal white stromal opacities, keratomalacia, and miosis[19,296] (Fig. 4-70). The cornea is usually opaque from edema with superficial burns or keratomalacia with collagenase activity. Epithelial loss can extend over the entire corneal surface, and some cases can be affected bilaterally.

Differential Diagnoses

Corneal ulceration including infected (bacteria, fungus, mixed) ulcers, sterile ulcers, and melting ulcers should all be included in the list of differential diagnoses.

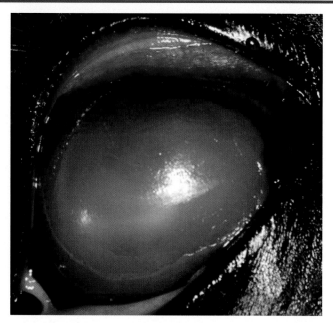

Fig. 4-70 Chemical keratitis in the left eye of a 16-year-old Thoroughbred mare. The owners had been applying a formalin mixture to the feet and inadvertently splashed some on the cornea. There is a large corneal ulcer, but no keratomalacia is evident.

Corneal degeneration, calcific band keratopathy, and ulcerated stromal abscess should also be included. Generally, the history can help to narrow the list of differential diagnoses.

Pathogenesis

Chemical burns that are acidic in nature (pH <7.0) tend to precipitate superficial corneal proteins but do not penetrate deeper.[19] However, alkali chemical burns (pH >7.0) are much more damaging and can penetrate all corneal layers[19] and cause severe protein denaturation. Much of the damage that occurs with alkali burns is due to neutrophilic response that appears in two peaks: at 12 to 24 hours after injury and then at 21 days.[297]

Medical Treatment

If possible, irrigation with eye wash or tap water should be performed immediately, and in cases of alkali burns, the irrigation should be prolonged (20 to 30 minutes).[19] Treatment with a topical broad-spectrum antibiotic, a mydriatic-cycloplegic agent, and anticollagenase(s) should be initiated. Systemic NSAIDs are used only if necessary because they will decrease corneal vascularization and potentially slow wound healing. Many topical and systemic medications have been used experimentally and clinically in corneal chemical burns in attempts to halt corneal destruction and prevent symblepharon and scarring. In alkali-injured rabbit eyes treated with 10% citrate, the incidence and severity of corneal ulceration were significantly reduced, and Haddox et al.[297] hypothesized that early use of 10% citrate diminished the initial peak of neutrophils, interfering with the release of inflammatory mediators and also decreasing the later accumulation of neutrophils, which causes ulceration. Oral and topical tetracyclines have been shown to inhibit collagen degradation after moderate and severe chemical injuries causing stromal ulceration in humans.[151] In rabbits, topical dexamethasone has been shown to potentially enhance endothelial healing after corneal alkali injuries,[298] but this is not usually recommended in equine corneal ulcers because topical corticosteroids predispose to secondary infection and also decrease epithelialization.

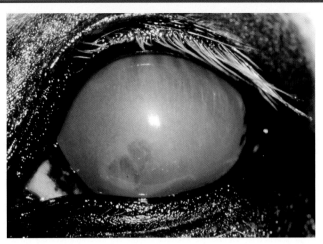

Fig. 4-71 Diffuse, dense corneal edema is present in this horse with late-stage progressive endothelial degeneration. Coalescing epithelial and stromal bullae are seen ventrally.

Surgical Treatment

Most chemical burns will heal with medical therapy alone. However, in cases presented late or those not treated with appropriate medical therapy, surgery may be warranted to save the eye. Placement of conjunctival pedicle grafts may be advised. Recently, amniotic membrane transplantation has been used for severe corneal burns in humans to promote reepithelialization and decrease inflammation by restoring corneal and conjunctival surfaces.[299]

Prognosis

Corneal and conjunctival scarring can be pronounced, especially with alkali burns. The treatment course is often prolonged (weeks to months), and corneas are often fairly opaque.

Corneal Degenerations/Dystrophies

Endothelial Degeneration

Prevalence and Literature Review

Primary endothelial degeneration may be unilateral or bilateral and can occur in adult horses of any breed.[300,301] Dystrophies and degenerations of the cornea accounted for 2.7% (165/6122) of corneal diseases tabulated by the VMDB,[70] but the specific breakdown of epithelial, stromal, and endothelial lesions was not recorded.

Clinical Appearance

Endothelial degeneration presents commonly as a gray-blue vertical band opacity in the central cornea. It is nonpainful in the early stages, although with progression and excess corneal edema, epithelial bullae can occur, which can produce painful ulcers if ruptured (Fig. 4-71).

Differential Diagnoses

Differential diagnoses for primary endothelial degeneration include other causes of corneal edema such as corneal ulceration, anterior lens luxation, increased IOP, and traumatic corneal endothelial injury. A thorough clinical examination may reveal indicators of most of these other differential diagnoses; however, the diagnosis of endothelial trauma requires a complete history to discern whether trauma may have occurred before the onset of the edema. Blunt trauma is the most common exogenous cause of endothelial dysfunction.

Pathogenesis

A sodium-potassium adenosine triphosphatase pump within the corneal endothelial cells actively removes corneal water, and the endothelial cells provide a physical barrier to electrolyte diffusion and therefore decrease fluid flow into the corneal stroma. Damaged tissue does not regenerate in adults of most species; therefore endothelial dysfunction and subsequent fluid imbibition into the stroma can result. Hypothesized causes of endothelial degeneration include aging, genetic predisposition, prior or current viral infection, and immune-mediated conditions.[301] Mean endothelial cell density in healthy horses is 3155 ± 765 cells/mm^2, and the density decreases with age.[11]

Treatment

Topical administration of hypertonic 5% sodium chloride ointment may be helpful to reduce the severity of corneal edema and minimize the incidence of corneal bullae. The frequency of administration may vary from one to six times daily, depending on the severity of the edema. Thermokeratoplasty involves the use of superficial thermal cautery placed over the corneal surface in multiple punctate applications to create a superficial scarring of the anterior stroma,[93] and successful results have been reported in dogs.[295] Thermokeratoplasty may be considered in cases refractory to topical treatment, although the results of this treatment for endothelial disease in the horse have not been reported. In the dog, complete resolution of the corneal edema is not expected; but bullae formation, erosions, and pain should be decreased or absent.[93]

Prognosis

The prognosis for horses with endothelial degeneration is guarded, because progressive corneal edema is likely, limiting vision and predisposing to bullous keratopathy and its sequelae.

Calcific Band Keratopathy

Prevalence and Literature Review

Calcific band keratopathy is a degenerative condition in which calcium hydroxyapatite is deposited in and adjacent to the basement membrane of corneal epithelium.[301] It has been reported in 21 horses in association with uveitis. Reports through the VMDB indicate that the prevalence of dystrophies was 2.7% (165/6122) during the period from 1964 to 2003.[70]

Clinical Appearance

The typical distribution of calcific band keratopathy is in the interpalpebral space of the cornea. These corneal lesions appear as variably dense, white, chalky plaques localized to the subepithelial and superficial stromal region of the cornea (Fig. 4-72). Frequently, there may be lucent zones within the dystrophic region. These clear areas are believed to correspond to the penetration of corneal nerves thorough the epithelial basement membrane.[302] Lesions can be may become dense enough to elevate the epithelium, creating ulceration. Horses

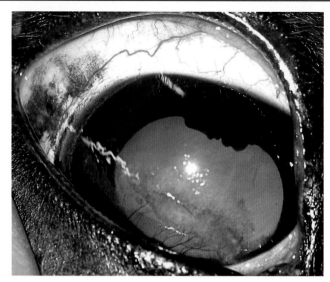

Fig. 4-72 Calcific band keratopathy was present in the interpalpebral space of this horse with concurrent equine recurrent uveitis. The location is typical, as is the associated corneal vascularization. The pupil was pharmacologically dilated.

with ulceration will demonstrate blepharospasm, lacrimation, and photophobia. Signs of active anterior uveitis or intraocular lesions associated with past uveitis may be present.

Histopathologic evaluation of keratectomy specimens from horses with calcific band keratopathy reveals amorphous, basophilic granular deposits at the level of the lamina propria of the corneal epithelium and the underlying superficial stroma. These corneal deposits stain positive with von Kossa and alizarin red stains, confirming the material to be calcium. Neovascularization is frequently present with an associated lymphocytic and neutrophilic cellular reaction commonly found around the calcium deposits.

Differential Diagnoses

Differential diagnoses considered in the horse that is presented with calcific band keratopathy include bacterial or fungal keratitis, eosinophilic keratitis, and lipid degeneration. The dull, gritty appearance of calcium is helpful in the diagnosis; however, because corneal ulceration is frequently present, corneal cytology and culture are warranted in the initial evaluation of the horse with calcific band keratopathy. The presence of calcium can be confirmed by staining keratectomy samples with von Kossa or alizarin red stains.

Pathogenesis

The exact pathogenesis of calcific band keratopathy is unknown. Alterations in corneal pH in the interpalpebral region may be a contributing factor.[302] Physiologic alterations that produce locally higher pH may predispose to the precipitation of calcium and phosphorus. The avascular nature of the cornea may prevent adequate buffering in the central region. A loss of carbon dioxide (CO_2) from the corneal epithelium is believed to allow a minor pH change, encouraging precipitation of calcium salts; the deeper cornea, which utilizes anaerobic glycolysis with subsequent lactic acid production, may have a pH low enough to preclude precipitation of these salts. Evaporation of tears has also been suggested as a mechanism for calcific band keratopathy.[303] Band keratopathy appears in the interpalpebral region of the central cornea and spares the limbus, where less evaporation occurs and where more vascular tissue may buffer the cornea and prevent the subtle increases in pH that can trigger calcium precipitation.[303] In horses, the lesion appears to be an occasional complication of uveitis, although the specific relationship between the two conditions is not clear.[302] Horses with severe corneal injuries or infection may have dystrophic calcific lesions, and although the calcium accumulates in the basement membrane or superficial corneal stroma, the location of lesions in the cornea coincides with the site of injury, rather than the interpalpebral space.[302] The use of steroid- and phosphate-containing topical solutions was postulated as a contributing factor in the development of calcific band keratopathy in five human patients.[304] All horses with calcific band keratopathy in the series presented by Rebuhn et al.[302] had a history of topical corticosteroid use to control signs of anterior uveitis; however, the effect of these preparations on the deposition of corneal calcium is unknown.

Treatment

Superficial keratectomy is recommended in horses with dense calcium deposits, chronic corneal ulceration, and pain. Postoperative prophylactic therapy with a topical broad-spectrum antibiotic is recommended in addition to topical atropine and a systemic NSAID until the cornea re-epithelializes. Despite topical antibiotic treatment, the rate of postkeratectomy infection may be high, potentially influenced by a compromised cornea from previous bouts of uveitis[302] or the prior long-term use of topical steroids in the control of intraocular inflammation. A solution of 0.4% to 1.38% EDTA in a neutral solution may be applied to the cornea to dissolve the calcium deposits after removal of the overlying epithelium, but its efficacy in horses is not well established.

Prognosis

Although treatment is indicated in horses with pain and ulceration associated with band keratopathy, the

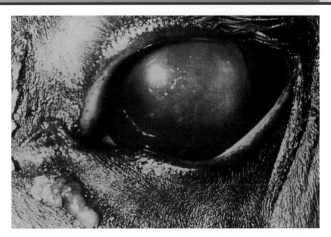

Fig. 4-73 Corneal vascularization, fibrosis, and superficial ulceration were present in this horse with keratoconjunctivitis sicca. Note the lackluster, dull appearance of the cornea and the mucoid periocular discharge.

long-term prognosis is related to the underlying cause. Horses with recurrent uveitis are at risk for additional corneal scarring and other vision-threatening sequelae if the uveitis cannot be specifically controlled.

Other Corneal Diseases

Keratoconjunctivitis Sicca

Prevalence and Literature Review

Tear deficiency disorders are not commonly recognized in horses according to the paucity of cases in the literature. Neurogenic KCS is the most common type of tear underproduction problem recognized in horses,[305] and it may also be associated with fractures in the region of the guttural pouch or of the mandible.[306,307] Toxic dacryoadenitis resulting from locoweed ingestion[308] and bilateral eosinophilic dacryoadenitis[309,310] are reported causes of KCS in the horse.

Clinical Appearance

Inadequate tear production should be considered whenever there are indicators of ocular surface disease, especially a cornea with a lackluster appearance, conjunctivitis and blepharospasm with an absence of epiphora, changes in the superficial cornea including epithelial defects or ulceration, and mucopurulent ocular discharge (Fig. 4-73). In chronic cases, corneal vascularization and pigmentation may be present in addition to active corneal surface or stromal infection. KCS is confirmed with a Schirmer tear test (STT) I result of 10 mm/min of wetting or less. If borderline values are obtained, the test should be repeated. A wide range of values and a lack of repeatability of the measurements were identified in a large study in which STT I and STT II results for horses and ponies were evaluated.[311] STT I (basal and reflex) results of 24.8 mm/min wetting have been recorded in a group of 50 healthy horses,[312] and a lower mean value of 12.7 mm/min was reported in a separate study in which Whatman No. 42 filter papers (reported to be larger in surface area than standard STT strips) were used.[313]

Differential Diagnoses

Conditions that may have a clinical appearance similar to KCS in the horse include evaporative dry eye or exposure keratopathy caused by eyelid abnormalities that result in inadequate blinking, lid margin incongruity caused by unrepaired eyelid injuries, and rarely, eyelid colobomas. Meibomianitis can be associated with a reduction of the lipid contribution to the tear film and a resultant evaporative dryness to the cornea.

Pathogenesis

Direct damage to the lacrimal gland can occur as a result of toxin exposure and was the reported cause of bilateral dacryoadenitis and KCS in a horse exposed to locoweed poisoning.[308] The cause of a bilateral granulomatous eosinophilic dacryoadenitis in a horse was not apparent through histologic demonstration of a parasite; however, migration of *Thelazia lacrimalis* through the lacrimal gland was suggested.[310] *Thelazia lacrimalis* has a tropism for lacrimal tissue. The authors speculated that larval death occurred after administration of an anthelmintic, resulting in a severe granulomatous reaction in the lacrimal tissues.[310] The bilateral dacryoadenitis diagnosed in an Oldenberg filly was eosinophilic in nature, but a granulomatous component was not observed.[309] The lesions seen supported the concept of an adverse drug reaction, parasitic infection, or another systemic condition initiating dacryoadenitis, but a specific cause was not determined. Trauma to the nerve supply to the lacrimal gland can result in neurogenic KCS.[305] The ophthalmic branch of the fifth cranial nerve forms the afferent arm of the trigeminal-lacrimal reflex pathway. The autonomic nervous system supplies the efferent arm.[314] The preganglionic parasympathetic neurons responsible for lacrimal secretion originate from the parasympathetic nucleus of the facial nerve. Damage to the nerves along this pathway can result in reduced stimulation to the lacrimal gland. Neurogenic KCS may also be associated with fractures in the guttural pouch or of the mandible,[306,307] which can occur in vestibular disease with facial paralysis if the lesion of the facial nerve is proximal to the geniculate ganglion within the facial canal.[305]

Treatment

Tear stimulatory and tear replacement therapy can be attempted in the horse, but the frequency and duration of administration required for an adequate response may be impractical. Topical 2% cyclosporine every 12 hours and pilocarpine (0.125% to 4%) every 8 to 12 hours have been used for their lacrimogenic effects with variable effects.[309,310,315] A positive response to cyclosporine therapy was seen in at least two horses.[309,315] Corneal lubricants and tear replacement products are recommended as frequently as possible, ideally every 2 to 6 hours in cases of severe dryness. Topical antibiotics are recommended if corneal epithelial defects are present. Systemic antiinflammatory therapy (flunixin meglumine or phenylbutazone) may be warranted if there is corneal ulceration and reflex anterior uveitis. Although topical atropine use can reduce tear production in the dog,[316] the effect of atropine on lacrimation in the horse is not reported. Judicious use to effect cycloplegia may be helpful in reducing pain in the horse with ulcerative keratitis associated with KCS. The logistics of treatment necessitated euthanasia of at least two of the horses reported.[309,310] Parotid duct transposition was reportedly successful in one horse.[317] Bilateral parotid duct transposition was avoided in one case of equine KCS because of the suggestion that this would impair the horse's ability to adequately lubricate and digest food.[310]

Prognosis

The prognosis for horses with KCS is related to the underlying cause and the tolerance of the patient to long-term treatment, if required. Although successful parotid duct transposition may be ideal for the long-term management of KCS in the horse, the rarity with which this technique is reported precludes a statement as to its potential in the management this condition.

Burdock Pappus Bristle Keratopathy

Prevalence and Literature Review

Plant material embedded in the conjunctiva, causing chronic ocular irritation and corneal ulcers, was reported in 10 horses in the Northeastern United States.[318] Corneal lesions were focal in nine horses and diffuse in one. Backyard horses, draft horses that have long forelock hair, and pleasure horses allowed access to ungroomed pastures and paddocks are at greatest risk. Of horses with corneal disease reported in the VMDB, 2.7% (164/6122) were presented with a foreign body affecting the cornea, although a distinction between foreign bodies embedded directly in the cornea and those embedded in the conjunctiva and causing corneal disease was not made.[70]

Clinical Appearance

Burdock pappus bristles are very small and difficult to detect without microscopic equipment. Typical clinical signs include blepharospasm; lacrimation; photophobia; and nonhealing, persistent, or recurrent ulceration of the cornea. The corneal lesions were variable in depth, and most had some degree of corneal vascularization. Some horses showed transient improvement with diminishing size of the corneal defects after treatment with topical medications (antibiotics, atropine, antibiotic-corticosteroids), only to experience relapse.

Differential Diagnoses

A complete ophthalmic examination is required to rule out other causes of chronic or recurrent corneal ulceration, such as eyelid abnormalities (distichiasis, trichiasis, ectopic cilia, or entropion), corneal dystrophies, corneal foreign bodies, neuroparalytic or neurotropic keratitis, and corneal microbial infection. Corneal cytology and microbial culture should be performed to rule out infection. Slit-lamp biomicroscopy is likely required to identify tiny foreign bodies embedded in the palpebral conjunctiva or in the bulbar side of the nictitating membrane. The topographic location of the corneal erosion or ulcer should be a clue to the location of the offending foreign body.

Pathogenesis

Burdocks are noxious weeds that have hooked bracts, which can become tangled within the facial hair and manes of horses. Numerous microscopic barbed pappus bristles are enclosed within the seeds of the burdocks, and these structures can migrate into the eyelids and conjunctiva.

Treatment

Conjunctivectomy is performed to remove a 5- to 8-mm zone around the identified pappus bristle.

This can be performed in the standing horse with the use of sedation, auriculopalpebral nerve block, and topical anesthetic. Hemorrhage from the initial incision can be controlled with dilute (1:10,000) topical epinephrine and gentle clamping of the conjunctival tissue. The authors of this chapter induced general anesthesia in one horse to remove more than 60 such bristles from the conjunctiva; removal was accomplished by using a distichia forceps and a gentle, continuous pull to avoid breaking the bristle and leaving remnants behind. Follow-up therapy is directed at the corneal ulcer with the administration of topical broad-spectrum antibiotics and atropine for cycloplegia, as well as systemic NSAIDs to control ocular pain and treat signs of reflex anterior uveitis.

Superficial, Nonhealing Ulcers (Indolent-like Corneal Ulcers)

Prevalence and Literature Review

Indolent ulcers are superficial ulcers that are refractory to healing despite an absence of detectable mechanical foreign body or infection. Their prevalence in horses is unknown, although ulcerative conditions of any variety accounted for more than 56% of the submissions to the VMDB between 1964 and 2003.[70] Indolent-like ulcers have been reported in horses.[95,121,271,295,319] Affected horses are typically older, and in one retrospective study of 23 cases, a mean age at presentation of 13.7 years was reported.[320] No breed or sex predilection has been reported.[320] Recurrent nonhealing ulceration may be seen in some horses.[320]

Clinical Appearance

Indolent ulcers are limited to the corneal epithelium, do not heal in the expected time frame, and are characterized by a redundant epithelial border that is easily removed with minimal debridement (Fig. 4-74).[320] The central or paracentral cornea appears to be the most common location. This may simply reflect the increased exposure of the central cornea in the horse.[320] The presence of corneal vascularization in affected eyes is variable; in some cases an absence of or minimal vascularization has been reported,[95,121] and a larger series documented that 34.8% of cases had some degree of vascularization.[320]

Differential Diagnoses

Other causes of epithelial ulceration should be ruled out before a diagnosis of indolence is made. Indolent ulcers

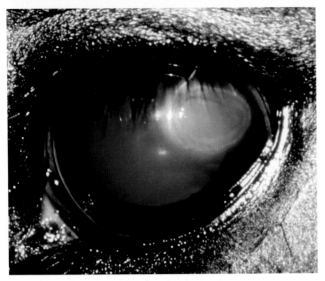

Fig. 4-74 This paracentrally located, superficial nonhealing ulcer was classified as an indolent ulcer after a complete evaluation was done to rule out mechanical and microbial influences. Note the circumferential lip of nonadherent epithelium within the ulcer bed.

are devoid of stromal involvement, microbial infection, inflammation, and an underlying mechanical cause. A thorough clinical examination is required to rule out the presence of ocular foreign bodies, including aberrant hairs, and eyelid margin defects that may be producing persistent mechanical erosion of the epithelium. Corneal infection is both common and potentially serious in horses, and therefore cytology and bacterial and fungal cultures are warranted in the horse with a nonhealing ulcer before the ulcer is categorized as indolent.

Pathogenesis

The cause of most indolent corneal ulcers is not known, although some may follow an observed trauma to the eye.[320] In both dogs and humans with nonhealing corneal ulceration, histologic and electron microscopic studies reveal basal cell and basement membrane abnormalities, such as a thick irregular basement membrane, degeneration of basal cells, and a decreased density of hemidesmosomes.[321-324] These changes have yet to be confirmed in horses with nonhealing ulcers.

Treatment

Treatment options reported in the horse include medical therapy with topical antimicrobials and atropine, epithelial debridement, chemical cautery of the cornea with 2% to 7% iodine, conjunctival graft, grid keratotomy, superficial keratectomy, and thermal cautery.[1,95,121,325] Debridement of all redundant tissue is the recommended treatment on initial presentation of an indolent ulcer. Topical anesthetic (0.5% proparacaine) is applied, and auriculopalpebral nerve block may be performed. Sterile, dry, cotton-tipped applicators are then used to manually débride the unattached and loosely attached epithelium. This procedure removes abnormal epithelium and may stimulate migration of adjacent epithelial cells. In a retrospective evaluation of treatment modalities for indolent ulcers in 23 horses, those treated with a single debridement at the initial evaluation healed in a significantly shorter period than those treated with grid keratotomy or superficial keratectomy.[320] Grid keratotomy or superficial keratectomy can be performed if an ulcer fails to heal after epithelial debridement. Grid keratotomy breaches the basement membrane, which can remain on the surface of the erosion. New corneal epithelial cells are then exposed to type I collagen in the anterior stroma, which may promote more effective cell attachment. Superficial keratectomy removes both abnormal epithelium and basement membrane to expose the underlying stroma.[55] Bentley and Murphy[325] hypothesized that superficially applied thermal cautery may alter the abnormal hyalinized stromal lamina associated with indolent ulcers and effect reepithelialization. Positive results were observed after thermal cautery in two horses with indolent ulcers that were unsuccessfully treated with epithelial debridement alone.[325]

Prognosis

Although therapy may be prolonged in some affected horses, intervention with debridement, grid keratotomy, thermal cautery, or superficial keratectomy improves the chance for more rapid resolution. However, indolent ulcers are potentially recurrent, as was demonstrated in 4 of the 23 horses described previously.

Adverse Effects of Radiation Therapy

Prevalence and Literature Review

Negative effects of radiation therapy for lesions involving facial or periocular structures are infrequently reported. Beta irradiation (strontium 90) of the cornea in conjunction with surgical excision for treatment of limbal SCC was presumed to be the stimulus for a progressive keratopathy in a 20-year-old Tobiano paint horse.[326] Ulcerative keratitis was observed in a horse with a periorbital fibrosarcoma treated with high-dose gamma irradiation (radioactive gold [^{198}Au]).[327]

Clinical Appearance

In the horse with SCC treated with ^{90}Sr, corneal opacification caused by edema reportedly began 10 weeks after keratectomy and radiation application, and by 18 weeks after surgery, had progressed to involve 90% of the cornea.[326] The edema was eventually accompanied by epithelial bullae, but the eye remained free of pain with no signs of inflammation throughout the follow-up period of 1 year. In the horse treated with ^{198}Au, corneal disease originated with a 3- to 4-mm central corneal epithelial ulcer that had been present for 4 weeks. A wide area of the inferior corneal epithelium was affected diffusely with minute, punctate, fluorescein-negative defects. A larger area of the cornea was dull in appearance and had reduced corneal sensitivity. Noncorneal lesions included iris swelling, miosis, and focal retinal atrophy.[327]

Differential Diagnoses

Differential diagnoses considered for corneal disease associated with radiation damage should include trauma, infection, and a recurrence of the original neoplastic lesion. These possibilities can be ruled out with history, thorough clinical examination, corneal culture, and cytology or biopsy of areas suggestive of recurrence.

Pathogenesis

Radiation damage to the cornea is likely related to radiolysis of cellular water, decreased renewal of enzyme systems, inhibition of DNA synthesis, and limited repair of the membrane structures of the affected cells.[328] The time lag observed between radiation exposure and clinically visible lesions may be related to cell turnover time.[329] An excessive radiation dose could be implicated in the horse treated with ^{198}Au, because high-dose radiation was chosen because of the aggressive nature of the neoplasm. The exact dose was not calculated but was approximated at 6000 to 7000 rad. In this horse, corneal exposure was associated with immobilization of the medial upper eyelid caused by postoperative fibrosis and decreased corneal sensitivity. Dry, cold winter air was also believed to contribute to the postradiation keratopathy.[327] Although the cornea treated with ^{90}Sr was exposed to a radiation dose within a reportedly acceptable range,[330] individual patient susceptibility to radiation damage may vary and could have been a factor in this horse.

Treatment

Symptomatic therapy is indicated for radiation-induced lesions of the cornea. In the case of corneal exposure with ulceration, topical lubricants and antimicrobials are indicated, as are systemic NSAIDs and topical cycloplegics. Corneal edema may respond to topical hyperosmotic 5% sodium chloride ointment, particularly if bullous keratopathy results.

Prognosis

The prognosis for eyes with radiation damage is guarded. Progressive disease necessitated enucleation in one horse. The cornea of the horse with ^{90}Sr damage remained stable but opaque and nonvisual during a follow-up period of 1 year.

Corneal Neoplasia

The corneoscleral limbus is predisposed to ocular neoplasia in horses. Neoplasia of any type accounted for 8% (489/6122) cases of equine corneal disease recorded by the VMDB since 1964.[70] The most common tumor types were SCC (447/489, 91.4%), hemangioma/hemangiosarcoma/vascular tumors (11/489, 2.2%), melanoma (9/489, 1.8%), and papilloma (7/489, 1.4%).[70] The most frequently affected breeds are the Appaloosa (140/489, 28.6%), American Quarter horse (82/489, 16.8%), and mixed breed horses (54/489, 11%).[70]

Squamous Cell Carcinoma

Prevalence and Literature Review

SCC is the most common tumor affecting the equine cornea. Horse breeds with the least ocular and periocular pigmentation, such as Appaloosas, paints, and pintos appear to be at increased risk for ocular SCC.[331] However, draft horses such as Belgians, Shires, Clydesdales, and some other breeds have a high incidence of corneal SCC despite having pigmented periocular skin and eyelid margins.[332] The prevalence of ocular and periocular SCC increases with age. One author reported that horses are presented initially between 7 and 10 years of age; however, he proposed that many of these horses were diagnosed months to years after the actual onset of the neoplasm or the precursor lesion.[331] Sex may be a contributing factor, with stallions reported to be five times less likely and mares two times more likely to have SCC than geldings.[332] Particular genetic influences may be obvious (as with coat color or ocular pigmentation) or unapparent (such as with genetic immunologic determinants).[331]

Clinical Appearance

The appearance of corneal SCC varies, depending on the duration of the lesion, the topographic location, and the extent of tissue involvement. The lateral limbal region is most commonly affected, although this site is not exclusive. SCC can appear at any limbal location. Lesions typically have a white-pink, rough or fleshy appearance (Fig. 4-75). Some tumors are firm with a smooth surface, whereas others may have a more friable surface topography with superficial necrosis and secondary bacterial infection. Extensive corneal SCC may also appear as nonraised, infiltrative lesions (Fig. 4-76).[48]

Differential Diagnoses

Corneal SCC must be differentiated from conditions that have a similar appearance and topographic distribution. These conditions include other corneal neoplasms, particularly mast cell tumors; amelanotic melanoma and angiosarcoma; eosinophilic keratitis; peripherally oriented infectious keratitis; NUKU; and corneal granulation tissue. Histologic confirmation of well-differentiated SCC is based on the malignant transformation of epithelial cells in the basilar layer and the stratum spinosum. Affected cells exhibit hyperchromatic nuclei, pleomorphism, increased mitotic index, loss of polarity, and keratin pearl formation (Fig. 4-77). Secondary changes such as surface necrosis of the mass with hemorrhage, ulceration, and inflammatory cell infiltration are very common.

Pathogenesis

SCC and its precursors such as epithelial dysplasia (Fig. 4-78) and carcinoma in situ should be thought of as progressive pathologic conditions, which start as nonneoplastic abnormalities (dysplasia) but may progress to neoplastic masses when neglected or modulated by a variety of intrinsic or environmental

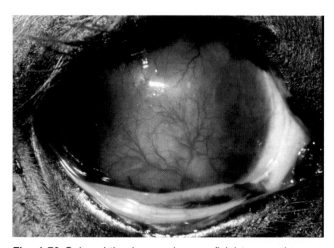

Fig. 4-76 Only subtle changes in superficial topography were present in this cornea with a less common, infiltrative manifestation of corneal squamous cell carcinoma. The lesion involved approximately 75% of the stroma in the deepest areas affected.

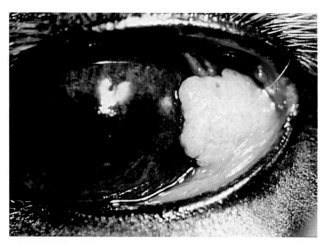

Fig. 4-75 The raised, cobblestone-like texture of this limbal corneal lesion had the typical appearance of squamous cell carcinoma in this region.

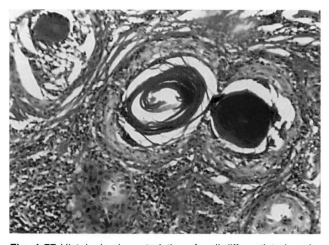

Fig. 4-77 Histologic characteristics of well-differentiated ocular squamous cell carcinoma include the presence of keratin pearls. (Hematoxylin and eosin stain; ×100.)

factors.[331] Ultraviolet radiation and resultant actinic tissue damage and chronic irritation or infection (as with chronic, untreated parasitic conditions) causing tissue metaplasia can also predispose to the development of ocular SCC.[331-333]

Surgical Treatment

Surgery is indicated for the treatment of corneal SCC. The depth of the lesion into the corneal stroma and involvement of the ocular adnexa are important determinants of the appropriate surgical treatment for corneal SCC. Corneal tumors that extend into the adjacent palpebral conjunctiva, eyelid, or orbit may not be amenable to complete excision; whereas those that involve only cornea and bulbar conjunctiva may be treated surgically with keratoconjunctivectomy and some form of adjunctive therapy, such as beta radiation, cryosurgery, or radiofrequency hyperthermia. Lamellar keratectomy has been described[93] and should facilitate complete removal of all abnormal appearing tissue. Beta radiation is delivered by a ^{90}Sr source. Tissue penetration is not typically greater than 1 to 2 mm, so it is a good option for corneal lesions.[334] A dose of 75 to 100 Gy per site is indicated with slight overlapping of successive sites. Reepithelialization may be delayed after application of beta radiation; therefore additional healing time should be expected if this is used in conjunction with keratectomy.[334] Excessive doses (total surface dose >500 Gy) could permanently damage the corneal endothelium and cause deep corneal necrosis.[334] Although significant adverse effects are rare, beta radiation was implicated in the development of progressive corneal edema and bullous keratopathy.[326] (See discussion of radiation therapy.) The primary disadvantage to beta radiation is its availability and the need for a radiation handling license; however, most strontium units are portable and easy to use and maintain. Cryoablation may be used for lesions not exceeding 2 mm in thickness. Cryogen sources include compressed nitrous oxide and liquid nitrogen, and optimal cryonecrosis of malignant epithelial cells is achieved between –20° C and –40° C by using a double freeze-thaw technique.[335] A fast freeze and slower thaw facilitate cryodestruction.[335] The major advantages of cryoablation are its relative accessibility and portability. Adverse effects are uncommon when cryoablation is used appropriately. Radiofrequency hyperthermia may be applied to superficial or shallow SCC lesions with a depth of less than 0.2 to 0.5 cm. Surface area is more important than depth when this technique is used.[336] Radiofrequency hyperthermia makes use of the greater sensitivity of malignant cells, compared with that of normal cells, to temperatures between 41° C and 45° C.[336] Thirty seconds of radiofrequency hyperthermia at 50° C is used to treat ocular SCC.[336] Radiofrequency hyperthermia is reported to have a synergistic effect with radiotherapy.[337] Tumor ablation with a CO_2 laser may be an appropriate primary treatment modality for limbal SCC.[338] The CO_2 laser emits radiation in the infrared spectrum (10,600 nm), which is absorbed by water molecules. Thermal tissue ablation occurs as cells are flash-boiled and vaporized. The incidence of tumor recurrence may be less after CO_2 laser ablation compared with sharp dissection.[338] Advantages of CO_2 laser ablation include rapid tumor removal with a zone of cellular destruction in the remaining tissue adjacent to the incision, effective hemostasis, and the provision of a dry surgical field, allowing constant visualization of tumor margins. Nerve endings and lymphatic vessels are also sealed, leading to less postoperative edema, exudation, and patient discomfort.[338] The sealing of capillaries and lymphatics may also decrease the incidence of metastasis of tumor cells liberated during surgery. Although infection is uncommon after other methods of removal of limbal SCC, vaporization by CO_2 laser may further decrease the incidence of postoperative microbial keratitis because the CO_2 laser vaporizes bacteria, viruses, and fungi.[338]

General anesthesia is recommended for all methods of surgical treatment for horses with limbal SCC, although in select cases, particularly very early, small lesions may be amenable to standing therapy if adequate analgesia, akinesia, and restraint can be provided with sedation and local anesthesia. Table 4-15 summarizes the available surgical methods for treatment of corneal SCC.

Medical Treatment

The effects of antineoplastic topical chemotherapeutic agents in the treatment of corneal and conjunctival

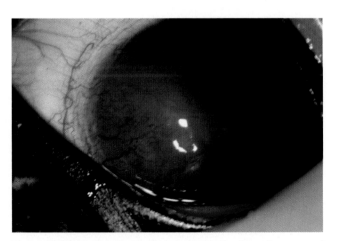

Fig. 4-78 Epithelial dysplasia is seen in the lateral cornea of this 22-year-old Arabian stallion. The condition was bilateral and diagnosed by means of cytologic scraping.

Table 4-15 Guidelines for Treatment of Limbal Squamous Cell Carcinoma With Various Modalities

Treatment Modality	Source	Surgical Specifics	Postoperative Care	Cautions
Keratectomy	Corneal blade, corneal dissector	Perform lamellar keratectomy to depth and circumference beyond visible infiltrated tissue; conjunctivectomy as required; re-apposition of conjunctiva to limbus may reduce granulation response	Topical antimicrobials and cycloplegics and oral NSAIDs until re-epithelialization of cornea is complete	Appropriate magnification required to accurately assess incisional depth; keratectomies deeper than one-half corneal thickness may require tectonic support with graft
Beta radiation	Strontium 90	Apply to contact affected tissue or to keratectomy site with slight overlap on adjacent regions; duration of contact dictated by age of unit to supply 75-100 Gy of radiation per site; tissue penetration 1-2 mm	As above if corneal epithelium removed	Avoid total surface dose >500 Gy; re-epithelialization may be prolonged
Cryoablation	Liquid nitrogen or compressed nitrous oxide	Apply to affected tissue or to keratectomy site in two freeze-thaw cycles; tissue temperature between −20° and −40° C achieves optimal necrosis of malignant epithelial cells; tissue penetration 2 mm	As above if corneal epithelium removed	Thermocouples not appropriate for corneal tissue; re-epithelialization may be prolonged
CO₂ laser ablation	Compressed carbon dioxide	3-6 W applied to affected region using continuous mode with a defocused beam to achieve vaporization of visibly abnormal tissue	Topical antimicrobials and cycloplegics and oral NSAIDs until re-epithelialization of cornea is complete	Surgeon requires eye protection; adequate smoke evacuation required; re-epithelialization may be prolonged
Radiofrequency hyperthermia	Radiofrequency thermal unit	Apply to affected tissue to achieve temperature between 41° and 45° C; tissue penetration 0.2-0.5 cm	As above if corneal epithelium removed	Avoid excessive heating of adjacent normal tissue

NSAIDs, Nonsteroidal antiinflammatory drugs.

SCC have not been evaluated in the horse. However, 5-fluorouracil has been used successfully to treat dermal SCC in the horse.[339,340] No systemic adverse effects were observed, but there was a localized inflammatory reaction in the skin in each case,[340] and this type of reaction in the cornea may have deleterious effects.

Prognosis

The prognosis for SCC of the cornea and conjunctiva is generally good for lesions less than or equal to 1 cm in diameter and less than 0.2 cm in depth.[334] Equine ocular SCC is typically locally aggressive but may eventually metastasize to regional lymph nodes, salivary glands, and rarely, the thorax.[341] Twenty of 24 horses with limbal SCC treated with keratectomy and beta radiation remained tumor-free after 2 years in one report.[334] One was lost to follow-up, and three had recurrences. The recurrences were retreated with subsequent cure (one horse), enucleation (one horse), and euthanasia (one horse). The risk of ocular SCC development may be reduced by deceasing exposure to ultraviolet radiation. Penetrating keratoplasty was used to treat a deep recurrence of corneal SCC after lamellar keratectomy, beta radiation, and radiofrequency hyperthermia.[342] Histologic examination revealed no neoplastic cells at the peripheral margins of the excised corneal button. The use of this technique preserved a visual eye in the affected horse.

Melanoma

Prevalence and Literature Review

Melanocytic neoplasms of the cornea and sclera are rare in horses. Benign epibulbar limbal melanocytomas that extend onto the cornea have been reported in the horse.[344,345] A corneal melanoma in association with a conjunctival melanoma has also been reported.[346] Although dermal melanoma has an increased incidence in gray horses,[346-348] coat color is not a known predisposing factor for the development of ocular melanoma.

Clinical Appearance

Limbal melanomas are typically seen in the dorsotemporal region of the limbus and can extend cranially into the cornea and caudally into the sclera (Fig. 4-79).[345] Pigmentation tends to be a prominent feature, although the corneal mass reported by Hamor et al.[345] was nonpigmented and raised and arose from the ventronasal corneal limbus, extending 6 to 8 mm into the cornea. It was associated with a darkly pigmented, raised,

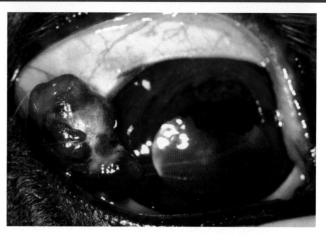

Fig. 4-79 A large melanoma can be seen in the lateral limbus of the right eye of a middle-aged, darkly pigmented horse.

pedunculated, and verrucous conjunctival mass arising from the limbal bulbar conjunctiva.

Differential Diagnoses

Differential considerations for a nonpigmented or variably pigmented mass on the cornea include melanoma, amelanotic melanoma, iris prolapse, a variably pigmented SCC, angiosarcoma, and granulation tissue. Definitive diagnosis is based on biopsy results.

Histologic examination of the epibulbar lesion, reported by Hirst et al.,[343] revealed a large submucosal collection of uniform cells with vesicular nuclei and paler eosinophilic cytoplasm. Cell margins had a polyhedral outline. Occasional intracytoplasmic light brown granules were present, and mitotic figures were absent. Several large tumor cells with extensive cytoplasm and dense pigment were scattered in the submucosa adjacent to the epithelium. The epithelium overlying the mass was heavily pigmented.[343] Histologic evaluation of the conjunctival mass, reported by Hamor et al.,[345] revealed coalescing cellular lobules formed by a heterogeneous population of cells that ranged from spindle to polygonal in shape. Nuclei were round to oval with prominent single or multiple nucleoli, and cellular cytoplasm was granular and eosinophilic, containing variable amounts of melanin. One to three mitotic figures per high-power field were evident. A lymphoplasmacytic inflammatory infiltrate was present throughout the mass, and melanophages were numerous. The overlying epithelium was hyperplastic. The corneal mass was similar in cellular arrangement and architecture to the conjunctival mass but contained little or no melanin. Warthin-Starry stain for melanin was positive in both the corneal and conjunctival masses. The masses were also positive for vimentin and neuron-specific enolase, supporting the diagnosis of conjunctival and corneal melanoma.

Pathogenesis

Epibulbar melanocytic lesions arise from the cells at the corneoscleral limbus. The stimulus for this growth is unknown. The mass reported by Hamor et al.[345] had a deep stromal extension at the limbus, but the limbus was not confirmed to be the site of origin.

Treatment

Epibulbar melanocytomas are amenable to lamellar corneosclerectomy; full-thickness resection followed by homologous corneoscleral, third eyelid, or synthetic grafting; cryotherapy; beta irradiation; laser photocoagulation; and enucleation in the case of intraocular extension.[343,349-353] Excision followed by adjunctive therapy, commonly cryosurgery, is the treatment of choice for corneal melanoma. Melanocytes are selectively sensitive to freezing, and regions in which recurrence is suspected may be treated repeatedly.[354,355] Alternative adjunctive therapies after excision of conjunctival melanomas in humans include application of brachytherapy, beta radiation, and mitomycin-C.[356] Systemically administered histamine antagonists have been reported to have in vivo and in vitro effects on melanoma[357,358]; however, their potential effect on corneal melanoma is unknown.

Prognosis

The lack of available data on epibulbar and corneal melanomas precludes an accurate statement pertaining to prognosis of affected horses. On the basis of the benign nature of equine epibulbar melanoma as revealed by histopathologic examination, although local extension may occur, its biologic behavior is believed to be benign, as is seen in the dog and cat.[349,350]

Hemangioma and Angiosarcoma

Prevalence and Literature Review

Hemangiosarcomas and lymphangiosarcomas are malignant tumors arising from the blood vascular system and the lymphatic system, respectively. The term *angiosarcoma* is used when the tissue of origin is uncertain. Hemangiomas are neoplasms of vascular origin that exhibit more benign characteristics. Both hemangiomas and angiosarcomas arising in ocular tissues of horses have been described,[359-363] and both can occur in the limbal region and extend onto the cornea.[359,362] Hemangiomas and angiosarcomas appear to be more common in middle-aged to older horses, although no sex or breed predilection is recognized.

Clinical Appearance

The clinical appearance of corneal hemangiomas and angiosarcomas varies, depending on the extent and duration of the lesion. Reported descriptions include a "blood shot" vessel at the corneoscleral limbus, focal thickening of the lateral aspect of the cornea caused by vascularization and edema, a cystic red mass in the limbal cornea associated with bulbar conjunctiva or nictitans masses, and a solid pink mass involving the cornea and conjunctiva (Fig. 4-80).

Hemangiomas are typically well circumscribed and are composed of variably sized vascular spaces lined with a single layer of uniform endothelial cells. Mitotic figures are rare. Hemangiosarcomas are more highly variable in their appearance. Some areas contain

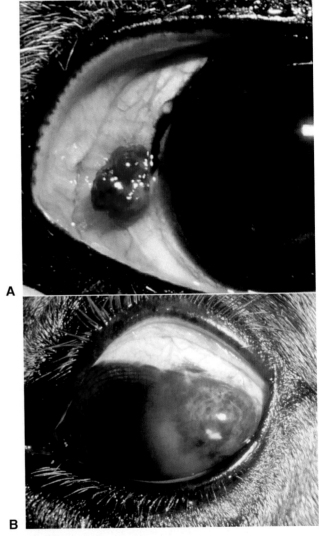

Fig. 4-80 A, A focal region of distended conjunctival blood vessels and vascular extension into the limbal cornea characterized this limbal hemangioma. **B,** Invasive extension into the cornea is seen with this large cornea lesion, confirmed by histologic examination to be a hemangiosarcoma.

vascular channels lined by pleomorphic endothelial cells, with bulging pleomorphic and hyperchromatic nuclei. Mitotic figures are frequent. Some tumors contain poorly differentiated regions, in which vascular channels are either rudimentary or absent. Red blood cells may be scarce in vascular structures formed by hemangiosarcomas, complicating the diagnosis. Differentiation between hemangiosarcoma and lymphangiosarcoma at the microscopic level, without the aid of immunohistochemical markers, is difficult, although the diagnosis of lymphangiosarcoma is usually made on the basis of clinical signs and a paucity of erythrocytes seen within endothelium-lined vascular channels. Factor VIII–related antigen (VIII: Rag), a blood vascular endothelial marker, may assist in the confirmation of hemangiosarcoma in questionable cases.[361]

Differential Diagnoses

Any of the corneoscleral neoplasms or inflammatory lesions should be considered in the differential diagnosis of hemangioma or angiosarcomas. SCC, corneoscleral LSA, mastocytoma, amelanotic melanoma, granuloma, and NUKU may be considered. Biopsy is required for a definitive diagnosis.

Pathogenesis

Most tumors of vascular origin appear initially on the conjunctiva or nictitans but can advance to a size at which definition of origin is precluded.[331] Ultraviolet light has been speculated as a causative agent because lesions in one group of horses tended to be first recognized on conjunctival surfaces that had been exposed to light.[360]

Treatment

In cases in which small hemangiomas were diagnosed with excisional biopsy, follow-up beta radiation and cryotherapy were successful in preventing tumor regrowth.[359,363] One horse with a lesion affecting 40% of the cornea underwent enucleation without evidence of complication by metastasis.[361] Angiosarcomas behave much more aggressively and do not appear to be radiosensitive.[359,360] Early and aggressive surgical debulking is recommended for angiosarcomas. Reported cases were locally invasive into the orbit and periorbital sinuses and metastasized through mandibular and cervical lymph nodes.[359,360] Orbital exenteration was performed on several horses, only one of

which was still alive at an 18-month postoperative follow-up examination.[359]

Prognosis

If cases are identified and treated early, the prognosis for small limbal or corneal hemangiomas appears favorable. Angiosarcomas are locally invasive and eventually metastasize. A biopsy should be performed on any lesion believed to be of vascular origin, and the lesion should be treated aggressively if it is confirmed to be an angiosarcoma.[331]

Lymphosarcoma

Prevalence and Literature Review

Corneoscleral masses were present in two horses in a series of 21 cases of horses with LSA and associated ocular lesions.[364] Compared with other ocular locations, this was an uncommon location for LSA. One horse was affected bilaterally, whereas the other had a unilateral lesion. Because of the obvious nature of ocular surface lesions, they may be the initial reason for examination of affected horses.

Clinical Appearance

Reported corneoscleral masses were raised, well-vascularized, pink or pink-white, smooth, nonulcerated firm masses in the temporal or ventrotemporal limbal region and extended more than 1 cm on either side of the limbus, involving both cornea and sclera.[364]

Differential Diagnoses

Corneal LSA must be differentiated from other conditions with a similar appearance and distribution such as SCC, hemangioma, angiosarcoma, amelanotic melanoma, NUKU, corneal granulation tissue, and eosinophilic keratitis.

Pathogenesis

Corneoscleral LSA, as with other ocular manifestations, is generally considered to represent a systemic disease, but the cause is unknown.

Treatment

Excisional biopsy of the ocular lesion, total body evaluation (blood work, lymph node aspiration or biopsy, and visceral imaging) is advised so that the disease may be staged.

Prognosis

Twenty of the 21 horses with ocular LSA reported by Rebuhn and Del Piero[364] were subsequently found to have LSA in other organs, and all died or were euthanized because of LSA within 6 months of the establishment of a definitive diagnosis. The two horses with corneoscleral LSA had detectable skin tumors, and one horse had peripheral lymph node tumors. Ocular lesions may precede or be more obvious than lymph node enlargement or signs of visceral involvement. Although the prognosis of LSA is grave, early recognition of ocular lesions suggestive of LSA may allow a more rapid diagnosis of LSA in horses and earlier aggressive treatment, thus increasing the potential for remission.

Mast Cell Tumor (Mastocytosis)

Prevalence and Literature Review

Proliferative mast cell lesions of the equine eye are rare but have been reported to involve the corneoscleral junction in several horses. The term *mastocytoma* was used to describe a pinkish-white proliferative lesion in the limbal cornea and sclera of a 12-year-old Quarter horse mare, and the term *mastocytosis* has been applied to a scleral mass observed in 9-month-old Arabian colt[365] and a 5-year-old pony[366] with lesions of similar character.

Clinical Appearance

One lesion was described as a flat, irregular, grayish-white lesion at the 12 o'clock limbus in one horse, with focal areas of yellow to brown regions of necrosis. The affected eye had a 3-week history of a seropurulent discharge before presentation.[366] A pinkish-white, rough mass of approximately 1 cm in diameter and projecting approximately 2 mm above the corneal surface in the 6 o'clock location of the peripheral cornea was described in another horse,[367] similar to the lesion shown in Fig. 4-81. Clinical findings in a young Arabian colt included a firm, 1.5-cm–diameter, raised, tan-colored protuberance on the limbal sclera in the 10 o'clock position.

Histologic examination of the masses revealed sheets of well-differentiated large round cells with predominantly hyperchromatic nuclei and finely granular, slightly eosinophilic to amorphous cytoplasm.

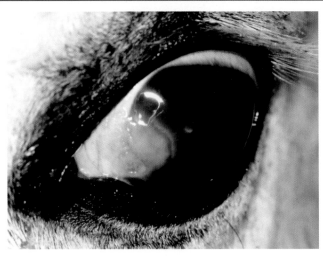

Fig. 4-81 Mast cells were the predominant cell type found on cytologic examination of this medial limbal corneal lesion that was histologically characterized as a mastocytoma.

Toluidine blue stained the cytoplasmic granules, identifying the cells as mast cells in all tumors. Rare mitotic figures were noted within the mast cell population of two masses[365,367] but were not noted in the histologic description of the other mass.[366] Large numbers of eosinophils were scattered irregularly throughout the section of two masses.[366,367] Some inflammation was present in the associated overlying conjunctiva and cornea.

Differential Diagnoses

Differential diagnoses may vary, depending on the extent and duration of the lesion. They include limbal SCC, eosinophilic keratitis, granuloma (e.g., parasitic), subconjunctival cyst, and prolapse of orbital fat.

Pathogenesis

The terms *mast cell tumor* and *mastocytoma* generally imply neoplastic change and are reserved for those cases in which invasive growth or definitive evidence of anaplasia is demonstrated.[368] In the horse, the term *mastocytosis* generally accompanies mast cell lesions in which neoplastic characteristics are not readily apparent.[369] These cases all fit the histologic description of mastocytosis.[365] A cause or specific stimulus was not elucidated in these cases.

Treatment

Surgical excision of the masses with a lamellar sclerectomy or corneosclerectomy was apparently curative.

One case was also treated with ^{90}Sr beta irradiation after excision of the mass.[367] One horse was available for follow-up with no sign of tumor recurrence 45 months after surgery.[365] Follow-up was limited to 3 months after surgery in the other reported cases.[367] No postsurgical recurrence was identified in one horse.[637] In the other horse, granulation tissue that suggested mastocytosis was present at the original surgical site, but biopsy was not performed for confirmation.

Prognosis

Cutaneous mastocytosis has been reported to undergo spontaneous remission,[370] and it has been proposed that similar ocular lesions may also spontaneously regress.[365] In spite of this, surgical removal is indicated if the tumor is large and interferes with eyelid function to the extent that corneal damage may occur during the regression period. Excision also allows for a histopathologic evaluation, thus differentiating the lesion from other potentially more problematic neoplasms. The prognosis appears to be favorable with excision, with or without adjunctive therapy.

FUTURE RESEARCH

A great deal of work still needs to be done regarding equine corneal diseases and the corneal response to healing. There is much to be learned in general about equine wound healing and scarring, as well as determination of specific methods to increase healing rates and to decrease associated scar tissue formation. Control of vascularization (both increasing and preventing) for various corneal diseases needs to be investigated with a primary focus on the study of graft rejection. More controlled studies on the use of growth factors and anticollagenolytics should be performed.

The degree of sensory nerve fiber innervation in the horse cornea compared with that of other species is unknown. Further studies need to be performed to determine whether the OGF-OGF receptor system can be manipulated to facilitate corneal wound healing in horses. Endothelial cell density changes that occur with diseases such as cornea globosa of Rocky Mountain horses, equine recurrent uveitis, anterior lens luxation, and equine glaucoma, as well as changes that occur after intraocular surgeries and corneal graft techniques should be investigated. Finally, some studies should also be directed at the prevention of corneal disease in horses.

REFERENCES

1. Neaderland MH et al: Healing of experimentally induced corneal ulcers in horses, *Am J Vet Res* 48:427-430, 1987.
2. Samuelson DA: Ophthalmic anatomy. In Gelatt KN, editor: *Veterinary ophthalmology*, ed 3, Philadelphia, 1999, Lippincott Williams & Wilkins, pp 31-150.
3. Gum GG, Gelatt KN, Ofri R: Physiology of the eye. In Gelatt KN, editor: *Veterinary ophthalmology*, ed 3, Philadelphia, 1999, Lippincott Williams & Wilkins, pp 151-181.
4. Biros DJ et al: Regional and zonal variations in the sulfation pattern of chondroitin sulfate in normal equine cornea, *Am J Vet Res* 63:143-147, 2002.
5. Pepose JS, Ubels JL: The cornea. In Hart WM, editor: *Adler's physiology of the eye*, St Louis, 1992, Mosby, pp 29-70.
6. Lavach JD: *The handbook of equine ophthalmology*, Ft Collins, 1987, Giddings Studio Publishing, pp 101-149.
7. Ramsey DT, Hauptman JG, Petersen-Jones SM: Corneal thickness, intraocular pressure, and optical corneal diameter in Rocky Mountain horses with cornea globosa or clinically normal corneas, *Am J Vet Res* 60:1317-1321, 1999.
8. Latimer CA, Wyman M, Hamilton J: An ophthalmic survey of the neonatal horse, *Equine Vet J Suppl* 2:9-14, 1983.
9. Plummer CE, Ramsey DT, Hauptman JG: Assessment of corneal thickness, intraocular pressure, optical corneal diameter, and axial globe dimensions in Miniature horses, *Am J Vet Res* 64: 661-665, 2003.
10. van der Woerdt A et al: Effect of auriculopalpebral nerve block and intravenous administration of xylazine on intraocular pressure and corneal thickness in horses, *Am J Vet Res* 56: 155-158, 1995.
11. Andrew SE et al: Density of endothelial cells and corneal thickness in eyes of euthanatized horses, *Am J Vet Res* 62: 479-482, 2001.
12. Ramsey DT et al: Refractive error in Rocky Mountain horses with cornea globosa and with normal corneas, *Invest Ophthalmol Vis Sci* 41:S135, 2000.
13. Roberts SM: Equine vision and optics, *Vet Clin North Am Equine Pract* 8:451-457, 1992.
14. Stuhr CM et al: The normal refractive state of the equine. Presented at the *30th Annual Meeting of the American College of Veterinary Ophthalmology*, Chicago, IL, October, 1999, p 74.
15. Miller PE: Equine vision and optics. In Robinson NE, editor: *Current therapy in equine medicine 5*, St Louis, 2003, Saunders, pp 454-457.
16. Moore CP et al: Prevalence of ocular microorganisms in hospitalized and stabled horses, *Am J Vet Res* 49:773-777, 1988.
17. Andrew SE et al: Seasonal effects on the aerobic and fungal conjunctival flora of normal thoroughbred brood mares in Florida, *Vet Ophthalmol* 6:45-50, 2003.
18. Cattabiani F et al.: Bacterial flora of the conjunctival sac of the horse, *Ann Sclavo* 18:91-119, 1976.
19. Riis RC: Equine ophthalmology. In Gelatt KN, editor: *Textbook of veterinary ophthalmology*, ed 1, Philadelphia, 1981, Lea & Febiger, pp 569-605.
20. Rosa M et al: Fungal flora of normal eyes of healthy horses from the state of Rio de Janeiro, Brazil, *Vet Ophthalmol* 6:51-55, 2003.
21. Samuelson DA, Andersen TL, Gwin RM: Conjunctival fungal flora in horses, cattle, dogs, and cats, *J Am Vet Med Assoc* 184: 1240-1242, 1984.

22. Chan-Ling T: Sensitivity and neural organization of the cat cornea, *Invest Ophthalmol Vis Sci* 30:1075-1082, 1989.

23. Brooks DE, Clark CK, Lester GD: Cochet-Bonnet aesthesiometer-determined corneal sensitivity in neonatal foals and adult horses, *Vet Ophthalmol* 3:133-137, 2000.

24. Kaps S, Richter M, Speiss BM: Corneal esthesiometry in the healthy horse, *Vet Ophthalmol* 6:151-155, 2003.

25. Robertson SA, Andrew SE: Presence of opioid growth factor and its receptor in the normal dog, cat and horse cornea, *Vet Ophthalmol* 6:131-134, 2003.

26. Zagon IS et al: Re-epithelialization of the human cornea is regulated by endogenous opioids, *Invest Ophthalmol Vis Sci* 41:73-81, 2000.

27. Zagon IS et al: Re-epithelialization of the rat cornea is accelerated by blockade of opioid receptors, *Brain Res* 798:254-260, 1998.

28. Tripathi RC, Raja SC, Tripathi BJ: Prospects for epidermal growth factor in the management of corneal disorders, *Surv Ophthalmol* 34:457-462, 1990.

29. Cintron C, Kublin CL, Covington H: Quantitative studies of corneal epithelial wound healing in rabbits, *Curr Eye Res* 1:507-516, 1981.

30. Cenedella RI, Fleschner CR: Kinetics of corneal epithelial turnover in vivo: studies of lovastatin, *Invest Ophthalmol Vis Sci* 31:1957-1962, 1990.

31. Schultz G, Khaw P: Growth factors and corneal wound healing, *Eye* 8:184-187, 1994.

32. Lemp MA et al: The precorneal tear film. I. Factors in spreading and maintaining a continuous tear film over the corneal surface, *Arch Ophthalmol* 83:89-94, 1970.

33. Doughman DJ et al: Human corneal endothelial layer repair during organ culture, *Arch Ophthalmol* 94:1791-1796, 1976.

34. Van Horn DL, Hyndiuk RA: Endothelial wound repair in primate cornea, *Exp Eye Res* 21:113-124, 1975.

35. Landshman N, Solomon A, Belkin M: Cell division in the healing of the corneal endothelium of cats, *Arch Ophthalmol* 107:1804-1808, 1989.

36. Befanis PJ, Peiffer RL Jr, Brown D: Endothelial repair of the canine cornea, *Am J Vet Res* 42:590-595, 1981.

37. Swank A, Hosgood, G: Corneal wound healing and the role of growth factors, *Comp Contin Educ Pract (Vet)* 18:1007-1016, 1996.

38. Schultz G et al: Effects of growth factors on corneal wound healing, *Acta Ophthalmol* 70:60-66, 1992.

39. Haber M et al: Effects of growth factors (EGF, PDGF-BB and TGF-beta 1) on cultured equine epithelial cells and keratocytes: implications for wound healing, *Vet Ophthalmol* 6:211-217, 2003.

40. Burling K et al: Effect of topical administration of epidermal growth factor on healing of corneal epithelial defects in horses, *Am J Vet Res* 61:1150-1155, 2000.

41. Ollivier FJ et al: Connective tissue growth factor in tear film of the horse: detection, identification and origin, *Graefes Arch Clin Exp Ophthalmol* 242:165-171, 2004.

42. BenEzra D: Possible mediation of vasculogenesis by products of the immune system. In Silverstein AM, O'Connor, editors: *Immunology and immunopathology of the eye*, New York, 1978, Masson, p 315.

43. Rochels R: Animal experiment studies on the role of inflammation mediators in corneal neovascularization, *Doc Ophthalmol* 57:215-262, 1984.

44. Hendrix DVH et al: Corneal stromal abscesses in the horse: a review of 24 cases, *Equine Vet J* 27:440-447, 1995.

45. Andrew SE et al: Posterior lamellar keratoplasty for treatment of deep stromal abscesses in nine horses, *Vet Ophthalmol* 3:99-103, 2000.

46. Welch PM et al: In vitro analysis of antiangiogenic activity of fungi isolated from clinical cases of equine keratomycosis, *Vet Ophthalmol* 3:145-151, 2000.

47. Kern TJ, Brooks DE, White MM: Equine keratomycosis: current concepts of diagnosis and therapy, *Equine Vet J Suppl* 2:22-38, 1983.

48. Brooks DE: Equine ophthalmology. In Gelatt KN, editor: *Veterinary ophthalmology*, ed 3, Philadelphia, 1999, Lippincott Williams & Wilkins, pp 1052-1116.

49. Price FW, Whitson WE, Marks RG: Progression of visual acuity after penetrating keratoplasty, *Ophthalmology* 98:1177-1185, 1991.

50. English RV: Immune responses and the eye. In Gelatt KN, editor: *Veterinary ophthalmology*, ed 3, Philadelphia, 1999, Lippincott Williams & Wilkins, pp 239-258.

51. Mader TH, Stulting RD: The high-risk penetrating keratoplasty, *Ophthalmol Clin North Am* 4:411-426, 1991.

52. Sano Y, Ksander BR, Streilein JW: Fate of orthotopic corneal allografts in eyes that cannot support anterior chamber-associated immune deviation induction, *Invest Ophthalmol Vis Sci* 37:2176-2185, 1995.

53. Gillette TE, Chandler JW, Greiner JW: Langerhans' cells of the ocular surface, *Ophthalmology* 89:700-711, 1982.

54. Streilein JW, Toews GB, Bergstresser R: Corneal allografts fail to express Ia antigens, *Nature* 282:325-327, 1979.

55. Whitley RD, Gilger BC: Diseases of the canine cornea and sclera. In Gelatt KN, editor: *Veterinary ophthalmology*, ed 3, Philadelphia, 1999, Lippincott Williams & Wilkins, 646-648.

56. Halenda RM et al: Congenital equine glaucoma: clinical and light microscopic findings in two cases, *Vet Comp Ophthalmol* 7:105-109, 1997.

57. Zadunaisky JA: Active transport of chloride ions across the cornea, *Nature* 209:1136-1137, 1977.

58. Twining SS et al: Alpha 2-macroglobulin is present in and synthesized by the cornea, *Invest Ophthalmol Vis Sci* 35:3226-3233, 1994.

59. Twining SS et al: Corneal synthesis of alpha 1-proteinase inhibitor (alpha 1-antitrypsin), *Invest Ophthalmol Vis Sci* 35:458-462, 1994.

60. Slansky HH et al: Cysteine and acetylcysteine in the prevention of corneal ulcerations, *Ann Ophthalmol* 2:488-491, 1970.

61. Fini ME, Girard MT: Expression of collagenolytic/gelatinolytic metalloproteinases by normal cornea, *Invest Ophthalmol Vis Sci* 31:1779-1788, 1990.

62. Fini ME, Girard MT, Matsubara M: Collagenolytic/gelatinolytic enzymes in corneal wound healing, *Acta Ophthalmol Suppl* 202:26-33, 1992.

63. Fini ME, Cook JR, Mohan R: Proteolytic mechanisms in corneal ulceration and repair, *Arch Dermatol Res* 290(Suppl):S12-S23, 1998.

64. Sivak JM, Fini ME: MMPs in the eye: emerging roles for matrix metalloproteinases in ocular physiology, *Prog Retin Eye Res* 21:1-14, 2002.

65. Strubbe DT et al: Evaluation of tear film proteinases in horses with ulcerative keratitis, *Vet Ophthalmol* 3:111-119, 2000.

66. Ollivier FO et al: Evaluation of various compounds to inhibit activity of matrix metalloproteinases in the tear film of horses with ulcerative keratitis, *Am J Vet Res* 64:1081-1087, 2003.

67. Brooks DE et al: MMP production by microbial isolates from equine corneal ulcers, *Vet Ophthalmol* 6:354, 2003.

68. Ollivier FO et al: Reduction in matrix metalloproteinase activity in the equine tear film during corneal healing, *Vet Ophthalmol* 6:350, 2003.

69. Rainbow ME et al: Effects of systemic flunixin meglumine, topical oxytetracycline, and topical prednisolone on tear film proteinases in normal horses, *Vet Ophthalmol* 6:357, 2003.

70. *Veterinary Medical Database (VMDB)*, W. Lafayette, Ind, Purdue University.

71. Ramsey DT et al: Congenital ocular abnormalities of Rocky Mountain horses, *Vet Ophthalmol* 2:47-59, 1999.

72. Latimer CA, Wyman M: Neonatal ophthalmology, *Vet Clin North Am Equine Pract* 1:235-259, 1985.

73. Mann I: *Developmental abnormalities of the eye,* London, 1957, JB Lippincott, p 352.

74. Townsend WM: Congenital anomalies of the cornea. In Kaufman HE et al, editors: *The cornea,* New York, 1988, Churchill Livingstone, pp 333-360.

75. Ewart SL et al: The horse homolog of congenital aniridia conforms to codominant inheritance, *J Hered* 91:93-98, 2000.

76. Barnett KC et al: *Color atlas and text of equine ophthalmology,* London, 1995, Mosby, pp 98-135.

77. Williams DL, Barnett KC: Bilateral optic disc colobomas and microphthalmos in a thoroughbred horse, *Vet Rec* 132:101-103, 1993.

78. Cook CS: Embryogenesis of congenital eye malformations, *Vet Comp Ophthalmol* 5:109-123, 1995.

79. Lewis DG, Kelly DF, Sansom J: Congenital microphthalmia and other developmental anomalies in the Doberman, *J Small Anim Pract* 27:559-566, 1986.

80. Narfstrom K, Dubielzig RR: Posterior lenticonus, cataracts, and microphthalmia: congenital ocular defects in the Cavalier King Charles spaniel, *J Small Anim Pract* 25:669-677, 1984.

81. Joyce JR et al: Iridal hypoplasia (aniridia) accompanied by limbic dermoids in a group of related quarterhorses, *Equine Vet J Suppl* 2:26-28, 1990.

82. McLaughlin SA, Brightman AH: Bilateral ocular dermoids in a colt, *Equine Pract* 5:10-14, 1983.

83. Munroe GA: Congenital corneal vascularization in a neonatal Thoroughbred foal, *Equine Vet J* 27:156-157, 1995.

84. Gelatt KN: The eye. In Mansmann RA, McAllister ES, Pratt PW, editors: *Equine medicine and surgery,* ed 3, Santa Barbara, Calif, 1982, American Veterinary Publications, pp 1280-1282.

85. Szutter L: Ophthalmoscopic examination of newborn domestic animals, *Acta Vet Acad Sci Hung* 11:183-193, 1961.

86. Burton H: Somatic sensations form the eye. In Hart WM, editor: *Adler's physiology of the eye,* ed 9, St Louis, 1992, Mosby, pp 71-100.

87. Massa KL et al: Usefulness of aerobic microbial culture and cytologic evaluation of corneal specimens in the diagnosis of infectious ulcerative keratitis in animals, *J Am Vet Med Assoc* 215:1671-1674, 1999.

88. Dantas PE et al: Antibacterial activity of anesthetic solutions and preservatives: an in vitro comparative study, *Cornea* 19:353-354, 2000.

89. Jacob P et al: Calcium alginate swab versus Bard Parker blade in the diagnosis of microbial keratitis, *Cornea* 14:360-364, 1995.

90. Andrew SE et al: Equine ulcerative keratomycosis: visual outcome and ocular survival in 39 cases (1987-1996), *Equine Vet J* 30:109-116, 1998.

91. Gaarder JE et al: Clinical appearance, healing patterns, risk factors, and outcomes of horses with fungal keratitis: 53 cases (1978-1996), *J Am Vet Med Assoc* 213:105-112, 1998.

92. Alexandrakis G et al: Corneal biopsy in the management of progressive microbial keratitis, *Am J Ophthalmol* 129:571-576, 2000.

93. Wilkie DA, Whittaker C: Surgery of the cornea, *Vet Clin North Am Small Anim Pract* 27:1067-1107, 1997.

94. Peiffer RL: Corneoconjunctival foreign body in a horse, *Vet Med Small Anim Clin* 12:1870-1871, 1977.

95. Rebhun WC: Chronic corneal epithelial erosions in horses, *Vet Med Small Anim Clin* 78:1635-1638, 1983.

96. Nasisse MP, Nelms S: Equine ulcerative keratitis, *Vet Clin North Am Equine Pract* 8:537-555, 1992.

97. Boulton C, Campbell K: Orbital bone sequestration as a cause of equine recurrent blepharitis and ulcerative keratitis, *Vet Med Small Anim Clin* 77:1057-1058, 1982.

98. Moore CP: Eyelid and nasolacrimal disease, *Vet Clin North Am Equine Pract* 8:499-519, 1992.

99. Vestre WA, Brightman AN: Correction of cicatricial entropion and trichiasis in the horse, *Equine Pract* 2:13-16, 1980.

100. Miller WW: Aberrant cilia as an aetiology for recurrent corneal ulcers: a case report, *Equine Vet J* 20:145-146, 1988.

101. Wilkinson JD: Distichiasis in the horse treated by partial tarsal lid excision, *Vet Rec* 94:128-129, 1974.

102. Stern GA, Weitzenkorn D, Valenti J: Adherence of *Pseudomonas aeruginosa* to the mouse cornea. Epithelial v stromal adherence, *Arch Ophthalmol* 100:1956-1958, 1982.

103. Rao NA et al: Adherence of *Candida* to corneal surface, *Curr Eye Res* 4:851-856, 1985.

104. Ramphal R, McNiece MT, Polack FM: Adherence of *Pseudomonas aeruginosa* to the injured cornea: a step in the pathogenesis of corneal infections, *Ann Ophthalmol* 13:421-425, 1981.

105. Sloop GD et al: Acute inflammation of the eyelid and cornea in *Staphylococcus* keratitis in the rabbit, *Invest Ophthalmol Vis Sci* 40:385-391, 1999.

106. McGregor MLK: Anticholinergic drugs (parasympatholytics). In Mauger TF, Craig EL, editors: *Havener's ocular pharmacology,* ed 6, St Louis, 1994, Mosby, pp 140-159.

107. Hardee MM, Moore JN, Hardee GE: Effects of flunixin meglumine, phenylbutazone and a selective thromboxane synthetase inhibitor (UK-38,485) on thromboxane and prostacyclin production in healthy horses, *Res Vet Sci* 40:152-156, 1986.

108. Halbert SP, Swick L, Sonn C: Characteristics of antibiotic-producing strains of the ocular surface bacterial flora, *J Immunol* 70:400-413, 1953.

109. Berman MB et al: Corneal ulceration and the serum anti-proteases. I. Alpha 1-antitrypsin, *Invest Ophthalmol Vis Sci* 12:759-770, 1973.

110. Berman M: Collagenase inhibitors: rationale for their use in treating corneal ulceration, *Int Ophthalmol Clin* 15:49-66, 1975.

111. Berman M et al: Corneal ulceration and the serum antiproteases. II. Complexes of corneal collagenases and alpha-macroglobulins, *Exp Eye Res* 20:231-244, 1975.

112. Woessner JF: Matrix metalloproteinases and their inhibitors in connective tissue remodeling, *FASEB J* 5:2145-2154, 1991.

113. Twining SS: Regulation of proteolytic activity in tissues, *Crit Rev Biochem Mol Biol* 29:315-383, 1994.

114. Woessner FJ: MMP inhibition. From the Jurassic to the third millennium, *Ann N Y Acad Sci* 878:388-403, 1999.

115. Pruzanski W et al: Inhibition of enzymatic activity of phospholipases A2 by minocycline and doxycycline, *Biochem Pharmacol* 44:1165-1170, 1992.

116. Solomon A et al: Doxycycline inhibition of interleukin-1 in the corneal epithelium, *Invest Ophthalmol Vis Sci* 41:2544-2557, 2000.

117. Kuzin II et al: Tetracyclines inhibit activated B cell function, *Int Immunol* 13:921-931, 2001.

118. Miller TR: Principles of therapeutics, *Vet Clin North Am Equine Pract* 8:479-497, 1992.

119. Moore CP: Diseases of the cornea. In Robinson NE, editor: *Current therapy in equine medicine II,* Philadelphia, 1987, WB Saunders, 450-456.

120. Wada S, Yoshinari M, Mizuno Y: Practical usefulness of a therapeutic soft contact lens for a corneal ulcer in a racehorse, *Vet Ophthalmol* 3:217-219, 2000.

121. Cooley PL, Wyman M: Indolent-like corneal ulcers in 3 horses, *J Am Vet Med Assoc* 188:295-297, 1986.

122. Tammeus J, Krall CJ, Rengstorff RH: Therapeutic extended wear contact lens for corneal injury in a horse, *J Am Vet Med Assoc* 182:286-286, 1983.

123. Gelatt KN: *Pseudomonas* ulcerative keratitis and abscess in a horse, *Vet Med Small Anim Clin* 69:1309-1310, 1974.

124. Divers TJ, George LW: Hypopyon and descemetocele associated with *Pseudomonas* ulcerative keratitis in a horse: a case report and review, *Equine Vet Sci* 2:104, 1982.

125. Moore CP et al: Bacterial and fungal isolates from Equidae with ulcerative keratitis, *J Am Vet Med Assoc* 182:600-603, 1983.

126. Moore CP, Collins BK, Fales WH: Antibacterial susceptibility patterns for microbial isolates associated with infectious keratitis in horses: 63 cases (1986-1994), *J Am Vet Med Assoc* 207:928-933, 1995.

127. Sweeney CR, Irby NL: Topical treatment of *Pseudomonas* sp-infected corneal ulcers in horses: 70 cases (1977-1994), *J Am Vet Med Assoc* 209:954-957, 1996.

128. Brooks DE et al: Ulcerative keratitis caused by beta-hemolytic *Streptococcus equi* in 11 horses, *Vet Ophthalmol* 3:121-125, 2000.

129. da Silva Curiel JMA, et al: Nutritionally variant streptococci associated with corneal ulcers in horses: 35 cases (1982-1988), *J Am Vet Med Assoc* 197:624-626, 1990.

130. Callegan MC et al: Corneal virulence of *Staphylococcus aureus*: roles of alpha-toxin and protein A in pathogenesis, *Infect Immun* 62:2478-2482, 1994.

131. Aarestrup FM, Scott NL, Sordillo LM: Ability of *Staphylococcus aureus* coagulase genotypes to resist neutrophil bactericidal activity and phagocytosis, *Infect Immun* 62:5679-5682, 1994.

132. Raus J, Love DN: Characterization of coagulase-positive *Staphylococcus intermedius* and *Staphylococcus aureus* isolated from veterinary clinical specimens, *J Clin Microbiol* 18:789-792, 1983.

133. Dajcs JJ et al: Corneal virulence of *Staphylococcus aureus* in an experimental model of keratitis, *DNA Cell Biol* 21:375-382, 2002.

134. Loeffler DA, Norcross NL: Enzyme-linked immunosorbent assay for detection of milk immunoglobulins to leukocidin toxin of *Staphylococcus aureus*, *Am J Vet Res* 46:1728-1732, 1985.

135. Reichert RW, Das ND, Zam ZS: Adherence properties of *Pseudomonas pili* to epithelial cells of the human cornea, *Curr Eye Res* 2:289-293, 1982-1983.

136. Stern GA, Lubniewski A, Allen C: The interaction between *Pseudomonas aeruginosa* and the corneal epithelium: an electron microscopic study, *Arch Ophthalmol* 103:1221-12251225, 1985.

137. Twining SS et al: Effect of *Pseudomonas aeruginosa* elastase, alkaline protease, and exotoxin A on corneal proteinases and proteins, *Invest Ophthalmol Vis Sci* 34:2699-2712, 1993.

138. Jones S et al: Ocular streptococcal infections, *Cornea* 7:295-299, 1988.

139. Bachman JA, Gabriel H: A 10-year case report and current clinical review of chronic beta-hemolytic streptococcal kerato-conjunctivitis, *Optometry* 73:303-310, 2002.

140. Schoster JV: The assembly and placement of ocular lavage systems in horses, *Vet Med* 87:460-471, 1992.

141. Sweeney CR, Russell GE: Complications associated with the use of a one-hole subpalpebral lavage system in horses: 150 cases (1977-1996), *J Am Vet Med Assoc* 211:1271-1274, 1997.

142. Giuliano EA et al: Inferomedial placement of a single-entry subpalpebral lavage tube for treatment of equine eye disease, *Vet Ophthalmol* 3:153-156, 2000.

143. McLaughlin SA et al: Pathogenic bacteria and fungi associated with extraocular disease in the horse, *J Am Vet Med Assoc* 182:241, 1983.

144. Goldstein M, Kowalski R, Gordon YJ: Emerging fluoro-quinolone resistance in bacterial keratitis, *Ophthalmology* 106:1313-1318, 1999.

145. Alexander G, Alfonso EC, Miller D: Shifting trends in bacterial keratitis in south Florida and emerging resistance to fluoro-quinolones, *Ophthalmology* 107:1497-1502, 2000.

146. Kowalski RP et al: Gatifloxacin and moxifloxacin: an in vitro susceptibility comparison to levofloxacin, ciprofloxacin, and ofloxacin using bacterial isolates, *Am J Ophthalmol* 136:500-505, 2003.

147. Sauer P et al: Changes in antibiotic resistance in equine bacterial ulcerative keratitis (1991-2000): 65 horses, *Vet Ophthalmol* 6:309-313, 2003.

148. Wilhelmus KR, Schlech BA: Clinical and epidemiological advantages of culturing bacterial keratitis, *Cornea* 23:38-42, 2004.

149. Brown S, Weller C, Akiya S: Pathogenesis of ulcers of the alkali-burned cornea, *Arch Ophthalmol* 83:205-208, 1970.

150. Aruoma OI et al: Apparent inactivation of alpha 1-antiproteinase by sulphur-containing radicals derived from penicillamine, *Biochem Pharmacol* 38:4353-4357, 1989.

151. Ralph RA: Tetracyclines and the treatment of corneal stromal ulceration, *Cornea* 19:274-277, 2000.

152. Frauenfelder H, McIlwraith W: Heparin treatment of an equine corneal ulcer, *Equine Vet J* 12:88-89, 1980.

153. Schultz GS et al: Treatment of alkali-injured rabbit corneas with a synthetic inhibitor of matrix metalloproteinases, *Invest Ophthalmol Vis Sci* 33:3325-3331, 1992.

154. Shams N, Hanninen L, Kenyon K: Increased gelatinolytic and caseinolytic activity in the thermally injured, nutritionally compromised rat cornea: detection of a 27-kDa lymphoreticular cell-associated caseinase, *Curr Eye Res* 13:11-19, 1994.

155. Haffner JC, Fecteau KA, Eiler H: Inhibition of collagenase breakdown of equine corneas by tetanus antitoxin, equine serum and acetylcysteine, *Vet Ophthalmol* 6:67-72, 2003.

156. Ueda Y, Homma JY, Abe C: Effects of immunization of horses with common antigen (OEP), protease toxoid, and elastase toxoid on corneal ulceration due to *Pseudomonas aeruginosa*, *Jpn J Vet Sci* 44:289-300, 1982.

157. Ueda Y, Sanai Y, Homma JY: Therapeutic effect of intracorneal injection of immunoglobulins on corneal ulcers in horses experimentally infected with *Pseudomonas aeruginosa*, *Jpn J Vet Sci* 44:301-308, 1982.

158. Williams MM et al: Systemic effects of topical and subconjunctival ophthalmic atropine in the horse, *Vet Ophthalmol* 3:193-199, 2000.

159. Imanishi J et al: Growth factors: importance in wound healing and maintenance of transparency of the cornea, *Prog Retin Eye Res* 19:113-129, 2000.

160. Blair MJ et al: Granulocyte macrophage colony stimulating factor: effect on corneal wound healing, *Vet Comp Ophthalmol* 7:168-172, 1997.

161. Lambiase A et al: Clinical application of nerve growth factor on human corneal ulcer, *Arch Ital Biol* 141:141-148, 2003.

162. Sosne G et al: Thymosin beta 4 promotes corneal wound healing and decreases inflammation in vivo following alkali injury, *Exp Eye Res* 74:293-299, 2002.

163. Sassani JW, Zagon IS, McLaughlin PJ: Opioid growth factor modulation of corneal epithelium: uppers and downers, *Curr Eye Res* 26:249-262, 2003.

164. Klippenstein K et al: The qualitative evaluation of the pharma-cokinetics of subconjunctivally injected antifungal agents in rabbits, *Cornea* 12:512-516, 1993.

165. Baum J, Barza M: Topical vs subconjunctival treatment of bacterial corneal ulcers, *Ophthalmology* 90:162-168, 1983.

166. Reichel MB et al: New model of conjunctival scarring in the mouse eye, *Br J Ophthalmol* 82:1072-1077, 1998.

167. Gelatt KN, Gelatt JP: *Handbook of small animal ophthalmic surgery, vol 1, Extraocular procedures*, New York, 1994, Pergamon, pp 165-188.

168. Collins MB, Ethell MT, Hodgson DR: Management of mycotic keratitis in a horse using a conjunctival pedicle graft, *Aust Vet J* 71:298-299, 1994.

169. Holmberg DL: Conjunctival pedicle grafts used to repair corneal perforations in the horse, *Can Vet J* 22:86-89, 1981.

170. Nasisse MP: Principles of microsurgery, *Vet Clin North Am Small Anim Pract* 27:987-1010, 1997.

171. Hacker DV et al.: Surgical repair of collagenolytic ulcerative keratitis in the horse, *Equine Vet J* 22:88-92, 1990.

172. Hekmati P: Lamellar corneal transplantation in the horse, *Vet Rec* 99:46-49, 1976.

173. McLaughlin SA, Brightman AH, Brogdon JD: Autogenous partial-thickness corneal graft for repair of a perforated corneal ulcer in a horse, *Equine Pract* 7:34-38, 1985.

174. Andrew SE, Tou S, Brooks DE: Corneoconjunctival transposition for the treatment of feline corneal sequestra: a retrospective study of 17 cases (1990-1998), *Vet Ophthalmol* 4:107-111, 2001.

175. Hacker DV: Frozen corneal grafts in dogs and cats: a report on 19 cases, *J Am Anim Hosp Assoc* 27:387-398, 1991.

176. Andrew SE et al: Comparison of Optisol-GS and neomycin-polymyxin B-gramicidin ophthalmic solution for corneal storage in the dog, *Vet Ophthalmol* 2:155-161, 1999.

177. Andrew SE. Corneal stromal abscess in a horse, *Vet Ophthalmol* 2:207-211, 1999.

178. Lassaline ME et al: Equine amniotic membrane transplantation for keratomalacia in three horses, *Vet Ophthalmol* 3:352, 2003.

179. Solomon A et al: Amniotic membrane grafts for nontraumatic corneal perforations, descemetoceles, and deep ulcers, *Ophthalmology* 109:694-703, 2002.

180. Kim JS et al: Amniotic membrane transplantation in infectious corneal ulcer, *Cornea* 20:720-726, 2001.

181. Madhavan HN et al: Preparation of amniotic membrane for ocular surface reconstruction, *Indian J Ophthalmol* 50:227-231, 2002.

182. Tseng SC et al: Amniotic membrane transplantation with or without limbal allografts for corneal surface reconstruction in patients with limbal stem cell deficiency, *Arch Ophthalmol* 116:431-441, 1998.

183. Lee SH, Tseng SC: Amniotic membrane transplantation for persistent epithelial defects with ulceration, *Am J Ophthalmol* 123:303-312, 1997.

184. Shimazaki J, Yang HY, Tsubota K: Amniotic membrane transplantation for ocular surface reconstruction in patients with chemical and thermal burns, *Ophthalmology* 104:2068-2076, 1997.

185. Grahn B et al: Equine keratomycosis: clinical and laboratory findings in 23 cases, *Vet Comp Ophthalmol* 3:2-7, 1993.

186. Barton MH: Equine keratomycosis, *Comp Contin Educ Pract (Vet)* 14:936-944, 1992.

187. Beech J, Sweeney CR: Keratomycoses in 11 horses, *Equine Vet J Suppl* 2:39-44, 1983.

188. Ball MA et al: Evaluation of itraconazole-dimethyl sulfoxide ointment for treatment of keratomycosis in nine horses, *J Am Vet Med Assoc* 211:199-203, 1997.

189. Jones BR: Principles in the management of oculomycosis. XXXI Edward Jackson Memorial Lecture, *Am J Ophthalmol* 79:719-751, 1975.

190. Coad CT, Robinson NM, Wilhelmus KR: Antifungal sensitivity testing for equine keratomycosis, *Am J Vet Res* 46:676-678, 1985.

191. Brooks DE et al: Rose bengal positive epithelial microerosions as a manifestation of equine keratomycosis, *Vet Ophthalmol* 3:83-86, 2000.

192. Kuonen VJ et al: A PCR-based assay for the diagnosis of equine fungal keratitis, *Vet Ophthalmol* 6:364, 2003.

193. Neary A et al: Diagnosis of equine fungal keratitis using polymerase chain reaction, *Vet Ophthalmol* 6:363, 2003.

194. Wu TG, Wilhelmus KR, Mitchell BM: Experimental keratomycosis in a mouse model, *Invest Ophthalmol Vis Sci* 44:210-216, 2003.

195. Gaudio PA et al: Polymerase chain reaction based detection of fungi in infected corneas, *Br J Ophthalmol* 86:755-760, 2002.

196. Ferrer C et al: Polymerase chain reaction diagnosis in fungal keratitis caused by *Alternaria alternate*, *Am J Ophthalmol* 133: 398-399, 2002.

197. Kercher L et al: Molecular screening of donor corneas for fungi before excision, *Invest Ophthalmol Vis Sci* 42:2578-2578, 2001.

198. Zhu WS et al: Extracellular proteases of *Aspergillus flavus*: fungal keratitis, proteases, and pathogenesis, *Diagn Microbiol Infect Dis* 13:491-497, 1990.

199. Sack RA et al: Changes in the diurnal pattern of the distribution of gelatinases and associated proteins in normal and pathological tear fluids: evidence that the PMN cell is a major source of MMP activity in tear fluid, *Adv Exp Med Biol* 506:539, 2002.

200. Isnard N et al: Effect of hyaluronan on MMP expression and activation, *Cell Biol Int* 25:735739, 2001.

201. Lassaline ME et al: Histologic analysis of keratectomy specimens from horses undergoing corneal transplantation for stromal abscess, *Vet Ophthalmol* 5:286, 2002.

202. Davis BD: Bacterial architecture. In Davis BD et al, editors: *Microbiology*, ed 4, Philadelphia, 1990, JB Lippincott, pp 38-39.

203. Alcamo IE: Fundamentals of microbiology. In Tortora GS, Funke BR, Case CL, editors: *Microbiology: an introduction*, Menlo Park, Calif, 1991, Benjamin Cummings.

204. Miller Michau T et al: Findings from 16 consecutive cases of penetrating keratoplasty for deep stromal abscess in the horse (2001-2002), *Vet Ophthalmol* 5 296, 2003.

205. Woo S et al: Synergism between fungal enzymes and bacterial antibiotics may enhance biocontrol, *Antonie Van Leeuwenhoek* 81:353-356, 2002.

206. Alexopoulos CJ, Mims CW, Blackwell M: In Alexopoulos CJ, Mims CW, Blackwell M, editors: *Introductory mycology,* ed 4, New York, 1996, John Wiley & Sons, pp 20-60.

207. Johns KJ, O'Day DM: Pharmacologic management of keratomycoses, *Surv Ophthalmol* 33:178-188, 1988.

208. O'Day DM et al: Influence of the corneal epithelium on the efficacy of topical antifungal agents, *Invest Ophthalmol Vis Sci* 25:855, 1984.

209. Foster CS, Stefanyszyn M: Intraocular penetration of miconazole in rabbits, *Arch Ophthalmol* 97:1703-1706, 1979.

210. Hemady RK, Chu W, Foster CS: Intraocular penetration of ketoconazole in rabbits, *Cornea* 11:329-333, 1992.

211. Foster CS et al: Ocular toxicity of topical antifungal agents, *Arch Ophthalmol* 99:1081-1084, 1981.

212. Ball MA et al: Corneal concentrations and preliminary toxicological evaluation of an itraconazole/dimethyl sulphoxide ophthalmic ointment, *J Vet Pharmacol Ther* 20:100-104, 1997.

213. Latimer FG et al: Pharmacokinetics of fluconazole following intravenous and oral administration and body fluid concentrations of fluconazole following repeated oral dosing in horses, *Am J Vet Res* 62:1606-1611, 2001.

214. Yee RW et al: Ocular penetration and pharmacokinetics of topical fluconazole, *Cornea* 16:64-71, 1997.

215. Ghannoum MA, Kuhn DM: Voriconazole: better chances for patients with invasive mycoses, *Eur J Med Res* 31:242-256, 2002.

216. Kappe R: Antifungal activity of the new azole UK-109,496 (voriconazole), *Mycoses* 42(Suppl 2):83-86, 1999.

217. Holmberg K: In vitro assessment of antifungal drug resistance, *Acta Derm Venereol Suppl (Stockh)* 121:131-138, 1986.

218. Brooks DE et al: Antimicrobial susceptibility patterns of fungi isolated from horses with ulcerative keratomycosis, *Am J Vet Res* 59:138-142, 1998.

219. Afonso EC, Rosa RH Jr: Fungal keratitis. In Krachmer JH, Mannis MJ, Holland EJ, editors: *Cornea, vol II, Cornea and external disease. Clinical diagnosis and management,* St Louis, 1997, Mosby, pp 1253-1265.

220. Roberts SM, Severin GA, Lavach JD: Antibacterial activity of dilute povidone iodine solutions used for ocular surface disinfection, *Am J Vet Res* 47:1207-1210, 1986.

221. Bates EE, McCartney DL: A study of the potential effect of povidone-iodine solution in treating ocular fungal pathogens, *Invest Ophthalmol Vis Sci* 37:S872, 1996.

222. Wlodkowski TJ, Rosenkranz HS: Antifungal activity of silver sulphadiazine, *Lancet* 29:739-740, 1973.

223. De Lucca AJ, Walsh TJ, Daigle DJ: N-acetylcysteine inhibits germination of conidia and growth of *Aspergillus* spp. and *Fusarium* spp., *Antimicrob Agents Chemother* 40:1274-1276, 1996.

224. Rahman MR et al: Trial of chlorhexidine gluconate for fungal corneal ulcers, *Ophthalmic Epidemiol* 4:141-149, 1997.

225. Scotty NC et al: Lufenuron: determination of antifungal activity in vitro and measurement of blood concentrations following oral administration in horses, *Vet Ophthalmol* 6:351, 2003.

226. Rebhun WC: Corneal stromal abscesses in the horse, *J Am Vet Med Assoc* 181:677-679, 1982.

227. Sweeney CR et al: Corneal stromal abscess in two horses: a case report, *Comp Contin Educ Pract (Vet)* 6:S595-S599, 1984.

228. Schmotzer WB, Riebold T, Holland J: Corneal stromal abscess in a horse, *Mod Vet Pract* 66:967-968, 1985.

229. Wolfer J, Grahn B: Diagnostic ophthalmology, *Can Vet J* 35: 450-451, 1994.

230. Whittaker CJG et al: Therapeutic penetrating keratoplasty for deep corneal stromal abscesses in eight horses, *Vet Comp Ophthalmol* 7:19-28, 1997.

231. Hamilton HL et al: Histological findings in corneal stromal abscesses of 11 horses: correlation with cultures and cytology, *Equine Vet J* 26:448-453, 1994.

232. Rebhun WC: Corneal stromal infections in horses, *Comp Contin Educ Pract (Vet)* 14:363-371, 1992.

233. Mondino BJ: Inflammatory diseases of the peripheral cornea, *Ophthalmology* 95:577-590, 1988.

234. Wilcock BP: The eye and ear. In Jubb KVF, Kennedy PC, Palmer N, editors: *Pathology of domestic animals,* ed 4, San Diego, 1990, Academic Press, pp 441-522.

235. O'Conner RG: Basic mechanism responsible for the initiation and recurrence of uveitis, *Am J Ophthalmol* 96:577-599, 1983.

236. Robert PY, Adenis JP: Comparative review of topical ophthalmic antibacterial preparations, *Drugs* 61:175-185, 2001.

237. O'Day DM et al: Efficacy of antifungal agents in the cornea. II. Influence of corticosteroids, *Invest Ophthalmol Vis Sci* 25:331-335, 1984.

238. Gilger BC, McLaughlin SA: Glaucoma and corneal stromal abscess in a horse treated by an intraocular silicone prosthesis and a conjunctival pedicle flap, *Equine Pract* 15:10-15, 1993.

239. Carson-Dunkerley S et al: Treatment of equine corneal stromal abscesses using frozen canine corneal grafts, *Vet Surg* 25:442, 1996.

240. Danjoux JP, Reck AC: Corneal sutures: is routine removal really necessary? *Eye* 8:339-342, 1994.

241. van Ee RT et al: Effects of nylon and polyglactin 910 suture material on perilimbal corneal wound healing in the dog, *Vet Surg* 15:435-440, 1986.

242. Melles GRJ et al: A surgical technique for posterior lamellar keratoplasty, *Cornea* 17:618-626, 1998.

243. Brooks DE et al: Deep lamellar endothelial keratoplasty (DLEK) in six horses, *Vet Ophthalmol* 6:354, 2003.

244. Jain S, Azar DT: New lamellar keratoplasty techniques: posterior keratoplasty and deep lamellar keratoplasty, *Curr Opin Ophthalmol* 12:262-268, 2001.

245. Krohne SG et al: Use of small intestinal submucosa (SIS) as a graft for corneal perforations and abscesses in horses, dogs and cats, *Vet Ophthalmol* 6:354, 2003.

246. Draeger J, Kohler L, Winter R: Technical aspects in ultra-large corneal grafts, *Ophthalmic Res* 17:266-268, 1985.

247. Inoue K et al: Risk factors for corneal graft failure and rejection in penetrating keratoplasty, *Acta Ophthalmol Scand* 79:251-255, 2001.

248. Andrew SE, Brooks DE: The success and complication rates of penetrating keratoplasty in the horse, *Invest Ophthalmol Vis Sci* 40:S253, 1999.

249. Banerjee S, Dick AD: Recent developments in the pharmacological treatment and prevention of corneal graft rejection, *Expert Opin Investig Drugs* 12:29-37, 2003.

250. Harkins JD, Carney JM, Tobin T: Clinical use and characteristics of the corticosteroids, *Vet Clin North Am Equine Pract* 9:543-562, 1993.

251. Murthy RC et al: Corneal transduction to inhibit angiogenesis and graft failure, *Invest Ophthalmol Vis Sci* 44:1837-1842, 2003.

252. Kershaw O et al: Detection of equine herpesvirus type 2 (EHV-2) in horses with keratoconjunctivitis, *Virus Res* 80:93-99, 2001.

253. Collinson PN et al: Isolation of equine herpesvirus type 2 (equine gammaherpesvirus 2) from foals with keratoconjunctivitis, *J Am Vet Med Assoc* 205:329-331, 1994.

254. Matthews AG, Handscombe MC: Superficial keratitis in the horse: treatment with the antiviral drug idoxuridine, *Equine Vet J Suppl* 2:29-31, 1983.

255. Miller TR et al: Herpetic keratitis in a horse, *Equine Vet J Suppl* 10:15-17, 1990.

256. Maggs DJ: Ocular manifestations of equine herpesviruses. In Robinson NE, editor: *Current therapy in equine medicine 5,* St Louis, 2003, Saunders, pp 473-476.

257. Telford EAR et al: Equine herpesvirus 2 and 5 are gammaherpesviruses, *Virology* 195:492-499, 1993.

258. Cello RM: Recent findings in periodic ophthalmia. In: *Proceedings of the 8th Annual Meeting of the American Association of Equine Practitioners, vol 123,* 1962, p 123.

259. Cello RM: Ocular onchocerciasis in the horse, *Equine Vet J* 3: 148-143, 1971.

260. Schmidt GM et al: Equine ocular onchocerciasis: histopathologic study, *Am J Vet Res* 43:1371-1375, 1982.

261. Hammond R, Severin GA, Snyder S: Equine ocular onchocerciasis: a case report, *Equine Vet J Suppl* 2:74-75, 1983.

262. Munger RJ: Equine onchocercal keratoconjunctivitis, *Equine Vet J Suppl* 2:65-70, 1983.

263. Stannard AA, Cello RM: *Onchocerca cervicalis* infection in horses from the western United States, *Am J Vet Res* 36:1029-1031, 1975.

264. Lloyd S, Soulsby EJL: Survey for infection with *Onchocerca cervicalis* in horses in eastern United States, *Am J Vet Res* 39: 1962-1963, 1978.

265. Moran CT, James ER: Equine ocular pathology ascribed to *Onchocerca cervicalis* infection: a re-examination, *Trop Med Parasitol* 38:287-288, 1987.

266. Collobert C, Bernard N, Lamidey C: Prevalence of *Onchocerca* species and *Thelazia lacrimalis* in horses examined post mortem in Normandy, *Vet Rec* 136:463-465, 1995.

267. French DD et al: Efficacy of ivermectin in paste and injectable formulations against microfilariae of *Onchocerca cervicalis* and resolution of associated dermatitis in horses, *Am J Vet Res* 49:1550-1554, 1988.

268. Lyons ET, Drudge JH, Tolliver SC: Verification of ineffectual activity of ivermectin against adult *Onchocerca* spp in the ligamentum nuchae of horses, *Am J Vet Res* 49:983-985, 1988.

269. Monahan CM et al: Efficacy of moxidectin oral gel against *Onchocerca cervicalis* microfilariae, *J Parasitol* 81:117-118, 1995.

270. Gilger BC: Equine recurrent uveitis. In Robinson NE, editor: *Current therapy in equine medicine 5,* St Louis, 2003, Saunders, pp 468-473.

271. Hakanson NE, Dubielzig RR: Chronic superficial corneal erosions with anterior stromal sequestration in three horses, *Vet Comp Ophthalmol* 4:179-183, 1994.

272. McLellan GL, Archer FJ: Corneal stromal sequestration and keratoconjunctivitis sicca in a horse, *Vet Ophthalmol* 3:207-212, 2000.

273. Brooks DE et al: Nonulcerative keratouveitis in five horses, *J Am Vet Med Assoc* 196:1985-1991, 1990.

274. Gratzek AT et al: Ophthalmic cyclosporine in equine keratitis and keratouveitis: 11 cases, *Equine Vet J* 27:327-333, 1995.

275. Matthews AG: Nonulcerative keratopathies in the horse, *Equine Vet Educ* 2000, pp 350-357.

276. Wada S et al: Nonulcerative keratouveitis as a manifestation of Leptospiral infection in a horse, *Vet Ophthalmol* 6:191-195, 2003.

277. Lucchesi PM, Parma AE: A DNA fragment of *Leptospira interrogans* encodes a protein which shares epitopes with equine cornea, *Vet Immunol Immunopathol* 71:173-179, 1999.

278. Ramsey DT et al: Eosinophilic keratoconjunctivitis in a horse, *J Am Vet Med Assoc* 205:1308-1311, 1994.

279. Yamagata M, Wilkie DA, Gilger BC: Eosinophilic keratoconjunctivitis in seven horses, *J Am Vet Med Assoc* 209:1283-1286, 1996.

280. Glaze MB: Equine adnexal habronemiasis, *Equine Vet J Suppl* 2:71-73, 1983.

281. McEwan BJ et al: The response of the eosinophil in acute inflammation in the horse. In von Tascharner C, Halliwell REW, editors: *Advances in veterinary dermatology,* London, 1990, Bailliere Tindall, pp 176-194.

282. Trocme SD et al: Eosinophilic granule major basic protein deposition in corneal ulcers associated with vernal keratoconjunctivitis, *Am J Ophthalmol* 115:640-643, 1983.

283. Rebhun WC: Conjunctival and corneal foreign bodies, *Vet Med Small Anim Clin* 68:874, 1973.

284. Lavach JD, Severin GA, Roberts SM: Lacerations of the equine eye: a review of 48 cases, *J Am Vet Med Assoc* 184:1243-1248, 1984.

285. Chmielewski NT et al: Visual outcome and ocular survival following iris prolapse in the horse: a review of 32 cases, *Equine Vet J* 29:31-39, 1997.

286. Scott WR et al: Ocular injuries due to projectile impacts, *Annu Proc Assoc Adv Automot Med* 44:205-217, 2000.

287. Gwin RM, Peiffer RL, Gelatt KN: Repair of a limbal laceration in a horse, *J Equine Med Surg* 1:413-417, 1977.

288. Riggs C, Whitley RD: Intraocular silicone prostheses in a dog and a horse with corneal lacerations, *J Am Vet Med Assoc* 196:617-619, 1990.

289. Riedl M et al: Intraocular ointment after small-incision cataract surgery causing chronic uveitis and secondary glaucoma, *J Cataract Refract Surg* 29:1022-1025, 2003.

290. Keller WF, Blanchard GL, Goble DO: Vesicle formation and scarring of a horse's cornea following whip injury, *J Am Anim Hosp Assoc* 9:252-255, 1973.

291. Moore CP et al: Post traumatic keratouveitis in horses, *Equine Vet J* 30:366-372, 1998.

292. Robin JB et al: The histopathology of corneal neovascularization. Inhibitor effects, *Arch Ophthalmol* 103:284-287, 1985.

293. Iniguez MA et al: Cyclooxygenase-2: a therapeutic target in angiogenesis, *Trends Mol Med* 9:73-78, 2003.

294. Thompson RW Jr, et al: Long-term graft survival after penetrating keratoplasty, *Ophthalmology* 110:1396-1402, 2003.

295. Michau TM et al: Use of thermokeratoplasty for treatment of ulcerative keratitis and bullous keratopathy secondary to corneal endothelial disease in dogs: 13 cases (1994-2001), *J Am Vet Med Assoc* 222:607-612, 2003.

296. Rebhun WC: Chemical keratitis in a horse, *Vet Med Small Anim Clin* 75:1537-1539, 1980.

297. Haddox JL, Pfister RR, Yuille-Barr D: The efficacy of topical citrate after alkali injury is dependent on the period of time it is administered, *Invest Ophthalmol Vis Sci* 30:1062-1068, 1989.

298. Chung JH et al: Effect of topically applied 0.1% dexamethasone on endothelial healing and aqueous composition during the repair process of rabbit corneal alkali wounds, *Curr Eye Res* 18:110-116, 1999.

299. Meller D et al: Amniotic membrane transplantation for acute chemical or thermal burns, *Ophthalmology* 107:980-989, 2000.

300. Millichamp NJ, Carter GK, Dziezyc J: Idiopathic corneal odema in a horse, *Equine Vet J Suppl* 10:12-14, 1990.

301. Rebhun WC: Corneal dystrophies and degenerations in horses, *Comp Contin Educ Pract (Vet)* 14:945-950, 1992.

302. Rebhun WC, Murphy CJ, Hacker DV: Calcific band keratopathy in horses, *Comp Contin Educ Pract (Vet)* 15:1402-1409, 1993.

303. O'Connor GR: Calcific band keratopathy, *Trans Am Ophthalmol Soc* 70:58-81, 1972.

304. Taravella MJ et al: Calcific band keratopathy associated with the use of topical steroid-phosphate containing preparations, *Arch Ophthalmol* 112:608-613, 1994.

305. Crispin SM: Tear-deficient and evaporative dry eye syndromes of the horse, *Vet Ophthalmol* 3:87-92, 2000.

306. Joyce JR, Bratton GR: Keratoconjunctivitis sicca secondary to fracture of the mandible, *Vet Med Small Anim Clin* 68:619-620, 1973.

307. Spurlock SL, Spurlock GH, Wise M: Keratoconjunctivitis sicca associated with fracture of the stylohyoid bone in a horse, *J Am Vet Med Assoc* 194:258-259, 1989.

308. Van Kampen KR, James LF: Ophthalmic lesions in locoweed poisoning of cattle, sheep, and horses, *Am J Vet Res* 32:1293-1295, 1971.

309. Collins BK et al: Immune-mediated keratoconjunctivitis sicca in a horse, *Vet Comp Ophthalmol* 4:61-65, 1994.

310. Spiess BM, Wilcock BP, Physick-Sheard PW: Eosinophilic granulomatous dacryoadenitis causing bilateral keratoconjunctivitis sicca in a horse, *Equine Vet J* 21:226-229, 1989.

311. Beech J et al: Schirmer tear test results in normal horses and ponies: effect of age, season, environment, sex, time of day and placement of strips, *Vet Ophthalmol* 6:251-254, 2003.

312. Marts BS, Bryan GM, Prieur DJ: Schirmer tear test measurements and lysozyme concentration of equine tears, *J Equine Med Surg* 1:427-430, 1977.

313. Williams RD, Manning JP, Peiffer RL Jr: The Schirmer tear test in the equine: normal values and the contribution of the gland of the nictitating membrane, *J Equine Med Surg* 3:117-119, 1979.

314. Scagliotti RH: Comparative neuro-ophthalmology. In Gelatt KN, editor: *Veterinary ophthalmology,* ed 3, Philadelphia, 1999, Lippincott, Williams & Wilkins, pp 1307-1400.

315. Reilly L, Beech J: Bilateral keratoconjunctivitis sicca in a horse, *Equine Vet J* 26:171-172, 1994.

316. Hollingsworth SR et al: Effect of topically administered atropine on tear production in dogs, *J Am Vet Med Assoc* 200:1481-1484, 1992.

317. Wolf ED, Merideth R: Parotid duct transposition in the horse, *Equine Vet Sci* 1:143-145, 1981.

318. Rebhun WC, Georgi M, Georgi JR: Persistent corneal ulcers in horses caused by embedded burdock pappus bristles, *Vet Med* 86:930-935, 1991.

319. Anderson BC: Indolent-like corneal ulcers, *J Am Vet Med Assoc* 188:1138-1139, 1986.

320. Michau TM et al: Superficial, non-healing corneal ulcers in horses: 23 cases (1989-2003), *Vet Ophthalmol* 6:291-297, 2003.

321. Tripathi RC, Bron A: Ultrastructural study of non-traumatic recurrent corneal erosions, *Br J Ophthalmol* 56:73-85, 1972.

322. Gelatt KN, Samuelson DA: Recurrent corneal erosions and epithelial dystrophy in the boxer dog, *J Am Anim Hosp Assoc* 18:453-460, 1982.

323. Kirschner SE, Niyo Y, Betts DM: Idiopathic persistent corneal erosions: clinical and pathological findings in 18 dogs, *J Am Anim Hosp Assoc* 25:84-90, 1989.

324. Bentley E et al: Morphology and immunohistochemistry of spontaneous chronic corneal epithelial defects (SCCED) in dogs, *Invest Ophthalmol Vis Sci* 42:2262-2269, 2001.

325. Bentley E, Murphy CJ: Thermal cautery of the cornea for treatment of spontaneous chronic corneal epithelial defects in dogs and horses, *J Am Vet Med Assoc* 224:250-253, 2004.

326. Moore CP, Corwin LA, Collier LL: Keratopathy induced by beta radiation therapy in a horse, *Equine Vet J Suppl* 2:112-116, 1983.

327. Slatter DH, Nelson A, Smith G: Ocular sequelae of high-dose periocular gamma irradiation in a horse, *Equine Vet J Suppl* 2:110-111, 1983.

328. Singer B: Ocular effects of ionizing radiation: past and present problems, *Br J Ophthalmol* 63:455-456, 1979.

329. Bergeder H, Rink H: Ionizing radiation. In Lerman S, editor: *Radiation energy and the eye,* New York, 1979, MacMillan, pp 281-285.

330. Frauenfelder HC, Blevins WE, Page EH: ^{90}Sr for treatment of periocular squamous cell carcinoma in the horse, *J Am Vet Med Assoc* 180:307-309, 1982.

331. Rebhun WC: Tumors of the eye and ocular adnexal tissues, *Vet Clin North Am Equine Pract* 14:579-606, 1998.

332. Dugan SJ et al: Prognostic factors and survival of horses with ocular/adnexal squamous cell carcinoma: 147 cases (1978-1988), *J Am Vet Med Assoc* 198:298-303, 1991.

333. Walker MA, Goble D, Geiser D: Two-year non-recurrence rates for equine ocular and periorbital squamous cell carcinoma following radiotherapy, *Vet Radiol* 27:146, 1986.

334. Rebhun WC: Treatment of advanced squamous cell carcinomas involving the equine cornea, *Vet Surg* 19:297-302, 1990.

335. Schoster JV: Using combined excision and cryotherapy to treat limbal squamous cell carcinoma, *Vet Med* 87:357, 1992.

336. Grier RL et al: Treatment of bovine and equine ocular squamous cell carcinoma by radiofrequency hyperthermia, *J Am Vet Med Assoc* 177:55-61, 1980.

337. Kim SH, Kim JH, Hahn EW: The radiosensitization of hypoxic tumor cells by hyperthermia, *Radiology* 114:727-728, 1975.

338. English RV, Nasisse MP, Davidson MG: Carbon dioxide laser ablation for treatment of limbal squamous cell carcinoma in horses, *J Am Vet Med Assoc* 196: 439-442, 1990.

339. Fortier LA, Mac Harg MA: Topical use of 5-fluorouracil for treatment of squamous cell carcinoma of the external genitalia of horses: 11 cases (1988-1992), *J Am Vet Med Assoc* 205:1183-1185, 1994.

340. Paterson S: Treatment of superficial ulcerative squamous cell carcinoma in three horses with topical 5-fluorouracil, *Vet Rec* 141:626-628, 1997.

341. Dugan SJ: Ocular neoplasia, *Vet Clin North Am Equine Pract* 8:609-626, 1992.

342. van der Woerdt A, Gilger BC, Wilkie DA: Penetrating keratoplasty for treatment of recurrent squamous cell carcinoma of the cornea in a horse, *J Am Vet Med Assoc* 208:1692-1694, 1996.

343. Hirst LW et al: Benign epibulbar melanocytoma in a horse, *J Am Vet Med Assoc* 183:333-334, 1983.

344. Lavach JD, Severin GA: Neoplasia of the equine eye, adnexa, and orbit: a review of 68 cases, *J Am Vet Med Assoc* 170:202-203, 1977.

345. Hamor RE et al: Melanoma of the conjunctiva and cornea in a horse, *Vet Comp Ophthalmol* 7:52-55, 1997.

346. Murphy J, Young S: Intraocular melanoma in a horse, *Vet Pathol* 16:539-542, 1979.

347. Valentine BA: Equine melanocytic tumors: a retrospective study of 53 horses (1988 to 1991), *J Vet Intern Med* 9:291-297, 1995.

348. Seltenhammer MH et al: Equine melanoma in a population of 296 grey Lipizzaner horses, *Equine Vet J* 35:153-157, 2003.

349. Martin CL: Canine epibulbar melanomas and their management, *J Am Anim Hosp Assoc* 17:83-90, 1981.

350. Harling DE, Peiffer RL Jr, Cook CS: Feline limbal melanoma: four cases, *J Am Anim Hosp Assoc* 22:795-802, 1986.

351. Blogg JR, Dutton AG, Stanley RG: Use of third eyelid grafts to repair full-thickness defects in the cornea and sclera, *J Am Anim Hosp Assoc* 25:505-512, 1989.

352. Wilkie DA, Wolf ED: Treatment of epibulbar melanocytoma in a dog, using full-thickness eyewall resection and synthetic graft, *J Am Vet Med Assoc* 198:1019-1022, 1991.

353. Sullivan TC et al: Photocoagulation of limbal melanoma in dogs and cats: 15 cases (1989-1993), *J Am Vet Med Assoc* 208: 891-894, 1996.

354. Jakobiec FA et al: Combined surgery and cryotherapy for diffuse malignant melanoma of the conjunctiva, *Arch Ophthalmol* 98: 1390-1396, 1980.

355. Jakobiec FA et al: The role of cryotherapy in the management of conjunctival melanoma, *Ophthalmology* 89:502-515, 1982.

356. Werschnik C, Lommatzsch PK: Long-term follow-up of patients with conjunctival melanoma, *Am J Clin Oncol* 25:248-255, 2002.

357. Goetz TE et al: Cimetidine for treatment of melanomas in three horses, *J Am Vet Med Assoc* 196:449-452, 1990.

358. Ucar K: The effects of histamine H2 receptor antagonists on melanogenesis and cellular proliferation in melanoma cells in culture, *Biochem Biophys Res Commun* 177:545-452, 1991.

359. Bolton JR et al: Ocular neoplasms of vascular origin in the horse, *Equine Vet J Suppl* 10:73-75, 1990.

360. Hacker DV, Moore PF, Buyukmihci NC: Ocular angiosarcoma in four horses, *J Am Vet Med Assoc* 189:200-203, 1986.

361. Moore PF, Hacker DV, Buyukmihci NC: Ocular angiosarcoma in the horse: morphological and immunohistochemical studies, *Vet Pathol* 23:240-244, 1986.

362. Crawley GR, Bryan GM, Gogolewski RP: Ocular hemangiosarcoma in a horse, *Equine Pract* 9:11-14, 1987.

363. Vestre WA, Turner TA, Carlton WW: Conjunctival hemangioma in a horse, *J Am Vet Med Assoc* 180:1481-1482, 1982.

364. Rebhun WC, Del Piero F: Ocular lesions in horses with lymphosarcoma: 21 cases (1977-1997), *J Am Vet Med Assoc* 212:852-854, 1998.

365. Ward DA, Lakritz J, Bauer RW: Scleral mastocytosis in a horse, *Equine Vet J* 25:79-80, 1993.

366. Hum S, Bowers JR: Ocular mastocytosis in a horse, *Aust Vet J* 66:32, 1989.

367. Martin CL, Leipold HW: Mastocytoma of the globe in a horse, *J Am Anim Hosp Assoc* 8:32-34, 1972.

368. Wilcock BP: Neoplastic diseases of the skin. In Jubb KVF, Kennedy PC, Palmer N, editors: *Pathology of domestic animals*, Orlando, Fla, 1985, Academic Press, pp 519-520.

369. Prasse KW, Lundvall RL, Cheville NF: Generalized mastocytosis in a foal, resembling urticaria pigmentosa of man, *J Am Vet Med Assoc* 166:68-70, 1975.

370. Altera K, Clark L: Equine cutaneous mastocytosis, *Pathol Vet* 7:43-45, 1970.

371. Lundvall RL: The bacteria and mycotic flora of the normal conjunctival sac in the horse. In: *Proceedings of the 13th Annual Meeting of the American Association of Equine Practitioners*, 1967, pp 101-107.

372. Whitley RD, Moore CP: Microbiology of the equine eye in health and disease, *Vet Clin North Am* 6:451, 1984.

373. Whitley RD, Burgess EC, Moore CP: Microbial isolates of the normal equine eye, *Equine Vet J Suppl* 2:138, 1983.

374. Ward D: Ocular pharmacology. In Gelatt KN, editor: *Veterinary ophthalmology*, ed 3, Philadelphia, 1999, Lippincott Williams & Wilkins, pp 336-354.

375. Barletta JP et al: Inhibition of pseudomonal ulceration in rabbit corneas by a synthetic matrix metalloproteinase inhibitor, *Invest Ophthalmol Vis Sci* 37:20-28, 1996.

376. Burns FR et al: The effect of a synthetic metalloproteinase inhibitor on corneal ulceration in alkali burns and pseudomonas keratitis, *Matrix Suppl* 1:317-318, 1992.

377. Kanao S et al: Clinical application of 3% N-acetylcysteine eye drops in corneal diseases in dogs, *J Japan Vet Med Assoc* 46: 487-491, 1993.

378. Petroutsos G et al: Effect of acetylcysteine (Mucomyst) on epithelial wound healing, *Ophthalmic Res* 14:241-248, 1982.

379. Rawal SY, Rawal YB: Non-antimicrobial properties of tetracyclines: dental and medical implications, *West Indian Med* 50: 105-108, 1984.

380. Golub LM et al: Tetracyclines inhibit tissue collagenase activity, *J Perdiodontal Res* 19:651-655, 1984.

381. Seedor JA et al: Systemic tetracycline treatment of alkali-induced corneal ulceration in rabbits, *Arch Ophthalmol* 105:268-271, 1987.

382. Perry HD et al: Effect of doxycycline hyclate on corneal epithelial wound healing in the rabbit alkali-burn model: preliminary observations, *Cornea* 12:379-382, 1993.

383. Rebhun WC et al: Presumed clostridial and aerobic bacterial infections of the cornea in two horses, *J Am Vet Med Assoc* 214:1519-1522, 1999.

384. Rebhun WC: Bacterial ulcers of the equine eye, *Equine Pract* 3:40-49, 1981.

385. Adamson PJ, Jang SS: Ulcerative keratitis associated with *Salmonella arizonae* infection in a horse, *J Am Vet Med Assoc* 186: 1219-1220, 1985.

386. Sanchez S et al: *Listeria* keratitis in a horse, *Vet Ophthalmol* 4: 217-219, 2001.

387. Cullen CL, Grahn BH: Diagnostic ophthalmology, *Can Vet J* 41:867-868, 2000.

388. Higgins R, Biberstein EL, Jang SS: Nutritionally variant streptococci from corneal ulcers in horses, *J Clin Microbiol* 20:1130-1134, 1984.

389. Gwin RM: Equine fungal keratitis: diagnosis and treatment, *Equine Vet Sci,* 1981, pp 66-68.

390. Bistner SI, Riis RC: Clinical aspects of mycotic keratitis in the horse, *Cornell Vet* 69:364-372, 1979.

391. Aho R, Tala M, Kivalo M: Mycotic keratitis in a horse caused by *Aspergillus fumigatus:* the first reported case in Finland, *Acta Vet Scand* 32:373-376, 1991.

392. Marolt J, Naglic T, Hajsig D: *Aspergillus oryzae* als ursache einer keratomykose beim pferd, *Tieraztl Prax* 12:489-492, 1984.

393. Hendrix DVH, Ward DA, Guglick MA: Disseminated candidiasis in a neonatal foal with keratomycosis as the initial sign, *Vet Comp Ophthalmol* 7:10-13, 1997.

394. Chopin JB et al: Keratomycosis in a Percheron cross horse caused by *Cladorrhinum bulbillosum, J Med Vet Mycol* 35:53-55, 1997.

395. Hendrix DVH et al: Keratomycosis in four horses caused by *Cylindrocarpon destructans, Vet Comp Ophthalmol* 6:252-257, 1996.

396. Hodgson DR, Jacobs KA: Two cases of *Fusarium* keratomycosis in the horse, *Vet Rec* 110:520-522, 1982.

397. Mitchell JS, Attleberger MH: *Fusarium* keratomycosis in the horse, *Vet Med Small Anim Clin* 68:1257-1260, 1973.

398. Richter M et al: Keratitis due to *Histoplasma* spp. in a horse, *Vet Ophthalmol* 6:99-103, 2003.

399. Foley JE, Norris CR, Jang SS: Paecilomycosis in dogs and horses and a review of the literature, *J Vet Intern Med* 16:238-243, 2002.

400. Friedman DS et al: *Pseudallescheria boydii* keratomycosis in a horse, *J Am Vet Med Assoc* 195:616-618, 1989.

401. Cooper SM, Sheridan A, Burge S: Mycosis fungoides responding to systemic itraconazole, *J Eur Acad Dermatol Venereol* 17:588-590, 2003.

402. Shah KB et al: Activity of voriconazole against corneal isolates of *Scedosporium apiospermum, Cornea* 22:33-36, 2003.

403. Varanasi NL et al: Novel effect of voriconazole on conidiation of *Aspergillus* species, *Int J Antimicrob Agents* 23:72-79, 2004.

404. Wlodkowski TJ, Rosenkranz HS: Antifungal activity of silver sulphadiazine, *Lancet* ii:739-740, 1973.

405. Fowler JD, Schuh JCL: Preoperative chemical preparation of the eye: a comparison of chlorhexidine diacetate, chlorhexidine gluconate, and povidone-iodine, *J Am Anim Hosp Assoc* 28: 451-457, 1992.

406. Hale LM: The treatment of corneal ulcer with povidone-iodine (Betadine), *N C Med J* 30:54-56, 1969.

407. Torres MA et al: Topical ketoconazole for fungal keratitis, *Am J Ophthalmol* 100:293-298, 1985.

408. Mohan M et al: Topical silver sulphadiazine: a new drug for ocular keratomycosis, *Br J Ophthalmol* 72:192-195, 1988.

409. Joyce JR: Thiabendazole therapy of mycotic keratitis in horses, *Equine Vet J Suppl* 2:45-46, 1983.

410. Korenek NL et al: Treatment of mycotic rhinitis with itraconazole in three horses, *J Vet Intern Med* 8:224-227, 1994.

5 Diseases of the Anterior Uvea

Steven R. Hollingsworth

With the exception of uveitis and neoplasia, abnormalities of the equine iris and ciliary body are relatively uncommon and often of minimal consequence to vision or comfort. However, some innocuous conditions can mimic serious disease, and therefore proper assessment is important to prevent misinterpretation and inappropriate clinical action. The purpose of this chapter is to characterize the diseases of the equine anterior uvea with the exception of the chronic, recurrent form of equine uveitis (equine recurrent uveitis or ERU), which is covered specifically in Chapter 7.

CLINICAL ANATOMY AND PHYSIOLOGY

The iris and ciliary body comprise the anterior uvea and are anatomically similar to that of other species in most clinically relevant aspects. As in most herbivores, the adult equine pupil is horizontally oval. The anterior surface of the iris is without a contiguous epithelial layer and is composed of connective tissue interspersed with fibroblasts and melanocytes. Beneath this surface layer is the iris stroma, which consists of chromatophores, fibroblasts, and collagen fibers that cradle a plexus of blood vessels. Within the central stroma and circumferentially oriented along the pupillary margin is the parasympathetically innervated iris sphincter muscle. Immediately posterior to the iris stroma is the iris dilator muscle, which is radially oriented and sympathetically innervated. The posterior aspect of the iris is lined with a double layer of densely melanotic epithelial cells (Fig. 5-1). The dorsal aspect of the pupillary margin is capped with a cystic extension of the posterior epithelium, the corpora nigra (or granula iridica) (Fig. 5-2).

The ciliary body is posterior to the base of the iris and is approximately triangular in cross-section.

As viewed from the vitreous cavity, the ciliary body is divided into the anteriorly positioned pars plicata and the posteriorly positioned pars plana. As the name suggests, the pars plicata is characterized by a folded or pleated appearance, although the number, prominence, and shape of the ciliary processes vary among species. In general, species with large anterior chambers, such as horses, have more processes than those with small anterior chambers. Carnivores' ciliary processes tend to be long and thin, whereas those of herbivores, including the horse, resemble blunted ridges.[1] From the ciliary processes, zonular fibers extend and connect to the equatorial region of the lens. The pars plana is a relatively smooth flat portion that extends from the pars plicata to the most peripheral extension of the retina (the ora ciliaris retinae). The width of the pars plana varies and is widest dorsolaterally.[2] The entire inner surface of the ciliary body (the surface in contact with the vitreous body) is lined with a double row of epithelial cells. The innermost epithelial cell layer (from the perspective of the vitreous cavity) is nonpigmented and is referred to as the nonpigmented epithelium (NPE) of the ciliary body. The NPE is confluent at the ora ciliaris retinae with the sensory retina and at the posterior base of the iris with the innermost layer of the posterior iris epithelium. The second epithelial cell layer is heavily melanotic and is referred to as the pigmented epithelium of the ciliary body. The pigmented epithelium lies immediately under the NPE and is contiguous with the retinal epithelium at the ora ciliaris retinae and at the posterior base of the iris with the outermost layer of the posterior iris epithelium. Tight junctions between NPE cells are thought to represent the epithelial portion of the blood-aqueous barrier.[3] Deep to the two-layer ciliary body epithelium, each ciliary process has a central portion of connective tissue and a vascular plexus, which is fenestrated, allowing leakage of

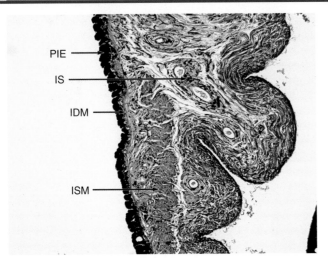

Fig. 5-1 Photomicrograph of normal equine iris. *PIE,* Posterior iris epithelium; *IS,* iris stroma; *IDM,* iris dilator muscle; *ISM,* iris sphincter muscle. (Original magnification ×4.)

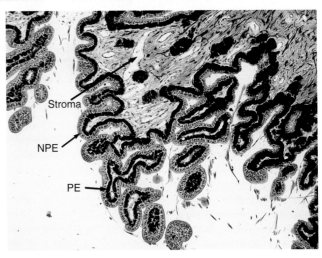

Fig. 5-3 Photomicrograph of normal equine ciliary body. *NPE,* Nonpigmented ciliary body epithelium; *PE,* pigmented ciliary body epithelium. (Original magnification ×4.)

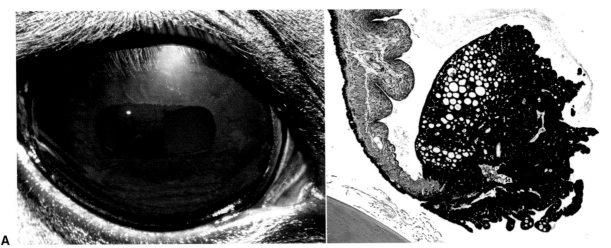

A   **B**

Fig. 5-2 A, Clinical photograph of the normal equine eye with normal large dorsal corpora nigra. **B,** Photomicrograph of normal equine corpora nigrum as a cystic extension of the posterior iris epithelium. (Original magnification ×2.)

plasma into the ciliary body stroma (Fig. 5-3). The epithelial portion of the blood-aqueous barrier filters this plasma, removing virtually all protein and cells. Thus the aqueous humor represents an ultrafiltrate of plasma. In addition to this filtration function, the NPE contains carbonic anhydrase, which catalyzes the active transport–mediated portion of aqueous humor production (Fig. 5-4).[1] Beneath the ciliary processes, lying on the internal surface of the sclera and forming the base of the ciliary body triangle, is the ciliary body musculature. Virtually all mammals have circumferentially oriented, parasympathetically innervated, smooth ciliary body muscles. When these muscles are contracted, the zonular fibers are relaxed, which in turn allows the lens to passively thicken. This mechanism is responsible for accommodation in mammals. However, most nonprimate mammals have poorly developed ciliary body musculature and therefore poor accommodative ability.

Anterior to the ciliary body musculature and visible at the juncture of the base of the anterior face of the iris and the limbus is the ciliary cleft. Spanning the opening of this cleft are strands of connective tissue called pectinate ligaments, which extend from the base of the iris to insert on the inner aspect of the limbus. The ciliary cleft is posterior to the pectinate ligaments and filled with a sponge-like network of connective tissue beams, the trabecular meshwork. In the horse, these beams are completely lined with endothelial cells called trabecular cells.[1] The ciliary cleft is the location of aqueous humor outflow. Any process that interferes with normal outflow can lead to increased intraocular pressure (see the discussion of equine glaucoma in Chapter 8).

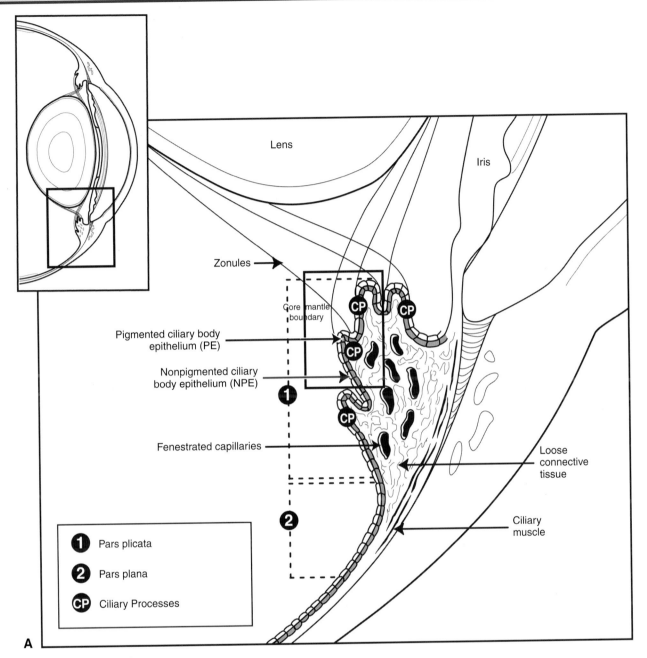

Fig. 5-4 A, Ciliary body anatomy.

Continued

IMPACT OF ANTERIOR UVEAL DISEASE ON THE EQUINE INDUSTRY

Complications associated with equine uveitis are the number one cause of blindness in horses worldwide, with annual costs in the United States estimated up to $1 billion.[4] The other conditions covered in this chapter occur infrequently and sporadically and have little impact on the equine industry from a strictly financial perspective. Therefore the importance of veterinarians correctly understanding and managing these

diseases is related to the well-being of the individual patient.

CONGENITAL DISEASES

Aniridia

Although the term *aniridia* implies a complete absence of an iris, it has been applied to a clinical condition reported in horses in which only a rudimentary,

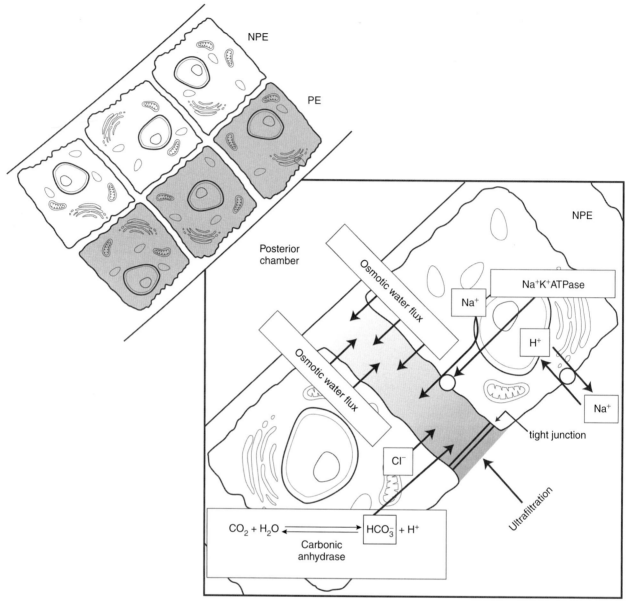

Fig. 5-4 B, Note the tight junctions between the lateral borders of the NPE, which represents the epithelial portion of the blood-aqueous barrier. Note the active transport of sodium and bicarbonate ions (by the action of the enzyme carbonic anhydrase), which contributes to the production of aqueous. These enzyme systems are located in the lateral wall of the ciliary body NPE.

nonfunctional ridge of iridal tissue is present (Fig. 5-5). Aniridia was first reported in 1955 in a Belgian Draft stallion and 65 of his offspring who were similarly affected.[5] The author concluded that aniridia was a heritable defect, which was passed via an autosomal dominant mode. Subsequently, aniridia was described in a Quarter horse stallion.[6] In an ensuing study, eight offspring of that stallion were followed up, and seven demonstrated aniridia.[7] These authors concluded that the mode of inheritance was similar to that of the Belgian draft stallion. Since then, aniridia has been observed sporadically, being specifically reported in a Thoroughbred colt[8] and a Welsh/Thoroughbred cross filly.[9]

Horses affected with aniridia are usually presented within the first few months of age because the client has noticed such signs as an unusual appearance of both eyes, excessive squinting in bright sunlight, and/or overreacting to flashes of light. On ophthalmic examination, the pupils are widely dilated and nonresponsive. The extent of the pupillary dilation is so marked that the lens equator and ciliary body processes are visible. The corpora nigra is absent. Virtually every reported case of aniridia has been accompanied by what is described as corneal vascularization and nodular changes along the dorsal and sometimes the ventral aspect of the limbus.[6-9] When affected globes have been available for histopathologic examination, fine hairs have been found

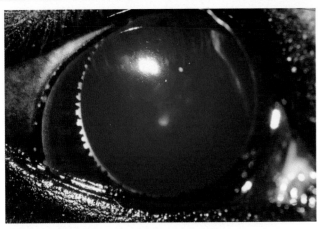

Fig. 5-5 Aniridia in a horse. Notice the ciliary body processes and edge of the lens, which are not visible in normal horses. (Photograph courtesy Dr. Michelle Willis.)

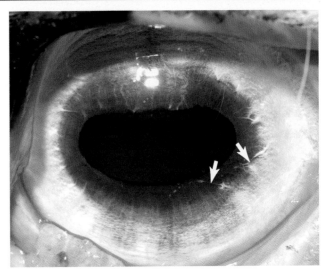

Fig. 5-6 Persistent pupillary membrane *(arrows)* in adult horse.

growing from the corneal nodules. These have been identified as dermoids. Cataractous changes are also a frequent accompanying sign with aniridia. The cataracts are usually focal and found in the anterior cortex. The cataracts are sometimes present at the time of initial examination but may not arise until later. They tend to be slowly progressive. Persistent pupillary membrane (PPM) was reported in one patient.[9] Findings on posterior segment examinations in horses with aniridia have been uniformly unremarkable.

The diagnosis of aniridia is straightforward and based on clinical signs alone (Fig. 5-5). No treatment is available. Many horses with aniridia have performed well in racing or other activities.[8,9]

Anterior Segment Dysgenesis/Persistent Pupillary Membrane

The term *anterior segment dysgenesis* is used to describe several syndromes with different clinical presentations. Ophthalmic structures potentially affected by anterior segment dysgenesis include the cornea, iridocorneal angle, iris, ciliary body, lens, and retina, as well as the globe itself as manifested by microphthalmos or buphthalmos.[10-13] The severity of signs associated with anterior segment dysgenesis varies greatly. Because most of the structures of the anterior segment are derived from the neural crest, alterations in the differentiation and migration of this layer lead to the signs associated with anterior segment dysgenesis.[12] Specific reported malformations involving the anterior uvea include miosis, iris hypoplasia, iris and ciliary body cysts, and persistent pupillary membranes (PPM). Of these, the most common clinical manifestation of anterior segment dysgenesis in domestic species, including the horse, is PPM.[12] During embryonic development, a vascular plexus called the pupillary membrane covers

the anterior surface of the iris and the pupillary aperture. This membrane rarifies near the end of gestation, but remnants can often be found in neonatal foals.[13,14] When such strands persist into adulthood, they are called PPMs. In adult horses, it is not uncommon to find small PPM strands, which originate from the collarette region of the iris and extend a few millimeters. Usually these strands terminate either as a free end in the aqueous or attach to the anterior surface of the iris (Fig. 5-6). Occasionally, PPMs attach to the anterior lens capsule or posterior surface of the cornea. In such instances, opacification is usually seen at the location of PPM attachment. Such opacities would be present from birth. However, in most equine patients, the distal end of the PPM is free floating or attached to adjacent iris. In such instances, no secondary signs are found. In a recent study the histopathologic changes of apparent PPMs extending from the iris to the posterior surface of the cornea in a 9-week-old Springer spaniel puppy were examined.[15] The area of attachment to the posterior cornea was characterized by disruption of Descemet's membrane and the corneal endothelium. These findings are identical to a developmental disease in humans referred to as Peters' anomaly. The authors suggested that this condition should be differentiated from PPM strands, which terminate by attaching to adjacent iris or as free floating in the aqueous.

The diagnosis of PPM is made on the basis of clinical appearance. In horses, opacities associated with PPM rarely cause significant visual deficits, and treatment is not usually indicated.

Anterior Uveal Cysts

The cysts discussed here may not be congenital but are included in this section because they have been noted

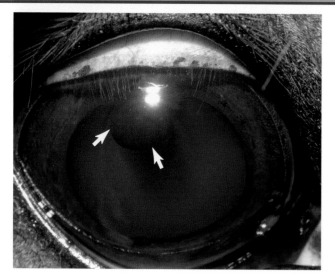

Fig. 5-7 Cystic corpora nigra *(arrows).*

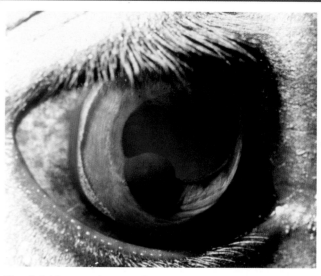

Fig. 5-8 Iris cyst along pupillary margin. (Photograph courtesy Dr. David J. Maggs.)

in horses of many different ages, including young horses, and may be present as very small cysts at birth, only to enlarge and become apparent later in life. Anterior uveal cysts may be found in four locations: (1) the corpora nigra, (2) along the margin of the pupil or free floating in the anterior chamber, (3) attached to the ciliary body, and (4) within the iris stroma.

The corpora nigra normally protrudes from the dorsal aspect and, to a lesser degree, the ventral aspect of the pupillary margin and is a vacuolated extension of the posterior iris epithelium. Because many horses that have cystic corpora nigra are middle-aged or older, it is believed that the condition is not congenital. The cause (or causes) of cystic corpora nigra is not known, but it does not seem to be related to past or present intraocular inflammation.[16]

When the corpora nigra becomes cystic, its normally roughened appearance becomes smooth and spherical (Fig. 5-7). The condition may be unilateral or bilateral, and the size of the cysts can vary markedly. Most are sufficiently small that they do not cause significant interference with vision. However, depending on the specific location, even moderate-sized cysts can partially inhibit the visual field, especially when the horse is in bright light and the pupil is miotic. For this reason, horses with cystic corpora nigra should be initially evaluated without pharmacologic dilation and under conditions of bright illumination, so that the extent of pupillary aperture blockage can be accurately assessed.

Differential diagnoses include inflammatory or neoplastic changes to the iris in the area of the corpora nigra. Although ultrasonography could be used to differentiate cystic corpora nigra from inflammatory or neoplastic infiltrates, this is rarely necessary because the clinical appearance is usually sufficiently characteristic.

Although treatment is not ordinarily necessary, the most effective and noninvasive treatment is deflation of the cystic corpora nigra with a laser. In a series of eight horses with signs including loss of vision, being startled when approached from the affected side, head shaking, and poor jumping performance, treatment with an ophthalmic Nd:YAG laser was effective in resolving the vision problems in all horses.[16] This procedure does not require general anesthesia; only sedation and an auriculopalpebral nerve block are needed. After surgery, some horses required a short course of topical antiinflammatory and mydriatic medication, but most of the horses were comfortable without treatment. An 810-nm diode laser delivered through an indirect ophthalmoscope headset has also been used successfully to shrink the cysts (Wilkie D. Personal communication, 2003).

Iridal cysts may be found distinctly separate from the corpora nigra along the margin of the pupil or free floating in the anterior chamber. These cysts are believed to develop in a manner similar to iridal cysts in dogs and represent a failure of the two layers of neuroectoderm to completely fuse, thus allowing fluid to accumulate in areas between the two-layered posterior iris epithelium. Because iridal cysts can enlarge, it has been theorized that some of the posterior iridal epithelial cells that comprise the lining of the cyst retain secretory ability.[17]

The clinical appearance of these cysts is spherical to oval and smooth. Although they can occasionally be transilluminated, most appear opaque (Fig. 5-8). Sometimes the cysts will spontaneously rupture and leave a circular area of pigmentation on the anterior lens capsule or the posterior surface of the cornea.

As with cysts of the corpora nigra, these must be differentiated from inflammatory or neoplastic masses,

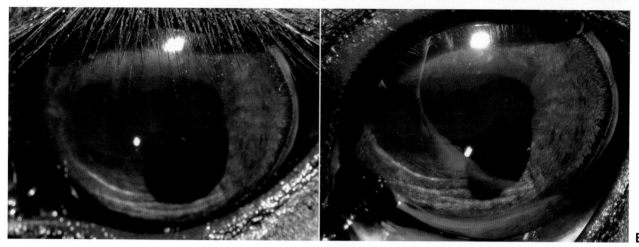

Fig. 5-9 A, Iris cyst in lower leaf of the iris immediately before application of an ophthalmic Nd:YAG laser. **B,** Iris cyst in lower leaf of the iris immediately after application of an ophthalmic Nd:YAG laser, demonstrating deflation of the cyst. (Photograph courtesy Dr. Brian Gilger.)

but this is rarely a problem because of the characteristic clinical appearance. Treatment is not commonly indicated because these iridal cysts seldom cause pain or visual impairment. Should removal be deemed necessary, they can be deflated with an Nd:YAG laser as described for cysts of the corpora nigra (Fig. 5-9).[16] Alternatively, a 25- to 27-gauge needle, attached to a tuberculin syringe, can be introduced into the anterior chamber at the limbus. The needle is used to perforate the cyst wall while gentle pressure from the syringe collapses the cyst.[17] This procedure is invasive and requires postoperative treatment with topical antiinflammatory and mydriatic medications for the resultant uveitis.

Ciliary body cysts are believed to originate in a manner similar to that of iridal cysts, except in this instance, the failure of the two layers of the neuroectoderm to fuse is in the area of the ciliary body, and so these cysts walls are made up of NPE (Fig. 5-10).[10,18] Other potential causes of ciliary body cysts include inflammatory processes, traction from zonules, anterior segment dysgenesis, and age.

Because the walls of these cysts are usually lined with NPE, they can be transilluminated. They tend to be oval and relatively large, often extending from the pars plicata to the ora ciliaris retinae (Fig. 5-11). Their most common location is ventrolaterally, and they can be difficult to detect without pharmacologic mydriasis.[10,18]

As with the other anterior uveal cysts discussed, differential diagnoses include inflammatory and neoplastic disease. Although ocular ultrasonography can be used to confirm the diagnosis of ciliary body cyst, the shape, contour, and ability to transilluminate make this differentiation straightforward on the basis of clinical signs alone. These cysts do not routinely cause pain or visual impairment, and treatment is not necessary.

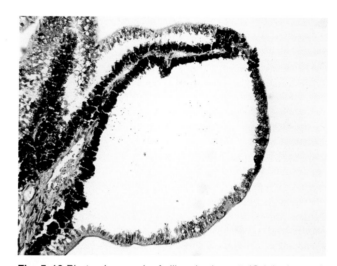

Fig. 5-10 Photomicrograph of ciliary body cyst. (Original magnification ×10.)

Cysts found within the iris stroma itself are probably not true cysts but represent thin, hypoplastic areas, which bulge forward as a result of aqueous pressure differences. This condition is covered in the following section.

Iris Hypoplasia

Historically, dark and bulging areas in the anterior surface of the iris have been interpreted as cysts within the iris stroma.[19] These dark, bulging areas are seen predominately in the dorsal region of eyes with blue irides, although they can be present in the ventral aspect of the iris and in eyes with brown irides. However, in one study, 15 horses with such lesions were examined, and histopathologic examination of lesions was performed for one horse with unilateral signs. The authors of that study concluded that these lesions represent areas of iridal stromal hypoplasia and that the resulting protrusion was the result of aqueous pressure pushing the relatively weaker portion of iris forward.[20]

The classic clinical picture of iris hypoplasia is a dark area, usually within the dorsal portion of the iris, that bulges forward (Figs. 5-12 and 5-13). Most of these eyes have blue irides, and the condition can be unilateral or bilateral. Age, breed, and sex predispositions do not seem to exist.[20] The affected eyes are not painful, and there is no discernable effect on vision. The dark, bulging areas are most evident when examined in bright light with the pupil miotic. The fact that these protruding areas actually represent thinning of the iris stroma is confirmed by passing a bright, focal beam of light through the pupil and observing the retroillumination of the fundic reflection through the lesion. When the pupil is subsequently dilated, either by the use of mydriatic agents or dark adaptation, the bulging area disappears, taking on a wrinkled appearance.

The most important condition to be ruled out for this clinical presentation is iridal neoplasia, specifically melanoma. Ocular ultrasonography can assist in making this differentiation, but careful examination under conditions of both miosis and mydriasis, as described previously, should allow for an accurate diagnosis. It is highly unlikely that a neoplasm, or inflammatory cell accumulation, would allow for retroillumination of the fundic reflection or would "deflate" under conditions of pupillary dilation. However, should there be confusion after careful ophthalmic examination, ocular ultrasonography would be indicated. Iris hypoplasia does not cause pain or vision impairment, and treatment is not indicated. Unfortunately, there are anecdotal reports suggesting that eyes demonstrating iridal hypoplasia have been removed because the presence of iridal melanoma was suspected.[20]

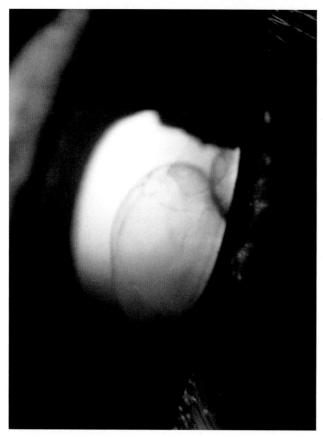

Fig. 5-11 Ciliary body cyst visible through pupil.

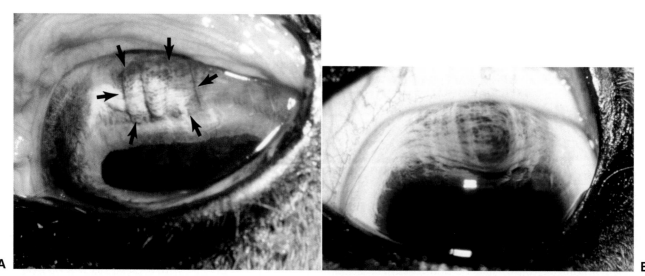

A   B

Fig. 5-12 A, Area of iris hypoplasia (outlined by *arrows*). B, Iris hypoplasia in a pony. (Photograph **[B]** courtesy Dr. Mike Davidson.)

Medulloepithelioma

Medulloepithelioma of the anterior uvea is infrequently reported in the horse.[21-24] These tumors arise from undifferentiated medullary epithelial cells that line the inner portion of the embryonic optic cup.[21,25] Normally, these cells differentiate into numerous epithelial cell lines in the adult eye, including the posterior iris epithelium, the ciliary body NPE, and the retinal epithelium. In individuals with this tumor, at least a portion of these cells fail to differentiate. In the horse, medulloepitheliomas most frequently arise from the ciliary body region. On histologic examination, medulloepitheliomas usually demonstrate nonpigmented neuroepithelial cells arranged in tubules and rosettes. They are classified as either teratoid[21] or nonteratoid,[22,23] depending on whether the neoplastic cell population is characterized by relatively homogeneous, undifferentiated primitive neuroepithelium or contains tissues not normally found in the eye such as cartilage, muscle, and brain tissue.[26]

Medulloepitheliomas are most frequently diagnosed in young adult horses presented because of a fleshly mass noted within the pupil[23] or anterior chamber.[22] Although these tumors are thought to grow slowly, they may be associated with other ophthalmic changes if they have been allowed to become large before presentation. Such changes would include corneal vascularization, corneal edema, corneal fibrosis, anterior uveitis, glaucoma, and buphthalmos (Fig. 5-14).[21]

Differential diagnoses include other intraocular neoplasms, such as melanoma, and cystic changes of the iris or ciliary body. The clinical characteristics of anterior uveal cysts have been described previously. Confirmation that an intraocular mass is solid tissue (as opposed to a cystic structure) and delineation of the specific location of the mass can be readily accomplished with ocular ultrasonography. Distinction between medulloepithelioma and intraocular melanoma is possible on the basis of clinical appearance. Melanomas are usually darkly pigmented and arise from the anterior surface of the iris, whereas medulloepitheliomas are most often fleshy masses apparent within the pupil. Although it is usually not necessary for determining appropriate clinical action, biopsy of a ciliary body medulloepithelioma has been described.[23]

Intraocular medulloepitheliomas are thought to grow slowly, with metastasis being a rare and late event. Extension into the orbit has been described in one horse.[24] The treatment of choice is enucleation, or exenteration if there is evidence that scleral integrity has been compromised.

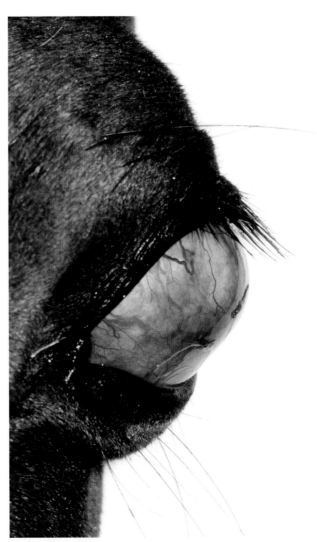

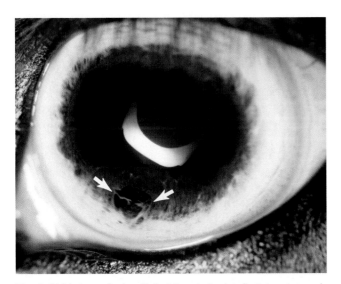

Fig. 5-13 Iris hypoplasia with bulging dark area (between *arrows*).

Fig. 5-14 Medulloepithelioma causing corneal vascularization, corneal fibrosis, and buphthalmos and completely filling intraocular space. (Photograph courtesy Dr. Carol M. Szymanski.)

Box 5-1	Signs Associated With Acute Anterior Uveitis

- Blepharospasm
- Epiphora
- Conjunctival hyperemia
- Episcleral injection
- Diffuse corneal edema
- Corneal vascularization
- Keratic precipitates
- Aqueous flare
- Fibrin clots in anterior chamber
- Hypopyon
- Hyphema
- Change in iris color
- Rubeosis iridis
- Miosis
- Inflammatory deposits on posterior lens capsule
- Hazy appearance to the anterior vitreous

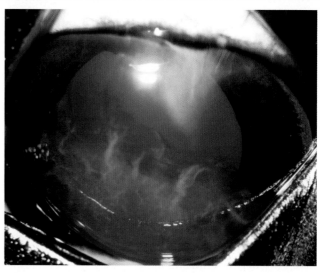

Fig. 5-15 Acute episode of anterior uveitis with fibrin clot in anterior chamber. (Photograph courtesy Dr. David J. Maggs.)

ACQUIRED DISEASES

Anterior Uveitis

As previously stated, anterior uveitis and its associated complications are the most common causes of blindness in horses worldwide. The prevalence of some manifestation of uveitis in the United States has been estimated to be between 8% and 25%.[4,27] As a clinical entity, acute anterior uveitis can be discussed separately from the chronic, recurrent form of equine uveitis (ERU), even though the two syndromes share some features. Furthermore, even though both forms of equine uveitis can affect the posterior uvea, this chapter deals with the anterior uveal manifestations.

Although draft breeds and Appaloosas are overrepresented in the group of horses with the chronic, recurrent form of uveitis, there is no age, breed, or sex predisposition for the acute form. Typical clinical signs associated with acute anterior uveitis are all due to damage of the anterior uvea and subsequent compromise of the blood-aqueous barrier. These signs are summarized in Box 5-1 (Figs. 5-15, 5-16, and 5-17).

The initial diagnosis of anterior uveitis is based on clinical signs. Because there is an almost endless list of proposed causes of anterior uveitis (Box 5-2),[4,14,27-31] in addition to a complete ophthalmic and physical examination, a number of laboratory tests have been proposed to help determine the underlying cause of a specific episode of acute anterior uveitis (see discussion of systemic diseases in Chapter 13).[14,27] These would include complete blood count, serum chemistry profiles, serologic tests for specific infectious causes such as leptospirosis, and conjunctival biopsies for detection of *Onchocerca* microfilaria (Fig. 5-18). Although tests for specific infectious agents can assist in ascertaining

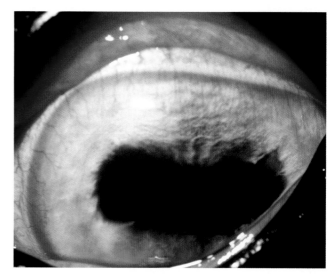

Fig. 5-16 Acute episode of anterior uveitis. Note episcleral injection, corneal vascularization, hazy aqueous, and miosis. (Photograph courtesy Dr. David J. Maggs.)

the underlying cause, the results must be interpreted with caution because horses without uveitis can often have positive test results for many of these agents (Fig. 5-18).[14]

The common denominator of all the proposed causes of anterior uveitis is damage to the uveal tract. This leads to the release of the mediators of inflammation such as prostaglandins, leukotrienes, and histamines.[17,32] Although the specific roles of the different mediators are still unclear and may vary between species, the overall effects of their release are iris sphincter muscle spasm, ciliary body muscle spasm, increased vascular permeability, and the breakdown of the blood-aqueous barrier. This is followed by leakage of protein, fibrin, and potentially cells into the aqueous, which

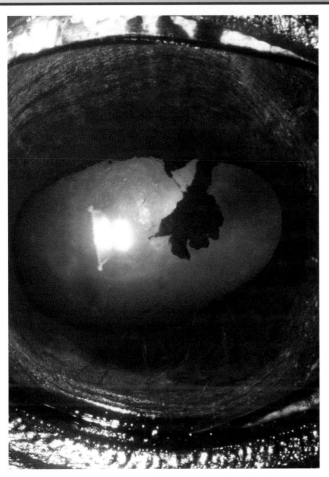

Fig. 5-17 Torn corpora nigra caused by blunt trauma. (Photograph courtesy Dr. David J. Maggs.)

accounts for the clinical signs most commonly associated with acute anterior uveitis: blepharospasm, epiphora, aqueous flare, fibrin clots in the anterior chamber, and miosis.

If a specific underlying cause can be identified, treatment centers on addressing that cause. Concomitant with treatment of the cause, or if no specific cause is found, the eye is treated symptomatically to reduce pain and minimize the intraocular damage associated with anterior uveitis. A list of common therapeutic agents with rationale for use, usual dosage, and precautions can be found in Table 5-1.[4, 14] The initial therapeutic approach for an acute episode of anterior uveitis is aggressive treatment in an attempt to rapidly counteract the inflammation. As the signs of acute uveitis begin to lessen, the frequency of medication can be slowly reduced. However, complete cessation of treatment is not advised until all clinical signs have resolved for at least 1 month. Surgical therapy is increasingly being used to combat the chronic, recurrent form of equine uveitis (ERU) and is covered in Chapter 7.

Most horses that are presented with acute uveitis initially respond well to symptomatic treatment. The long-term prognosis can often be problematic because recurrence is common and each inflammatory episode causes further intraocular damage. Long-term adverse sequelae for uveitis include corneal scarring, cataract formation, glaucoma, and retinal degeneration.

Melanoma

Although melanoma is relatively rare in horses and is certainly less common than in the dog, the literature contains numerous case reports of equine intraocular melanoma.[33-39] A review of these cases reveals some interesting trends. In older gray horses, cutaneous melanoma is a common finding. Most reported intraocular melanoma cases also occurred in gray or partially gray horses, but most of the horses were young adults, between 5 and 10 years of age. Only one of these horses also had skin lesions, which were described as "inguinal nodules." These nodules were not removed and did not change during the 6-month period during which the horse was followed up and therefore cannot be assumed to be melanomas.[38] Although none of the reported cases documented metastasis and the neoplasms were generally not judged to be malignant on histopathologic examination, rapid growth within the eye was common. One patient may have had a primary intraocular uveal melanoma extend through the cornea, but the originating tissue of that neoplasm could not be determined.[39] The most common site of origin was the iris, but melanomas arising from the ciliary body were also reported.

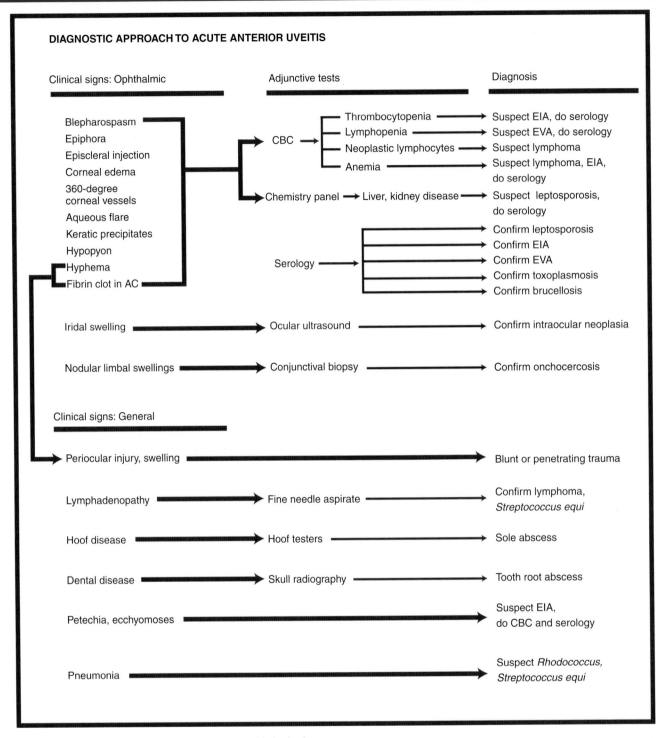

Fig. 5-18 Algorithm for the diagnosis of acute uveitis in the horse.

The initial clinical appearance of anterior uveal melanomas differs according to whether the ciliary body or the iris is the tissue of origin, how rapidly the neoplasm is growing, and the length of time before a medical evaluation was sought. When a horse with melanoma is presented early in the course of the disease, common clinical signs include focal corneal edema with a dark mass filling the anterior chamber, which is often in contact with the posterior surface of the cornea (Figs. 5-19 and 5-20). Depending on the location and extent of the mass, dyscoria may be present. The rest of the cornea in these patients is usually clear, and there is no aqueous flare. Evidence of pain is usually absent. As the neoplasm gets larger over time, common clinical

Table 5-1   Medical Therapy for Uveal Diseases[4,14]

Topical Medications	Frequency	Mode of Action	Adverse Effects
Prednisolone acetate, 1%	q1h-bid	Powerful antiinflammatory with excellent penetration	Can compromise ocular surface immunity
Dexamethasone, 0.1%	q1h-bid	Powerful antiinflammatory with excellent penetration	Can compromise ocular surface immunity
Flurbiprofen, 0.03%	q1h-bid	Nonsteroidal with good penetration	May prolong corneal ulcer healing
Diclofenac, 0.1%	q1h-bid	Nonsteroidal with good penetration	May prolong corneal ulcer healing
Cyclosporine A, 0.2%-2.0%	qid-bid	Immunosuppressive, but poor penetration	
Atropine, 1%	q6h-q48h	Relieves ciliary muscle spasm, provides pain relief, decreases synechia	May decrease gut motility

Systemic Medications	Dose	Mode of Action	Adverse Effects
Flunixin meglumine	0.5 mg/kg IV, IM, PO initially, then 0.25 mg/kg PO	Powerful antiinflammatory	Long-term use can lead to gastric and renal problems.
Phenylbutazone	4.4 mg/kg IV or PO q24h, or 1g IV or 1 g PO bid	Antiinflammatory	Long-term use can lead to gastric and renal problems.
Aspirin	Mature horses: 2 to 4, 240 grain boluses PO or 10-25 mg/kg PO q24h-bid	Antiinflammatory	Long-term use can lead to gastric problems.
Dexamethasone	5-10 mg/day PO or 2.5-5.0 mg IM q24h	Powerful antiinflammatory	Laminitis, must use with caution
Prednisolone	100-300 mg/day IM, PO	Powerful antiinflammatory	Laminitis, must use with caution
Triamcinolone	1-2 mg subconjunctival	Powerful antiinflammatory, 7-10 days' duration of action	Can compromise ocular surface immunity

bid, Twice a day; *IM,* intramuscularly; *IV,* intravenously; *PO,* orally; *qid,* four times a day.

signs include blindness, blepharospasm, epiphora, buphthalmos, diffuse corneal edema, aqueous flare, anterior chamber masses that often obliterate any normal architecture and prevent visualization of deeper structures. When structures deep to the iris can be seen, the lens is usually cataractous. If the tissue of origin is the ciliary body, a dark mass may be seen on the posterior surface of the lens extending into the vitreous cavity.[36]

Differential diagnoses for a dark mass in the anterior chamber include a uveal cyst and iris hypoplasia.[20,34] The distinction is usually not difficult to make on the basis of clinical appearance because cysts of the ciliary body, iris, and corpora nigra are all smooth and oval to spherical. Additionally, some cysts can be transilluminated. This clinical presentation would be contrasted to that of melanoma, which most frequently appears as an irregularly shaped mass arising from the anterior aspect of the iris and filling most, if not all, of the anterior chamber. On those occasions when there is doubt on the basis of clinical presentation, ocular ultrasonography can be used to differentiate cystic structures from

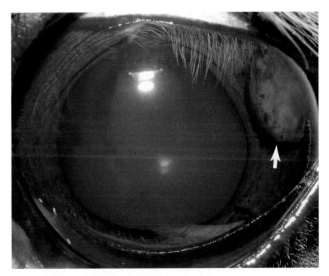

Fig. 5-19 Intraocular melanoma *(arrow)* arising from anterior surface of iris, filling the anterior chamber, and in contact with the posterior surface of the cornea.

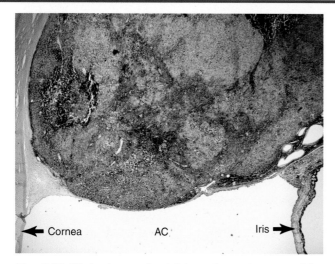

Fig. 5-20 Photomicrograph of intraocular melanoma arising from anterior surface of iris, filling the anterior chamber, and in contact with the posterior surface of the cornea. (Original magnification ×2.)

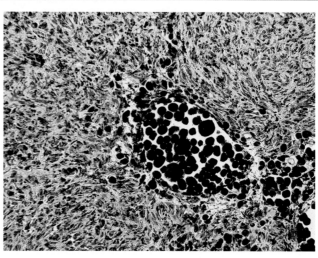

Fig. 5-21 Photomicrograph of intraocular melanoma. Note central area of plump, spherical, highly melanotic cells surrounded by pleomorphic, spindle-shaped cells. (Original magnification ×10.)

solid masses.[33] As discussed previously, horses with iris hypoplasia usually have either completely blue irides or exhibit heterochromia irides. Although the bulging forward of dark tissue characteristic of iris hypoplasia can mimic a melanoma, a number of characteristics allow for differentiation between the two conditions. These include ability to transilluminate, deflation of the bulging area with mydriasis, and absence of significant enlargement over time.

The pathogenesis of melanoma has been debated for years in both human and veterinary medicine.[40-42] Although differences exist in regard to intraocular melanoma among species, many believe that melanomas in general arise from preexisting nevi.[33,36,43] This theory is based in part on the fact that histopathologic examination of anterior uveal melanomas commonly reveals two cells types: (1) plump, spherical cells with abundant melanin granules and (2) smaller, pleomorphic, spindle-shaped cells, which may have a relatively higher nucleus to cytoplasm ratio (Fig. 5-21).[33,35,37] Mitotic figures are rare. One theory is that the plump, spherical cells represent a melanocytoma or nevus, which is the precursor of the melanoma portion of the mass represented by the spindle-shaped cells.[33,36,43]

In human medicine, a number of factors have been considered in determining the most appropriate treatment modality for intraocular melanoma. Considerations include whether excision or enucleation is the most efficacious therapy and whether enucleation promotes metastasis.[44-46] In veterinary medicine, there is one reported series of the use of a diode laser on 23 dogs with isolated masses believed to represent iridal melanoma.[47] The results of that study were encouraging in that the dogs were able to maintain

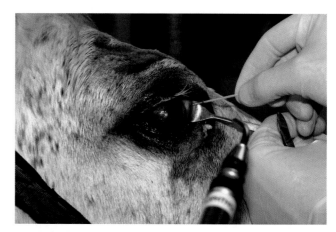

Fig. 5-22 Surgical Nd:YAG laser treatment of uveal melanomas in an equine eye. (Photograph courtesy Dr. Brian Gilger.)

comfortable, visual eyes as long as 4 years after treatment. Surgical Nd:YAG laser treatment of uveal melanomas in equine eyes has caused shrinkage of the masses (Gilger B. Personal communication); however, corneal edema and secondary uveitis are common adverse effects of laser therapy (Fig. 5-22). Among equine patients, there is one reported instance in which sector iridectomy was successfully used in the treatment of an intraocular melanoma.[37] Oral cimetidine (dose 2.5 mg/kg body weight, administered orally [PO] every 8 hours) has been used to shrink nonocular melanomas in horses, but no studies have been done to determine the effect of cimetidine on uveal masses.[48] Generally, intraocular melanoma in horses has been treated by enucleation or exenteration. Success with these procedures has been high, and metastasis has not been reported.[33,36,38,39]

Lymphoma

Lymphoma is the most common systemic neoplastic disease with an ocular manifestation in the horse.[49,50] Ocular manifestation of lymphoma has been documented in many species, but the specific ophthalmic structure most commonly affected varies among species. In cattle, exophthalmos caused by orbital masses is the most common ocular manifestation of lymphoma,[51] whereas in dogs and cats with systemic lymphoma, anterior uveal involvement is the most common ocular sign.[52,53] In one study of 79 horses with confirmed systemic lymphoma, 21 had ocular lesions. In these horses, eyelid swelling and inflammation were the most common ocular signs (11/21), with anterior uveal involvement being the next most common sign (4/21).[54]

The signs associated with anterior uveal manifestation of systemic lymphoma are nonspecific and include blepharospasm, episcleral injection, corneal edema and vascularization, aqueous flare, hypopyon, hyphema, iridal congestion, and swelling. Frequently, these nonspecific signs are accompanied by a history of chronicity and poor response to antiinflammatory medication. In addition, the ophthalmic signs are usually accompanied by nonspecific signs of systemic disease such as fever, respiratory disorders, weight loss, peripheral lymphadenopathy, and anemia.[55]

Intraocular lymphoma cannot usually be differentiated from other potential causes of anterior uveitis on the basis of ocular signs alone (Box 5-2). The diagnosis of systemic lymphoma should be considered in any horse with anterior uveitis, especially when it is accompanied by systemic signs of illness such as fever, weight loss, lethargy, and swollen lymph nodes. The diagnosis of lymphoma can be confirmed by identification of neoplastic lymphocytes from samples of solid tissues such as the spleen, lymph nodes, or skin nodules or by centesis of affected body cavities (thoracic or abdominal). In spite of this, diagnosis can be challenging, and confirmation occurs in less than 60% of cases.[49]

The pathogenesis of systemic equine lymphoma remains obscure. There are currently no known risk factors. Most affected horses are young adults between 4 and 10 years of age. No breed or sex predisposition has been demonstrated.[49]

The systemic treatment of lymphoma is outlined in equine medicine texts.[49] In general, success rates have been low for systemic lymphoma. The ocular portion of the treatment regimen would be the same as that previously described for anterior uveitis.

FUTURE RESEARCH

Many of the conditions described in this chapter are classified as developmental with a suspected heritable element. Although in the last 10 years significant advances have been made in the elucidation of the genetic details of canine heritable eye diseases, the same cannot be said for ophthalmic conditions with a suspected heritable component in horses. There are at least a couple of reasons for this. First, test matings in horses are more difficult than in dogs because of the longer gestation period and much smaller progeny number. Second, the suspected inherited ocular diseases in horses are frequently not blinding (especially those involving the anterior uvea) and so the motivation to eliminate these conditions is not as great as it is for dogs.

Another area in which great improvements have been made over the last 10 years is the use of imaging techniques in the diagnosis of ocular disease. Specifically, ocular ultrasonography has become increasingly useful in the diagnosis of intraocular conditions. Of particular benefit is the development of high-resolution, high-frequency probes that allow for ever-increasing detail in the evaluation of intraocular structures, particularly anterior uveal structures. As the detail and resolution of imaging techniques continue to improve, diagnoses can be made earlier, allowing for intervention sooner in the course of disease.

As mentioned previously in this chapter, medical laser technology has become a valuable addition to the treatment options for eye disease. In the future, it is anticipated that lasers will be even better at targeting specific diseased intraocular tissues and sparing adjacent normal tissue.

REFERENCES

1. Samuelson DA: Ophthalmic anatomy. In Gelatt KN, editor: *Veterinary ophthalmology*, ed 3, Philadelphia, 1999, Lippincott, Williams, & Wilkins, pp 31-150.
2. Miller TL et al: Description of ciliary body anatomy and identification of sites for transscleral cyclophotocoagulation in the equine eye, *Vet Ophthalmol* 4:183-190, 2001.
3. Gum GG, Gelatt KN, Ofri R: Physiology of the eye. In Gelatt KN, editor: *Veterinary ophthalmology*, ed 3, Philadelphia, 1999, Lippincott, Williams, & Wilkins, pp 151-181.
4. Gilger BC: Equine recurrent uveitis. In Robinson NE, editor: *Current therapy in equine medicine 5*, Philadelphia, 2003, Saunders, pp 468-473.
5. Eriksson K: Hereditary aniridia with secondary cataract in horses, *Nord Vet Med* 7:773-779, 1955.
6. Joyce JR: Aniridia in a quarterhorse, *Equine Vet J Suppl* 2:21-22, 1983.
7. Joyce JR et al: Iridial hypoplasia (aniridia) accompanied by limbic dermoids and cataracts in a group of related quarterhorses, *Equine Vet J Suppl* 10:26-28, 1990.

8. Ueda Y: Aniridia in a thoroughbred horse, *Equine Vet J Suppl* 10:29, 1990.

9. Irby NL, Aguirre GD: Congenital aniridia in a pony, *J Am Vet Med Assoc* 186:281-283, 1985.

10. Ramsey DT et al: Congenital ocular abnormalities of rocky mountain horses, *Vet Ophthalmol* 2:47-59, 1999.

11. Barnett KC et al: Buphthalmos in a thoroughbred foal, *Equine Vet J* 20:132-135, 1988.

12. Cook CS: Ocular embryology and congenital malformations. In Gelatt KN, editor: *Veterinary ophthalmology,* ed 3, Philadelphia, 1999, Lippincott, Williams, & Wilkins, pp 3-30.

13. Crispin SM: Developmental anomalies and abnormalities of the equine iris, *Vet Ophthalmol* 3:93-98, 2000.

14. Brooks DE: Equine ophthalmology. In Gelatt KN, editor: *Veterinary ophthalmology,* ed 3, Philadelphia, 1999, Lippincott, Williams, & Wilkins, pp 1053-1116.

15. Swanson HL et al: A case of Peters' anomaly in a Springer spaniel, *J Comp Pathol* 125:326-330, 2001.

16. Gilger BC et al: Neodymium:yttrium-aluminum-garnet laser treatment of cystic granula iridica in horses: eight cases (1988-1996), *J Am Vet Med Assoc* 211:341-343, 1997.

17. Collins BK, Moore CP: Diseases and surgery of the canine anterior uvea. In Gelatt KN, editor: *Veterinary ophthalmology,* ed 3, Philadelphia, 1999, Lippincott, Williams, & Wilkins, pp 755-795.

18. Dziezyc J, Samuelson DA, Merideth R: Ciliary cysts in three ponies, *Equine Vet J Suppl* 10:22-25, 1990.

19. Rubin LF: Cysts of the equine iris, *J Am Vet Med Assoc* 149:151-154, 1966.

20. Buyukmihci NC, MacMillan A, Scagliotti RH: Evaluation of zones of iris hypoplasia in horses and ponies, *J Am Vet Med Assoc* 200:940-942, 1992.

21. Szymanski CM: Malignant teratoid medulloepithelioma in a horse, *J Am Vet Med Assoc* 190:301-302, 1987.

22. Bistner SI: Medullo-epithelioma of the iris and ciliary body in a horse, *Cornell Vet* 64:88-95, 1974.

23. Riis RC, Scherlie PH, Rebhun WC: Intraocular medulloepithelioma in a horse, *Equine Vet J Suppl* 10:66-68, 1990.

24. Blodi FC, Ramsey FK: Ocular tumors in domestic animals, *Am J Ophthalmol* 64:627-633, 1967.

25. Peiffer RL et al: Fundamentals of veterinary ophthalmic pathology. In Gelatt KN, editor: *Veterinary ophthalmology,* ed 3, Philadelphia, 1999, Lippincott, Williams, & Wilkins, pp 355-425.

26. Broughton WL, Zimmerman LE: A clinicopathologic study of 56 cases of intraocular medulloepitheliomas, *Am J Ophthalmol* 85:407-418, 1978.

27. Schwink KL: Equine uveitis, *Vet Clin North Am Equine Pract Ophthalmol* 8:557-574, 1992.

28. Blogg JR et al: Blindness caused by *Rhodococcus equi* infection in a foal, *Equine Vet J Suppl* 2:25-26, 1983.

29. Faber NA et al: Detection of *Leptospira* spp. in the aqueous humor of horses with naturally acquired recurrent uveitis, *J Clin Microbiol* 38:2731-2733, 2000.

30. Grahn BH, Cullen CL: Equine phacoclastic uveitis: the clinical manifestations, light microscopic findings, and therapy of 7 cases, *Can Vet J* 41:376-382, 2000.

31. Maggs DJ: Ocular manifestations of equine herpesviruses. In Robinson NE, editor: *Current therapy in equine medicine 5,* Philadelphia, 2003, Saunders, pp 473-476.

32. Millichamp NJ, Dziezyc J: Mediators of ocular inflammation, *Prog Comp Vet Ophthalmol* 1:41, 1991.

33. Davidson HJ et al: Anterior uveal melanoma, with secondary keratitis, cataract and glaucoma in a horse, *J Am Vet Med Assoc* 199:1049-1050, 1991.

34. Barnett KC, Platt H: Intraocular melanomata in the horse, *Equine Vet J Suppl* 10:76-82, 1990.

35. Matthews AG, Barry DR: Bilateral melanoma of the iris in a horse, *Equine Vet J* 19:358-360, 1987.

36. Murphy J, Young S: Intraocular melanoma in a horse, *Vet Pathol* 16:539-542, 1979.

37. Latimer CA, Wyman M: Sector iridectomy in the management of iris melanoma in a horse, *Equine Vet J Suppl* 2:101-104, 1983.

38. Neumann SM: Intraocular melanoma in a horse, *Mod Vet Pract* 66:559-560, 1985.

39. Ramadan RO: Primary ocular melanoma in a young horse, *Equine Vet J* 7:49-50, 1975.

40. Albert DM: Ocular melanoma: a challenge to visual science, *Invest Ophthalmol Vis Sci* 23:550-579, 1982.

41. Lerner AB, Cage GW: Melanomas in horses, *Yale J Biol Med* 46:646-649, 1973.

42. Wilcock BP, Peiffer RL: Morphology and behavior of primary ocular melanomas in 91 dogs, *Vet Pathol* 23:418-424, 1986.

43. Yanoff M, Fine MS: Ocular melanotic tumors. In Ganoff M, Fine MS, editors: *Ocular pathology,* Hagerstown, Md, 1975, Harper & Row, pp 619-683.

44. Reese AB, Jones IS, Cooper WC: Surgery for tumors of the iris and ciliary body, *Am J Ophthalmol* 66:173-184, 1968.

45. Niederkorn JY: Enucleation in consort with immunologic impairment promotes metastasis of intraocular melanomas in mice, *Invest Ophthalmol Vis Sci* 25:1080-1086, 1984.

46. Zimmerman LE, McLean IW: An evaluation of enucleation in the management of uveal melanomas, *Am J Ophthalmol* 87:741-760, 1979.

47. Cook CS, Wilkie DA: Treatment of presumed iris melanoma in dogs by diode laser photocoagulation: 23 cases, *Vet Ophthalmol* 2:217-225, 1999.

48. Goetz TE et al: Cimetidine for treatment of melanomas in three horses, *J Am Vet Med Assoc* 196:449-452, 1990.

49. Schneider DA: Lymphoproliferative and myeloproliferative disorders. In Robinson NE, editor: *Current therapy in equine medicine 5,* Philadelphia, 2003, Saunders, pp 359-362.

50. Stiles J: Ocular manifestation of systemic disease. Part III. The horse. In Gelatt KN, editor: *Veterinary ophthalmology,* ed 3, Philadelphia, 1999, Lippincott, Williams, & Wilkins, pp 1473-1492.

51. Rebhun WC: Orbital lymphosarcoma in cattle, *J Am Vet Med Assoc* 180:149-152, 1982.

52. Krohne SG et al: Prevalence of ocular involvement in dogs with multicentric lymphoma: prospective evaluation of 94 cases, *Vet Comp Ophthalmol* 4:127-135, 1994.

53. Corcoran KA, Peiffer RL, Koch SA: Histopathologic features of feline ocular lymphosarcoma: 49 cases (1978-1992), *Vet Comp Ophthalmol* 5:35-41, 1995.

54. Rebhun WC, Del Piero F: Ocular lesions in horses with lymphosarcoma: 21 cases (1977-1997), *J Am Vet Med Assoc* 212:852-854, 1998.

55. Rebhun WC, Bertone A: Equine lymphosarcoma, *J Am Vet Med Assoc* 184:720-721, 1984.

6 Diseases and Surgery of the Lens

R. David Whitley

CLINICAL ANATOMY AND PHYSIOLOGY

Diseases of the equine lens may be congenital or acquired and generally involve malformation, malposition, or lens opacity (cataract). The most common and perhaps most significant lens disorder is cataract formation. This chapter discusses congenital and acquired lens disorders, then focuses on cataract evaluation and treatment. Although most practicing veterinarians may never perform cataract removal, general knowledge is important for appropriate client communication, case selection for specialty referral, and follow-up after surgery.

The equine lens is biconvex with a steeper curvature on the posterior surface.[1-3] The axial length varies from 11 to 13.5 mm, and the diameter is 20 mm (Fig. 6-1).[2-4] The total lens volume is approximately 2.5 to 3.2 ml. The refractive power of the equine lens is 14.88 diopters.[3-6] The lens is transparent because of the configuration of lens fibers, lack of fluid, lack of innervation, and lack of postnatal blood vessels. The anterior lens capsule, anterior cortex, lens nucleus, posterior cortex, and posterior lens capsule can be visualized by slit-lamp examination. The lens consists of surrounding outer capsule (basement membrane), lens epithelial cells, and lens fibers.

The lens capsule is the lens epithelium's basement membrane; it is thicker anteriorly than posteriorly. The anterior capsule continues to be produced by lens epithelium throughout life.[7] Zonular fibers insert on the lens capsule and connect to the pars plana region near the equator of the globe.[2,4,7] This insertion allows contraction of the ciliary muscle to relax zonular tension on the lens capsule, allowing increased axial length, which results in visual accommodation.

In postnatal life, lens epithelium normally exists beneath the anterior capsule and at the equator (lens bow). Epithelial cell mitosis crowds the cells to the equator, where cell elongation occurs, producing new lens fibers.[2,7] This continual fiber production leads to increased lens fiber density with age as fibers are compressed toward the lens nucleus (center of the lens). With slit-lamp biomicroscopy, different zones are visible within the lens (zones of discontinuity); these zones correspond to the embryonal nucleus, fetal nucleus, adult nucleus, and cortex of the lens (Fig. 6-2). Lens fibers do not extend from pole to pole, but rather, meet fibers from the opposite side to form lens suture lines. Usually, the anterior lens suture pattern is an upright Y configuration and the posterior lens suture is an inverted Y.[1-4] In many horses, alternate configurations, such as sawhorse or stellate patterns, may occur (Fig. 6-3).[3] Suture patterns may not be identical in both eyes of the same horse.[8-10] The lens nucleus or cortex may contain fain "dust-like" or "dot-like" opacities (imperfections) that do not represent a true cataract.[3,11] Small, short, refractile linear bodies may be present in the cortex. In many cases these are considered lens imperfections and not cataracts.[3]

IMPACT OF LENS DISEASE ON THE EQUINE INDUSTRY

Cataracts, or opacities of the lens, are the most common congenital ocular anomaly in horses, and development of cataracts in adult horses is a common cause of vision loss, with or without associated uveitis.

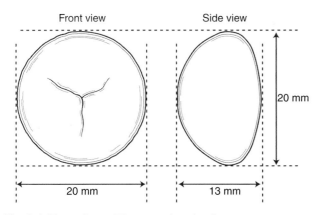
Fig. 6-1 Dimensions of the normal equine lens.

Front view — Side view — 20 mm — 20 mm — 13 mm

269

Therefore the economic impact of this disease on the equine industry may be quite significant. In a review of the Veterinary Medical Data Base records from January 1986 through December 1990, examination data on 79,037 horses were obtained.[12] Diagnoses of uveitis and cataract were made in 860 (1.1%) and 437 (0.6%) instances, respectively, with 145 (0.18%) horses recorded as having both uveitis and cataracts. In the population examined, the relative risk of cataract development in a horse with uveitis versus the risk of cataract development in a horse without uveitis was 42.5.[12] Appaloosas were significantly more likely than the total population to have uveitis ($P < 0.001$) and cataracts, with or without uveitis ($P < 0.005$).[12] Standardbreds and Thoroughbreds were significantly less likely to have uveitis ($P < 0.01$, Standardbred; $P < 0.05$, Thoroughbred) and cataracts, with or without uveitis ($P < 0.05$, Standardbred; $P < 0.05$, Thoroughbred) than the total population (Table 6-1).[12]

CONGENITAL DISEASES

Ocular anomalies account for 3% of all congenital defects in horses.[12,13] Cataracts (lens opacities) are the most commonly reported of these congenital ocular anomalies.[14-19] In one report, 13 of 34 (38%) congenital ocular defects involved the lens, and 12 of 13 [92%] lens anomalies were cataracts (Box 6-1).[14]

Congenital Cataracts

Cataracts, which are opacities of the eye's crystalline lens or lens capsule, occur as congenital or acquired defects in horses. In reports of congenital ocular defects in horses, the most common anomalies are congenital cataracts.[13-15,20-35] Congenital cataracts usually occur as the only ocular defect but may be associated with other congenital anomalies such as persistent pupillary membranes, persistent hyaloid vascular structures, aniridia, microphthalmia, and multiple ocular anomalies.[8-10,14,36] Anomalies must be present at birth to be termed congenital lesions, but anomalies recognized within the first few months of life are frequently presumed to be congenital. Cataracts in horses may be present at birth or occur in early neonatal life.

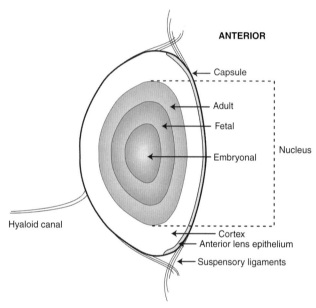

Fig. 6-2 Schematic cross-section of the adult equine lens.

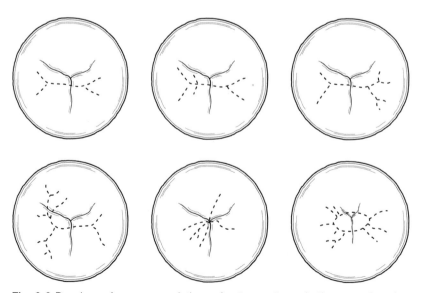

Fig. 6-3 Drawings of common variations of suture patterns in the normal equine lens.

Clinical Appearance

Cataracts are classified according to age at onset (congenital, juvenile, senile), cause (e.g., hereditary, secondary to uveitis, trauma, metabolic disease), or location within the lens: anterior polar, anterior subcapsular, anterior cortical, equatorial, peripheral cortical, nuclear, posterior cortical, posterior subcapsular, and posterior polar (Fig. 6-4). Congenital cataracts may be unilateral or bilateral and they may be focal (Fig. 6-5) or diffuse (Fig. 6-6). Focal opacities involving the anterior or posterior suture lines (Fig. 6-7) are often nonprogressive,[15,18,23,37,38] but progression does occur in some cases.[37,38] A nuclear cataract may appear as a ring-like opacity, a hollow sphere, or a solid opacity in the center (nucleus) of the affected lens. These cataracts rarely progress and often decrease in size relative to total lens size as new layers of normal cortical fiber are produced throughout life.[15,23,25,39] The location, density, and size of a focal cataract determine its effect on vision. Mydriasis (1% atropine ointment or solution applied topically twice a day until the pupil dilates, then twice a week to maintain dilatation) may improve vision in individuals with dense cataracts in the visual axis.[3,23]

Table 6-1 Uveitis and Cataracts in Selected Breeds

Breed	Individuals Examined	Uveitis*	Cataracts*	Uveitis and Cataracts*
Paint	2029	8	5	2
American Saddlebred	1801	13	8	3
Appaloosa[†]	3379	42	26	14
Arabian	7047	12	7	2
Belgian	107	10	4	1
Morgan	1121	19	12	2
American Quarter horse	24,909	10	6	1
Standardbred[‡]	8318	2	1	0.4
Tennessee Walking horse	1789	11	3	1
Thoroughbred[‡]	15,826	7	2	0.7
Mixed breed	6220	15	6	2
All horses	79,037	11	6	2

*Prevalence per 1000 cases.
[†]Prevalence of cataracts and uveitis was significantly greater than in the total population (uveitis: $P < 0.001$, cataract: $P < 0.005$).
[‡]Prevalence of cataracts and uveitis was significantly less than that in the total population (Standardbred: uveitis, $P < 0.01$; cataracts, $P < 0.05$; Thoroughbred: uveitis, $P < 0.05$; cataracts, $P < 0.05$).
From McLaughlin, Whitley, and Gilger.[12]

Box 6-1 Breed Predispositions to Lens Abnormalities in Horses

Cataracts
American Saddlebred
Appaloosa
Arabian
Belgian Draft horse
Kentucky Mountain Saddle horse
Miniature horse
Morgan horse
Mountain Pleasure horse
Rocky Mountain horse (presumed to be a semidominant trait)
Quarter horse
Shetland pony
Thoroughbred

Lens Subluxation
Kentucky Mountain Saddle horse
Miniature horse
Mountain Pleasure horse
Rocky Mountain horse
Shetland pony

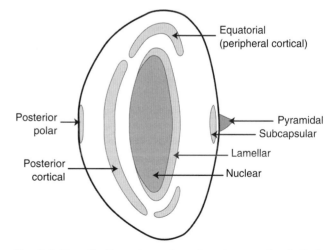

Fig. 6-4 Classification scheme for cataracts according to their location within the lens.

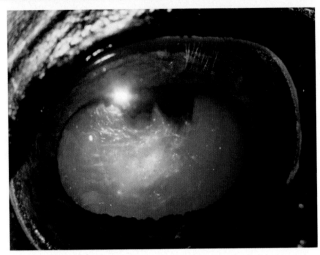

Fig. 6-5 Anterior cortical cataract in a foal. (Photograph courtesy Dr. Riccardo Stoppini.)

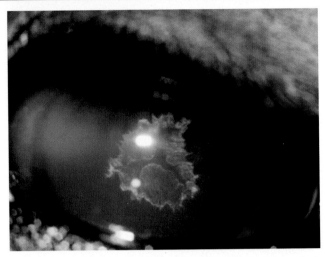

Fig. 6-7 Anterior cortical and suture-line cataract in a foal. (Photograph courtesy Dr. Riccardo Stoppini.)

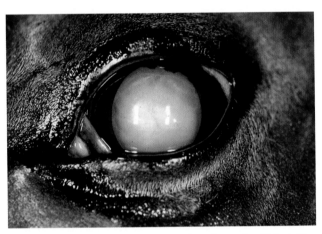

Fig. 6-6 Diffuse congenital cataract in a 3-month-old foal. The pupil has been dilated with 1% tropicamide.

Common Differential Diagnoses

Congenital cataracts are often complete and cause visual impairment or blindness in foals. Although the cause of congenital cataracts in horses can rarely be determined and no cause other than a heredity one has ever been proven, perinatal trauma and other maternal or environmental influences such as poor nutrition, in utero infection, exposure to toxic substances, and radiation have been proposed as possible causes.[15,31,39] Other considerations include radiation, systemic metabolic alterations, and toxic lens changes.[31,40,41]

Cataracts of presumed hereditary origin have been reported in several breeds. Cataracts that are inherited as a dominant trait have been reported in Belgian horses[28] and have been suggested in Quarter horses[3,39] and Thoroughbreds.[8] Anterior subcapsular cortical cataracts were observed in a Welsh-Thoroughbred cross-breed filly with aniridia.[21] Beech et al.[25] and Beech and Irby[42] described congenital nuclear cataracts in two groups of related Morgan horses. The cataracts were not associated with other ocular defects and did not impair vision or change in appearance with age. Pedigree analysis suggested an autosomal dominant mode of inheritance. Slatter[8,9] mentions a congenital cataract with dominant inheritance in the Thoroughbred but provides no details. Millichamp and Dziezyc[43] mention cataracts in two separate families of Arabians. Lavach[3] reported nuclear and cortical cataracts in three consecutive offspring of one Quarter horse mare. The foals were sired by three different stallions, suggesting a dominant mode of inheritance. Cataracts have been seen in two foals from an affected Quarter horse mare (Whitley, unpublished data, 2003). Erikson[28] described congenital aniridia and cataract in a Scandinavian Belgian stallion and all 65 of his offspring. A similar condition was seen in four of eight offspring of an affected Quarter horse stallion,[26] in a Thoroughbred colt,[27] and in a Welsh-Thoroughbred cross-breed filly.[21] The cataracts seen with aniridia are probably more accurately called juvenile, because they developed at about 2 months of age in the Belgians and at sometime between birth and 3 years of age in the Quarter horses. Schwink[44] has reported cataracts and dorsolateral strabismus in a 7-month-old color-dilute pony. Cataracts and lens luxations are associated with anterior segment dysgenesis in Rocky Mountain horses.[32]

Treatment

Treatment of congenital cataracts in foals depends on the severity and intended use of the horse. Extensive cataracts can be surgically removed with good success.

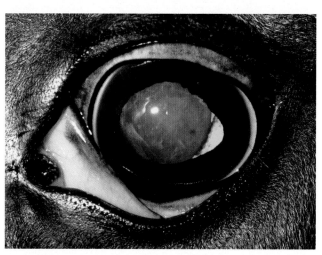

Fig. 6-8 Lateral lens coloboma in a foal with microphthalmia. The pupil is dilated with 1% tropicamide. (Photograph courtesy Dr. David Wilkie.)

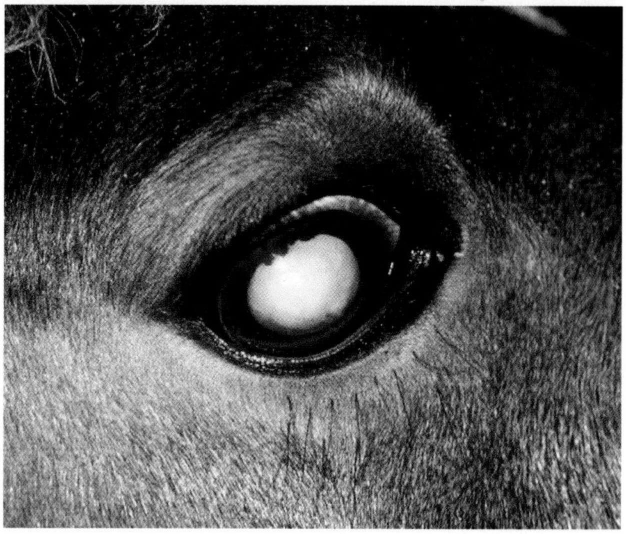

Fig. 6-9 Typical appearance of a diffuse mature cataract in an adult horse.

Other Congenital Abnormalities

Congenital anomalies of the lens other than cataract are uncommon in horses. Individual reports of aphakia, microphakia, lens coloboma (Fig. 6-8), lenticonus, lentiglobus, and ectopia lentis (congenital lens luxation) have been cited; but none of these defects occur with sufficient frequency to permit evaluation of their causes or the efficacy of treatment.*

ACQUIRED DISEASES

Acquired diseases of the lens include luxation, rupture, laceration or puncture, and opacity of the lens or lens capsule (cataract). The most common acquired disease of the lens is cataracts caused by immune-mediated inflammation (equine recurrent uveitis [ERU]). Senile cataracts that interfere with sight do occur in horses and ponies older than 20 years.[38,46]

Cataracts

Cataracts are a common complication of many forms of uveitis in humans and other species. Cataracts also are known to develop at an accelerated rate in many forms of uveitis, especially ERU (immune-mediated uveitis). It is generally believed that inflammation of the anterior uvea, such as that seen with immune-mediated uveitis (ERU, periodic ophthalmia), is the most common cause of acquired cataracts in horses.[3,37,45-58]

Clinical Appearance

Cataracts in adult horses are classified in a manner similar to that described in the discussion of congenital cataracts. In brief, cataracts are classified according to age at onset (congenital, juvenile, or senile), cause (e.g., hereditary, secondary to uveitis, trauma, or metabolic disease), or location within the lens: anterior polar, anterior subcapsular, anterior cortical, equatorial, peripheral cortical, nuclear, posterior cortical, posterior subcapsular, or posterior polar (Fig. 6-4). The location, density, and size of a focal cataract determine its effect on vision (Fig. 6-9).

Common Differential Diagnoses

In horses, acquired cataracts are often caused by immune-mediated uveitis (ERU) (Fig. 6-10) or trauma.[12,43,47-59] Cataracts of juvenile onset occur in many canine breeds but are uncommon in horses.[31,38,43] Senile cataracts that interfere with vision are uncommon in horses. Nuclear lenticular sclerosis is common in aged horses, but vision is clinically normal.[3,38,46]

Lens suture lines (Y sutures) are visible in most foals and adult horses and must be differentiated from cataracts. In a group of 144 foals, ranging in age from 5 days to 19.5 weeks (mean age, 9.4 weeks), lens sutures were visible in 137.[14]

Treatment

Historically, horses with cataracts associated with immune-mediated uveitis (ERU) have not been

---

*References 3, 13, 15-18, 23-24, 36, 45.

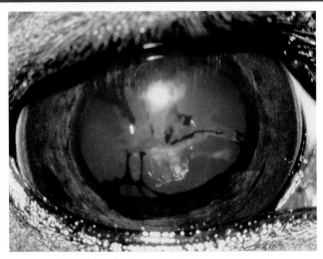

Fig. 6-10 Posterior synechia and anterior cortical cataract caused by chronic equine recurrent uveitis. (Photograph courtesy Dr. Riccardo Stoppini.)

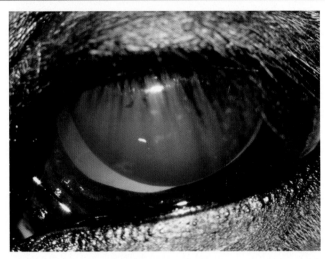

Fig. 6-11 Subluxated lens caused by blunt trauma in an adult horse. Note the ventromedial aphakic crescent and edge of the lens. (Photograph courtesy Dr. Riccardo Stoppini.)

considered appropriate candidates for cataract surgery because of the concurrent pathologic changes in the eye and the high rate of postoperative complications, both of which result in a very low surgical success rate.[35,37,54-56] Evidence from several reports on humans suggests that newer surgical techniques and careful medical management allow many patients with uveitis to undergo successful cataract removal.[60] Cataracts associated with trauma may be candidates for lens removal. See later in chapter for information on cataract extraction.

Lens Luxation

Lens luxation or subluxation may be caused by congenital anomalies of the zonules, chronic uveitis, or possibly trauma.[48,59,61] The luxated lens usually becomes cataractous.*

Clinical Appearance

Lens subluxations or luxations, in general, are rare in horses. A subluxated lens is partially broken free from its zonular attachments, but the lens is within its normal location, behind the iris and within the patellar fossa (Fig. 6-11). However, the lens may be slightly displaced, allowing the edge of the lens to be visible in the pupil and producing the appearance of an aphakic crescent. A lens luxation, which is the complete displacement of the lens either into the anterior chamber (i.e., anterior lens luxation) (Fig. 6-12) or into the

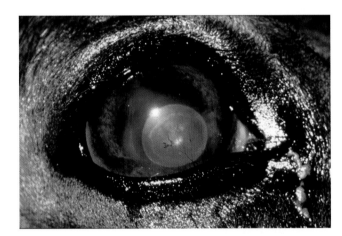

Fig. 6-12 Anterior lens luxation, corneal edema and keratitis, and microphthalmic in a foal. (Photograph courtesy Dr. David Wilkie.)

vitreous body (i.e., posterior lens luxation), is very rare in the horse. Both subluxations and luxations of the lens only occur as a result of other ocular damage, such as trauma, advanced glaucoma, or chronic cataract formation. Therefore the prognosis for vision and retention of the globe depends on the nature and severity of the primary ocular disease.

Common Differential Diagnoses

When a horse with lens luxations or subluxations is evaluated, the primary underlying condition in the eye must be determined. Cataract formation (either primary or as a result of chronic uveitis), glaucoma, severe trauma, intraocular neoplasia, and endophthalmitis are common causes of lens displacement.

---

*References 25, 37, 38, 50, 54, 60.

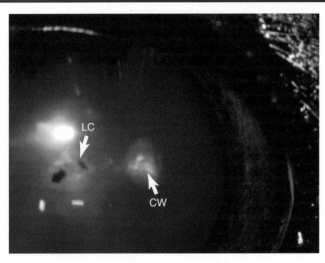

Fig. 6-13 Corneal laceration and lens capsule rupture. A corneal wound *(CW)* overlies the lens capsule *(LC)* trauma and cataract. It is likely that this cataract will progress. Lens-induced uveitis is possible, and lens extraction should be considered. (Photograph courtesy Dr. Riccardo Stoppini.)

Treatment

Intracapsular lens extraction has been recommended in cases of lens luxation.[25,38,39,62] Because uveitis or trauma of severity to cause lens displacement usually also causes severe uveal tissue damage, resulting in phthisis bulbi or blindness as a result of retinal degeneration, insertion of an intrascleral silicone prosthesis should be considered as an alternative to lens removal in blind eyes with acquired lens luxation.[63-67]

Lens Capsule Rupture

Lens capsule rupture, laceration, or puncture may be caused by blunt or penetrating trauma. These injuries usually occur in association with rupture, laceration, or puncture of the cornea or sclera. Severe uveitis and subsequent blindness may result from exposure of uveal or retinal tissue to lens material.[25,68,69]

Clinical Appearance

Any penetrating ocular injury can cause a lens capsular rupture. The most common injury is a corneal laceration. The integrity of the lens capsule should be evaluated in all cases of corneal perforation or penetrating injury (Fig. 6-13). Generally, thorough ocular examination coupled with careful ocular ultrasonography is required for assessment of the anterior lens capsule. The anterior chamber may be collapsed, and lens material may or may not be emanating from the lens capsule or

corneal laceration. In many cases, severe ocular inflammation, fibrin formation, and miosis make complete evaluation of the lens capsule difficult. If the laceration is being surgically repaired, evaluation of the lens capsule should be done by removing intraocular fibrin, flushing the anterior chamber, and dilating the pupil with dilute (1:10,000) intracameral epinephrine. If the lens capsule is ruptured, lens extraction is recommended.

Common Differential Diagnoses

Persistent intraocular inflammation after ocular penetration can be caused by endophthalmitis (i.e., bacterial or fungal infection), severe uveitis, or deposition of foreign material in addition to liberated lens protein. For proper management of these severe injuries, careful diagnostic workup consisting of a thorough ocular examination, aerobic bacterial and fungal culture and sensitivity of intraocular fluids, and ocular ultrasonography should be done; ocular exploratory surgery or irrigation to remove foreign material may be required.

Treatment

Although no studies have been done in horses, results in dogs suggest that lens removal should be performed in conjunction with repair of the corneoscleral injury.[60,63,68] The prognosis for vision is poor in eyes that have sustained blunt trauma sufficient to rupture the lens and in eyes with large lacerations that involve the limbus or sclera.[63] Placement of an intrascleral silicone prosthesis provides a cosmetic alternative to enucleation in some of these eyes.[64-67]

EVALUATION AND TREATMENT OF CATARACTS

Evaluation of the Equine Patient With Cataracts

Examination of the eye should be a routine part of prepurchase and insurance examinations and the physical examination of all newborn foals.[69] Brisk, complete pupillary light reflexes and a blink response to bright light usually indicate adequate retinal function.[39] Diffuse or focal axial cataracts may be identified during simple penlight examination (Figs. 6-5 and 6-6); however, complete evaluation of the lens requires dilation of the pupil.[69] Topical application of 1% tropicamide, twice at 5-minute intervals, usually results in adequate mydriasis for ophthalmic examination in the horse within

15 to 30 minutes. Focal cataracts will not prevent ophthalmoscopic examination of the ocular fundus. If complete, diffuse cataracts are present, ocular ultrasonography and electroretinography (see Chapter 1 for more information) are recommended to rule out concurrent retinal abnormality.[38,69]

Medical Management of Cataracts

Currently, no medical therapy will eliminate or prevent the progression of cataracts. Pharmacologic mydriasis may improve vision in eyes with focal axial or nuclear cataracts. One percent atropine ointment or solution is applied twice daily until the pupil is fully dilated, then twice weekly to maintain mydriasis.[12,23,25] Mydriasis is occasionally associated with photophobia manifested by lacrimation and blepharospasm. In individuals with photophobia, the mydriatic should be discontinued, and shelter from bright light should be provided until the atropinization effect is gone. Lavach[53] recommends oral administration of aspirin (30 mg/kg per day) to control any lens-induced uveitis that may be present.

Selection of Patients for Cataract Surgery

The decision to treat cataracts in horses presents philosophic and ethical concerns because of liability incurred if riders are injured as a result of a horse's less-than-optimal vision after lens removal. The treatment of cataracts in horses represents surgical and therapeutic challenges because of the nature and size of the patient and the expected performance of the horse after lens removal.

Few studies document visual perception in horses with aphakia, but some veterinary ophthalmologists believe that aphakia should be considered an unsoundness.[25,37,38,70] Retinoscopy, performed in one pony 6.5 years after removal of cataractous, subluxated lenses, suggested 9 to 10 diopters (D) of hyperopia. Despite this degree of ametropia, the pony was ridden regularly, was shown, and jumped "consistently well."[70]

Follow-up information was obtained by telephone from owners or veterinarians for six of seven foals 1 month to 3.5 years after cataract surgery.[71] All were reported to be doing well, with no visual difficulties. Eight months to 3 years after cataracts were removed from six eyes of five adult horses, follow-up information was obtained by telephone for four of the horses.[71] All horses were being used regularly: three for roping and one as a polo pony. All owners thought that the horses were working as well as they had before cataracts developed. The owner of one horse reported

that the animal's day vision was "fine" but that the horse had difficulty seeing dark-colored steers at night. In one horse, a superior retinal detachment developed after an episode of increased intraocular pressure (IOP) and corneal edema.[71]

The age of the patient may influence the postoperative success rate. The potential for deprivation amblyopia has not been documented in horses but should be considered and would dictate early surgical intervention in foals with congenital cataracts.[37,72,73] Deprivation amblyopia is decreased vision in one or both eyes subsequent to central fixation disuse caused by ocular opacities.[72] The condition occurs in children with congenital cataracts and in laboratory animals deprived of early vision.[72-75] The incidence of deprivation amblyopia has not been ascertained in older foals after extraction of congenital cataracts. Congenital cataracts may become hypermature as the animal ages, increasing the likelihood of lens-induced uveitis and postoperative complications caused by inflammation.[38,39] Patient selection is important. Because younger foals are smaller and easier to restrain, early surgery makes postoperative medication of the eye easier and less stressful for all concerned. A foal's temperament must be amenable to handling and frequent administration of medication.[24,31,38] Patients that are halter-broken are preferred. The presence of systemic problems or additional ocular anomalies might justify delay or refusal of surgery. *Rhodococcus* pneumonia is seen in some cases after foals have been anesthetized for cataract removal. Older foals should be halter-broken and handled around the head sufficiently to allow postoperative treatment without danger of injury to the foal or to personnel medicating the eye.*

If a cataract is present, the eye should be examined carefully for evidence of other congenital or acquired abnormalities. Foals with complete congenital cataracts and blindness are potential candidates for surgery. The eyelids, conjunctiva, and cornea should be evaluated carefully. Any blepharitis, conjunctivitis, or keratitis must be treated and controlled before cataract surgery is performed.[31,38,39] Brisk pupillary responses and a blink response to bright light (dazzle response) usually indicate a functional retina.[38,39,69,77] Because genetic nyctalopia (night blindness) has been reported in Appaloosas, preoperative electroretinography should be considered in treatment of this breed.[78,79]

Microphthalmia is generally considered a contraindication to cataract surgery, as are other congenital defects, such as retinal detachment and optic nerve hypoplasia, which may result in blindness, regardless of the condition of the lens.[16,37,38] Foals with microphthalmos and cataracts are usually not suitable candidates

---

*References 37,38,63,64,71,76.

for surgery.[31,37,38] However, cataract removal in mildly microphthalmic eyes can be successful.

In three studies of cataract treatment, surgery was most successful in foals younger than 6 months.[31,80,81] Older foals were more difficult to medicate topically; the cataracts were often hypermature, which increased the likelihood of lens-induced uveitis. The best post-operative prognosis is reserved for foals that are halter-broken and tolerant of handling and that have docile temperaments.[31,71,81] Owners of surgical candidates must be informed of the possible genetic implications of congenital cataracts and the uncertain visual perception related to uncorrected aphakia.[31,39,43] In foals, phacoemulsification and aspiration or aspiration alone of congenital cataracts can restore functional vision; however, phacoemulsification and aspiration is the preferred technique.

Presurgical Diagnostic Testing

Foals and adult horses being considered for cataract removal should be healthy and tractable. Major health problems and ophthalmic abnormalities should be addressed before elective cataract extraction is pursued. In foals, a careful pulmonary examination should be completed, and thoracic radiographs may be required to rule out inapparent, low-grade, or insidious pulmonary diseases. A complete ophthalmic examination should always be performed, which includes a thorough history, physical examination, and ocular examination. An appropriate preanesthetic evaluation would include a complete blood count and serum chemistry profile.

This animal's temperament is an important concern in the screening of potential cataract surgery patients. Intractable or poorly manageable horses or foals are poor candidates for elective cataract removal. Serious ocular injury can result when postoperative treatment is attempted in such animals. No less serious is the concern and possible liability for injuries to personnel and owners attempting to examine or medicate horses presented or hospitalized for elective surgery.

If the cataracts are congenital, the possibility of other general or ocular congenital defects should be considered. Likewise, if trauma or uveitis is suspected as the cause, evaluation of the uveal tract, vitreous, and retina is paramount.

A detailed history should reveal when the animal's vision is most severely affected. Poor vision in daylight may occur with cataracts, whereas poor light or dim-light vision may indicate retinal degeneration. In some cases, foals and horses with visual impairment and cataracts may be presented to the veterinarian with repeated cuts and abrasions of the face, chest, and forelegs.

A complete ophthalmic examination should be performed, beginning with an evaluation of vision; in such an examination, each eye is frequently blindfolded individually. The orbit and eyelids should be examined, followed by a systematic examination of the nictitating membrane, conjunctiva, cornea, anterior chamber, iris, and lens. If the vitreous, retina, and optic disc are visible through or around lens opacities, they are evaluated as well. The ophthalmic examination should be carried out in a quiet, semidark area with a 3.5-V transilluminator and portable slit lamp. Pupillary light responses, tear test, and IOP measurements with a tonometer (Tonopen XL; Dan Scott and Associates) should be performed before the pupils are dilated.

A short-acting mydriatic, tropicamide 1%, is essential for dilating the pupil to evaluate the lens, vitreous, retina, and optic nerve. One-quarter milliliter of tropicamide is deposited on the cornea with a 1-ml syringe with a 25-gauge needle hub (needle broken off at the hub); application may be repeated at 5- or 10-minute intervals; the normal (nonuveitic pupil) will dilate maximally (adequately) in 20 to 30 minutes. A darkened room, slit-lamp biomicroscope, magnifying loupes, and binocular indirect ophthalmoscope are very helpful in performing an adequate equine ocular examination.

Various eye diseases can complicate or obviate the recommendation for elective lens removal. These include but are not limited to distichiasis, entropion, keratoconjunctivitis sicca, keratitis, corneal ulcer, uveitis, glaucoma, lens subluxation, presence of vitreous in the anterior chamber, and retinal diseases (retinal detachment or retinal degeneration).

Additional diagnostic testing is indicated to obtain necessary information regarding the posterior segment before elective cataract removal is recommended. When substantial cataract formation prevents direct visualization or examination of the fundus, it is prudent to determine that the posterior segment is normal anatomically and physiologically. Electroretinography and ocular ultrasonography are standard diagnostic tests used in small animal ophthalmology and are being used more often in the horse when substantial opacification of the ocular medic impedes direct visualization of the vitreous, retina, and optic nerve.

Lenses with anterior capsular opacities can also have posterior capsular densities. Such opacities should be noted by slit-lamp biomicroscopy before surgery, and the owner should be informed. Posterior capsular opacities tend to intensify after surgery and can result in secondary cataracts or opacification of the posterior capsule, which can compromise vision.

B-mode ultrasonography is routinely performed in dogs as part of the pre-phacoemulsification procedure.[81-87] Ultrasonography should be considered as part of a diagnostic evaluation before cataract surgery is performed in horses.

PREOPERATIVE CARE

Preoperative management is critical to the surgical result. Mydriasis is mandatory and is achieved before surgery with topical 1% atropine solution. Lens-induced uveitis, iridocyclitis, or posterior synechiae can cause eyes to dilate incompletely. Topical antibiotics are used to prevent secondary infection. Topical and systemic antiinflammatory drugs are administered to decrease preoperative and postoperative uveitis; systemic prostaglandin inhibitors effectively perform this function in horses. Preoperative preparation of patients includes dilation of the pupils, topical application of antibiotics or corticosteroids, and administration of systemic prostaglandin inhibitors and corticosteroids. The preoperative protocol in Box 6-2 has been successfully used to manage congenital cataracts in foals.[31,39,43,76]

ANESTHESIA

General anesthesia is induced and maintained with inhalant anesthetics. The patient is placed in lateral recumbency, and the head is elevated with sandbags and inflatable ring-shaped cushions. Inhalation anesthesia with halothane alone lowers IOP enough for successful cataract aspiration. Muscle relaxants (e.g., atracurium) are used to maintain eye position and prevent anterior vitreous presentation. The use of muscle relaxants such as atracurium (Tracrium), vecuronium (Norcuron), or pancuronium (Pavulon) allows for a motionless eye during phacoemulsification with minimal vitreal and posterior capsule movement, contributing to a shortened operative time, decreased incidence of posterior capsule tearing with vitreous prolapse, and decreased amount of irrigating solution and drainage to corneal endothelium and iris. Topical anesthetics may be used to block the corneal reflex, which can persist through stage III of inhalation anesthesia in horses. In an effort to reduce intraoperative and postoperative uveitis, topical anesthetics might also be used to block the reflex between the conjunctiva-cornea and the iris. A retrobulbar lidocaine injection has also been used for intraocular surgery (see Chapter 1 for protocol).

Box 6-2	Example of a Cataract Surgery Preoperative Medication Protocol

Preoperative Protocol

Day 1
- Physical and ocular examination
- Intravenous or oral flunixin meglumine, 1.1 mg/kg, once daily
- Prednisolone, 1 to 2 mg/kg, once daily
- Topical ophthalmic antibiotic solution, three times daily
- Topical ophthalmic corticosteroid (1.0% prednisolone acetate or 0.1% dexamethasone), three times daily
- Topical 1% atropine solution, three times daily
- For weaned foals, no food for 12 hours before surgery
- For unweaned foals, milk only
- Systemic antibiotics
- Immunization with tetanus toxoid if needed

Day 2 (the day of surgery)
- Intravenous flunixin meglumine, 1.1 mg/kg, once daily
- Topical ophthalmic corticosteroid, three times daily
- Topical ophthalmic antibiotic solution, three times daily
- Topical 1% atropine solution, three times daily
- Topical 2% homatropine ophthalmic solution, 30 minutes before surgery
- Topical ophthalmic anesthetic after induction of anesthesia

---

SURGERY

Eyelid hair and lashes are clipped from the patient's eye, and the clipped hair is removed with a light vacuum and adhesive tape. The periorbital area is scrubbed with povidone-iodine solution diluted 50% with sterile saline solution and is then rinsed with sterile saline solution. The eyelid margins are carefully swabbed with povidone-iodine solution (with a sterile cotton-tipped applicator) and not rinsed. The cornea and conjunctiva are irrigated with 10 to 20 ml of sterile saline solution, and the upper and lower conjunctival fornices are cleaned with sterile cotton-tipped applicators.

The eye is draped with sterile towels and an ophthalmic drape so that only the palpebral fissure is exposed. An eyelid speculum is inserted to maintain an open palpebral fissure. An adhesive ophthalmic drape may be used to drape the eyelid margins. A lateral canthotomy may be performed, if necessary to increase exposure.

SURGICAL TECHNIQUES

Four surgical techniques have been described for the removal of equine cataracts: aspiration, extracapsular extraction, intracapsular extraction, and phacofragmentation with aspiration.[31,38,43,88-94] The surgical approaches used with these techniques are clear corneal incision or limbal incision beneath a conjunctival flap. Because cataracts in foals are usually soft and liquid, use of either aspiration or phacofragmentation with aspiration is recommended.

Aspiration

In the past, before the availability of phacofragmentation, two-needle discission aspiration was the most common technique for removal of congenital cataracts. This technique involves inserting needles through the clear cornea or at the limbus beneath a limbus-based conjunctival flap. If such a flap is used, electrocautery is helpful in controlling conjunctival hemorrhage.

A 5-mm limbal groove at three fourths of the depth of the cornea is formed with a No. 64 microsurgical blade. The incision into the anterior chamber is made with a No. 65 microsurgical blade or a 3.2-mm slit blade and can be extended with corneal scissors or Steven's tenotomy scissors. If the irrigating needle is to be inserted directly through the clear cornea, an incision is made 2 mm from the limbus and 120 to 180 degrees from the first incision. After the initial corneal (stab) incision, a split-thickness corneal suture can be placed to minimize the escape of aqueous humor and to facilitate wound closure after aspiration. The anterior lens capsule is incised with a cystotome or a No. 65 microsurgical blade. A 14- or 16-gauge hypodermic needle attached to a 12-ml syringe by polyethylene tubing is used to aspirate the lens material.[31,95]

The advantages of the clear corneal incision are speed and the elimination of the need for hemostasis. Disadvantages include corneal ulceration and increased postoperative corneal edema and scarring. The advantages of a properly performed conjunctival flap approach are the avoidance of corneal scarring and the added strength of a two-layer closure. Disadvantages include increased operation time and the need for hemostasis. The techniques are equally successful; selection is the surgeon's prerogative.

After removal of the lens, a simple interrupted pattern of 6-0 or 7-0 absorbable sutures is used to close the incisions. The incisions must be sealed, and the anterior chamber must be re-formed. Conjunctival incisions are closed with 6-0 absorbable sutures in a simple continuous pattern. If necessary, the lateral canthotomy is closed with 3-0 nonabsorbable sutures. The anterior chamber is re-formed with ophthalmic balanced salt solution or lactated Ringer's solution.

Phacofragmentation With Aspiration

Phacofragmentation with aspiration is much preferred to aspiration of soft cataracts.[31,81,96,97] In phacofragmentation, high-frequency ultrasonic vibrations are used to fragment the lens; aspiration is performed through a single needle to remove the cortex and nucleus.

Phacofragmentation with aspiration is most commonly performed through a single port or with a single cannula that infuses irrigating solution, aspirates, and provides ultrasonic phacoemulsification. In a second, two-needle technique, the anterior chamber is maintained with fluid via a second needle at a remote site. Use of the technique is limited by the expense and availability of instrumentation.

Phacofragmentation is the preferred technique for the removal of cataracts in foals. The technique has also been used to remove acquired cataracts in adult horses.[43] Ultrasonic phacofragmentation of the lens is accompanied by aspiration.[39,76,93-103] If a two-needle technique is used, a 19- or 20-gauge, sterile, disposable hypodermic needle is introduced under the conjunctiva and through the limbus; an intravenous drip set is used for infusion of balanced saline solution or lactated Ringer's solution to maintain the anterior chamber. If a single-needle technique is used, the irrigating solution is infused through the phacoemulsification machine.

In horses, several different fluid types have been used to irrigate and re-form the anterior chamber.[31,43,97] Warmed (37° C; 98.6° F) balanced saline solution and lactated Ringer's solution are most satisfactory. Sterile physiologic saline solution or lactated Ringer's solution with the addition of heparin, epinephrine, and sodium bicarbonate has also been used during intraocular surgery in horses. Antiprostaglandin antiinflammatory agents (before and after surgery) reduce intraocular fibrin formation and thus decrease the need for addition of anticoagulants (e.g., heparin) or vasopressors to irrigating solutions

A viscoelastic substance is used to reestablish the anterior chamber.[104-106] A 23- or 25-gauge sterile needle is used to make small punctures in the anterior lens capsule. Utrata forceps were then used to tear the anterior lens capsule by continuous curvilinear capsulorrhexis. In the single-needle technique, the ultrasonic needle for fragmentation and aspiration is then inserted through the capsule opening (Fig. 6-14). The lens cortex and nucleus are fragmented and aspirated. Penetration of the posterior lens capsule should be avoided.

The ultrasonic needle is removed. A 0.5-mm irrigation/aspiration tip is used to remove all remaining cortical material from the equator. Although the standard phacoemulsification needles easily fragment the equine lens, a custom-designed, longer-length irrigation/aspiration cannula is considered essential for adequate irrigation and aspiration of the entire equine lens. The corneal incision is closed with 7-0 absorbable sutures placed in a simple interrupted pattern at two thirds to three fourths of the depth of the cornea. The entrance site of the irrigation needle is grasped with toothed forceps, and the needle is withdrawn. Pressure at the site for 1 minute is usually adequate to seal

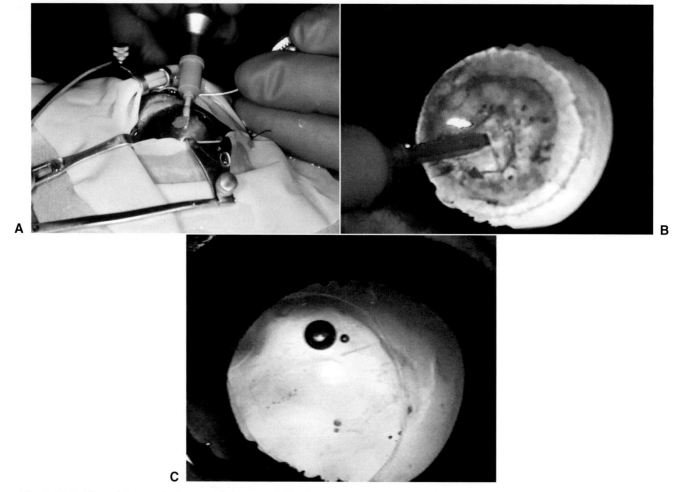

Fig. 6-14 A, View of the surgical setup of phacoemulsification and aspiration of a cataract in a horse. **B,** Intraoperative photograph. The anterior capsule has been partially removed by a continuous curvilinear capsulorrhexis; the nucleus and cortex are being broken up with ultrasonic phacoemulsification and aspirated from the eye. **C,** Intraoperative photograph immediately after removal of the cataract. (Photographs courtesy Dr. Brian Gilger.)

the wound. If leakage occurs, the site can be sutured with 6-0 absorbable material. A figure-of-eight suture is used to appose the canthal tissues, and 3-0 nonabsorbable sutures in a simple interrupted pattern are used to complete skin closure.

A temporary tarsorrhaphy can be performed by suturing the eyelids with 3-0 nylon or silk material in a horizontal mattress pattern to protect the eye during anesthesia recovery.[4,96] A protective helmet or eye shield may also be used during recovery from anesthesia and for 3 to 5 days after surgery; however, proper fit and tolerance of the devices by the horse should be monitored.[31,107-111]

EXTRACAPSULAR AND INTRACAPSULAR LENS EXTRACTION

Extracapsular and intracapsular techniques have been used to remove acquired mature cataracts.[38,70] These

techniques are not usually necessary for treating soft congenital cataracts in foals. The phacofragmentation with aspiration technique is recommended if cataract removal is indicated in an adult horse. Intracapsular extraction is used only for removal of luxated or subluxated lenses, and results are often poor in the horse. It is not indicated for routine lens removal.

POSTOPERATIVE MANAGEMENT

Postoperative therapy must include mydriatics, topical antibiotics, and topical and systemic antiinflammatory preparations (Box 6-3). Mydriasis and control of uveitis are essential. In controlling surgically induced uveitis in horses, prostaglandin inhibitors are valuable adjuncts to preoperative and postoperative therapy. Long-term use of flunixin meglumine must be avoided in foals.[48,112] Foals should be monitored for gastric and oral ulceration.

Box 6-3	Example of a Medication Protocol After Cataract Surgery in a Horse

Postoperative Protocol

Day 1—First day after surgery
- Physical and ocular examination
- Intravenous or oral flunixin meglumine, 1.1 mg/kg, once or twice daily
- Topical ophthalmic antibiotic solution, four times daily
- Topical ophthalmic corticosteroid (1.0% prednisolone acetate or 0.1% dexamethasone), four times daily
- Topical 1% atropine solution, two times daily
- Gastric protectants for foals

Day 3 after surgery
- If inflammation is minimal and no complications, release from hospital
  - Oral flunixin meglumine, 1.1 mg/kg, once daily for 5 to 7 days
  - Topical ophthalmic antibiotic solution, three times daily
  - Topical ophthalmic corticosteroid (1.0% prednisolone acetate or 0.1% dexamethasone), three times daily
  - Topical 1% atropine solution, every 48 hours
  - Gastric protectants for foals

Recheck 7 to 10 days after surgery
- Physical and ocular examination
- If eye is minimally inflamed, then:
  - Oral flunixin meglumine, 1.1 mg/kg, once every other day for 7 days
  - Topical ophthalmic antibiotic solution, two times daily
  - Topical ophthalmic corticosteroid (1.0% prednisolone acetate or 0.1% dexamethasone), two times daily
  - Topical 1% atropine solution—discontinue if pupil fully dilated

Recheck 4 to 6 weeks after surgery
- Physical and ocular examination
- If eye is noninflamed, then:
  - Topical ophthalmic antibiotic solution—discontinue
  - Topical ophthalmic corticosteroid (1.0% prednisolone acetate or 0.1% dexamethasone), once daily for 14 days, then discontinue
  - Topical 1% atropine solution—discontinue

Recheck 3 months after surgery
- Physical and ocular examination

Recheck 6 months after surgery
- Physical and ocular examination

Recheck 12 months after surgery
- Physical and ocular examination

Annual rechecks if no complications

After surgery, antibiotic or corticosteroid ophthalmic ointment and 1% atropine ophthalmic ointment are topically applied three or four times daily. Direct application of these ointments is facilitated by the use of a tuberculin syringe. The syringe plunger is removed, and 0.25 ml of each ointment is infused into the syringe barrel. The plunger is reinserted, and the air is expelled. The blunt syringe tip is gently inserted into the medial canthus over the lacrimal caruncle, and the medication is deposited anterior to the nictitating membrane. As the ointment is warmed by contact with the conjunctival membranes, the movements of the nictitating membrane and palpebrae distribute the medication over the eye.

If topical ointments cannot be satisfactorily instilled, a subpalpebral lavage system should be placed.[77,108] Subpalpebral lavage systems facilitate frequent topical application of medication to adult horses.[4,108,109,113] By allowing instillation of medication from a site distal to the painful eye, these systems minimize the risk to veterinary personnel and decrease the possibility of damage to the horse's eye. The value of these devices is offset by the possibility of ocular irritation if the devices are improperly positioned or maintained.

Oral flunixin meglumine (0.5 to 1.0 mg/kg, twice daily) and prednisolone (1.0 to 2.0 mg/kg) are administered for 1 to 2 weeks in decreasing doses. If a tarsorrhaphy was performed, the sutures are removed within 1 to 4 days after surgery, and fluorescein stain is applied to the cornea. If the cornea retains the stain, a topical ophthalmic antibiotic (without corticosteroids) is used until the cornea heals. Topical corticosteroid therapy is then restarted.

Frequently, corneal edema is present 24 hours after surgery and intensifies for 48 to 72 hours. A moderate amount of fibrin can be present in the anterior chamber for 7 to 10 days. Dilute tissue plasminogen activator (25 µg/µl) may be injected into the anterior chamber to dissolve large fibrin clots.[114] Corneal edema should clear 7 to 10 days after surgery.[31,43,71,76] The pupil should be dilated, and there should be a blink response to bright light.

Three weeks after surgery, the eye should be noninflamed and nonpainful and should have normal IOP. The patient should be able to negotiate a simple obstacle course. The pupil should be dilated, and the ocular media should be clear. A few strands of contracted fibrin might be present in the anterior chamber.

The intensity and duration of postoperative uveitis varies among patients; therefore the postoperative therapeutic regimen must be tailored to the individual. The duration of medical therapy usually ranges from 3 to 8 weeks after surgery.

COMPLICATIONS AND SEQUELAE

Common complications of equine cataract surgery include uveitis and synechiae. Keratopathy, secondary cataracts, and intraocular infections are other potentially significant sequelae (Fig. 6-15).[31,105,106]

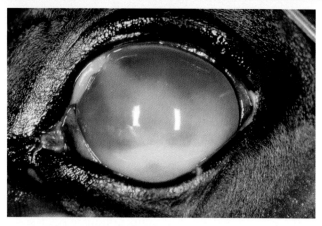

Fig. 6-15 Septic endophthalmitis, a rare complication, 1 week after phacoemulsification and aspiration of cataracts.

Most complications in foals occur as a result of intraoperative corneal damage or surgery-related uveitis. During surgery, care must be taken to avoid contacting or damaging the corneal endothelium or iris with the needle tip. Reducing postoperative uveitis depends on removal of all lens material. Synechiae of the pupillary margins can occur, but vision will not be compromised if the pupil is moderately dilated.

Sequelae of persistent or recurring postoperative uveitis can include intraocular fibrosis and phthisis bulbi. A regimented, deliberate withdrawal of ocular and systemic antiinflammatory drugs is essential to restore intraocular homeostasis. Evidence that postoperative iridocyclitis is controlled includes clarity of the ocular media, a nonpainful eye without photophobia or epiphora, a well-dilated pupil, and a normotensive globe.

After lens aspiration, secondary cataracts can develop from opacification of remnants of the anterior lens capsule, retained cortical material, migration of pigmented cells and fibroblasts on the posterior lens capsule, or posterior capsular opacities.[24,31,71,80] The degree of visual impairment depends on the location and extent of opacification.[39,43,71] This lens capsular fibrosis is particularly severe in foals that have undergone lens removal; therefore a planned primary posterior capsulotomy is generally recommended for these patients.

Other complications include self-trauma, periorbital edema, corneal ulceration, mycotic keratitis, superficial or deep corneal fibrovascular infiltrates, chronic corneal edema, ERU, and retinal detachment. Systemic illness, which can follow cataract surgery, is often related to the stress of anesthesia and surgery.

After cataract surgery, the soundness of the patient is of concern to the surgeon and owner. Vision is evaluated by means of an obstacle course negotiated by the patient in bright and dim light. Streak retinoscopy has been performed in horses with aphakia. Additional factors that determine whether a patient can perform riding exercises after cataract surgery are the horse's temperament, whether the condition is unilateral or bilateral, the experience of the rider, and the complexity of the maneuvers required.

FUTURE RESEARCH ON LENS DISEASES IN HORSES

Because of the high incidence of congenital cataracts in horses and many instances of suspected heritability of these cataracts, the genes and genetic causes of these defects need to be determined to allow testing of mares and stallions (see Chapter 11). As more information on the equine genome becomes available, these defects will become more likely to be determined.

Improving the cataract removal techniques and management of the preoperative and postoperative uveitis will improve the long-term outcome of cataract surgery. Understanding the formation and progression of lens capsule opacities in horses will also lead to methods to decrease or eliminate the development of "after-cataract" formation in horses.

The development of an intraocular lens (IOL) for horses has been discussed for years. Currently, in dogs, the IOL consists of either a one-piece, all-polymethylmethacrylate, rigid optic (7 mm), biconvex, posterior chamber lens of approximately 41.5 D or a foldable and injectable IOL made of hydroxyethyl methacrylate and methylmethacrylate copolymer of 41.5 D[62] As the obstacles in manufacturing lightweight, small-incision IOLs of sufficient dioptric strength are overcome, veterinary ophthalmologists should proceed with the design of an IOL for the equine eye, once the appropriate size and power of the equine prosthetic lens has been determined.[115,116]

REFERENCES

1. Cooley PL: Normal equine ocular anatomy and eye examination, *Vet Clin North Am Equine Pract* 8:427-449, 1992.
2. Martin CL, Anderson BG: Ocular anatomy. In: Gelatt KN, editor: *Textbook of veterinary ophthalmology*, Philadelphia, 1981, Lea & Febiger, pp 12-22.
3. Lavach JD: Lens. In JD Lavach, editor: *Large animal ophthalmology* St Louis, 1990, Mosby, pp 185-201.
4. Severin GA: *Severin's veterinary ophthalmology notes*, ed 3, Ft Collins, Colo, 1996, pp 379-406.
5. Murphy CJ, Howland HC: The optics of comparative ophthalmoscopy *Vis Res* 27:599-607, 1987.

6. Roberts SM: Equine vision and optics, *Vet Clin North Am Equine Pract* 8:451-457, 1992.

7. Samuelson DA: Ophthalmic anatomy. In Gelatt KN, editor: *Veterinary ophthalmology*, ed 3, Baltimore, 1999, Lippincott Williams & Wilkins, pp 31-150.

8. Slatter DH: Lens. In Douglas Slatter, editor: *Fundamentals of veterinary ophthalmology*, Philadelphia, 1990, WB Saunders, pp 365-393.

9. Slatter DH: *Fundamentals of veterinary ophthalmology*, ed 3, Philadelphia, 2001, WB Saunders, pp 21-33.

10. Blogg JR: Embryology and developmental anomalies. In Blogg JR, editor: The eye in veterinary practice, vol 1, extraocular disease, Philadelphia, 1980, WB Saunders, pp 80-89.

11. Garner A, Griffiths P: Bilateral congenital ocular defects in a foal, *Br J Ophthalmol* 53:513-517, 1969.

12. McLaughlin SA, Whitley RD, Gilger BC: Diagnosis and treatment of lens diseases, *Vet Clin North Am Equine Pract* 8:575-585, 1992.

13. Priester WA: Congenital ocular defects in cattle, horses, cats, and dogs, *J Am Vet Med Assoc* 160:1504-1511, 1972.

14. Latimer CA, Wyman M, Hamilton J: An ophthalmic survey of the neonatal horse, *Equine Vet J (Suppl)* 2:9-14, 1983.

15. Munroe GA, Barnett KC: Congenital ocular disease in the foal, *Vet Clin North Am Large Anim Pract* 6:519-537, 1984.

16. Riis RC: Equine ophthalmology. In Gelatt KN, editor: *Textbook of veterinary ophthalmology*, Philadelphia, 1981, Lea & Febiger, pp 569-605.

17. Wilcock BP: Ocular anomalies. In Peiffer RL, editor: *Comparative ophthalmic pathology*, Springfield, IL, 1983, Charles C. Thomas, pp 3-46.

18. Roberts SM: Congenital ocular anomalies. *Vet Clin North Am Equine Pract* 8:459-478, 1992.

19. Cook CS: Ocular embryology and congenital malformations. In Gelatt KN, editor: *Veterinary ophthalmology*, ed 3, Baltimore, 1999, Lippincott Williams & Wilkins, pp 3-30.

20. Huston R, Saperstein G, Leipold HW: Congenital defects in foals, *J Equine Med Surg* 1:146-161, 1977.

21. Irby NL, Aguirre GD: Congenital aniridia in a pony, *J Am Vet Med Assoc* 186:281-282, 1985.

22. Joyce JR: Aniridia in a Quarterhorse, *Equine Vet J (Suppl)* 2:21-22, 1983.

23. Latimer CA, Wyman M: Neonatal ophthalmology, *Vet Clin North Am Equine Pract* 1:235-259, 1985.

24. Matthews AG, Handscombe MC: Bilateral cataract formation and subluxation of the lenses in a foal: a case report, *Equine Vet J (Suppl)* 2:23-24, 1983.

25. Beech J, Aguirre G, Gross S: Congenital nuclear cataracts in the Morgan horse, *J Am Vet Med Assoc* 184:1363-1365, 1984.

26. Joyce JR et al: Iridial hypoplasia (aniridia) accompanied by limbic dermoids and cataracts in group of related Quarterhorses, *Equine Vet J (Suppl)* 10:26-28, 1990.

27. Ueda Y: Aniridia in a Thoroughbred horse, *Equine Vet J (Suppl)* 10:29, 1990.

28. Erikson R: Hereditary aniridia with secondary cataract in horses, *Nord Vet Med* 7:773-779, 1955.

29. Koch SA et al: Ocular disease in the newborn horse: a preliminary report, *J Equine Med Surg* 2:167-170, 1978.

30. Walde I: Some observations on congenital cataracts in the horse, *Equine Vet J (Suppl)* 2:27-28, 1983.

31. Whitley RD, Moore CP, Slone DE: Cataract surgery in the horse: a review, *Equine Vet J (Suppl)* 2:127-134, 1983.

32. Ramsey DT et al: Congenital ocular abnormalities of Rocky Mountain Horses, *Vet Ophthalmol* 2:47-59, 1999.

33. Dziezyc J, Kern TJ, Wolf ED: Microphthalmia in a foal, *Equine Vet J* 15:15-17, 1983.

34. Mosier DA et al: Bilateral multiple congenital ocular defects in quarter horse foals, *Equine Vet J* 15:18-20, 1983.

35. Barnett KC: The eye of the newborn foal, *J Reprod Fertil* 23:701-703, 1975.

36. Rubin LF: The horse fundus. In Lionel F. Rubin, editor: *Atlas of veterinary ophthalmoscopy*, Philadelphia, 1974, Lea & Febiger, pp 289-325.

37. Davidson MG: Equine ophthalmology. In Gelatt KN, editor: *Veterinary ophthalmology*, ed 2, Philadelphia, 1991, Lea & Febiger, pp 576-610.

38. Brooks DE: Equine ophthalmology. In Gelatt KN, editor: *Veterinary ophthalmology*, ed 3. Baltimore, 1999, Lippincott Williams & Wilkins, pp 1053-1116.

39. Whitley RD, Meek LA: Cataract surgery in horses, *Comp Contin Educ Pract Vet* 11:1396-1401, 1989.

40. Luntz MH: Clinical types of cataracts. In Duane TD, editor: *Clinical ophthalmology, vol 1*, Philadelphia, JB Lippincott Co, 1984, pp 1-20.

41. Cotlier E: The lens. In Moses RA, Hart WM, editors: *Adler's physiology of the eye*, ed 8. St Louis, 1987, Mosby, pp 268-290.

42. Beech J, Irby N: Inherited nuclear cataracts in the Morgan horse, *J Hered* 76:371-372, 1985.

43. Millichamp NJ, Dziezyc J: Cataract phacofragmentation in horses, *Vet Ophthalmol* 3:157-164, 2000.

44. Schwink K: Cataract and strabismus in a color-dilute pony foal, *Equine Pract* 12:9-12, 1990.

45. Saunders LZ, Rubin LF: The lens. In L Z Saunders and L F Rubin, editor: *Ophthalmic pathology of animals*, Basel, 1975, S Karger, pp 82-99.

46. Matthews AG: Lens opacities in the horse: a clinical classification, *Vet Ophthalmol* 3:65-71, 2000.

47. Cook CS, Peiffer RL, Harling DE: Equine recurrent uveitis, *Equine Vet J (Suppl)* 3:57-60, 1983.

48. Whitley RD, Miller TR, Wilson JH: Therapeutic considerations for equine recurrent uveitis, *Equine Pract* 15:16-23, 1993.

49. Miller TR, Whitley RD: Equine uveitis, *Mod Vet Pract* 68:351-357, 1987.

50. Schwink KL: Equine uveitis, *Vet Clin North Am Equine Practice* 8:557-574, 1992.

51. Turner LM, Whitley RD, Hager D: Management of ocular trauma in horses. Part II. Orbit, eyelids, uvea, lens, retina, and optic nerve, *Mod Vet Pract* 67:341-347, 1986.

52. Bistner S, Shaw D: Uveitis in the horse, *Comp Contin Educ Pract Vet* 2:S35-S43, 1980.

53. Lavach JD: Pupil, iris, and ciliary body. In J D Lavach, editor: *Large animal ophthalmology*, St Louis, 1990, Mosby, pp 150-177.

54. Rebhun WC: Diagnosis and treatment of equine uveitis, *J Am Vet Med Assoc* 175:803-808, 1979.

55. Saunders LZ, Rubin LF: Equine recurrent uveitis. In L Z Saunders and L F Rubin, editor: Ophthalmic pathology of animals, Basel, 1975, S Karger, pp 78-81.

56. Gilger BC et al: Use of an intravitreal sustained-release cyclosporine delivery device for treatment of equine recurrent uveitis, *Am J Vet Res* 62:1892-1896, 2001.

57. Whitley RD, Gelatt KN: Ocular manifestations of systemic disease. In Gelatt KN, editor: *Veterinary ophthalmology*, Philadelphia, 1981, Lea & Febiger, pp 724-741.

58. Angelos J et al. Evaluation of breed as a risk factor for sarcoid and uveitis in horses, *Anim Genet* 19:417-425, 1988.

59. Brooks DE, Wolf ED: Ocular trauma in the horse, *Equine Vet J (Suppl)* 2:141-146, 1983.

60. Hooper PL, Rao NA, Smith RE: Cataract extraction in uveitis patients, *Surv Ophthalmol* 35:120-144, 1990.

61. Barros PSM, Feitosa FLF, Alvarengna J: Lens subluxation in a horse, *Equine Pract* 12:16, 1990.

62. Nasisse MP, Davidson MG: Surgery of the lens. In Gelatt KN, editor: *Veterinary ophthalmology*, ed 3. Baltimore, 1999, Lippincott Williams & Wilkins, pp 827-856.

63. Lavach JD, Severin GA, Roberts SM: Lacerations of the equine eye: a review of 48 cases, *J Am Vet Med Assoc* 184:1243-1248, 1984.

64. Meek LA: Intraocular silicone prosthesis in a horse, *J Am Vet Med Assoc* 193:343-345, 1988.

65. Riggs C, Whitley RD; Intraocular silicone prostheses in a dog and a horse with corneal lacerations, *J Am Vet Med Assoc* 196:617-619, 1990.

66. McLaughlin SA et al. Intraocular silicone prosthesis, *Comp Contin Educ Vet Pract* 17:945-950, 1995.

67. Hamor RE et al: Ocular cosmetic and prosthetic devices, *Vet Clin North Am Equine Pract* 8:637-654, 1982.

68. Davidson MG et al: Traumatic anterior lens capsule disruption, *J Am Anim Hosp Assoc* 27:410-414, 1991.

69. Davidson MG, Nelms SR: Diseases of the lens and cataract formation. In Gelatt KN, editor: *Veterinary ophthalmology*, ed 3, Baltimore, 1999, Lippincott Williams & Wilkins, pp 797-825.

69. Lavach JD: Examination. In J D Lavach, editor: *Large animal ophthalmology*, St Louis, 1990, Mosby, pp 29- 41.

70. Farrall H, Handscombe MC: Follow-up report of a case of surgical aphakia with an analysis of equine visual function, *Equine Vet J (Suppl)* 10:91-93 1990.

71. Dziezyc J, Millichamp NJ, Keller CB: Use of phacofragmentation for cataract removal in horses: 12 cases (1985-1989), *J Am Vet Med Assoc* 198:1774-1778, 1991.

72. Crewther SG, Crewther DP, Mitchell DO: The effects of short-term occlusion therapy on reversal of the anatomical and physiological effects of monocular deprivation in the lateral geniculate nucleus and visual cortex of kittens, *Exp Brain Res* 51:206-216, 1983.

73. Tytla ME et al: Stereopsis after congenital cataract, *Invest Ophthalmol Vis Sci* 34:1767-1773, 1993.

74. Birch EE, Stager DR: Prevalence of good visual acuity following surgery for congenital unilateral cataract, *Arch Ophthalmol* 106:40-43, 1988.

75. Robb RM, Mayer DL, Moore BD: Results of early treatment of unilateral cataracts, *J Pediatr Ophthalmol Strabismus* 24:178-181, 1988.

76. Whitley RD et al: Cataract surgery in the horse: a review of six cases, *Equine Vet J (Suppl)* 2:85-90, 1990.

77. Meredith RE, Wolf ED: Ophthalmic examination and therapeutic techniques in the horse, *Comp Contin Educ Pract Vet* 3:S426-S433, 1981.

78. Witzel DA, Joyce JR, Smith EL: Electroretinography of congenital night blindness in an Appaloosa, *J Equine Med Surg* 1:226-229, 1977.

79. Witzel DA et al. Night blindness in the Appaloosa: sibling occurrence, *J Equine Med Surg* 1:383-386, 1977.

80. Gelatt KN, Myers VS, McClure JR: Aspiration of congenital and soft cataracts in foals and young horses, *J Am Vet Med Assoc* 165:611-616, 1974.

81. Gelatt KN, Kraft WE: A technique for aspiration of cataracts in young horses, *Vet Med* 64:415-421, 1969.

82. Adams R, Mayhew IG: Neurologic disease, *Vet Clin North Am Equine Pract* 1:209-234, 1985.

83. van der Woerdt A, Wilkie DA, Myer CW: Ultrasonographic abnormalities in the eyes of dogs with cataracts: 147 cases (1986-1992), *J Am Vet Med Assoc* 203:838-841, 1993.

84. Wilkie DA et al: Spontaneous lens capsule rupture secondary to diabetes mellitus: surgical outcome in canine eyes, *Vet Ophthalmol* 5:298, 2002 (abstract 53).

85. Williams DL: Lens morphometry determined by B-mode ultrasonography of the normal and cataractous canine lens, *Vet Ophthalmol* 7:91-95, 2004.

86. Whitley RD et al: Cataract removal in dogs. The presurgical considerations, *Vet Med* 9:848-858, 1993.

87. Scotty NC et al: Diagnostic ultrasonography of equine lens and posterior segment abnormalities, *Vet Ophthalmol* 7:127-139, 2004.

88. Fraser AC: An operation for the treatment of bilateral total cataracts in a Thoroughbred colt, *Vet Rec* 73:587-591, 1961.

89. Van Kruiningen HJ: Intracapsular cataract extraction in the horse, *J Am Vet Med Assoc* 145:773-777, 1964.

90. Gelatt KN: The eye. In Mansmann RA, McAllister ES, Pratt PW, editors: *Equine medicine and surgery*, ed 3, vol 2, Santa Barbara, Calif, 1982, American Veterinary Publications, pp 1253-1303.

91. Gelatt KN: Ocular surgery. In Catcott EJ, Smithcors JF, editors: *Equine medicine and surgery*, ed 2, Wheaton, Ill, 1972, American Veterinary Publications, pp 791-801.

92. Gelatt KN, Kraft WE: A technique for aspiration of cataracts in young horses, *Vet Med* 64:415-421, 1969.

93. Kelman CH: Phacoemulsification in the anterior chamber, *Ophthalmology* 86:1980-1982, 1979.

94. Glover TD, Constantinescu GM: Surgery for cataracts, *Vet Clin North Am Small Anim Pract* 27:1143-1173, 1997.

95. Gelatt KN, Myers VS, McClure JR: Aspiration of congenital and soft cataracts in foals and young horses, *J Am Vet Med Assoc* 165:611-616, 1974.

96. Bistner SI, Aguirre G, Batik G: *Atlas of veterinary ophthalmic surgery*, Philadelphia, 1977, WB Saunders, pp 206-215.

97. Gilger BC: Phacoemulsification technology and fundamentals, *Vet Clin North Am Small Anim Pract* 27:1131-1141, 1997.

98. Seibel BS: *Phacodynamics: mastering the tools and techniques of phacoemulsification surgery*, Thorofare, NJ, 1995, Slack.

99. Troutman RC: *Microsurgery of the eye, vol 1*, St Louis, 1974, Mosby, pp 105-106.

100. Kelman CD: Phacoemulsification and aspiration: the Kelman technique of cataract removal. In Duane TD, editor: *Clinical ophthalmology, vol 5*, Philadelphia, 1984, JB Lippincott, pp 1-13.

101. Weinstein GW: Cataract surgery. In Duane TD, editor: *Clinical ophthalmology, vol 5*, Philadelphia, 1984, JB Lippincott, pp 1-52.

102. Weinstein GW: Cataracts. In Spaeth GL, editor: *Ophthalmic surgery*, Philadelphia, 1982, WB Saunders, pp 131-190.

103. Whitley RD: Cataracts in the horse. In Robinson NE, editor: *Current therapy in equine medicine*, ed 2, Philadelphia, 1987, WB Saunders, pp 456-458.

104. Wilkie DA, Willis AM: Viscoelastic materials in veterinary ophthalmology, *Vet Ophthalmol* 2:147-153, 1999.

105. Jaffe NS: *Cataract surgery and its complications*, ed 4. St Louis, 1984, Mosby, pp 530-559.

106. Liesegang TJ: Viscoelastic materials in veterinary ophthalmology, *Vet Ophthalmol* 2:147-153, 1999.

107. Manning JP: An equine eye shield, *Vet Med* 70:822-824, 1975.

108. Whitley RD, Lavach JD, Gelatt KN: Subpalpebral lavage system for administering frequent topical medications to the equine eye, *Florida Vet J* 8:10-14, 1979.

109. Miller TR et al. Phacofragmentation and aspiration for cataract extraction in dogs, *J Am Vet Med Assoc* 190:1577-1580, 1987.

110. Brooks DE: *Ophthalmology for the equine practitioner*, Jackson WY, 2002, Teton New Media.

111. Millichamp NJ: Principles of ophthalmic surgery. In: Auer JA, editor: *Equine surgery*, Philadelphia, 1992, WB Saunders, pp 588-598.

112. Traub-Dargatz JL et al: Chronic flunixin meglumine therapy in foals, *Am J Vet Res* 49:7-12, 1988.

113. Giuliano EA et al: Inferomedial placement of a single-entry subpalpebral lavage tube for treatment of equine eye disease, *Vet Ophthalmol* 3:153-156, 2000.

114. Martin CL et al: Ocular use of tissue plasminogen activator in companion animals, *Prog Vet Comp Ophthalmol* 3:29-36, 1992.

115. Gaiddon J et al. Use of biometry and keratometry for determining optimal power for intraocular lens implants in dogs, *Am J Vet Res* 52:781-783, 1991.

116. Gilger BC, Davidson MG, Colitz CMH: Experimental implantation of posterior chamber prototype intraocular lenses for the feline eye, *Am J Vet Res* 59:1339-1343, 1998.

7 Equine Recurrent Uveitis

Ann Dwyer and Brian C. Gilger

With contributions from Carolyn Kalsow, Hartmut Gerhards, and Bettina Wollanke

Equine recurrent uveitis (ERU) (also known as moon blindness, iridocyclitis, and periodic ophthalmia) is a major ophthalmic disease and is the most common cause of blindness in horses.[1-4] This immune-mediated panuveitis has a reported prevalence of 8% to 25% in horses in the United States[2,5]; however, field observations suggest that 1% to 2% of American horses have clinical disease serious enough to threaten vision.[6] Fortunately, recent advances in the treatment of horses with ERU have led to an improvement in management of this disease. In this chapter some important facts about ERU, its causes, and treatment options for affected horses are discussed.

ERU is characterized by episodes of intraocular inflammation that develop weeks to months after an initial uveitis episode subsides.[1-4] Horses can have ERU at any age, but the initial uveitis episode frequently occurs in horses 4 to 8 years of age, a time when most horses are at or nearing their prime performance years.[1-4] Not every case of initial equine uveitis will develop into ERU (see discussion of differential diagnoses later in this chapter), but each horse that has signs consistent with uveitis is considered at risk for recurrence until several years without relapse have passed.

ERU-like diseases have been described in horses since Vegetius wrote about recurrent eye inflammation in the fourth century AD.[7] Initially, the syndrome was thought to be caused by the changes in the moon, hence, the descriptive term *moon blindness* still prevalent today. Much speculation occurred in the eighteenth, nineteenth, and early twentieth centuries as to the cause(s) of ERU. Before 1940, prevailing theories included various infectious causes, hereditary predisposition, thyroid deficiency, riboflavin deficiency, climate, toxin hypersensitivity, and parasites.[7-9] In early reviews describing the clinical examination and pathologic findings of ERU,[7-9] investigators speculated further on infectious causes, and ensuing research swung toward investigating bacterial causes. In 1947 Rimpau[10] presented evidence connecting some cases of the syndrome with leptospirosis, and the next year, Heusser[11] published data linking positive serum agglutinin titers to *Leptospira interrogans* serovars *grippotyphosa*, *pomona*, and *australis* in German horses. Although prevalence has varied with the geographic region, leptospirosis has been linked to spontaneous ERU around the world.[6,12-28] Correlations of serologic and ocular fluid agglutinin reactivity to various leptospiral serovars have been monitored by analysis of leptospiral DNA in ocular fluids[27] and culture of leptospires from the eyes of affected horses.[17,27,28]

Although leptospirosis has been linked to ERU in many horses, other bacterial, viral, protozoan, and parasitic causes—as well as noninfectious causes—have been associated with the syndrome. The pathophysiology of uveitis is far more complex than a simple systemic infection or traumatic episode. Research in horses, humans, and laboratory and domestic animals has shown that recurrent intraocular inflammation is multifactorial in origin, related to the genetic makeup of the individual, and strongly immune-mediated. Numerous pathologic investigations have provided descriptions of the variety of changes that accompany the syndrome in the anterior and posterior segments at the cellular level.[7,8,29-33] Recent work has centered on the immunohistopathology and immunohistochemistry of the disease complex.[31,33-38] Studies probing immune mechanisms responsible for triggering inflammatory episodes and tissue destruction and relationships between the equine major histocompatibility complex (MHC) and ERU susceptibility are ongoing.[39] Decades of work from laboratories around the world have demonstrated that ERU is an intricate disease complex, and defining the pathogenesis and risk factors will continue to challenge scientists and clinicians as research for effective therapies continues.

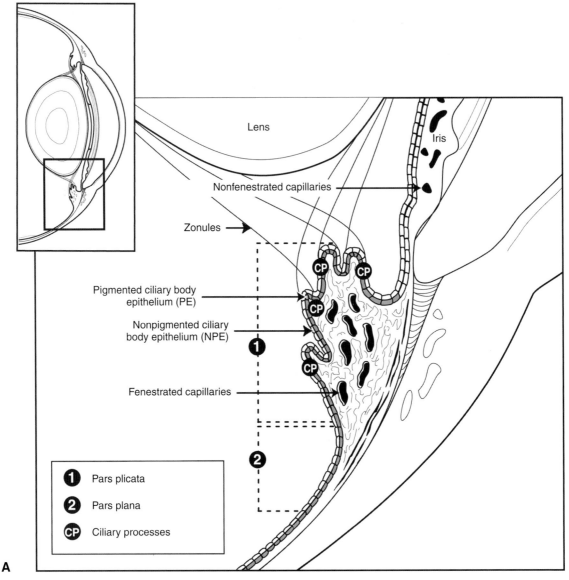

Fig. 7-1 A, Schematic diagram of the iris and ciliary body.

CLINICAL ANATOMY AND PHYSIOLOGY

ERU is a disease that involves all aspects of the equine eye. However, the origin of the inflammation and most of the initial manifestations of the disease are centered in the uveal tract (Fig. 7-1). The uveal tract consists of the iris and ciliary body (the anterior uvea) and the choroid (posterior uvea).

Anatomy and Physiology of the Uveal Tract

The two components of the anterior uvea, the iris and the ciliary body, contain heavily pigmented connective, vascular, and muscle tissue. The iris functions as a

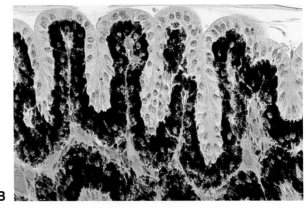

Fig. 7-1 cont'd. B, Normal histologic section of ciliary processes demonstrating pigmented and nonpigmented ciliary epithelium.

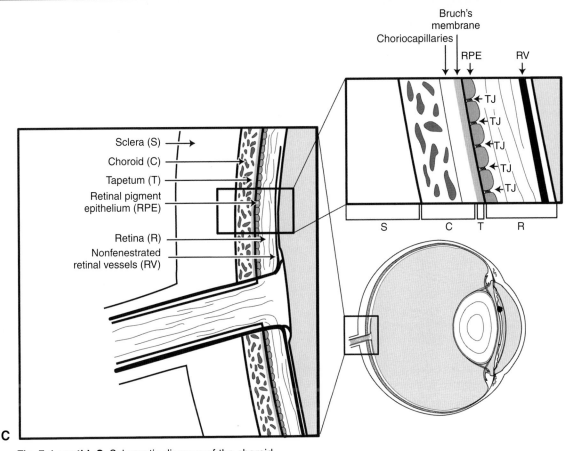

Fig. 7-1 cont'd. C, Schematic diagram of the choroid.

shutter that responds to prevailing light conditions, and the ciliary body produces aqueous humor through active secretion and ultrafiltration of plasma. Both the iris and ciliary body have many blood vessels within their connective tissue, and the inner aspect of both structures is lined by a double layer of epithelium, which has an important role in the pathogenesis of ERU. The layer of epithelium closest to the connective tissue is pigmented, and the boundary layer closest to the vitreous is nonpigmented. The clinical anatomy and microanatomy of the anterior portion of the uvea are described in Chapter 5.

The choroid, or posterior part of the uvea, functions as the primary vascular supply of the horse retina (see Chapter 10). It lies between the sclera and the retina and contains the tapetum, the fibrous reflective layer (see Chapter 10 for a complete description of the choroid).

The uveal tract contains most of the blood supply of the eye and is in direct contact with peripheral vasculature. Therefore diseases of the systemic circulation (e.g., septicemia and bacteremia) will also affect the uveal blood circulation. There is a barrier between this blood circulation and the internal aspects of the eye, called the *blood-ocular barrier* (Fig. 7-2). The blood-ocular barrier consists of the blood-aqueous barrier (i.e., tight junctions between the nonpigmented epithelial cells of

the ciliary body and nonfenestrated iridal blood vessels) and the blood-retinal barrier (i.e., tight junctions between the cells of the retinal pigmented epithelium [RPE] and nonfenestrated retinal vessels). These semipermeable barriers normally prevent large molecules and cells from entering the eye and help the intraocular fluids remain clear. The blood-ocular barrier also limits the immune response to the internal aspects of the eye, causing the eye to be considered an immune-privileged site.[40] In cases of trauma or inflammation, these barriers can be disrupted, allowing blood products and cells to enter the eye. Flare, cell accumulations, and haze in the aqueous or vitreous are clinically observable signs of the disruption of the blood-ocular barrier that occurs in ERU. Disruption of the barrier enables activation of various host immune responses, including production of antibodies to self-antigens not normally recognized by the horse's own immune system, as well as production of antibodies to foreign antigens inside the eye.

Physiology of Equine Recurrent Uveitis

Because all the uveal tissues are abundantly populated with blood vessels, the physiology of early inflammation

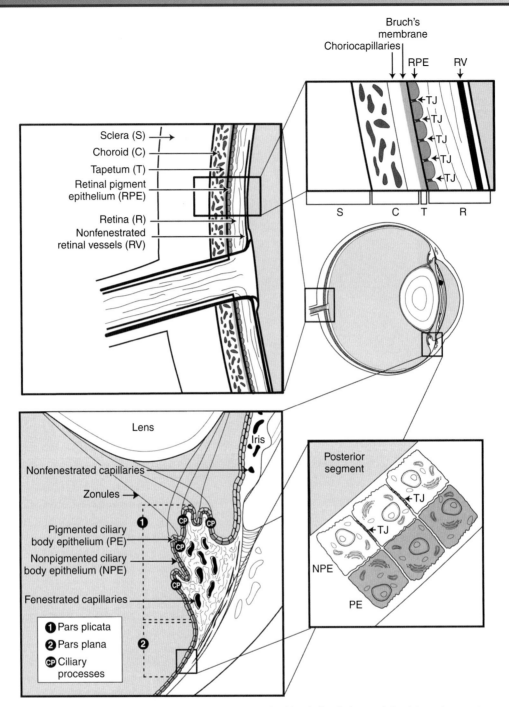

Fig. 7-2 Blood-ocular barrier. The barrier between the blood circulation and the internal aspects of the eye is called the blood-ocular barrier. This barrier normally prevents large molecules and cells from entering the eye, which helps the eye chambers and fluids remain clear. *TJ,* Tight junctions.

involves vascular *congestion*. This congestion causes dilation of the overlying limbal blood vessels, resulting in the "limbal flush" of scleral and conjunctival vessels that causes the characteristic "red eye" appearance of uveitis. Congestion and inflammatory activity of the uveal vessels cause leakage of protein and fluid into the surrounding connective tissues as the blood-ocular barrier is disrupted. Infiltration of mononuclear cells

into the uveal perivascular space is facilitated by vascular permeability, particularly in the ciliary body.

One hallmark of ERU is the accumulation of noncellular *exudates* adjacent to inner boundaries of the uveal tract. Exudates contribute to uveal tissue dysfunction and hypotony of the globe because the ciliary body produces less aqueous humor. Nourishment of the photoreceptor layer of the retina with oxygen and other nutrients from the choriocapillaris is decreased. In addition, iris sphincter muscle spasms cause miosis and block the ability of the iris to adjust to prevailing light conditions.

The uvea and aqueous humor nourish a number of anatomic and functionally dissimilar components in the eye. Inflammation in uveitis is thus associated with inflammation, dysfunction, or both in, variably, the cornea, sclera, lens, retina, and optic nerve. The physiology of inflammation in the nonuveal parts of the eye is dependent on the anatomy and physiology of each affected area (see Chapters 5 [uveal disease], 6 [lens], and 9 [retina]).

Transparency of the *cornea* is compromised when swelling of the corneal endothelium and stroma occurs. Resultant edema causes focal or diffuse opacity and general "steaminess" of the cornea. Infiltration of inflammatory cells in the tissue layers further hinders light passage. Disruption of the endothelial sodium-potassium pump that normally keeps the cornea relatively dehydrated further contributes to opacity changes. Edema can become permanent if endothelial dysfunction is severe.

Function of the *lens* is compromised when it becomes opacified or dislocated. Cataract occurs as the lens increases in water, electrolyte, and mineral content in response to changes in the adjacent media or synechial adhesions. Normal uptake of oxygen into the lens is reduced, contributing further to loss of transparency. Luxation of the lens occurs when the zonular fibers, normally attached to the ciliary processes of the ciliary body, become detached or degenerate.

Function of the *retina* is disrupted if the photoreceptors are deprived of oxygen and other nutrients normally supplied by the choriocapillaris, if inflammatory toxins from the vitreous damage cellular components, or if the retina is detached as a result of subretinal exudates and cellular infiltrate from the inner choroid. Optic nerve function is disturbed if the blood supply to the nerve is compromised as a result of choroidal inflammation, infarcts, or secondary glaucoma with resultant ischemia of the nerve.

The *ocular media* serve as collecting chambers for infiltrating cells and inflammatory by-products. Their physiology is often altered in ERU. The anterior chamber changes transparency in instances of fibrin accumulation, flare, hyphema, or hypopyon. Endothelial metabolism of the cornea is altered if the aqueous constitution is abnormal. Accumulation of inflammatory cells and by-products in the aqueous may obstruct the trabecular meshwork or uveoscleral region, resulting in secondary glaucoma.

The *posterior segment* of the eye may have altered clarity caused by leakage of blood cells, macromolecules, and plasma components from the choroid and ciliary body into the vitreous. Infiltrating mononuclear cells and inflammatory cytokines can alter waste removal and contribute to liquefaction of the normally gel-like framework of the vitreous. Loss of the viscoelastic properties, combined with traction from the collapsing collagen network of the vitreous, may exert pull on the sparsely anchored retina and contribute to detachments and vision loss.

IMPACT OF EQUINE RECURRENT UVEITIS ON THE EQUINE INDUSTRY

The equine industry in the United States has an estimated annual worth of 112 billion dollars and provides approximately 1.4 million full-time jobs across the country.[41] Because ERU has a high prevalence rate across horse breeds in the United States, the financial impact of this disease on the equine industry could be as high as 100 to 250 million dollars a year. ERU causes these large economic losses in the equine industry because it disrupts training, decreases performance, and disqualifies horses from competition (e.g., because of medication use). Horses with ERU have decreased value as a result of vision deficits, and many horses that are blinded by ERU must be euthanized for practical and economic reasons. Finally, treatment, veterinary care, and personnel costs add to the economic impact of the disease.

CLASSIFICATION OF EQUINE UVEITIS

Horses experiencing an initial episode of uveitis from any cause are at risk for recurrent uveitis but are not considered to have ERU until two or more episodes have been observed. If several (i.e., two or more) years have passed without occurrence of a second episode of uveitis, the risk of development of ERU in a horse is diminished.

It is useful to describe equine uveitis cases according to observable major anatomic location of inflammation (see Table 7-1). *Anterior uveitis* is inflammation localized primarily in the iris, ciliary body, and anterior chamber (Fig. 7-3), with the posterior chamber remaining clear and the retina showing minimal changes. Chronic changes occur in the cornea, iris, and lens (Fig. 7-4). To date, no breed predilection for anterior uveitis has been identified. *Posterior uveitis* is inflammation predominantly in the vitreous, retina, and choroid. Clinical signs include bouts of vitreal inflammation, cloudiness, and retinal degeneration (Fig. 7-5). Anterior uveitis is not present or is very mild. Over the long term, cataracts, retinal detachments, and vitreal degeneration may develop in horses with posterior uveitis.

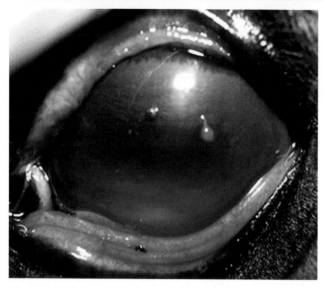

Fig. 7-3 Acute onset, active anterior uveitis—which is inflammation localized primarily in the iris, ciliary body, and anterior chamber—demonstrating conjunctival hyperemia, corneal edema, mild hypopyon, intense miosis, and iris swelling.

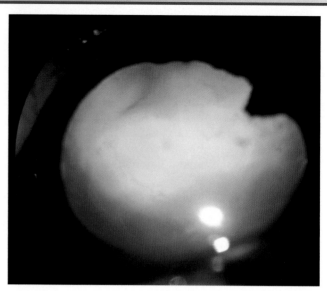

Fig. 7-5 Dense vitreous opacities and yellow discoloration of the vitreous in an eye with primarily posterior uveitis, although a small posterior synechia is present at the 2 o'clock position (see Fig. 7-32). (Photograph courtesy Hartmut Gerhards and Bettina Wollanke.)

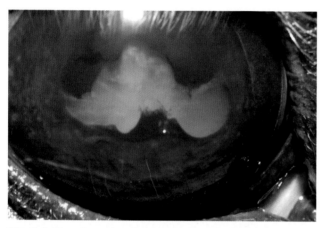

Fig. 7-4 Chronic ocular changes in an eye with multiple recurrent episodes of uveitis. Mild corneal edema, multifocal posterior synechia, corpora nigra atrophy, iris hyperpigmentation, and dense cataract are visible and are all signs typical of chronic equine recurrent uveitis.

This syndrome is most common in Warmbloods, draft breeds, and European horses. *Panuveitis* is inflammation that occurs in all segments of the uveal tract with sequelae in both the anterior and posterior segments. Clinically, it may not be possible to distinguish anterior uveitis from panuveitis with certainty, and some cases that begin as apparent anterior uveitis develop into panuveitis.

Another common classification divides equine uveitis into "classic cases" and "insidious cases" (Table 7-1). *Classic ERU* is most common and is characterized by active inflammatory episodes in the eye, followed by periods of minimal observable ocular inflammation. The acute, active phase of ERU predominantly involves inflammation of the iris, ciliary body, and choroid, with concurrent involvement of the cornea, anterior chamber, lens, retina, and vitreous (Fig. 7-3). After variable periods, the quiescent phase is generally followed by further and increasingly severe attacks of uveitis. In many horses, the repeated episodes of inflammation cause development of cataract, intraocular adhesions and phthisis bulbi and vision loss (Fig. 7-4).[1-4,29]

Insidious ERU is characterized by a low-grade intraocular inflammation that does not manifest as outwardly painful episodes. Internal ocular inflammation persists and leads to degeneration of ocular structures and chronic clinical signs of ERU. This type of uveitis is most commonly seen in Appaloosa and draft breed horses.

Classic cases may be further separated according to stage of chronicity, with cases labeled as "acute," "quiescent," or "end-stage" (Table 7-1). Horses with *acute cases* show active pain and observable internal inflammation, as well as extensive microscopic inflammation. Horses with *quiescent cases* are outwardly comfortable and show little active acute internal inflammation on clinical inspection. However, horses with quiescent cases do show ongoing inflammation at the microscopic level and may be presented with chronic inflammatory sequelae such as synechiae or cataracts. In *end-stage cases* eyes have a severe and often blinding deformity such as phthisis bulbi, dense cataract, luxated lens, detached retina, or loss of normal pupillary architecture (Fig. 7-4).

Table 7-1 Clinical Classification of Equine Recurrent Uveitis

Classification Schemes		Description
Anatomic location of inflammation	Anterior uveitis	Inflammation localized primarily in the iris, ciliary body, and anterior chamber
	Intermediate uveitis	Inflammation primarily of the ciliary body—not specifically described in horses, but is common in humans
	Posterior uveitis	Inflammation primarily in the vitreous, retina, and choroid
	Panuveitis	Inflammation of all segments of the uveal tract
Type of recurrence	Classic	Active inflammatory episodes followed by periods of minimal ocular inflammation
	Insidious	Persistent low-grade intraocular inflammation without overt signs of discomfort
Stage of chronicity	Acute	Active pain and observable internal inflammation
	Quiescent	Comfortable eye with no active internal inflammation visible clinically
	End-stage	Usually blind eyes, with phthisis bulbi, dense cataract, luxated lens, detached retina, and/or loss of normal pupillary architecture
Cause	Leptospiral MAT serology	Seropositive or negative for *L. pomona* spp.
	ELA typing	Positive for (ELA)-9 haplotype may indicate increase genetic susceptibility to ERU

ELA, Equine leukocyte antigen; *ERU,* equine recurrent uveitis; *MAT,* microagglutination test.

Clinicians in areas endemic for leptospirosis may find it useful to separate cases into those horses seropositive for pathogenic serovars of *L. interrogans* and those that are seronegative. Breed classification is also practical because increasing evidence has shown that Appaloosas and certain Warmblood horses are at risk for uveitis.

Uveitis cases should be classified as primary or recurrent, once the history of a case is known (see more information in Chapter 5). Recurrent cases can further be classified as to observable anatomic involvement, pattern of classic or insidious inflammation, stage of chronicity, and breed. *Recurrent uveitis is not one disease, but a whole complex of diseases with many subsets related to cause and presenting pattern.* It is expected that as understanding of the pathogenesis and etiology of ERU in horses grows, refined classification schemes will evolve as well.

CLINICAL APPEARANCE OF EQUINE RECURRENT UVEITIS

No sex predilection has been reported for ERU. Age at the initial episode is variable. One study of 160 horses with ERU revealed that half presented before 12 years of age, a time when horses experience prime performance.[42] Clinical signs are variable and depend on the acuteness of the episode, preexisting chronic ocular changes, the nature of the inflammation, and the anatomic location of most of the inflammation.

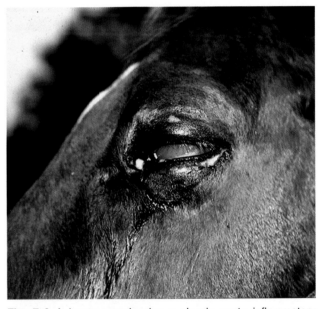

Fig. 7-6 A horse experiencing a classic acute inflammatory episode of equine recurrent uveitis. Periocular swelling, lacrimation, corneal edema, and blepharospasm are visible.

Anterior Segment

A horse experiencing a *classic acute inflammatory episode* is presented with pain, lacrimation, and blepharospasm (Fig. 7-6). The severity of the outward signs varies from a horse with a slightly closed eye to one that will not tolerate any manipulation of the periocular structures without sedation. Observable acute signs will depend on the severity of the episode, the duration of the episode at the time of examination, and preexisting changes from previous episodes. Diffuse edema of the eyelids may make globe inspection difficult. The cornea may be edematous, with the resultant haze being most marked at the periphery. Circumlimbal vascularization is frequent, and the length of the vessels provides a clue as to the duration of the episode. Fluorescein dye uptake will be negative, unless the horse has had a secondary ulcer caused by self-trauma. The anterior chamber may appear cloudy or hazy because of aqueous flare, and hypopyon or hyphema may be present in the ventral anterior chamber. Keratic precipitates may be visible as focal white spots on the endothelium of the cornea. *The cardinal sign of classic uveitis is miosis.*[1] Miosis is always present in an acute episode, unless mydriatics have been administered or synechiae distort the pupillary border. The iris may be dull in color or show mottled pigmentation, changes in color, or

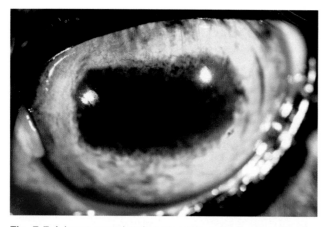

Fig. 7-7 A horse experiencing an acute episode of uveitis. The pupil is miotic and the iris is dull, slightly yellow in color, and has mottled pigmentation and hyperemia.

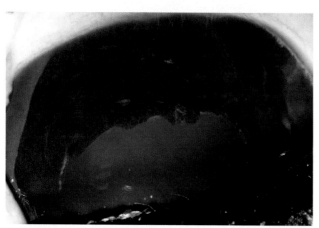

Fig. 7-8 Corpora nigra degeneration and/or thinning, depigmentation of the iris margin, and hyperpigmentation of the iris stroma are typical of chronic recurrent uveitis.

fibrosis (Fig. 7-7). Corpora nigra degeneration and/or thinning and depigmentation of the iris margin may be apparent after multiple episodes (Fig. 7-8).

A horse with *insidious uveitis* does not appear to be in pain, but close inspection of the eyes often shows inflammatory changes suggestive of chronic irritation: the conjunctiva may be inflamed, and mild to moderate blepharitis is often observed (Fig. 7-9). The cornea may be mildly edematous, dull, or hazy and may show scars or striae. Fluorescein dye uptake will usually be negative, but some Appaloosa horses with insidious uveitis may have an irregular epithelial surface that has faint staining properties. Focal limbal vascularization may be discernible. Subtle aqueous flare may be detectable in the anterior chamber. The iris is often a muddy grayish brown, and degeneration of the corpora nigra is common. The pupil may be slightly miotic and show a sluggish pupillary light reflex. Corpora nigra degeneration and thinning of the pupillary border (iris atrophy) are common.

Inflammatory sequelae and scarring from secondary problems are often apparent in the anterior segment of both classic and insidious uveitis cases. If the horse has had previous corneal disease (such as a corneal ulcer), old scars or discolorations may be present. Calcific band keratopathy is occasionally seen in the corneal subepithelium or outer stroma (Fig. 7-10). Posterior synechiae, pigment rests on the anterior lens capsule, and pupillary occlusion are common manifestations of previous damage in both classic and insidious cases. Focal or diffuse cataracts may be apparent (Fig. 7-11). Dense cataracts may obscure visualization of the posterior segment. Lens luxation or subluxation with an aphakic crescent is seen occasionally.

Most eyes with acute uveitis are hypotensive, and anterior chambers are shallow. Tonometry reveals ocular

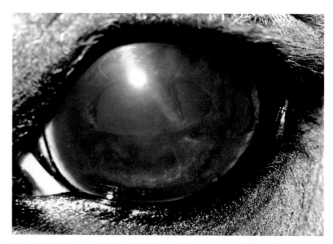

Fig. 7-9 A horse with insidious uveitis. A horse with this condition does not appear to be in pain, but close inspection of the eyes often shows inflammatory changes suggestive of chronic irritation (i.e., corneal edema, iris fibrosis, corpora nigra degeneration, and cataract formation).

pressures of 5 to 12 mm Hg. Some classic cases that have had numerous recurrences and insidious cases that are longstanding may develop secondary glaucoma (see Chapter 8). Horses with acute uveitis will demonstrate elevated pressures on digital and applanation tonometry and may have buphthalmos.

Posterior Segment

Observable signs in the posterior segment are variable. Changes in the posterior segment may be observed in both classic and insidious cases of uveitis. Cases belonging to the ERU subset of posterior uveitis will lack easily observable gross changes in the anterior segment, but slit-lamp biomicroscopic examination may reveal aqueous flare.

Some horses have no observable vitritis but show chorioretinal scarring of the peripapillary region or other evidence of retinal degeneration. The most common patterns of chorioretinal scarring are seen in the nontapetal area near the disc and present as either multiple small circular focal areas of depigmentation with a central area of hyperpigmentation ("bullet hole" scarring) or wing-shaped areas of hypopigmentation nasal and temporal to the optic disc ("butterfly" lesions) (Figs. 7-12 and 7-13).

Other horses demonstrate severe vitritis in which detail of the fundus is obscured and the optic disc appears orange-red because of the vitreal inflammation and haze. Liquefaction of the vitreous is common, as are visible strands of clumped infiltrating mononuclear cells and inflammatory products (floaters). These opacities appear to float and move easily in the vitreous in response to eye movements. Fibrinous traction bands may be apparent as white spike-like structures that radiate from the perimeter of the optic disc. Retinal detachments may be present and appear as a veil-like transparency that obscures fundic detail.

Bilateral Versus Unilateral Ocular Involvement

The initial episode of uveitis may be bilateral or unilateral. Recurrences may occur in one or both eyes. Sometimes one eye has initial inflammation, and the other eye becomes inflamed later. In other instances,

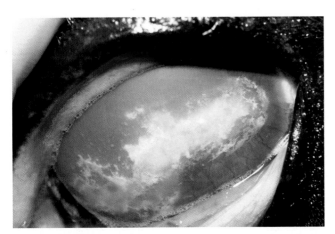

Fig. 7-10 Calcific band keratopathy in a horse with chronic recurrent uveitis (see Chapter 4, Corneal Diseases). (Photograph courtesy Dr. Stacy Andrew).

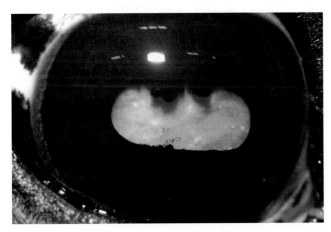

Fig. 7-11 Cataract formation in a horse with chronic recurrent uveitis. Notice the iris hyperpigmentation, corpora nigra degeneration, and pigment on the anterior lens capsule—all typical signs of multiple recurrent episodes of uveitis.

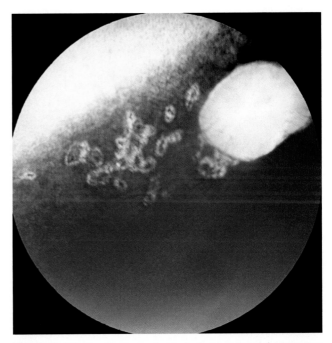

Fig. 7-12 Chorioretinal scarring is in the nontapetal area near the disc and appears as multiple small circular focal areas of depigmentation with a central area of hyperpigmentation ("bullet hole" scarring). These lesions are suggestive of previous uveitis.

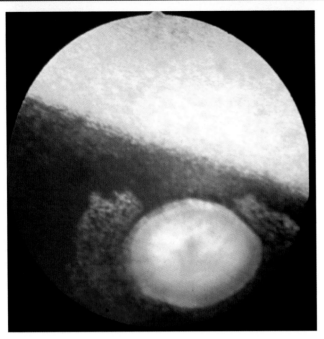

Fig. 7-13 Wing-shaped areas of hypopigmentation nasal and temporal to the optic disc ("butterfly" lesions) suggestive of previous uveitis.

inflammation remains in just one eye. A horse that has had unilateral ERU for 2 or more years, but has had no inflammation in the fellow eye during that time, has a greatly reduced chance of development of ERU in the second eye. The majority of cases of insidious uveitis are bilateral, but one eye may be more severely affected than the other.

One study demonstrated that about half of a series of 100 horses with leptospirosis-associated cases had unilateral disease and the other half had bilateral disease.[42] The same study revealed that of 42 Appaloosas with uveitis, 81% had bilateral involvement and 19% had unilateral disease. In a small series of 32 non-Appaloosa horses that were seronegative to *L. interrogans* serovar *pomona*, 38% had bilateral involvement and 62% had unilateral disease (Table 7-2).[42]

Quiescent Uveitis

Horses in the quiescent period between uveitis episodes will be comfortable. Careful ophthalmoscopic examination may reveal inflammatory sequelae from previous

| Table 7-2 | Outcome, Chronic Ocular Changes, and Concurrent Ocular Problems in Appaloosa and Non-Appaloosa Horses That Are Seropositive or Seronegative to *Leptospira Pomona* Over an 11-Year Observation Period |

	Appaloosa Horses				Non-Appaloosa Horses				Total	
Serology to *L. pomona*	Positive		Negative		Positive		Negative		Total	%
Total No. with Uveitis	14		28		86		32		**160**	**100**
Unilateral ERU	5	36%	3	11%	48	56%	20	62%	**76**	**48**
Bilateral ERU	9	64%	25	89%	38	44%	12	38%	**84**	**52**
Vision loss	14	100%	20	72%	44	51%	11	34%	**89**	**56**
(one or both eyes)										
Bilateral vision loss	7	50%	8	29%	15	17%	2	6%	**32**	**20**
Chronic ocular changes										
Corneal striae	2	14%	5	18%	4	5%	2	6%	**13**	**8**
Corneal scars	4	29%	10	36%	22	26%	6	7%	**42**	**26**
Corneal Ca$^+$ deposits	1	7%	1	4%	8	9%	0		**10**	**6**
Corneal streaks	6	43%	4	14%	5	19%	0		**15**	**9**
Corneal opacity, other	0		0		3		0		**3**	**8**
Corpora Nigra—excess	0		4	14%	5	19%	3	9%	**12**	**2**
Iris atrophy	7	50%	16	67%	16	19%	2	6%	**41**	**26**
Iris color change	5	36%	12	43%	13	22%	3	9%	**33**	**21**
Anterior synechiae	1	7%	0		3	3%	0		**4**	**3**
Posterior synechiae	6	43%	11	39%	23	27%	5	16%	**45**	**28**
Lens luxation	4	29%	8	29%	6	7%	4	13%	**22**	**14**
Diffuse cataract	10	71%	21	75%	26	30%	9	28%	**66**	**41**
Focal cataract	5	36%	4	14%	16	19%	3	9%	**23**	**14**
Vitritis	0		6	21%	23	27%	7	22%	**41**	**26**
Vitreal traction bands	0		2	7%	7	8%	2	6%	**11**	**7**
? Detached retina	0		2	7%	9	10%	0		**11**	**7**
Peripapillary alar depigmentation	1	7%	5	18%	5	19%	8	25%	**19**	**12**
Peripapillary focal depigmentation	3	21%	1	4%	11	13%	9	28%	**24**	**15**

episodes of ERU, including pigment rests on the anterior lens capsule, synechiae, iris atrophy, cataracts, and peripapillary scarring. Slit-lamp biomicroscopic examination may reveal flare in the aqueous or vitreous.

Chronic End-Stage Equine Recurrent Uveitis

Horses with *chronic end-stage* ERU show variable degrees of comfort and inflammatory sequelae. Recurrent episodes of inflammation generally subside but may be replaced by constant low-grade discomfort from blepharitis, mucopurulent lacrimation, conjunctivitis, and ocular irritation (Fig. 7-14). Other horses appear comfortable. Ocular structures often become severely scarred if phthisis bulbi has developed. In these eyes, corneal scarring may be dense and show folding and anterior synechiae (Fig. 7-15). Iris architecture may be lost or indistinct. Cataracts and lens luxations are common, and the lens may become yellow. Complete retinal detachment with collapse of the globe is common. The nictitans may prolapse as the globe becomes phthisical, and the mucosa may show chronic inflammation. A head-tilt or star-gazing head posture

| Table 7-2 | Outcome, Chronic Ocular Changes, and Concurrent Ocular Problems in Appaloosa and Non-Appaloosa Horses That Are Seropositive or Seronegative to *Leptospira Pomona* Over an 11-Year Observation Period—cont'd |

	Appaloosa Horses				Non-Appaloosa Horses				Total	
Serology to *L. pomona*	Positive		Negative		Positive		Negative		Total	%
Glaucoma	1	7%	8	29%	6	7%	3	9%	**18**	**11**
Phthisis bulbi	7	7%	3	11%	13	15%	1	3%	**24**	**15**
Concurrent problems										
Corneal ulcers	4	29%	12	42%	19	22%	8	25%	**43**	**27**
COPD (heaves)	1	7%	6	21%	0		1	3%	**8**	**5**
Laminitis	2	14%	3	11%	2	2%	0		**7**	**4**
Abortion	0		0		2	2%	0		**2**	**1**
Fever in past	0		0		7	8%	0		**7**	**4**
Night blindness	0		3	11%	0		0		**3**	**2**
Neoplasia	1	7%	1	4%	2	2%	3	9%	**7**	**4**
Cushing's disease	0		1	4%	0		0		**1**	**0**
Enucleations	0		3	11%	2	2%	1	3%	**6**	**4**
Injuries secondary to blindness	1	7%	3	11%	6	7%	4	13%	**14**	**9**
Died or euthanized because of blindness	2	14%	6	22%	7	8%	0		**15**	**9**

COPD, Chronic obstructive pulmonary disease; *ERU*, equine recurrent uveitis.

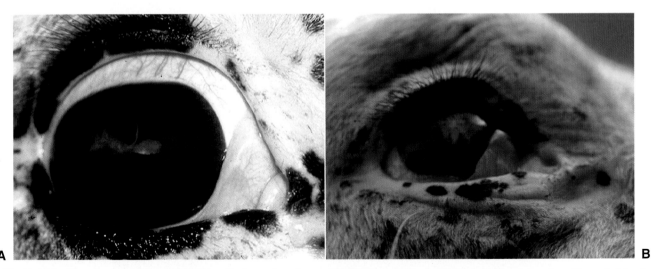

Fig. 7-14 A, Chronic end-stage recurrent uveitis in an Appaloosa. This horse had the insidious form of recurrent uveitis and did not demonstrate discomfort. **B,** Chronic end-stage recurrent uveitis in an eye, demonstrating phthisis bulbi, mild blepharitis, mucopurulent lacrimation, conjunctivitis, and ocular irritation.

is sometimes observed in blind horses with end-stage ERU (Fig. 7-16).

PATHOLOGIC AND IMMUNOPATHOLOGIC FEATURES OF EQUINE RECURRENT UVEITIS

Anterior Uvea

The manifestations of *early ERU* include congestion of the vessels of the anterior uvea and infiltration of the

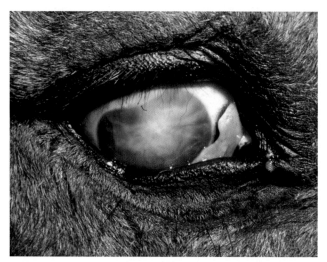

Fig. 7-15 Chronic end-stage recurrent uveitis in an eye with phthisis bulbi, dense corneal scarring and wrinkling, and extensive anterior synechiae.

uveal tract with inflammatory cells. The iris and ciliary body are infiltrated first by neutrophils. The neutrophils, which may escape into the anterior chamber to cause visible hypopyon, are soon replaced by large numbers of lymphocytes, as well as some plasma cells and macrophages. Exudates of fibrin, serum proteins, and other substances are a predominant feature. Gross or histopathologic examination of eyes acutely affected with ERU reveals notable exudates on the surface of the iris, ciliary body, and ciliary processes and over the lenticular capsule. Serous and cellular exudates are also noted in the iridic stroma, in trabecular meshwork, and in the aqueous and vitreous humors. Simultaneous congestion and infiltration occur in the conjunctiva. The retina is relatively unaffected in the first few attacks of inflammation.

With time and further recurrences, organization of the lymphocyte infiltrate is evident. The ciliary body and base of the iris regularly demonstrate prominent lymphocytic nodules (Fig. 7-17). Histologic analysis of both spontaneous and experimental leptospirosis-associated cases of ERU has shown that the lymphocytes in the center of the nodules are B lymphocytes, whereas those on the periphery of the nodules, as well as most of the diffuse infiltrating population, are T lymphocytes.[31,34] Many of the resident cells in the ciliary body show immunoreactive MHC II antigen expression, and a high percentage of the infiltrating lymphocytes are CD4+.[33,36] Also, the ocular media show high concentrations of interferon-γ and interleukin (IL)–2.[36] These observations suggest that the predominant

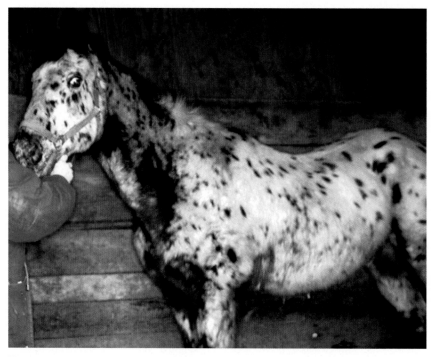

Fig. 7-16 A head-tilt or star-gazing head posture is sometimes observed in blind horses with end-stage equine recurrent uveitis.

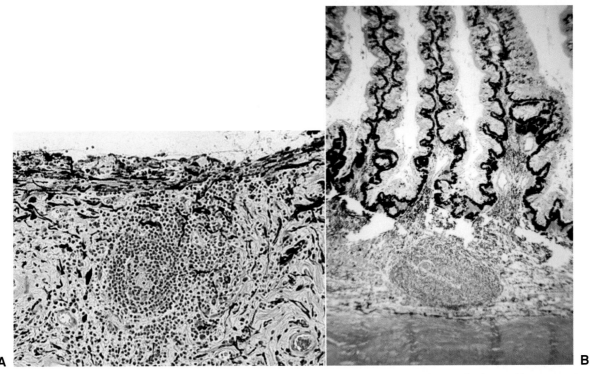

Fig. 7-17 A, Lymphocytic follicle or nodule formation at the base of the iris, a common feature in eyes with recurrent uveitis. (Hematoxylin and eosin stain; approximately ×400.) **B,** Lymphocytic follicle or nodule formation at the base of the ciliary body, a common feature in eyes with recurrent uveitis. (Hematoxylin and eosin stain; approximately ×400.) (Photograph courtesy Dr. Carolyn Kalsow.)

lymphocytic response in the eye is one of a T_H1 subset, of the T helper–type response. This kind of immune response is a proinflammatory one typical of many diseases of chronic inflammation. T_H1 memory lymphocytes secrete proinflammatory cytokines that activate macrophages and increase local cytotoxicity in response to resident or foreign antigens in T_H1 responses. Lymphocytic follicles may also be seen in the conjunctiva adjacent to the limbus.

As pathologic damage continues, the epithelium of the ciliary processes and uveal blood vessel walls thickens. Exudation occurs in the uvea, and exudates are easily seen occupying space over the ciliary processes and on the posterior epithelium of the iris. Studies on the histopathology of the ciliary body of both experimental leptospirosis-associated[32] and spontaneous ERU[32,43] have demonstrated the following three distinct features:

1. Presence of a thick noncellular hyaline membrane tightly adherent to the inner aspect of the nonpigmented ciliary epithelial (NPE) cells

2. Eosinophilic linear inclusions in the cytoplasm of the NPE cells

3. Accumulation of clusters of lymphocytes and plasma cells directly within the NPE layer of the posterior iris and ciliary body

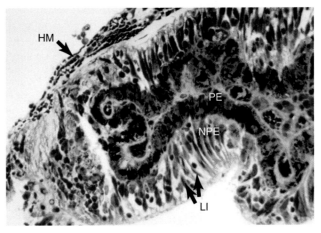

Fig. 7-18 Ciliary process from an eye with chronic equine recurrent uveitis. *PE,* Pigmented epithelium; *NPE,* nonpigmented epithelium; *LI,* linear cytoplasmic inclusions in the NPE; *HM,* hyaline membrane. (Hematoxylin and eosin stain; ×400.) (Photograph courtesy Dr. Penny Coolie.)

The finding of the hyaline membrane adjacent to the posterior aspect of the iris (Fig. 7-18) (characteristically staining orange-red with Congo red stain), coupled with the presence of the linear cytoplasmic inclusion bodies in the adjacent NPE cells (Fig. 7-19), is considered pathognomonic for ERU.[32,43]

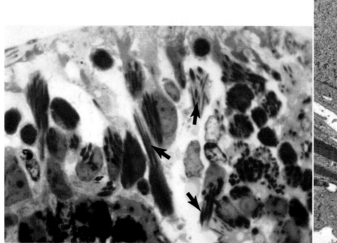

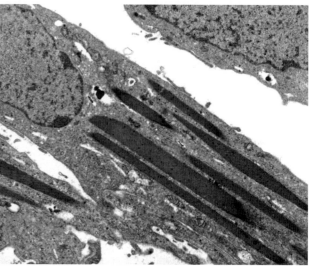

Fig. 7-19 A, Linear cytoplasmic inclusions *(arrows)* in the nonpigmented epithelium from an eye with chronic recurrent uveitis. (Hematoxylin and eosin stain; ×1000.) **B,** Transmission electron microscope image of the nonpigmented epithelium linear cytoplasmic inclusions (×5000.) (Photographs courtesy Dr. Penny Coolie.)

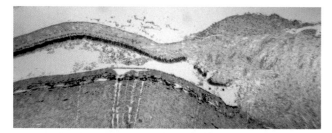

Fig. 7-20 Serofibrinous exudate is commonly seen between the retinal pigmented epithelium and the photoreceptors. This photograph shows optic nerve involvement and retinal detachment with exudates in a 9-year-old gelding Thoroughbred with a *Leptospira pomona* titer of 1:3200. The horse was blind and had had severe uveitis for 14 months with the last recurrence at 11 months. (Hematoxylin and eosin stain; ×31.25.) (Photograph courtesy Dr. Carolyn Kalsow.)

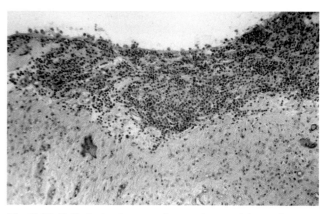

Fig. 7-21. Pathologic changes observed around the optic nerve head in horses with equine recurrent uveitis include surface infiltrate, occasional lymphocyte nodule formation, and retinal traction folds around the margin of the nerve. This photograph shows optic nerve infiltrate. This is the same horse as shown in Fig. 7-20. (Hematoxylin and eosin stain; ×31.25.) (Photograph courtesy Dr. Carolyn Kalsow.)

Posterior Segment

Although acute cases of ERU have manifestations that are most distinct in the anterior uvea, recurrence and chronicity of inflammation bring many changes to the retina and adjacent choroid. Scattered foci of T-lymphocyte infiltration are seen, particularly near the ora ciliaris retinae and optic nerve head. B lymphocytes have been demonstrated in the retinas of horses with known leptospirosis-associated ERU.[31] The RPE may undergo focal hypertrophy or degeneration. Serofibrinous exudate is commonly seen between the RPE and the photoreceptors and can be so extensive that it replaces the vitreous in a portion of the posterior chamber (Fig. 7-20). Loss of rods and cones caused by macrophage activity, destruction of the inner nuclear layer,[33] and detachment of the retina may follow, with the RPE remaining attached to Bruch's membrane of the choroid and the rest of the retina collapsing into the posterior chamber. Retinal changes that have been studied in spontaneous cases are similar to those observed in ponies with experimental leptospirosis-associated ERU, and severity of the experimental disease generally parallels the severity of the clinical disease in the individual.[31]

Pathologic changes observed around the optic nerve head of horses with ERU include surface infiltrate (Fig. 7-21), occasional lymphocyte nodule formation, and retinal traction folds around the margin of the nerve. Infiltrating cells in the perivascular and parenchymal space of the nerve are immunoreactive. The optic

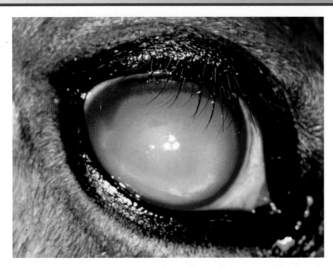

Fig. 7-22. Circumlimbal vascularization of an eye with chronic recurrent uveitis. These peripheral vessels are common with chronic equine recurrent uveitis and may only be present on the inferior limbus, or they may extend all around the periphery in a radial pattern. Corneal edema and a corneal ulcer are also present. (Photograph courtesy Dr. Stacy Andrew.)

nerve itself can show swelling, or it may be cupped or atrophied if secondary glaucoma is present.[31]

Accessory Structures

The lens often shows thick exudates adherent to the capsule, particularly on the posterior aspect, in early ERU. The lens capsule proliferates, and over time, capsular cataracts develop. Luxation of the lens is common as deterioration of the zonules occurs. Wrinkling of the lens capsule (caused by a hypermature, resorbing cataract) or osseous metaplasia occasionally occurs.

Many cases of ERU will show vascularization of the cornea that begins at the limbus. Histologic examination of the cornea in these cases shows that the new vessels start out as tiny capillary offshoots from the scleral vessels that grow into the lamina propria of the cornea below the epithelium (see the discussion of the cornea in Chapter 4). They may only be present on the inferior limbus, or they may extend all around the periphery in a radial pattern (Fig. 7-22). Cellular infiltrate is rarely present in the stroma of the cornea in horses with ERU. If the cellular infiltrate is prominent, then the uveitis may be caused by primary corneal disease, such as stromal abscessation or immune-mediated keratitis.

Several studies have shown that ERU is accompanied by inflammation in the pineal gland of the brain. The inflammation is variable and may be transient. It involves immunoreactive cells and is similar to inflammation seen in experimentally induced recurrent uveitis in laboratory animals.[30,44]

Acute classic ERU episodes are followed by periods of quiescence when the eye is outwardly comfortable and gross disease evidence is restricted to observable sequelae (synechiae, cataract, peripapillary scarring) from previous episodes and occasionally subtle aqueous flare. Histopathologic and immunohistopathologic examination of specimens obtained from quiescent eyes reveals that inflammation does persist in these eyes at the cellular level. Lymphocyte nodules are frequently present in the ciliary body, and infiltrating lymphocytes are identifiable in the uveal stroma and in many accessory eye structures. Immunoreactivity is demonstrable during periods of quiescence as well.

Many old eyes with chronic ERU develop phthisis bulbi (Fig. 7-14). Others maintain normal globe size but show extensive posterior synechiae, loss of normal iris shape and motility, and dense cataract. Histologic examination of a specimen from an eye with end-stage ERU with blinding consequences reveals a shrunken globe with thickened sclera, cataracts with posterior and anterior synechiae, and a torn distorted iris (Fig. 7-23). The lens may be luxated and may be surrounded by thick exudates. Iris vessels are thick walled, and the ciliary body is filled with organized exudates. The retina is detached, and exudates may fill the posterior chamber. Other eyes retain a functional ocular structure with fewer inflammatory sequelae.

DIFFERENTIAL DIAGNOSES AND DIAGNOSTIC METHODS

The clinical diagnosis of ERU is based on the presence of characteristic clinical signs and history of documented recurrent or persistent episodes of uveitis. Both features are required for this clinical diagnosis to be made, especially in differentiating ERU from nonrecurrent equine uveitis and other causes of recurrent or persistent ocular inflammation, such as herpesvirus or immune-mediated keratitis (Tables 7-3 and 7-4). These and many other primary conditions of the eye present with signs typical of uveitis, particularly pain, blepharospasm, photophobia, miosis, and altered corneal transparency. Any clinician presented with a horse with an acute, painful "red" eye must ask the following question:

Is the inflammation coming from inside of the eye, or does the primary problem involve a different part of the eye that is inducing a secondary uveitis?

The question must be answered because standard therapy for uveitis (topical corticosteroids) is contraindicated for most primary corneal problems, and failure to properly treat ulcers or other problems (corneal ulcer or foreign body, stromal abscess, unusual keratitis,

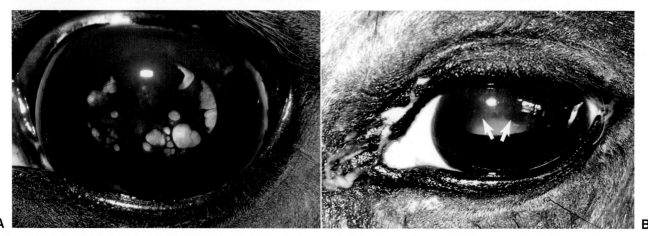

A   **B**

Fig. 7-23 A, Many eyes with chronic ERU develop phthisis bulbi; other eyes maintain normal globe size, as seen in this photograph, but show extensive posterior synechiae, loss of normal iris shape and motility, and dense cataract. **B,** Other eyes with chronic ERU may demonstrate lens luxation (*arrows* = edge of lens) and cataracts.

Table 7-3	Causes of Uveitis in Horses
Classification	**Causes**
Trauma	Blunt or penetrating injury
Bacterial organisms	*Leptospira*
	Brucella
	Streptococcus
	Rhodococcus equi
	Borrelia bergdorferi (Lyme disease)
Viral organisms	Equine influenza
	Equine viral arteritis
	Parainfluenza type 3
	Equine herpes virus type 1 and 2
Parasites	*Onchocerca*
	Strongylus
	Toxoplasma
Miscellaneous	Endotoxemia
	Septicemia
	Tooth root abscesses
	Neoplasia

glaucoma, or corneal or intraocular neoplasia) may have disastrous consequences. These diseases are referred to as masquerading syndromes of ERU (Table 7-4).

A thorough ocular examination with careful inspection of the eyelids and cornea is needed to rule out primary corneal disease (see discussion of ocular examination in Chapter 1 and discussion of corneal diseases in Chapter 4). In horses with extreme swelling or pain, lid blocks and heavy sedation may be required for complete visual inspection of the entire cornea. If swelling still obstructs a portion of the cornea, a repeat examination may need to be scheduled for the next day, after nonsteroidal antiinflammatory drug (NSAID) therapy has reduced pain and swelling. Evaluation for other

differential diagnoses requires a careful inspection of all accessory anatomic structures of the eye; the clinician should look for masses, pigment changes, scars, opacities, accumulation of fluid in the ocular media, and changes of the fundus, particularly the peripapillary region. The clinician should examine both eyes of the animal with all ophthalmologic equipment available: most field clinicians will use a direct ophthalmoscope and a penlight; and specialists will add examination with an indirect ophthalmoscope, magnifying equipment, and biomicroscope. Tonometry is a valuable stall-side test for ruling out glaucoma or documenting the hypotony that often accompanies ERU. Digital or standard film photographs of both eyes provide valuable baselines for assessment of future changes.

The other scenario in which prudent diagnostic skills are needed is the quiet, comfortable eye that shows one or more signs of ERU. A clinician who discovers ocular abnormalities consistent with previous uveitis (e.g., synechiae, pigment rests on the anterior lens capsule, diffuse cataract, peripapillary scarring) must take a careful history. If the owner reports that a horse has had brief or protracted episodes of ocular pain or swelling in the past, the scenario is strongly suggestive of ERU. However, owners often report that a horse has had no observable eye inflammation, or they may not know the history of the animal. Such a case is more problematic and could represent a horse with insidious disease (especially if the horse is an Appaloosa, draft horse, or European Warmblood) or a horse that has classic ERU but has not had an episode that was witnessed by the owner. Such a case could also represent a horse that has had a single episode of uveitis that has not recurred. In cases in which the history is unknown but recurrent uveitis is suspected, at least *three signs of disease* (corneal edema, vascularization, pigment rests, synechiae, iris

Table 7-4 Equine Recurrent Uveitis: Masquerade Syndromes

Syndrome	Comment	Diagnosis Aid
Nonrecurrent uveitis	Anterior or posterior uveitis	History of no recurrence of uveitis
Corneal ulcer	Self-trauma, corticosteroids contraindicated	Fluorescein dye positive, focal opacity or defect
Stromal abscess	Past trauma, corticosteroids contraindicated	Fluorescein dye negative, focal yellow-white opacity
Immune-mediated keratitis	Appearance may change often, severity varies, recurrent inflammation possible	Fluorescein dye negative, multiple opacities, variable pattern
Herpes keratitis	Variable pain, may retain rose bengal	Fluorescein dye variable, multiple punctate or linear opacities
Corneal foreign body	May be vascularized focally, may be visible	Fluorescein dye variable
Corneal neoplasia	Squamous cell carcinoma, melanoma	Mass or cellular infiltrate visible on corneal surface or through epithelium
Intraocular neoplasia	Melanoma, medulloepithelioma, anterior or posterior segments	Ocular ultrasonography, or may be visualized in anterior chamber
Glaucoma	Often caused by ERU, persistent corneal edema	Tonometry

ERU, Equine recurrent uveitis.

atrophy or color change, cataract, lens luxation or subluxation, vitreal densities, retinal detachment or traction bands, peripapillary scarring in a focal or alar pattern) should be observed before a presumptive diagnosis of previous ERU is made.[2] *Leptospiral serology* is useful for determining previous exposure to this well-known risk factor. Equine leukocyte antigen (ELA) typing may also help determine whether the animal is susceptible to ERU.[39]

Candid counseling is indicated whenever signs of uveitis are detected during a routine ophthalmic examination. The owner should be educated about the disease syndrome, and a frank discussion of visual prognosis should occur. It is best to stress the possible scenarios early and to prepare owners for the expense, treatment effort, and progression associated with overt future attacks. Frequent veterinary follow-up examinations should be recommended. In cases in which the veterinarian suspects either insidious uveitis or classic disease that has been unobserved by the current owner, biannual examination, coupled with immediate evaluation if the horse has pain in one or both eyes, should help sort out the diagnosis. Referral to a board-certified veterinary ophthalmologist may be helpful in evaluation of cases of uncertain etiology.

Other tests that may be used in assessing the horse that is presented with acute uveitis or signs compatible with previous disease include complete blood count and blood chemistry. In addition to a leptospiral microagglutination test (MAT), blood tests for exposure to Lyme disease (serum titer and Western blot analysis) and equine viral arteritis may be done. Fecal parasite analysis is indicated, as well as a full physical examination of other body systems to check for concurrent problems (Tables 7-3 and 7-4).

PATHOGENESIS OF DISEASE PROCESS AND PROGRESSION

ERU is a nonspecific immune-mediated condition that results in recurrent or persistent inflammatory episodes in the eye. Many infectious and noninfectious agents can cause acute uveitis in the horse. Although any of these causes of uveitis may allow ERU to develop in horses, not all of these acute uveitis cases will develop into ERU. To diagnose the syndrome of ERU, the clinician must differentiate it from nonrecurrent equine uveitis. The recurrent episodes typical of ERU are thought to develop because of one of the following three pathogeneses:

1. Incorporation of an infectious agent or antigen into the vitreous or uveal tract after the initial uveitis episode. Such an inciting antigen becomes established in the ocular tissues, and its continued presence causes periodic episodes of inflammation. Recent studies have suggested that *Leptospira* organisms may be sequestered antigens.[26-28] However, in these studies, only 26% to 70% of the eyes had *Leptospira* organisms detected, suggesting that other antigens or organisms also play a role.

2. Deposition of antibody/antigen complexes into the uveal tract that incites later inflammation.

3. Persistence of an immune-competent sensitized T lymphocyte in the uveal tract that reactivates when given a signal. T lymphocytes have been demonstrated to be the predominant infiltrating cell type in eyes with chronic ERU,[33,34,36] and cell-mediated immunity to uveal antigens has been demonstrated in horses with ERU.[37,45-47] In these

eyes, possibly, a systemic re-exposure to the original antigen, exposure to a self-protein that is similar to the original antigen (i.e., "molecular mimicry"), or a decreased immunologic feedback downregulation of the T lymphocyte may be the inciting signal for reactivation of the T lymphocyte and inflammation.

Immunologic Aspects of Equine Recurrent Uveitis

Carolyn Kalsow

The immune system has been documented to participate in the pathogenesis of ERU. Initial indications of a genetic predisposition to ERU through recognition of breed-associated increased risk have recently been solidified by studies of immune response gene (MHC) association with ERU.[6,48] Just as human leukocyte antigen (HLA) haplotype and uveitis are strongly associated in some autoimmune uveitides in humans,[49] so recent equine studies have shown an increased risk of uveitis in horses with the ELA-9 haplotype.[39] Hence, the association is not simply genetic, but genetic through genes associated with the immune system, and could even involve cross-reactivity between self-antigens and HLA peptides.[50] The control of uveitis by antiinflammatory treatments,[2] including immunosuppressive action of cyclosporine implants,[51] further supports some form of immunologic pathogenesis of ERU.

The immune system is activated during ERU. Both T and B lymphocytes, sometimes organized into follicles,[33,52] have been demonstrated in the eyes and pineal glands of horses with ERU.[31,34,35] The preponderance of T lymphocytes that are mainly CD4+ and the presence of cytokines IL-2 and interferon-γ indicate that ERU is a T_H1-like lymphocyte-mediated disease,[36] which suggests that the recurrent inflammation is an immune-mediated delayed-type hypersensitivity reaction.

In immune-mediated disease, an inciting antigen is required to induce the pathologic immune response. In ERU, the inciting antigen has yet to be identified. It may be an autoantigen to the horse's own ocular tissues, or it could be a microbial antigen from an ocular or a systemic infection. The intraocular fluids of horses with ERU contain autoantibodies against retinal autoantigens (S-antigen or interphotoreceptor binding protein [IRBP])[45,53] and T lymphocytes that respond to S-antigen.[45] This degree of increased intraocular reactivity is not seen systemically in serum autoantibody levels[45,46,54] or in activation of T lymphocytes recovered from peripheral blood lymphocytes[45] of horses with ERU as compared with control horses without ERU. Although intraocular antibodies and T lymphocytes reactive to ocular autoantigens indicate that there is an

autoimmune response, they do not reveal whether that autoimmunity is involved in the pathogenesis or is a result of the ERU.

Although there are multiple infectious causes of ERU, uveitis as a sequela to leptospiral infection is well documented.[55] Many studies throughout the world have correlated ERU to the presence of serum antibodies to *L. interrogans* serovars, especially *pomona*.[2,28] High titers of antileptospiral antibody in ocular fluids[2] are suggestive of intraocular infection, as well as intraocular antibody production to antigens in the eye. A potential concern with present antibody studies lies with the use of laboratory-cultured leptospires as antigens in accepted serologic tests such as the MAT. New genetic techniques allow the detection of antibodies to antigens that are *only* expressed when the bacteria are growing in the horse.[56] Hence, testing sera for reactivity to laboratory-cultured strains of leptospires may not reveal antibodies to these molecules. Identification of the exact relevant antigen is critical to defining immunopathogenesis of the disease syndrome.

Leptospiral bacteria have been avidly sought in ocular tissues. Evidence of their presence has been intriguing yet sparse. Direct detection of leptospiral bacteria in the eye has, on occasion, been accomplished by culture of ocular fluids,[26,57] and more recently, by polymerase chain reaction (PCR), which is used to identify small fragments of DNA unique to *Leptospira* spp.[27,58] Relative roles of bacterial pathogenesis and immunopathogenesis in this intraocular inflammation are not clear.[59] Equine post leptospirosis uveitis could result from direct bacterial toxicity to ocular structures, or it could result from inflammation originating in a local immune response to bacteria in the eye. Leptospiral infection could induce the autoimmune reactions discussed previously, if leptospiral antigens were cross-reactive with ocular autoantigens. Such a relationship has been demonstrated between *Leptospira* organisms and equine cornea.[60,61] Alternatively, autoimmunity could be induced by the release of retinal autoantigens as a result of bacterial toxicity.

In summary, there is evidence that the pathogenesis of ERU involves a genetic predisposition for a T_H1-type lymphocyte immune response involving autoantigens, microbial infection, or both. Clarification of precise mechanisms of immune involvement, as well as specific inciting antigens, is a current area of research interest.

EXPERIMENTAL INDUCTION OF RECURRENT UVEITIS

Laboratory animal models of an experimental autoimmune uveitis were developed to study the autoimmune etiology of uveitis and have consequently formed the foundation for hypotheses concerning naturally occurring uveitides.[62] Rats or mice systemically sensitized with retinal autoantigens in adjuvant consistently have a uveitis and accompanying pinealitis in which the specific immune components of antibodies, activated cells, and cytokines have been identified so as to delineate immunopathogenic mechanisms.[63] Extensive study has, in most cases, detailed a T_H1-type cytokine response that is operative in the experimental model, and by inference, applicable to naturally occurring uveitis.[64] This in turn has led to identification of new, more specific strategies for treatment, which can be evaluated in the animal model before they are used in clinical practice. Experimental autoimmune uveitis studies were a factor in successful development of treatment strategies for humans, such as induction of tolerance to retinal autoantigens by oral presentation (feeding) of autoantigens and use of monoclonal antibodies against the IL-12 receptor (Daclizumab), a critical cytokine receptor involved in the immunopathogenic cascade.[65]

Adaptation of the experimental autoimmune uveitis model to ERU has been met with limited success. Ponies or horses injected with S-antigen did not show signs of uveitis, even though they showed an immune response to the autoantigen.[46] However, horses sensitized with IRBP did have signs of uveitis.[37] This dichotomy is similar to that seen in mice in which IRBP is uveitogenic but S-antigen is not,[63] although rats are responsive to both IRBP and S-antigen.

In a direct experimental investigation of leptospiral pathogenesis of ERU, all nine Shetland ponies systemically infected with the *L. interrogans* serovar *pomona* subsequently had signs of recurrent uveitis.[66] These results closely parallel those of the initial field studies that linked leptospiral infection to ERU.[12] This experimental model has the potential to be extended to evaluate the molecular relationship of infection to immune response.

Equine Recurrent Uveitis and Leptospirosis

Ann Dwyer
Although many different endogenous and exogenous inciting factors have been associated with uveitis in horses, leptospiral infection has been linked to a very large number of spontaneous cases of ERU around the world and has been studied extensively.

Features of Leptospirosis

Leptospirosis is a bacterial disease affecting domestic animals, wildlife, and humans. It has been reported to be the most common zoonosis worldwide.[67] Leptospirae are the smallest spirochete bacteria, measuring less than 0.3 μm in width and 6 to 30 μm in length. They have a tightly wound spiral shape with a distinctive hook on one or both ends (Fig. 7-24). Other genera of related pathogenic spirochetes include *Treponema* (agents of syphilis and swine dysentery) and *Borrelia* (agents of relapsing fever and Lyme disease). The organisms are motile and able to enter hosts by penetrating mucous membranes or abraded skin mechanically. Leptospirae do not stain with conventional pathology stains and require special silver impregnation stains for identification. Clinical tests available to diagnose leptospiral infections include direct culture of infected organs or body fluids, microscopic agglutination testing of sera or ocular fluids, PCR analysis of ocular fluids, and fluorescent antibody testing of urine samples.

Leptospirae are aquatic unicellular organisms found in river and lake waters and in sewage. *L. interrogans* is host adapted, and infective strains are maintained in a variety of mammalian species. The principle reservoirs for the serovars associated with ERU are deer, cattle, swine, and rats. The organisms multiply in the kidneys of adapted hosts and are shed in the urine. Pathogenic leptospires can only survive for short periods in soil outside a host but are able to live for up to 6 weeks in groundwater if environmental conditions include slightly alkaline conditions (pH 6.2 to 8.0), low salinity, and moderate temperatures above 22° C.

Leptospirosis in Horses

Exposure to the organism occurs when horses drink contaminated groundwater that contains urine shed from a host-adapted species. Horses pastured next to unvaccinated cattle or pigs and horses that live on farms frequented by deer or infested with rats are at increased risk for exposure. Ponds on the property, the

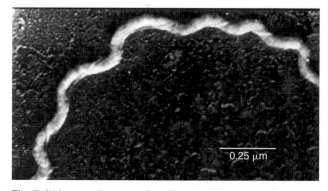

Fig. 7-24 Leptospirae organism. These organisms are the smallest spirochete bacteria, measuring less than 0.3 μm in width and 6 to 30 μm in length. They have a tightly wound spiral shape with a distinctive hook on one or both ends.

use of pond water as piped drinking water, and proximity to a river are other frequently observed risk factors (Fig. 7-25).[68] Clinical infections are thought to be most prevalent during rainy periods in the spring and fall. The inciting organisms enter the body through mechanical penetration of mucous membranes or abraded skin and rapidly gain access to the vascular space. Bacteremia persists for about 8 days. Invasion of many internal organs occurs, and infection induces a strong host antibody response that is first detectable in the serum 4 to 8 days after exposure.[69] Organisms are eliminated rapidly from the blood and most organs by host mechanisms. However, localization of organisms in the genital tract and renal tubules[68,70] may occur, and the infected horse may shed pathogenic leptospires in the urine for up to 3 months.[69] Organisms may also localize in the anterior and posterior chambers of the eyes.[17,25,27]

Acute signs of leptospirosis in the horse include transient depression, fever, icterus, anemia and anorexia. Sporadic reports of severe disease in neonates or adult horses exist,[71,72] and the disease has been associated with many equine abortions in Kentucky,[73,74] but most infections are outwardly self-limiting. Clinical diagnostic tests that would confirm acute infection in the horse are rarely performed because observable initial illness is generally mild and brief. Serologic surveys in horses have shown that exposure to leptospires is common but variable according to geographic region and climate. Seropositivity rates tend to be highest in tropical climates[70] and in river valleys in temperate climates, especially in the Ohio, Delaware,[13,75,76] Genesee, and Mississippi[24] river valleys in North America. These regions have high rates of ERU in resident horse populations. Other regions with arid, dry climates have lower rates of ERU.

Classification and Clinical Testing for Leptospirosis

Biologically, leptospirae are classed into two large species: L. bireflexa, the nonpathogenic, free-living, and saprophytic complex and L. interrogans, the parasitic species complex that causes disease. L. interrogans is further classified into more than 20 serovars. Diagnostic laboratories distinguish exposure to these serovars by performing serial MATs on equine sera or ocular fluids, looking for antibodies to leptospiral surface antigens. The L. interrogans serovars most often incriminated in equine disease are pomona and grippotyphosa.*

The serovar most often associated with ERU in North America and South America is pomona.[6,16,17,24,27]

---

*References 6, 11, 15-17, 19, 24, 26-28, 72-74.

The serovar grippotyphosa predominates in horses in central Europe, but disease associated with the serovar pomona is seen in Europe as well.[26,28,68] Sporadic reports have also associated serovars autumnalis[2] and icterohemmorrhagiae[24] with ERU.

Most public diagnostic laboratories perform MATs for five to seven serovars (pomona, icterohaemorrhagiae, grippotyphosa, canicola, hardjo, and sometimes bratislava and autumnalis). Interpreting serology for leptospiral reactivity can be confusing, because many horses that live in temperate or tropical climates demonstrate low titers to one or more serovars. Furthermore, exposure analysis is often not performed in horses until years after episodes of ERU have begun, when titer levels in these animals are usually low. However, the diagnostic picture is clearer in acute infection.

Acute infections are characterized by high-titer seroreactivity to at least one serovar by the eighth day.[69] Cross-reactivity to one or more other serovars is common because of surface antigen overlap and is usually detectable at the same time, but at reduced titer levels. Over time, the titer to the predominant serovar falls to lower dilution levels, but positive seroreactivity to the original panel of serovars persists for many years and probably for life. Usually, the predominant serovar titer will be elevated above the cross-reacting serovars for the first several years after infection and will be identifiable if serologic testing is performed during an early episode of ERU (Dwyer AE. Unpublished data, 2004). Reactivity to serovar pomona is often associated with seroreactivity to serovar icterohaemorrhagiae (Dwyer AE. Unpublished data, 2004).[24,77] The horse has been shown to be an adapted host that can maintain the bratislava serovar,[68] but this serovar has not been associated with ERU.

One study has shown that in 56% of ERU cases occurring in a New York river valley, horses were seropositive for pomona, whereas only 9% of healthy horses were seropositive for pomona.[6] Other studies have demonstrated leptospiral seroreactivity[11,24] or presence in ocular media[11,24,26-28] in a majority of the affected populations. These data imply that any positive pomona titer in a horse (i.e., ≥1:400) should be considered a risk factor for ERU. Analysis of the ocular fluids of affected horses has shown that, occasionally, leptospiral organisms or leptospiral DNA can be isolated from horses with ERU that are seronegative for leptospiral reactivity.[27,28] This means that although positive seroreactivity to pathogenic groups of leptospires, particularly pomona and grippotyphosa, is often linked to the cause of ERU, negative seroreactivity does not rule out leptospirosis as a contributing factor to the disease. University and research diagnostic laboratories are capable of further classifying the leptospiral serovars into more than 170 different serovars.

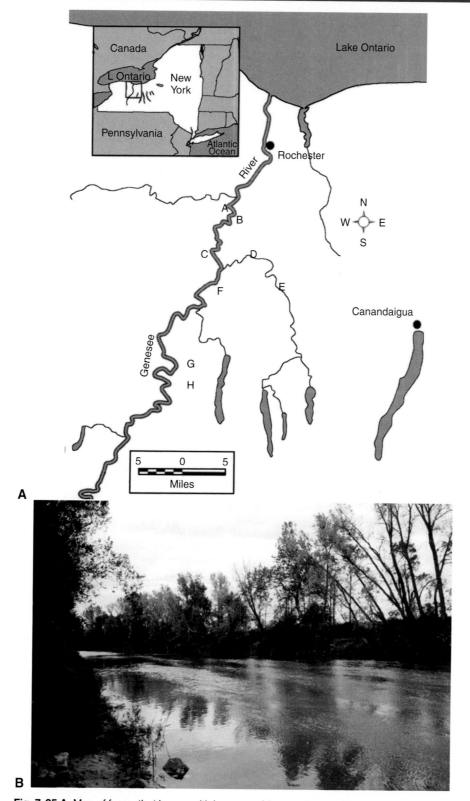

Fig. 7-25 A, Map of farms that have multiple cases of *Leptospira pomona*–associated equine recurrent uveitis, showing proximity to the Genesee River of New York State. **B,** Genesee River. See Table 7-5, p. 306.

Table 7-5   Horses With Equine Recurrent Uveitis Near the Genesee River of New York State

Farm ID	Distance to River (miles)	No. of horses	Seropositive	Horses With Uveitis	Farm Conditions or History
A	0.5 W	33	9 (27%)	4 (44%)	Many blind horses in past years before survey
B	1.0 E	8	3 (38%)	2 (66%)	Pastures very muddy with standing water in rainy season
C	0.8 W	8	3 (38%)	3 (100%)	Additional blind horse died before survey
D	0.5 N	6	4 (66%)	3 (75%)	Several cows mixed with horses on the property
E	0.8 E	5	2 (40%)	2 (100%)	Pastures very muddy seasonally
F	1.3 E	5	2 (40%)	2 (100%)	Dairy farm with many cows in adjacent pasture
G	1.5 E	37	10 (27%)	5 (50%)	Pond water used for drinking
H	2.0 E	5	3 (60%)	3 (100%)	Cows and pigs on property
Total	**Mean 1.05 miles**	**107**	**36 (34%)**	**24 (67%)**	

The Role of Leptospirosis in Equine Recurrent Uveitis

The initial association of leptospirosis with ERU, reported in Germany in the 1940s by Rimpau[10] and Heussler,[11] was followed by case reports of an outbreak of acute leptospirosis on two horse farms in Ithaca, New York.[12,14-16,78] Analysis of events on one of the Ithaca farms showed that in the spring of 1952, 6 of 15 resident horses had acute systemic disease confirmed as infection with *L. interrogans* serovar *pomona*.[12] All horses recovered, but one of the six horses had intraocular inflammation during acute disease, which later become recurrent.[15] In most of the remaining horses, ERU developed 18 to 24 months after the initial infection. This pattern is typical of leptospirosis-associated ERU. Ocular signs at the time of acute infection are generally absent or mild, but overt ocular inflammation develops months to years later. Recurrence of uveitis is typical, with subsequent episodes of inflammation often increasing in severity and threatening vision.

Experimental work to try to reproduce this unusual pattern ensued in the 1960s at Purdue University. Morter et al.[69] succeeded in inducing leptospirosis-associated uveitis by injecting guinea pig blood containing live *L. interrogans* serovar *pomona* organisms subcutaneously into a group of ponies. All the ponies had systemic-leptospiral infections that resolved but were followed by the development of ocular inflammation in the ensuing 15 months after exposure.[66,69,79] The ponies had recurrent uveitis that varied in intensity but resulted in blinding sequelae in many cases. Subsequent analysis of the ocular tissues of this same set of ponies in recent studies has shown that the pathology and immunohistopathology of the experimental disease were quite similar to those of spontaneous cases of leptospirosis-associated ERU.[32,59]

Pathogenesis of Leptospirosis-Associated Equine Recurrent Uveitis

Although a large body of research has been stimulated by the early reports of clinical and experimental leptospirosis-related ERU, the precise pathogenesis of recurrent inflammation is still poorly understood. Much progress has been made recently. In 1985, clinicians at the University of Florida used an enzyme-linked immunosorbent assay to detect antibodies specific to *L. interrogans* serovar *pomona* in the sera and aqueous and vitreous humors of horses with ERU. Their data suggested that antibodies in the ocular media may be synthesized in the eye rather than just leaking across the blood-ocular barrier.[80-82] Recent analysis of aqueous and vitreous humor samples have continued to support the concept of intraocular antibody synthesis.[22,26,45,83]

In 1985, Argentinean researchers demonstrated an antigenic relationship between *Leptospira* and the equine cornea, suggesting that molecular mimicry occurs between the bacteria and host tissues.[84] Subsequent work has demonstrated that tears and aqueous humor from horses inoculated with *Leptospira* spp. contain antibodies that bind to the cornea[85] and that the antigenic relationship between the bacteria and ocular tissues includes the lens as well and involves a peptide fragment.[86] Recent work has shown that a leptospiral DNA fragment encodes cross-reacting epitopes toward equine cornea. This fragment was found in several pathogenic *L. interrogans* subgroups but not in the nonpathogenic *L. bireflexa*.[61] Subcutaneous injection of fractions of equine cornea in adjuvant has been shown to induce corneal opacities in horses.[84]

Isolation of *L. interrogans* serovar *pomona* from the aqueous humor of horses affected with ERU was reported in 1977.[17] Since then, researchers in California[27] and Germany[28] have succeeded in culturing leptospires from the eyes of several horses with ERU and have found leptospiral DNA in many cases that were culture negative.[26,27] These studies demonstrate that leptospiral organisms frequently persist in the eyes of horses with ERU. However, the precise role that the organisms play in mediating recurrences remains to be clarified.

In 1993, a case report was published showing that a horse with a medical history consistent with previous infection with *L. interrogans* serovar *pomona* and ERU had pinealitis that was coincident with severe, blinding uveitis.[30] In subsequent studies investigators have described the immunohistopathology of this and similar cases and have demonstrated MHC type II reactivity on resident cells and infiltration of T and B lymphocytes in both the eyes and pineal glands of horses with spontaneous leptospirosis-associated ERU. Similar MHC II reactivity has been demonstrated by the same laboratory in slides of the eyes of the ponies from Purdue University with experimentally induced leptospirosis-associated ERU. Horses with leptospirosis-associated ERU were also found to have seroreactivity to retinal proteins,[31] suggesting that the retinal disease may be a primary event in leptospirosis-associated uveitis.

The exact interaction that occurs between bacterial infection and the host immune system in ERU is a subject of debate. Culture of organisms from horses with chronic ERU and organization of infiltrating lymphocytes indicate a direct interaction of the bacteria with the immune system. Evidence of antibodies against *Leptospira* spp. in the eye, coupled with demonstration of molecular mimicry between leptospiral DNA fragments and equine cornea and lens, supports an autoimmune component, as does the existence of antiretinal seroreactivity in horses with leptospirosis-related ERU. The presence of MHC class II expression and immunoglobulin deposition on resident and infiltrating cells in the eyes and pineal glands of these horses suggests that leptospiral infection may modulate the immune response of the eye. Because the disease has an immune pathogenesis, it is likely that the genetic makeup of the individual, specifically the MHC, also plays a role in determining both susceptibility to leptospirosis as an inciting trigger and severity of subsequent inflammatory episodes. Further studies, coupled with advances in ocular immunology and molecular biology and greater understanding of the equine immune system, should refine our knowledge

of how leptospiral infections cause such a devastating disease in the horse and may lead to novel therapies for this common cause of equine vision loss.

Equine Recurrent Uveitis in Appaloosa Horses

Ann Dwyer

Early equine uveitis literature indicated that there was no breed predilection for ERU. However, in 1988, clinicians at Cornell analyzed admission records of 16,242 horses with ERU and found that the Appaloosa breed had a significantly higher risk for development of uveitis compared with Thoroughbreds and that Standardbreds had a reduced risk for the syndrome.[48] This study supported the observations of many equine practitioners who had diagnosed insidious uveitis in a large number of their Appaloosa patients, many of which became blind or had other secondary complications. A field study of a large number of cases in New York confirmed the breed predilection and indicated that the odds of finding uveitis were 8.3 times greater in Appaloosas than in all other breeds combined.[6]

Uveitis in the Appaloosa breed is often clinically distinct from classic ERU reported in other breeds. Many affected horses show an insidious course of disease without overt recurrent episodes of pain, so lumping these cases together with horses that exhibit classic recurrences may be misleading. In fact, uveitis in the Appaloosa horse may have a different cause and pathogenesis than classic ERU. Age at onset is variable and often difficult to determine because the owner of an affected horse may be unaware of a problem until a veterinary examination is done or the horse shows overt vision loss.

Secondary complications and severe degeneration of ocular tissues are common sequelae of uveitis in Appaloosas. Analysis of case records of 160 horses with uveitis in New York showed that 25%, or 42, of these cases occurred in Appaloosas and that this subset of 42 horses had many characteristic chronic ocular changes and concurrent medical problems (Table 7-2).[42] More than 80% of cases were bilateral. Corneal striae or streaks were seen in nearly one quarter of the Appaloosas with uveitis. During an 11-year period of observation, 38% of the affected horses were treated for acute corneal ulcers; and corneal scars, indicating previous ulcers, were apparent in one third of the cases. Glaucoma signs were present in 21%. More than half of the Appaloosas that were followed up showed iris atrophy, and slightly less than half had evidence of or presented with posterior synechiae. Diffuse cataract developed in nearly three quarters of the group, and one third experienced lens luxation or subluxation.

Posterior changes such as vitritis, chorioretinitis, or detached retina were common but hard to quantify because so many of the horses had cataracts that obscured visualization of these structures. In nearly one quarter of the cases, phthisis bulbi later developed in one or both eyes (Table 7-2).[42]

Coat color pattern of affected horses trended toward overall light hair coats and focal darker spots. Appaloosas in the same practice population that had dark basic coat patterns with a light "blanket" over the rump were often spared from uveitis. Affected horses often showed annual coat color changes, with their base coat becoming lighter as they aged (Fig. 7-26). Night blindness was only rarely associated with uveitis, being confirmed in just 3 of 42 cases. Seventeen percent of affected Appaloosas showed signs of recurrent obstructive airway disease (heaves), which were often severe.[42]

Appaloosas that live in river valleys or other temperate areas may contract leptospirosis because of environmental risks. One study showed that Appaloosa horses seropositive to *L. interrogans* serovar *pomona* have a particularly severe clinical course with a nearly 100% incidence of blindness in one or both eyes.[6] These horses often showed clinical disease that was a hybrid between classic and insidious forms of uveitis: the horses would experience recurrent episodes of fulminant ocular inflammation and severe pain and also show signs of progressive deterioration in the interludes between episodes.

Any disease that has a breed proclivity likely has a genetic basis. In Appaloosas, it is believed that the equine MHC may play a role in susceptibility (Antczak DF et al. Unpublished data, 1989). A recent report has shown that ERU is strongly associated with the MHC class I haplotype ELA-A9 in a population of German Warmblood horses.[39]

MANAGEMENT OF EQUINE RECURRENT UVEITIS

The main goals of therapy for ERU are to preserve vision, reduce and control ocular inflammation in an attempt to limit permanent damage to the eye, and relieve pain. In horses in which a definite inciting cause has been identified, treatment is directed at eliminating the primary problem, and initial tests to isolate an inciting agent are performed. These tests may consist of a complete blood count, biochemistry profile, conjunctival biopsy, and serology for bacterial and viral agents, particularly an MAT for seroreactivity to a panel of *L. interrogans* serovars. However, often, one particular cause cannot be isolated. In these instances, therapy is directed at treatment of symptoms and reduction of ocular inflammation.

Practical and Stable Management Practices to Decrease Equine Recurrent Uveitis

Practices that decrease ocular injury or minimize the inflammatory stimuli may decrease or eliminate the development of ERU (Table 7-6, p. 310). It may be possible to eliminate environmental triggers (e.g., allergens, antigens) of recurrent episodes of uveitis by changing the horse's pasture, pasture mates, or stable; increasing insect and rodent control; decreasing sun exposure; or changing bedding type. Trauma to the eyes can also be decreased by eliminating sharp edges, nails, and hooks from the stable; taping up exposed handles on feed and water buckets; removing low tree branches in the pasture; reducing the training and show schedule; minimizing trailering; and constant use of a quality fly mask. Ensuring that the horse has proper hoof care, an optimal anthelmintic schedule, and proper diet may also reduce uveitis episodes by minimizing infectious disease occurrence and optimizing systemic health.

Anecdotal reports have suggested that vaccination with multivalent vaccines or administration of a number of different individual vaccines on the same day is sometimes associated with a relapse and signs of ocular inflammation. For this reason, it is recommended that horses with ERU be given their annual vaccinations in at least two sessions, spaced 1 week or more apart, rather than all at once. Optimal immunization schedules vary with geographic area and the use of the animal. The attending veterinarian should determine the appropriate immunizations and the route and frequency of administration of the products.

VACCINATION OF HORSES AGAINST LEPTOSPIROSIS

Vaccination of horses with a leptospiral bacterin has been proposed as a preventative measure for leptospirosis-associated ERU.[16] Several vaccines that contain bacterins of pathogenic leptospiral serovars are available commercially. However, *none* of these vaccines have undergone testing in horses, and all are labeled solely for use in bovine or porcine species. Moreover, because ERU has been shown to have a strong immune-mediated component and research has demonstrated molecular homology between equine cornea and lens and certain leptospiral proteins, it is not known whether vaccination carries any risk of exacerbating the immune response or precipitating inflammation.

Anecdotal reports suggest that selective use of a bacterin on farms with demonstrated risk of exposure to

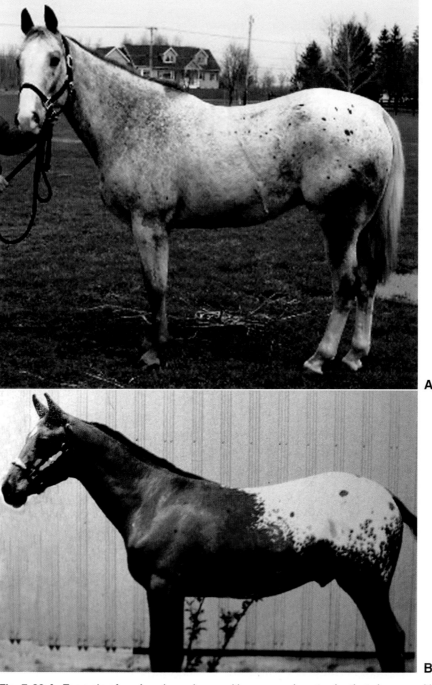

Fig. 7-26 A, Example of an Appaloosa horse with an annual coat color that changes with its base coat and becomes lighter as the horse ages. This type of Appaloosa horse may be more likely to have equine recurrent uveitis. **B,** Example of an Appaloosa horse with a dark basic coat pattern with a light "blanket" over the rump. This type of Appaloosa horse is less likely to have recurrent uveitis.

Leptospira spp. has reduced incidence of eye disease.[16] However, acute uveitis signs have also been observed shortly after vaccine administration in a few horses who had unknown previous exposure to the bacteria (Dwyer AE. Unpublished data, 2004). *No recommendations can be made regarding vaccine use in horses because no clinical trials have been done with the available products, and any use of these produces in horses is off label.*

The vaccine has occasionally been used in situations in which the possible benefit has been judged worthy of the unknown risks; that is, vaccination has been done only on farms in the known geographic risk zones that have had multiple cases of ERU in the past. Before any decision was made to immunize, all horses on those farms had leptospiral serology. Vaccine administration was limited to horses with normal eyes that were

Table 7-6	Practical and Stable Management Practices to Decrease Equine Recurrent Uveitis
Classification	**Practice to Institute**
Environmental	Change pasture/stable/pasture mates
	Increase insect and rodent control
	Decrease dust
	Decrease sun exposure
	Change bedding type
Health maintenance	Proper hoof and dental care
	Optimal anthelmintic and vaccination schedule
	Avoid large multivalent vaccines; split up immunizations
	Proper diet/minimize weeds in pasture
Decrease ocular trauma	"Soften" stable (eliminate sharp objects), tape up bucket handle hooks
	Eliminate low tree branches and burdock plants in pasture
	Decrease training an show schedule
	Minimize trailering
	Do not feed from hay nets
	Use quality fly mask

seronegative to *L. interrogans* serovar *pomona*. Informed consent was obtained from owners, and no other drugs or vaccines were administered on the same day as the bacterin. This conservative approach seems to have reduced the incidence of new cases of ERU on the at-risk farms and, to date, has not resulted in any ocular inflammation that has been associated with vaccine administration with this protocol (Dwyer, Unpublished data, 2004).

Several universities are pursuing research on leptospiral vaccines for horses and their effect on ERU. A preliminary study of the effect of an inactivated bovine vaccine against six serovars of *L. interrogans* in a small group of horses with ERU demonstrated no significant increase or decrease in recurrent episodes of inflammation after vaccination compared with control groups receiving adjuvant only.[87] No commercial equine product is currently being developed.

MEDICAL THERAPY FOR EQUINE RECURRENT UVEITIS

Because vision loss is a common long-term manifestation of ERU, initial therapy must be aggressive (Table 7-7). The two main goals of therapy are to reduce discomfort, which is achieved through use of mydriatic-cycloplegics (e.g., topical atropine), and to

decrease inflammation (e.g., by means of corticosteroids and NSAIDs). Topical atropine 1% is generally given to effect and then continued as required to maintain pupil dilation, usually once a day. If the pupil does not dilate after topical atropine use, then addition of 10% phenylephrine hydrochloride, applied topically every 6 hours for 24 to 48 hours, may help to achieve mydriasis. Phenylephrine is an α-agonist but has poor mydriatic and cycloplegic effect in horses.[88] When it is used in combination with topical atropine, there may be a slightly improved mydriatic effect as compared with that observed with atropine alone. Poor response to mydriatics in general suggests that severe intraocular inflammation is present. Therefore control of the inflammation is required to allow the mydriatics to function. Increasing the frequency of topical atropine application (e.g., more often than every 6 hours) or an increased concentration of atropine (e.g., 2% to 4%) is rarely indicated and could predispose the horse to colic.[89]

Topical corticosteroids are most commonly used to decrease inflammation. Prednisolone acetate 1% and dexamethasone hydrochloride 0.1% are the most commonly used topical corticosteroids. Both medications have excellent ocular penetration, and frequency of therapy varies according to the severity of the disease and ranges from hourly topical application to once-daily application. Dexamethasone is used most often in clinical situations because it is available in an ointment form and is inexpensive. Topical corticosteroids have adverse effects, including the ability to potentiate infections, collagenase ulceration (melting of the cornea), delay of epithelialization of corneal ulcers, and possibly the potentiation of calcific band keratopathy.

Topical NSAIDs (e.g., 0.03% flurbiprofen or 0.1% diclofenac sodium) can also be used. Their main advantage is that they can be administered without concern for potentiating infections; however, they do delay epithelialization of corneal ulcers.

Systemic therapy is the most potent therapy for management of ERU. Flunixin meglumine, which can be administered orally, intramuscularly, or intravenously, is one of the most potent antiinflammatory medications for the eye (Table 7-7). Phenylbutazone and aspirin are much less effective. Systemic dexamethasone and prednisolone are also effective but generally are only used in severe cases that will not respond to other antiinflammatory medications (Table 7-7).

Initial therapy is instituted for at least 2 weeks and should be tapered off over an additional 2 weeks after the resolution of clinical signs. In severe cases, local subconjunctival injections of corticosteroids may be indicated as an adjunct to therapy. The steroid of choice for subconjunctival administration is 2 mg of triamcinolone acetamide (0.2 ml of 10 mg/ml solution). Triamcinolone injections will deliver medication for

Table 7-7 Medical Therapy for Equine Recurrent Uveitis

Medications	Dose	Indication	Caution
Topical Medications			
Prednisone acetate 1%	q 1-6h	Potent antiinflammatory medication with excellent ocular penetration	Predisposes to corneal fungal infection
Dexamethasone HCl 0.5-1%	q1-6h	Potent antiinflammatory medication with excellent ocular penetration	Predisposes to corneal fungal infection
0.03% Flurbiprofen, 0.1% diclofenac (or other topical NSAIDS)	q1-6h	Antiinflammatory medications with good ocular penetration	Decreases corneal epithelialization
Cyclosporine A 0.02%-2%	q6-12h	Strong immunosuppressant	Poor eye penetration, weak antiinflammatory effect
Atropine HCl 1%	q6-48h	Cycloplegic, mydriatic (provides pain relief and minimizes synechia formation)	May decrease gut motility and predispose to colic
Phenylephrine HCl 10%	q6-12h	Use with atropine, primarily as a mydriatic	
Systemic Medications			
Flunixin meglumine	0.5 mg/kg PO, IV, or IM bid for 5 days, then 0.25 mg/kg PO bid	Potent ocular antiinflammatory medication	Long-term use may predispose to gastric and renal toxicity
Phenylbutazone	4.4 mg/kg PO or IV bid	Antiinflammatory medication	Long-term use may predispose to gastric and renal toxicity
Prednisolone	100-300 mg/day PO or IM	Potent antiinflammatory medication	Frequent adverse effects, laminitis formation (use with caution and only as a last resort). Must taper off dose.
Dexamethasone (Azium)	5-10 mg/day PO or 2.5-5 mg daily IM	Potent antiinflammatory medication	Frequent adverse effects, laminitis formation (use with caution and only as a last resort); must taper off dose
Subconjunctival triamcinolone	1-2 mg	Potent antiinflammatory medication with a duration of action of 7 to 10 days	Severe predisposition for bacterial or fungal keratitis, cannot stop therapy once given

IM, Intramuscularly; IV, intravenously; PO, orally.

7 to 10 days and will not result in the granuloma or abscess formation that other steroids, such as methylprednisolone acetate, will cause. However, once the injections are given, the steroid treatment cannot be withdrawn. The long-term presence of corticosteroids may delay healing of corneal ulcers and substantially predispose the eye to fungal keratitis. In some instances, treatment with the use of a subpalpebral lavage catheter is preferred to facilitate delivery of topical medications.

RESPONSE TO THERAPY AND VISUAL PROGNOSIS OF HORSES WITH EQUINE RECURRENT UVEITIS IN CLINICAL PRACTICE

Response to treatment of clinical cases of ERU is variable and difficult to predict. Acute attacks of inflammation may last a few days or several weeks. Some recurrences are mild and respond quickly to simple treatment with mydriatics, topical corticosteroids, and systemic NSAIDs; whereas other episodes are severe and highly refractive to treatment. Subsequent bouts of inflammation may not show the same response to therapy as the initial episode.

Repeat episodes of ocular inflammation may be progressively more severe and refractive to therapy in some horses. These horses usually go blind in the affected eye or eyes, despite all attempts at therapy. Other horses experience a few mild relapses then never have another episode. Still others (primarily Appaloosas and horses of draft breeding) experience insidious disease that progresses quietly but relentlessly, regardless of treatment. The multiple factors that contribute to the onset of the syndrome in a particular horse (inciting cause, specific immune system, and genome of the host) probably play a key role in determining susceptibility to recurrence, response to therapy, and eventual visual outcome.

Incidence of Inflammatory Sequelae in Equine Recurrent Uveitis

Long-term outcome of horses with ERU has received scant attention in the literature, and extensive data regarding occurrence of sequelae are unavailable. However, the visual prognoses for 112 cases of ERU that were followed up for a 7-year period in the Genesee River Valley were reviewed[6]; and the visual outcome, chronic ocular changes, and concurrent medical problems in a group of 160 cases (including the original 112) were followed up over 11 years.[42] The horses were segregated by breed and by seroreactivity to *L. interrogans* serovar *pomona*. Of the total group of 160 horses, 20% (32) had no known risk factor for ERU; that is, they were seronegative and non-Appaloosas. Of the remaining 128 horses, 86 were leptospiral seropositive non-Appaloosa horses, 28 were Appaloosa horses with insidious uveitis, and 14 were horses that were both Appaloosas and seropositive to *L. pomona*. Table 7-2 summarizes the chronic ocular changes observed in these four groups, concurrent medical problems observed, and the eventual visual outcomes. Several interesting findings were noted in this series, which are representative of sequelae seen in horses with ERU in other geographic regions of the world. The findings are as follows:

1. *Cornea:* Focal scars, streaks, calcium deposits, and other corneal opacities were common. The seropositive horses experienced a high rate of calcific band keratopathy. Striae and dense corneal streaks were common in Appaloosas and were highly correlated with blindness.

2. *Iris:* Iris atrophy and color change were common, especially in Appaloosas and seropositive horses. Anterior synechia were rare unless phthisis bulbi was present, but posterior synechia occurred in nearly one third of all cases and in 40% of Appaloosas.

3. *Lens:* Diffuse cataract(s) developed in 41% of all cases and in nearly three fourths of the Appaloosas. These were a common cause of blindness. Lens luxation was common in Appaloosas (29%).

4. *Posterior segment:* Severe vitritis was observed in nearly one third of the cases. Peripapillary scarring (focal or alar) was also present in about one third of the horses. Cataracts and synechiae often obstructed posterior segment evaluation, so inflammatory changes were probably underreported.

5. *Glaucoma and phthisis bulbi:* Appaloosas had the highest rate of glaucoma (21%). Phthisis bulbi developed most often in Appaloosas and seropositive horses.

Owners are often concerned that horses with ERU will require enucleation. In the previously mentioned series, only 4% (6/160) underwent enucleation because of complications from corneal infection or glaucoma. Of more concern is the fact that 43 of the 160 horses (27%) were treated for corneal ulcers during the observation period. Risk of corneal ulcers in horses with ERU should be stressed, because owners often choose to medicate horses with painful eyes themselves, and they may potentiate serious infections by applying corticosteroids and delaying proper diagnosis. Ten horses had calcific band keratopathy. This is a troublesome complication that limits therapeutic options for ERU.

Ocular Involvement

Few data have been tabulated relating ocular involvement to specific equine uveitides. In the New York study, ocular involvement was compared with the presence of known risk factors of Appaloosa breeding and MAT seroreactivity to *L. pomona* in a group of 160 horses. Appaloosas usually had bilateral disease (81%, including a few horses that were also seropositive to *L. pomona*). About half of seropositive horses had ERU in just one eye, and the other half had bilateral disease. Horses with no known risk factor for disease (seronegative non-Appaloosas) showed unilateral involvement more often than bilateral involvement.

Visual Prognosis of Equine Recurrent Uveitis

The overall prognosis for sight in horses with uveitis has been described as poor.[9,90] Limited data have been published regarding actual rates of vision loss in horses with ERU. In the New York study, complete blindness was noted in 20% (32/160) of all the horses followed up on a long-term basis. Unilateral blindness occurred in 36% (57/160). Overall, 56% of all horses experienced blindness in one or both eyes.

Appaloosas and seropositive horses were at increased risk for blindness in this study: Seropositive Appaloosas had the poorest visual prognosis: all lost vision in at least one eye, and half became completely blind. Appaloosas that had never been exposed to *L. pomona* and those that had insidious disease fared a little better: the rate of vision loss in one or both eyes was 72%, with 29% experiencing total blindness. Horses that had been exposed to *L. pomona* but were not Appaloosas lost vision in one or both eyes about half the time and had a total blindness rate of 17%. Horses that had idiopathic uveitis (i.e., horses that were seronegative to *L. pomona* and were not Appaloosas) had the best visual prognosis: just 34% became blind in one or both eyes, and total blindness occurred in only 6%.

The central question in the mind of any owner of a horse with ERU is: *"Will my horse go blind?"* The presenting signs, response to treatment, and recurrence rate of the various equine uveitides are highly variable and likely related to a variety of environmental, genetic, and immune factors, as well as inciting triggers that produce disease. Future efforts should be directed toward defining the specific visual prognosis that is associated with the subsets of disease that comprise the syndrome of ERU, and evolution of classification schemes should include assessment of the prognoses associated with the various uveitic entities.

NEW THERAPIES FOR EQUINE RECURRENT UVEITIS

Traditional treatments used for ERU (i.e., corticosteroids, mydriatics, and NSAIDs) are aimed at reducing inflammation and minimizing permanent ocular damage during each active episode. They are not effective in preventing recurrence of disease. Other medications used to prevent or decrease severity of recurrent episodes—such as aspirin, phenylbutazone, and various herbal treatments—have limited efficacy and potential detrimental effects on the gastrointestinal and hematologic systems when used on a long-term basis in the horse.

However, several anecdotal reports of benefit in which antibiotics were used as a primary treatment for ERU have emerged. In cases of suspected leptospiral infections (e.g., an elevated leptospiral serum or ocular fluid titer), a 4-week course of oral doxycycline (10 to 20 mg/kg, given orally every 12 hours) may minimize or eliminate recurrent episodes of uveitis (Gilger BC. Unpublished data, 2004). Single injections of 4 mg of gentamicin into the vitreous cavity have also been reported anecdotally to help minimize or eliminate recurrent episodes of uveitis in cases of leptospirosis-associated ERU (Neaderland M, Lindley D. Personal communication, 2002). *However, the effectiveness, mode of action, complications, and long-term results of these therapies have not been determined; and until these studies are done, it is recommended that these treatments be used with caution.* It is thought that these therapies may kill residual organisms that may be responsible for recurrent uveitis episodes, but no studies have been done to determine whether this is the mode of action or whether these medications are having another effect.

Acupuncture, herbal, Methyl-sulfonyl-methane (MSM), and holistic therapies may be worth an attempt, as long as their use is concurrent with traditional medications or in cases in which traditional medication is poorly effective.

SUSTAINED-RELEASE MEDICATION DEVICES IN THE TREATMENT OF EQUINE RECURRENT UVEITIS

Ocular sustained-release medication devices or implants have many advantages over more traditional methods of drug administration to the eye.[91] These advantages include delivery of constant therapeutic levels of drug directly to the site of action, bypassing some of the blood-ocular barriers and eliminating the need to depend on owners to treat their horses. Release rates are typically well below toxic levels of the drug, and therefore higher concentrations of the drug are achieved in the eye without any systemic adverse effects. Devices also have the benefit of being more convenient for the patient and reducing the risk involved with frequent intravitreal injections. Ocular implants should be sterile and made from a biocompatible, preferably biodegradable, noninflammatory material.[91]

Cyclosporine is a 1.2-kd cyclic peptide that blocks the transcription of IL-2 production and the responsiveness of the T lymphocyte[92,93]; therefore, it may be the ideal drug for prevention of the activation of T lymphocytes and recurrence of uveitis. However, currently available methods of delivery to the eye are inadequate. Cyclosporine is hydrophobic and does not penetrate the eye when it is applied topically.[94-96] Systemic treatment may promote serious adverse effects such as renal, hepatic, and neurologic toxicity[97] and is also very costly to administer to a horse.

Originally, a polyvinyl alcohol/silicone–coated intravitreal cyclosporine sustained delivery device that had been shown previously to produce a sustained level of cyclosporine in ocular tissues (rabbit)[98,99] was evaluated for use in horses. A cyclosporine device was implanted into normal horse eyes for up to 1 year and was not associated with ocular inflammation or complications.[100] In equine eyes with experimentally induced uveitis, the cyclosporine decreased the duration and severity of inflammation, cellular infiltration, tissue destruction, and level of transcription of proinflammatory cytokines.[101] In a study in which cyclosporine devices were used in horses with naturally occurring ERU,[51] horses with frequent recurrence of uveitis without vision-threatening ocular changes (e.g., cataracts, retinal degeneration) or systemic illnesses were selected to receive the devices. Although the devices prevented the development of recurrent episodes in 81% of horses,

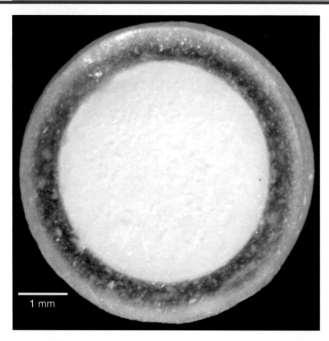

Fig. 7-27 A reservoir/matrix device designed for long-term release of cyclosporine to the eye. (Photograph courtesy Dr. Mike Robinson.)

1 mm

complications that included intraocular hemorrhage, progression of cataract, and retinal detachment were noted after surgery.[51] Surgical intervention in fragile eyes with ERU was thought to be the source of the observed complications, so less invasive methods for the constant release of cyclosporine were evaluated.

A device (Fig. 7-27) that allows constant release of cyclosporine (or other selected immunosuppressive medications) directly to the ciliary body was developed to be inserted in the suprachoroidal space. Horses with documented chronic ERU, as determined after complete ophthalmic examination, that have little or no active inflammation but are experiencing frequent recurrences or early relapse of active ERU after medications have been stopped are appropriate candidates for surgical placement of a cyclosporine implant. Horses with active inflamed eyes that cannot be controlled with antiinflammatory medications are *not* candidates for cyclosporine implantation because cyclosporine has poor antiinflammatory properties (its immunosuppressive properties help prevent new recurrent episodes) and inflamed eyes are prone to postoperative complications. Control of active inflammation with traditional antiinflammatory medications is critical for success of the cyclosporine implantation technique. Evidence of significant cataract formation or other ocular condition (e.g., glaucoma) makes an animal a poor candidate for surgery.

The suprachoroidal implant surgical technique requires induction of general anesthesia in the horse. A 1-cm conjunctival incision is made in the dorsolateral bulbar conjunctiva. A 7-mm–wide scleral flap is created, exposing the uveal tract (the black uvea is just visible through the sclera) approximately 8 mm posterior to the limbus and just lateral to the insertion of the dorsal rectus muscle (Fig. 7-28, *A*). The cyclosporine-containing device is placed into the incision, in contact with the uveal tract (Fig. 7-28, *B*). The scleral flap and incision are closed with 5-0 to 6-0 Vicryl (Fig. 7-28, *C*). Postoperative medications include flunixin meglumine (500 mg, given orally every 24 hours) for 5 days, topical triple antibiotic ophthalmic ointment applied every 12 hours for 10 days, and topical atropine ointment applied every 24 hours for 7 days. Approximately 25% of the horses have had a mild flare after discontinuation of the flunixin meglumine.

Preliminary results from the clinical trial suggest that it takes 30 to 45 days after implantation of the device for adequate ocular levels of cyclosporine to be achieved. If recurrent episodes occur, traditional treatment with systemic NSAIDs, topical steroids, and atropine, is recommended. Approximately 25% of horses have had recurrent episodes after surgery, but less medication for control of the active inflammation is needed, and the durations of the inflammatory episodes are shorter. More importantly, early results suggest that the suprachoroidal implant is not associated with any vision-threatening complications such as retinal detachment. The duration of medication delivery from the current devices is approximately 24 months. Evaluation of results from a multicenter clinical trial is currently underway, and if the evaluation is favorable, Food and Drug Administration approval and commercial manufacture of the device will follow. Other immunosuppressive medications such as tacrolimus (FK506), sirolimus, or rapamycin may also be evaluated in similar devices.[102,103]

Surgical Treatment of Equine Recurrent Uveitis: Trans-Pars-Plana-Vitrectomy in Horses

Hartmut Gerhards and Bettina Wollanke

In 1989, Werry and Gerhards introduced vitrectomy via pars plana sclerotomy as a surgical treatment for horses with ERU.[104,105] Since then, surgical technique and perioperative management have been improved step by step.[106,107] To date, more than 1200 equine eyes in varying stages of the disease have been subjected to vitrectomy at the University of Munich, Germany. The indications and contraindications for vitrectomy and the technique currently used for pars plana vitrectomy in horses at the University of Munich are described. Typical problems and complications with the surgery, as well as some long-term surgical outcomes, are reported.

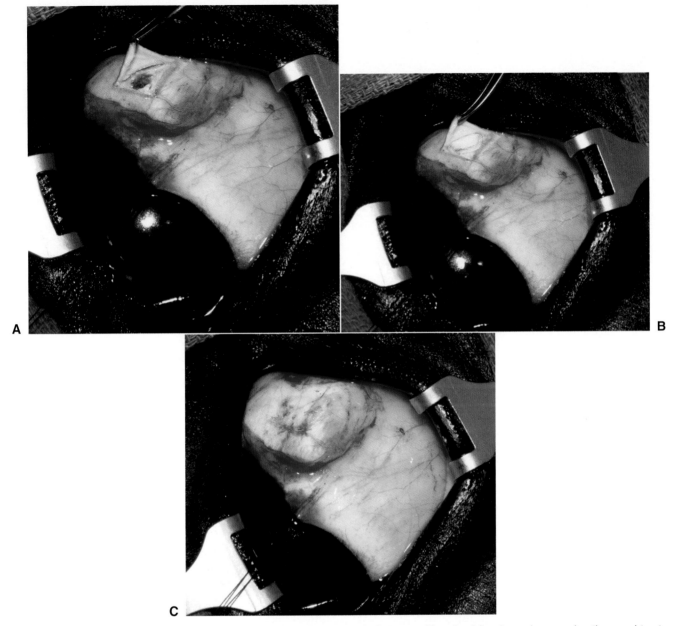

Fig. 7-28 Suprachoroidal cyclosporine-releasing device implantation. **A,** A 7-mm wide scleral flap is made, exposing the uveal tract (the black uvea is just visible through the sclera) approximately 8 mm posterior to the limbus and just lateral to the insertion of the dorsal rectus muscle. **B,** The cyclosporine-containing device is placed into the incision, in contact with the uveal tract. **C,** The scleral flap and conjunctival incision are closed with 6-0 polyglactin 910 sutures.

Criteria for Selection of Cases

The typical candidate for vitrectomy is a horse that continues to have recurrent uveitis, despite careful medical treatment. Horses with a history of two or three attacks of uveitis that have been treated conservatively and have only minor intraocular changes are considered "ideal" surgical patients (Fig. 7-29). Eyes with anterior uveitis are reported to gain as much from surgery as eyes with predominantly posterior uveitis.[108]

Also included among surgical candidates are horses with unknown or incomplete histories, for example, horses pastured without close observation or recently purchased horses with characteristic uveitic changes. Other cases in which vitrectomy can be indicated are horses with painless (i.e., not noted by horse owners) posterior uveitis.

Horses with ERU caused by a persistent intraocular leptospiral infection are suitable candidates for surgery. A diagnostic paracentesis can be performed in quiescent

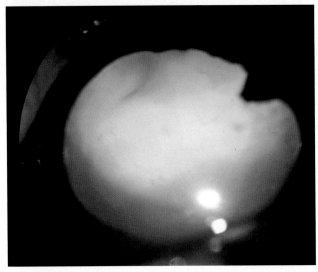

Fig. 7-29 Eye with equine recurrent uveitis, dense vitreous opacities, and yellow-murky discoloration. Vision can be improved by vitrectomy because the lens is still transparent and the pupil is dilated (only small posterior synechia at 2 o'clock position). (Photograph courtesy Hartmut Gerhards and Bettina Wollanke.)

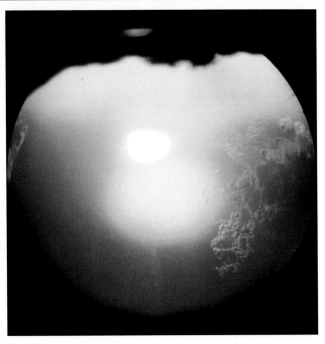

Fig. 7-30 Eye with equine recurrent uveitis (ERU), beginning diffuse cataract, and numerous vacuoles under the posterior lens capsule. Vitrectomy can still be performed, and further ERU attacks may be prevented, but the cataract will progress. (Photograph courtesy Hartmut Gerhards and Bettina Wollanke.)

cases or cases in which infection is suspected, and aqueous can be tested for leptospiral antibodies by MAT and for leptospiral DNA by PCR. The decision for vitrectomy in horses with questionable ERU should be based on the results of these tests.

Vitrectomy is also performed in eyes that have dense vitreous opacities, such as substantial accumulations of cellular debris, to improve vision. Surgery is also sometimes performed on horses with considerable opacities in the refractory media. However, the goal of vitrectomy in an eye with changes such as early cataract is *not* to preserve vision, but to terminate the inflammatory bouts and to preserve the globe (Fig. 7-30). In these cases, vitrectomy can be regarded as "cosmetic" surgery, but it also prevents pain in affected horses, keeps horses serviceable, and reduces costs and treatment time for the owner. Good communication with the client is necessary to explain the expected success (cessation of uveitic attacks) and limitations (no more vision) of the surgical treatment. In selected cases, vitrectomy combined with lens removal by phacoemulsification and aspiration can be considered as a last-resort attempt to preserve vision in eyes with dense (complicated) cataract or lens luxation that still have an intact retina, as confirmed by ophthalmoscopy, functioning consensual pupillary reflexes, and normal ultrasonography and electroretinography findings. Other, more rare indications for vitrectomy are vitreous hemorrhage, septic uveitis, and foreign bodies in the vitreous chamber. Finally, surgery can be performed in blind eyes that still have painful inflammations to "save" the globe and to stop uveitis and medical treatment, but of course not to restore vision.

Contraindications

Noninfectious forms of uveitis (e.g., phacogenic and traumatic uveitis), as well as other recurrent eye problems (e.g., keratitis and conjunctivitis)—the symptoms of which can be similar to those of ERU—do not respond to vitrectomy. Acute inflammatory signs, ulcerative keratitis, and infectious conjunctivitis are regarded as contraindications for vitrectomy. Extensive posterior synechiae, mature cataract, and retinal detachment are regarded as relative contraindications for vitrectomy, whereas moderate hypotony is not. Vitrectomy is generally contraindicated in eyes with glaucoma because elevated intraocular pressure is only temporarily relieved after surgery. However, in selected cases of glaucomatous eyes with severe vitreous opacities, vision can be improved by vitrectomy for some time.

Preoperative Medication

All animals are examined (see Chapter 1) and hospitalized at least 3 days before surgery. Treatment is initiated with antibiotic and corticosteroid eye ointments (two to three times a day). Atropine eye ointment (1%) is given to effect mydriasis. If mydriasis is achieved immediately, one application per day can be sufficient. In cases with extensive posterior synechia, atropine is given up to six times a day. Additionally, the frequency of application of topical medication depends on the level of pretreatment before hospitalization. Systemic NSAIDs (e.g., antiprostaglandin) are administered in recommended dosages. On the day of surgery, gentamicin eye drops and NSAIDs are given. Ointments are not applied to the eye immediately before surgery so that good visualization of the surgical field can be maintained during the vitrectomy.

Surgery

After induction of general anesthesia, the animal is positioned in lateral recumbency with the affected eye uppermost. The eye is prepared for aseptic surgery by thorough irrigation of the conjunctival sac and the periocular skin with a gentamicin-balanced salt solution mixture (20 mg of gentamicin sulfate in 250 ml of balanced salt solution). Next, the closed eye and the area around the eye are dressed with adhesive sterile impermeable drapes. The head and neck are covered with sterile cloth drapes. The adhesive drape is incised along the palpebral fissure, and care must be taken so that the cilia from the upper eyelid remain below the adhesive drape. A custom-built eyelid speculum is used to open the palpebral fissure. At this point, the depth of anesthesia is increased to provide ocular immobility and corneal analgesia. After the bulbar conjunctiva has been exposed by gently rotating the globe with an instrument placed in the ventral conjunctival sac, one or two scleral incisions are made with a carbon dioxide laser at 20 W in the continuous wave mode, with the laser beam being directed toward the center of the globe and activated by a foot switch. A single incision is made at the 12 o'clock position when a combined irrigation/suction instrument is used. When separate incisions are used for the vitreous cutter and the infusion line, two sclerotomies are made at the 11 o'clock and 1 o'clock positions. The incisions are placed 14 mm away from the limbus in large horses and 12 mm away from the limbus in smaller horses; the distance is measured with calipers. With the use of two ports, the first incision is for an irrigation tip, which is introduced and secured in place with the help of a pre-placed suture of monofilament polyglecaprone (1 metric or United States Pharmacopeia [USP] 5-0). Then the second laser incision is made. Again, a suture is pre-placed, and a custom-built vitrectomy cutter is inserted through the incision (Fig. 7-31). The instrument is controlled transpupillarly with the aid of a head-mounted binocular indirect ophthalmoscope.

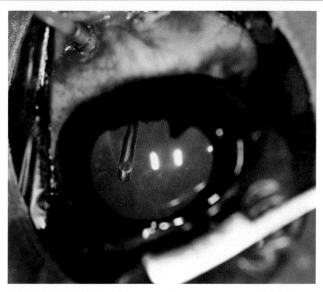

Fig. 7-31 Surgeon's view during vitrectomy surgery. The infusion tip is fixed in the sclera at the 11 o'clock position; the cutter is introduced at the 1 o'clock position and observed through the pupil. (Photograph courtesy Hartmut Gerhards and Bettina Wollanke.)

Vitrectomy is performed with a microprocessor-controlled unit (*Erbe Phakotom E* and *Erbe Aspimat E*; Erbe, Tübingen, Germany) with automatic aspiration pumps. Gravitation irrigation maintains an intraocular pressure of about 40 mm Hg. The vitrectomy device operates with a magnet-driven cutting head (600 cuts/min), which is controlled by the surgeon with a foot pedal. The cutting head (*Vitrectom Pferd*, H. P. Braem AG, Ophthaltech, Moerschwil, Switzerland) has a diameter of 1.6 mm and a length of 65 mm. Twenty milligrams of gentamicin is added to 250 ml of balanced salt solution and is used as lavage fluid. Vitrectomy is started in the center of the vitreous and is gradually extended toward the periphery. Undiluted sterile vitreous samples for further examinations can be obtained from the suction line at the beginning of surgery. A small muscle hook is used to dent the sclera carefully to make the ciliary body inflammatory membranes visible from this region. Great care must be taken to avoid touching the posterior lens capsule and the retina. In horses with dense opacities of cornea and lens, a small endoscope ("vitroptic") is introduced through an additional scleral incision, and the vitrectomy cutter is controlled via a screen as is done in arthroscopy. This is, of course, for special indications and not performed routinely.

After as much vitreous as possible (estimated >90%) has been removed from the vitreous chamber, the vitrectomy device is withdrawn from the eye, and the pre-placed suture for the sclera incision for the cutter is tied. After removal of the infusion tip and closure of the second scleral incision, the conjunctiva is closed with 0.7 or 1 metric (USP 6-0 or 5-0) polyglecaprone.

The intraocular surgery takes approximately 7 minutes, and the duration of anesthesia is approximately 35 minutes.

Postoperative Medication

After closure of the conjunctiva, a subconjunctival injection of 20 mg of gentamicin sulfate and 2 mg of aqueous dexamethasone is given, and antibiotic eye ointment is administered to the conjunctival sac. No other topical treatment is used on the day of surgery. Medical treatment starts on the first postoperative day and includes topical atropine ointment (as needed), antibiotics (gentamicin eye ointment), and corticosteroids (dexamethasone ointment) or a combination of tetracycline/dexamethasone eye ointment (every 4 hours) and oral phenylbutazone (4.0 mg/kg, every 12 hours). This treatment regimen is continued for at least 3 days, and the eye ointments are administered for an additional 5 to 7 days. Discharge from the clinic is usually on the fifth postoperative day.

Prognosis

In 98% of the more than 1200 eyes that were operated on at the University of Munich, no further attack of ERU occurred.[108] Vision was preserved in operated eyes that had clear lenses, normal retinas, and little or no observable ocular inflammatory damage at the time of surgery. Cataract formation and retinal detachment in these eyes were rare: cataract developed in less than 3% of these cases and retinal detachment occurred in less than 1% (Gerhards H, Wollanke B. Unpublished data, 2004).[108]

In eyes that showed ocular inflammatory changes at the time of surgery, the prognosis for preserving vision was guarded to poor. Posterior synechia, as well as inflammatory products adherent to the posterior lens capsule, often initiate cataract formation that progresses even when inflammatory products have been removed from the eye. Thus in these eyes, surgery was performed to stop painful attacks and eliminate the need for medical treatment, *not* to preserve vision. Eyes with early retinal detachment have an increased risk for retinal detachment during surgery. Cataract formation and continued retinal detachment can be expected in these cases before surgery. These risks must be explained to owners before surgery. Owners should also be informed that horses that are presented with chronic ERU sequelae (e.g., synechiae, cataract) at the time of vitrectomy may have signs of ocular discomfort or pain later as a result of lens luxation or other problems not related to acute ERU, even though the problem of overt recurrent uveitis attacks should subside after surgery.

Complications

Small amounts of fibrin can be observed in the anterior chamber in 10% of the eyes after surgery, but this is usually absorbed by the time that the horse is discharged from the clinic. Blepharospasm, epiphora, and photophobia are usually absent in horses that have undergone vitrectomy. Intraocular hemorrhage occurs very rarely (in less than 1% of operations) and can be treated with a second operation, if necessary. The risk for postoperative endophthalmitis caused by *Streptococcus* or *Staphylococcus* spp. is less than 0.5%. If this occurs, a second lavage of the vitreous chamber should be performed as soon as possible. In these cases, infectious endophthalmitis is complicated by rapid cataract formation, which causes blindness, but there is a chance for preserving the globe.

The use of surgical instrumentation other than that described, especially for the scleral incisions (e.g., knife or high-frequency unit instead of a carbon dioxide laser), leads to more complications including intraocular hemorrhage, postoperative traumatic uveitis, retinal detachments, and even endophthalmitis. The custom-built irrigation tip and vitrectomy cutter are absolutely essential for the surgery because instruments for human eyes are too small and too short for efficient removal of the equine vitreous and will increase surgery time and complications considerably.

Other complications that may occur include those associated with general anesthesia in horses (e.g., anesthetic complications, injuries sustained during recovery, postoperative colitis, thrombophlebitis, and pneumonia). Pneumonia seems to occur more frequently after vitrectomy than after other operations. An explanation for this may be the long-distance transport often required to have access to specialized clinics, because this is a known risk factor for pneumonia in horses.

Lower success rates with vitrectomy for treatment of ERU reported in other studies may reflect different preoperative and operative protocols than those described earlier. Frühauf et al.[109] performed vitrectomy in 38 equine eyes at the University of Hannover, Germany. Most of these eyes had posterior synechia and capsular cataracts and thus were not optimal candidates for surgery. Cataract formation could be expected to progress in these eyes with or without vitrectomy. Other reasons for different outcomes might be different surgery techniques, different and possibly inadequate instrumentation for horses, insufficient removal of vitreous material, and inadequate case selection. For example, Frühauf et al.[109] used a knife rather than a carbon dioxide laser for the scleral incision, and this technique may have contributed to the reported vitreal hemorrhage in 3 of 38 eyes. Finally, there is a learning curve for vitrectomy, and the results described from our clinic at the University of Munich reflect careful case selection and use of specialized instrumentation. The results given previously were obtained by a very experienced, well-trained team of surgeons and anesthetists performing every operation under optimized conditions.[104-107,110]

How Vitrectomy May Improve Equine Recurrent Uveitis

Many studies have demonstrated intraocular leptospiral infection in horses with ERU.[26-28,108] In horses, antibodies against leptospires could be detected in more than 90% of the vitreous samples, PCR for leptospires was positive in 70% of the vitreous samples, and leptospires could be cultured from 53% of the vitreous samples.[28] The Goldmann-Witmer coefficient (relationship between immunoglobulin G and antibodies in serum and vitreous samples) strongly suggested intraocular antibody production in 97% of the vitreous samples.[108] Vitreous samples from horses with positive MAT results at the time of surgery, reexamined at different intervals after vitrectomy (horses died for reasons other than eye diseases, e.g., colic, mediastinal tumor, chronic lameness) showed decreasing MAT after surgery and negative MAT results 1 year after surgery.[108]

Selected equine eyes with ERU benefit from the removal of the vitreal inflammatory products and activated immune cells, but the main effect of vitrectomy is thought to be removal of persistent intraocular leptospiral infection. Persistence of leptospiral organisms in the posterior segment may play a role in the occurrence of the autoimmune reactions that have been studied in ERU. Only vitreous material is removed by vitrectomy, not the intraocular antigens (e.g., retinal S-antigen and IRBP) commonly associated with autoimmune uveitis in experimental models of uveitis.

FUTURE RESEARCH ON EQUINE RECURRENT UVEITIS

Future understanding of recurrent uveitis in all species will revolve around the investigation of the following key questions[111]:

1. What genetic makeup predisposes individuals to develop disease?

2. If the disease is autoimmune, which autoantigens participate in the initiation and perpetuation of inflammation?

3. What immune mechanisms initiate the immune response and mediate tissue destruction?

Research to determine the genetic predisposition for the syndrome in certain horse breeds (i.e., Appaloosas and German Warmbloods) is ongoing. If a genetic marker is associated with susceptibility, then horses with this genotype could be identified and excluded from use for reproduction, thus decreasing the prevalence of the disease. New immunosuppressive therapies, such as tacrolimus (FK506), may provide improved medical management. Perfecting a device to deliver such a medication may also be feasible. Studies are also being done to determine the role of leptospires or other microorganisms in the initiation and pathogenesis of ERU. Effort continues to further quantify the immune events that characterize inflammation and mediate recurrence. Vaccine research is ongoing at several universities.

Although there is a perplexing range of clinical syndromes in both horses and humans, certain common features of intraocular inflammation are observed in all cases. The result of severe unchecked recurrent uveitis is vision loss. Blindness or reduced vision is inarguably an unacceptable outcome for humans or horses, and uveitis is a cause of large economic losses worldwide. Continued research on ERU should provide better understanding of the clinicopathologic features of uveitis in all species, and new therapies under development for horses may lead to improved therapy for humans, with subsequent reduction in the incidence of blindness in both species worldwide.[111]

Future Study Opportunities in Human and Equine Uveitis

Carolyn Kalsow

Experimental studies in laboratory animals and horses complement each other in that laboratory studies can involve immunologic reagents, numbers of animals, and multiple experimental parameters not feasible in equine studies; whereas equine studies are directly relevant to control of ERU. Equine experimental studies directly examine the equine immune system, whereas rodent studies provide a fully controlled environment and reagents to define precise immunopathogenic mechanisms.

Because ERU is similar to human uveitides in manifestation, incidence, lack of effective therapy, and resulting loss of vision,[2] parallel clinical and laboratory studies in rodents, horses, and humans would increase current understanding of the immunopathogenesis of recurrent uveitis and could determine appropriate targets for prevention and treatment in both horses and humans. Clinical studies of ERU present a unique opportunity to study a uveitis that (1) is naturally occurring rather than laboratory-induced, (2) has an established link between bacterial infection and immune-associated uveitis, (3) involves a relatively homogenous population, (4) allows identification and tracking of individuals at risk, (5) permits acquisition of relevant tissues and serum, and (6) provides a more controlled setting than the study of human uveitis. Likewise, outbreaks of leptospirosis-associated uveitis in humans[112-114] provide collaborative insight from an identifiable population in which human-specific reagents, not available for equine studies, are available to evaluate precise immunopathogenic mechanisms.

Future studies should correlate the microbial and autoimmune responses to define a specific cause and pathogenesis for ERU. Specific studies may further define the genetic relationship of specific ELA haplotypes to various forms of equine uveitis, identify precise antigens and immunologic responses involved in immunopathogenesis of uveitis, and determine the relationship of infectious agents to immune response. Knowledge of such mechanisms will indicate the "magic bullet" for appropriate targets for prevention and treatment of ERU through immunoregulation of an identifiable immune response.

REFERENCES

1. Rebhun WC: Diagnosis and treatment of equine uveitis, *J Am Vet Med Assoc* 175:803-808, 1979.
2. Schwink KL: Equine uveitis, *Vet Clin North Am Equine Pract* 8:557-574, 1992.
3. Abrams K, Brooks DE: Equine recurrent uveitis: current concepts in diagnosis and treatment, *Equine Pract* 12:27-35, 1990.
4. Davidson MG: Anterior uveitis. In: Robinson N, editor: *Current therapy in equine medicine*, ed, 4, Philadelphia, 1992, WB Saunders, pp 593-592.
5. Nelson M: Equine recurrent uveitis, a report of 68 horses in the United States and Canada, *ERU Network Newsletter*, 1995.
6. Dwyer AE, Crockett RS, Kalsow CM: Association of leptospiral seroreactivity and breed with uveitis and blindness in horses: 372 cases (1986-1993), *J Am Vet Med Assoc* 207:1327-1331, 1995.
7. Jones T: Equine periodic ophthalmia, *Am J Vet Res* 3:45-70, 1942.
8. Schlotthauer C: Recurrent ophthalmia, *North Am Vet* 14:18-29, 1933.
9. Lavach JD: *Large animal ophthalmology*, St Louis, 1990, Mosby.
10. Rimpau W: Leptospirose beim Pferde (periodische Augenentzundung), *Tierarztliche Umschau, Nr* 20:15-16, 1947.
11. Heusser H: Die periodische augenentzundung, eine Leptspirose? *Schweiz Arch Tierheilkd* 90:288-312, 1948.
12. Roberts SR, York C, Robinson J: An outbreak of leptospirosis in horses on a small farm, *J Am Vet Med Assoc* 121:237-242, 1952.
13. Yager R, Gochenour W, Wetmore P: Recurrent iridocyclitis (periodic ophthalmia) of horses, *J Am Vet Med Assoc* 117:207-209, 1952.
14. Bryans J: Studies on equine leptospirosis, *Cornell Vet* 45:16-50, 1955.
15. Roberts SJ: Sequela of leptospirosis in horses on a small farm, *J Am Vet Med Assoc* 133:189-194, 1958.
16. Roberts SJ: Comments on equine leptospirosis, *J Am Vet Med Assoc* 155:442-445, 1969.
17. Gelatt KN et al: The status of equine ophthalmology, *J Equine Med Surg* 1:13-19, 1977.
18. Trap D: Leptospirose equine. Enquete sur la presence d'agglutinines antileptospires chez les chevaux en France, *Pratique Veterinaire Equine XI* 3:149-153, 1979.
19. Hathaway S et al: Leptospiral infection in horses in England: a serological study, *Vet Rec* 108:396-398, 1981.
20. Kemenes F: Studies on equine leptospirosis with emphasis on eye-lesions/equine periodic ophthalmia, *Ann Immunol Hung* 24:345-355, 1984.
21. Egan J, Yearsley D: A serologic survey of leptospiral infection in horses in the Republic of Ireland, *Vet Rec* 119:306-310, 1986.
22. Davidson MG, Nasisse MP, Roberts SM: Immunodiagnosis of leptospiral uveitis in two horses, *Equine Vet J* 19:155-157, 1987.
23. Matthews AG, Waitkins SA, Palmer MF: Serological study of leptospiral infections and endogenous uveitis among horses and ponies in the United Kingdom, *Equine Vet J* 19:125-128, 1987.
24. Sillerud CL et al: Serologic correlation of suspected *Leptospira interrogans* serovar *pomona*-induced uveitis in a group of horses, *J Am Vet Med Assoc* 191:1576-1578, 1987.
25. Wollanke B et al: [Intraocular and serum antibody titers to *Leptospira* in 150 horses with equine recurrent uveitis (ERU) subjected to vitrectomy]. *Berl Munch Tierarztl Wochenschr* 111: 134-139, 1998.
26. Brem S et al: 35 Leptospirenisolationen aus Glaskörpern von 32 Pferden mit rezidivierender Uveitis (ERU), *Berl Munch Tierarztl Wochenschr* 112:390-393, 1999.
27. Faber NA et al: Detection of *Leptospira* spp. in the aqueous humor of horses with naturally acquired recurrent uveitis, *J Clin Microbiol* 38:2731-2733, 2000.
28. Wollanke B, Rohrbach BW, Gerhards H: Serum and vitreous humor antibody titers in and isolation of *Leptospira interrogans* from horses with recurrent uveitis, *J Am Vet Med Assoc* 219: 795-800, 2001.
29. Cook CS, Harling DE: Equine recurrent uveitis, *Equine Vet J* 2(Suppl):2-15, 1983.
30. Kalsow CM et al: Pinealitis accompanying equine recurrent uveitis, *Br J Ophthalmol* 77:46-48, 1993.
31. Kalsow CM, Dwyer AE: Retinal immunopathology in horses with uveitis, *Ocul Immunol Inflamm* 6:239-251, 1998.
32. Dubielzig R, Render J, Morreale R: Distinctive morphologic features of the ciliary body in equine recurrent uveitis, *Vet Comp Ophthalmol* 7:163-167, 1997.
33. Deeg CA et al: Immunopathology of recurrent uveitis in spontaneously diseased horses, *Exp Eye Res* 75:127-133, 2002.
34. Romeike A, Brugmann M, Drommer W: Immunohistochemical studies in equine recurrent uveitis (ERU), *Vet Pathol* 35:515-526, 1998.

35. Kalsow CM, Dubielzig RR, Dwyer AE: Immunopathology of pineal glands from horses with uveitis, *Invest Ophthalmol Vis Sci* 40:1611-1615, 1999.

36. Gilger BC et al: Characterization of T-lymphocytes in the anterior uvea of eyes with chronic equine recurrent uveitis, *Vet Immunol Immunopathol* 71:17-28, 1999.

37. Deeg CA et al: Uveitis in horses induced by interphotoreceptor retinoid-binding protein is similar to the spontaneous disease, *Eur J Immunol* 32:2598-2606, 2002.

38. Gilger BC et al: Expression of a chemokine by ciliary body epithelium in horses with naturally occurring recurrent uveitis and in cultured ciliary body epithelial cells, *Am J Vet Res* 63:942-947, 2002.

39. Deeg CA et al: Equine recurrent uveitis is strongly associated with the MHC class I haplotype ELA-A9, *Equine Vet J* 36:73-75, 2004.

40. Bellhorn RW: An overview of the blood-ocular barriers, *Prog Vet Comp Ophthalmol* 1:205-217, 1990.

41. Geller S, Paul R. Public Sector Gaming Study Commission: Economic impact of the equine racing industry, *Public Sector Gaming Study Commission*, Tallahassee, FL 1999.

42. Dwyer AE: Visual prognosis in horses with uveitis, Presented at the American Society of Veterinary Ophthalmology Annual Meeting, Chicago, Ill, 1998.

43. Cooley PL, Wyman M, Kindig O: Pars plicata in equine recurrent uveitis, *Vet Pathol* 27:138-140, 1990.

44. Kalsow CM et al: Pinealitis coincident with recurrent uveitis: immunohistochemical studies, *Curr Eye Res* 11(Suppl):147-151, 1992.

45. Deeg CA et al: Immune responses to retinal autoantigens and peptides in equine recurrent uveitis, *Invest Ophthalmol Vis Sci* 42:393-398, 2001.

46. Hines M, Halliwell R: Autoimmunity to retinal S-antigen in horses with equine recurrent uveitis, *Prog Vet Comp Ophthalmol* 1:283-290, 1991.

47. Hines MT: Immunologically mediated ocular disease in the horse, *Vet Clin North Am Large Anim Pract* 6:501-512, 1984.

48. Angelos J et al: Evaluation of breed as a risk factor for sarcoid and uveitis in horses, *Anim Genet* 19:417-425, 1988.

49. Dick A: Immune mechanisms of uveitis: insights into disease pathogenesis and treatment, *Int Ophthalmol Clin* 40:462-466, 2002.

50. Thurau SR, Wildner G: An HLA-peptide mimics organ-specific antigen in autoimmune uveitis: its role in pathogenesis and therapeutic induction of oral tolerance, *Autoimmun Rev* 2:171-176, 2003.

51. Gilger BC et al: Use of an intravitreal sustained-release cyclosporine delivery device for treatment of equine recurrent uveitis, *Am J Vet Res* 62:1892-1896, 2001.

52. Kalsow C, Turpin L, Dwyer A: Immunopathology of eyes and pineal glands in equine recurrent uveitis, *Regional Immunol* 6:14-20, 1994.

53. Hines MT, Jarpe A, Halliwell RE: Equine recurrent uveitis: immunization of ponies with equine retinal S antigen, *Prog Vet Comp Ophthalmol* 2:3-10, 1992.

54. Maxwell SA et al: Humoral responses to retinal proteins in horses with recurrent uveitis, *Prog Vet Comp Ophthalmol* 1:155-161, 1991.

55. Duke-Elder S, Perkins S: Disease of the uveal tract. In Duke-Elder S, editor: *System of ophthalmology*, St Louis, 1966, CV Mosby.

56. Palaniappan RU et al: Cloning and molecular characterization of an immunogenic LigA protein of *Leptospira interrogans*, *Infect Immun* 70:5924-5930, 2002.

57. Brem S et al: [Demonstration of intraocular leptospira in 4 horses suffering from equine recurrent uveitis (ERU)], *Berl Munch Tierarztl Wochenschr* 111:415-417, 1998.

58. Wada S et al: Nonulcerative keratouveitis as a manifestation of leptospiral infection in a horse, *Vet Ophthalmol* 6:191-195, 2003.

59. Kalsow CM, Dwyer AE: Role of leptospiral infection in equine recurrent uveitis. Presented at the One Hundred and first Annual Meeting of the United States Animal Health Association, Frankfort, KY, October 21, 1997.

60. Lucchesi PM, Parma AE, Arroyo GH: Serovar distribution of a DNA sequence involved in the antigenic relationship between *Leptospira* and equine cornea, *BMC Microbiol* 2:3, 2002.

61. Lucchesi PM, Parma AE: A DNA fragment of *Leptospira interrogans* encodes a protein which shares epitopes with equine cornea, *Vet Immunol Immunopathol* 71:173-179, 1999.

62. Wacker WB: Proctor Lecture. Experimental allergic uveitis. Investigations of retinal autoimmunity and the immunopathologic responses evoked, *Invest Ophthalmol Vis Sci* 32:3119-3128, 1991.

63. Caspi RR: Regulation, counter-regulation, and immunotherapy of autoimmune responses to immunologically privileged retinal antigens, *Immunol Res* 27:149-160, 2003.

64. Forrester JV: Duke-Elder Lecture: new concepts on the role of autoimmunity in the pathogenesis of uveitis, *Eye* 6:433-446, 1992.

65. Nussenblatt RB et al: Humanized anti-interleukin-2 (IL-2) receptor alpha therapy: long-term results in uveitis patients and preliminary safety and activity data for establishing parameters for subcutaneous administration, *J Autoimmun* 21:283-293, 2003.

66. Williams RD et al: Experimental chronic uveitis. Ophthalmic signs following equine leptospirosis, *Invest Ophthalmol* 10:948-954, 1971.

67. Sperber SJ, Schleupner CJ: Leptospirosis: a forgotten cause of aseptic meningitis and multisystem febrile illness, *South Med J* 82:1285-1288, 1989.

68. Ellis WA et al: Leptospiral infection in aborted equine foetuses, *Equine Vet J* 15:321-324, 1983.

69. Morter RL et al: Experimental equine leptospirosis (*Leptospira pomona*), *Proc Annu Meet US Anim Health Assoc* 68:147-152, 1964.

70. Myers DM: Serological studies and isolation of serotype hardjo and *Leptospira biflexa* (sic) strains from horses of Argentina, *J Clin Microbiol* 3:548-555, 1976.

71. Bernard WV: Leptospirosis, *Vet Clin North Am Equine Pract* 9:435-444, 1993.

72. Divers TJ, Byars TD, Shin SJ: Renal dysfunction associated with infection of *Leptospira interrogans* in a horse, *J Am Vet Med Assoc* 201:1391-1392, 1992.

73. Giles RC et al: Causes of abortion, stillbirth, and perinatal death in horses: 3,527 cases (1986-1991), *J Am Vet Med Assoc* 203:1170-1175, 1993.

74. Poonacha KB et al: Leptospirosis in equine fetuses, stillborn foals, and placentas, *Vet Pathol* 30:362-369, 1993.

75. Smith RE, Williams IA, Kingsbury ET: Serologic evidence of equine leptospirosis in the northeast United States, *Cornell Vet* 66:105-109, 1976.

76. Cross RS: Equine periodic ophthalmia, *Vet Rec* 78:8-13, 1966.

77. Verma BB, Biberstein EL, Meyer ME: Serologic survey of leptospiral antibodies in horses in California, *Am J Vet Res* 38:1443-1444, 1977.

78. Roberts SR: Chorioretinitis in a band of horses, *J Am Vet Med Assoc* 158:2043-2046, 1971.

79. Morter RL et al. Equine leptospirosis, *J Am Vet Med Assoc* 155:436-442, 1969.

80. Halliwell RE, Hines MT: Studies on equine recurrent uveitis. I. Levels of immunoglobulin and albumin in the aqueous humor of horses with and without intraocular disease, *Curr Eye Res* 4:1023-1031, 1985.

81. Halliwell RE et al: Studies on equine recurrent uveitis. II. The role of infection with *Leptospira interrogans* serovar *pomona*, *Curr Eye Res* 4:1033-1040, 1985.

82. Halliwell RE et al: Studies on equine uveitis. II. The role of infection with *Leptospira interrogans* serovar *pomona*, *Curr Eye Res* 2:1033-1040, 1985.

83. Eule JC et al: [Occurrence of various immunoglobulin isotopes in horses with equine recurrent uveitis (ERU)], *Berl Munch Tierarztl Wochenschr* 113:253-257, 2000.

84. Parma AE et al: Experimental demonstration of an antigenic relationship between *Leptospira* and equine cornea, *Vet Immunol Immunopathol* 10:215-224, 1985.

85. Parma AE et al: Tears and aqueous humor from horses inoculated with *Leptospira* contain antibodies which bind to cornea, *Vet Immunol Immunopathol* 14:181-185, 1987.

86. Parma AE, Cerone SI, Sansinanea SA: Biochemical analysis by SDS-PAGE and Western blotting of the antigenic relationship between *Leptospira* and equine ocular tissues, *Vet Immunol Immunopathol* 33:179-185, 1992.

87. Rohrbach BW et al: Effect of an inactivated vaccine against *Leptospira interrogans* on the frequency and severity of uveitis in horses with equine recurrent uveitis, Presented at the Annual Meeting of the American College of Veterinary Ophthalmologists, Denver, CO, October 9-13, 2002;52.

88. Hacker DV et al: Effect of topical phenylephrine on the equine pupil, *Am J Vet Res* 48:320-322, 1987.

89. Williams MM et al: Systemic effects of topical and subconjunctival ophthalmic atropine in the horse, *Vet Ophthalmol* 3:193-199, 2000.

90. Brooks D: Equine ophthalmology. In Gelatt KN, editor: *Veterinary ophthalmology*, ed 3, Philadelphia, 1999, WB Saunders. (Neaderland M, Lindley D. Personal communication, 2002).

91. Davis J, Gilger BC, Robinson M: Novel approaches to ocular drug delivery, *Curr Opin Mol Ther* 6:44-54, 2004.

92. Kay JE: Inhibitory effects of cyclosporin A on lymphocyte activation. In Thomson AW, editor: *Cyclosporine: mode of action and clinical application*. Dordrecht, 1989, Kluwer Academic Publishers, pp 1-23.

93. Granelli-Piperno A: Cellular mode of action of cyclosporin A. In Bach JF, editor: *T-cell directed immunointervention*, Oxford, 1993, Blackwell Scientific Publishers, pp 3-24.

94. BenEzra D, Maftzir G: Ocular penetration of cyclosporine A in the rat eye, *Arch Ophthalmol* 108:584-587, 1990.

95. BenEzra D, Maftzir G: Ocular penetration of cyclosporin A, the rabbit eye, *Invest Ophthalmol Vis Sci* 31:1362-1366, 1990.

96. BenEzra D et al: Ocular penetration of cyclosporin A. III. The human eye, *Br J Ophthalmol* 74:350-352, 1990.

97. Svenson K, Bohman SO, Hallgren R: Renal interstitial fibrosis and vascular changes. Occurrence in patients with autoimmune diseases treated with cyclosporine, *Arch Intern Med* 146:2007-2010, 1986.

98. Jaffe GJ et al: Intravitreal sustained-release cyclosporine in the treatment of experimental uveitis, *Ophthalmology* 105:46-56, 1998.

99. Enyedi LB, Pearson PA, Ashton P, et al: An intravitreal device providing sustained release of cyclosporine and dexamethasone, *Curr Eye Res* 15:549-557, 1996.

100. Gilger BC et al: Long-term effect on the equine eye of an intravitreal device used for sustained release of cyclosporine A, *Vet Ophthalmol* 3:105-110, 2000.

101. Gilger BC et al: Effect of an intravitreal cyclosporine implant on experimental uveitis in horses, *Vet Immunol Immunopathol* 76:239-255, 2000.

102. Kulkarni P: Review: uveitis and immunosuppressive drugs, *J Ocul Pharmacol Ther* 17:181-187, 2001.

103. Sakurai E et al: Scleral plug of biodegradable polymers containing tacrolimus (FK506) for experimental uveitis, *Invest Ophthalmol Vis Sci* 44:4845-4852, 2003.

104. Werry H, Gerhards H: Moglichkeiten der und indikationen zur chirurgishen behandlung der euinen rezidivierenden uveitis (ERU), *Pferdeheilkunde* 7:321-331, 1991.

105. Werry H, Gerhards H: Zur operativen therapie der equinen rezidivierended uveitis (ERU), *Tierarztl Prax* 1992;20:178-186.

106. Gerhards H, Wollanke B, Brem S: Vitrectomy as a diagnostic and therapeutic approach for equine recurrent uveitis, Presented at the 45th Annual Meeting of the American Association of Equine Practitioners, Albuquerque, NM, November 1999;89-93.

107. Gerhards H et al: Technique for and results with surgical treatment of equine recurrent uveitis (ERU), Presented at the 29th Annual Meeting of the American College of Veterinary Ophthalmologists, Seattle, WA, October, 1998;30.

108. Wollanke B: Die equine rezidivierende Uveitis (ERU) als intraokulare Leptospirose, Tieraerztliche Fakultaet, Muenchen, 2002, Ludwig-Maximilians-Universitaet.

109. Frühauf B et al: Surgical management of equine recurrent uveitis with single port pars plana vitrectomy, *Vet Ophthalmol* 1:137-151, 1998.

110. Winterberg A, Gerhards H: Langzeitergebnisse der Pars-plana-Vitrektomie bei equiner rezidivierender Uveitis, *Pferdeheilk* 13:377-383, 1997.

111. Dick AD: Understanding uveitis through the eyes of a horse: relevance of models of ocular inflammation to human disease, *Ocul Immunol Inflamm* 6:211-214, 1998.

112. Zaki SR, Shieh WJ: Leptospirosis associated with outbreak of acute febrile illness and pulmonary haemorrhage, Nicaragua, 1995.The Epidemic Working Group at Ministry of Health in Nicaragua, *Lancet* 347:535-536, 1996.

113. Rathinam SR et al: Uveitis associated with an epidemic outbreak of leptospirosis, *Am J Ophthalmol* 124:71-79, 1997.

114. Katz AR et al: Leptospirosis on Oahu: an outbreak among military personnel associated with recreational exposure, *Mil Med* 162:101-104, 1997.

8 Equine Glaucoma

Mary E. Lassaline and Dennis E. Brooks

Glaucoma is a disorder of aqueous humor outflow that results in phases of elevated intraocular pressure (IOP). It is a common but poorly understood eye disease of horses and is related in many aspects to equine recurrent uveitis (ERU). In this chapter the clinical signs, pathogenesis, and therapy of glaucoma in the horse are discussed.

CLINICAL ANATOMY AND PHYSIOLOGY

Aqueous Humor Dynamics

Aqueous humor provides nutrition to the avascular cornea, trabecular meshworks, and lens. Knowledge of aqueous humor formation and the structure of the aqueous humor drainage apparatus are critical to understanding glaucoma in horses. Aqueous humor is formed primarily by active secretion through the ciliary body epithelia into the posterior chamber by utilizing energy and the enzyme carbonic anhydrase. A small portion of aqueous humor production arises from ultrafiltration of blood in the ciliary body circulation. Aqueous humor then percolates through the pupil into the anterior chamber and finally exits through the highly specialized tissues of the iridocorneal angle (ICA) (conventional outflow pathway) or through the more primitive pathways of the iris, ciliary body, and sclera (unconventional outflow pathway).[1-3]

The ICA or ciliary cleft is bordered anteriorly by the peripheral cornea and perilimbal sclera and posteriorly by the peripheral iris and ciliary body. Stout pectinate ligaments separate the anterior chamber from the ICA in the equine eye, and these are visible at the limbus in many horses.[1-3] Aqueous humor moves between the pectinate ligaments into and through the cell-lined trabecular beams of the uveal trabecular meshwork (UTM), the corneoscleral trabecular meshwork (CSTM), the angular aqueous plexus (AAP), and then the intrascleral plexus (ISP) in the conventional outflow pathway (Figs. 8-1 and 8-2).[1-3] The aqueous humor then drains from the ISP into the vortex veins that empty into the choroid. The UTM, CSTM, and AAP comprise 74.3%, 21.5%, and 4.2% of the equine ICA area, respectively.[1-3] The intertrabecular spaces of the UTM are very wide, and the spaces of the CSTM are very narrow. The AAP is a plexus of radially oriented, narrow-diameter vessels.[1-3] The ISP consists of an extensive network of anastomosing circumferential channels that drain aqueous humor to the vortex venous system (Fig. 8-3). The ISP and vortex systems have a rich collateralization. Aqueous humor thus follows a path of low resistance in the UTM and CSTM, high resistance to outflow in the narrow tributaries of the AAP and ISP and low resistance to outflow again in the vortex systems. Resistance to outflow is focused at the AAP and ISP in the conventional outflow system of the horse. The CSTM acts as a sieve or filter for large particles, but it may or may not restrict aqueous flow directly.[1,2]

Morphologic studies indicate a potentially extensive unconventional aqueous humor outflow pathway in the horse.[1-3] The large ICA provides a large trabecular contact area with the iris and ciliary body. Aqueous humor enters the anterior iris face to drain into the vortex veins and leaves the UTM through the interstitial spaces of the ciliary body musculature to drain into the supraciliary and suprachoroidal spaces and choroids.[1-3] Microsphere perfusion studies have shown the suprachoroidal and supraciliary spaces to provide an extensive unconventional outflow pathway to the sclera and choroid in the horse (Fig. 8-4).[2]

Intraocular Pressure

The balance between the rate of production of aqueous humor and the rate of exit of aqueous humor from the eye results in the tissue pressure of the eye, the IOP. Obstruction to the outflow of aqueous humor causes an elevation in IOP. Persistent IOP elevation causes a reduction in blood flow in the eye and induces degeneration of optical and neural structures in the eye.

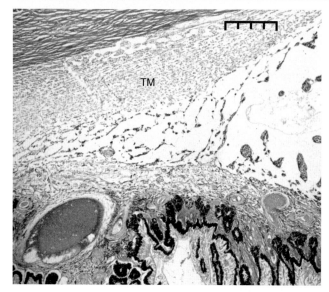

Fig. 8-1 The trabecular meshworks *(TM)* of the iridocorneal angle of the horse are very large, wide, and open for the conventional outflow of aqueous humor. (Periodic acid-Schiff stain. Bar equals 70 μm.)

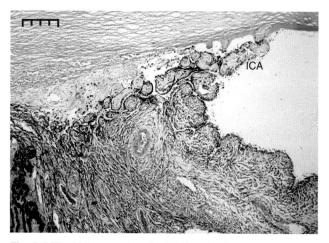

Fig. 8-2 The iridocorneal angle *(ICA)* and trabecular meshworks of this horse with glaucoma have collapsed. (Periodic acid-Schiff stain. Bar equals 80 μm.)

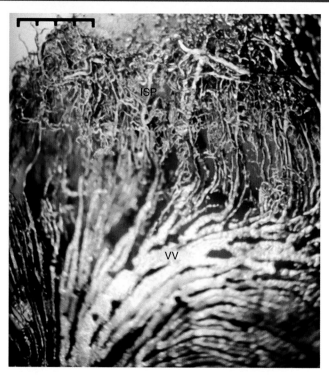

Fig. 8-3 This vascular cast of an equine eye reveals the tremendous plexiform nature of the intrascleral plexus *(ISP)* and its extensive connections to the posterior vortex veins (VV). (Bar equals 330 μm.)

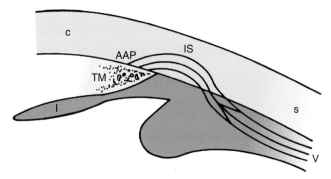

Fig. 8-4 Aqueous humor outflow pathways in the horse. Aqueous humor moves through the trabecular meshworks *(TM)*, to the angular aqueous plexus *(AAP)*, to the intrascleral plexus *(IS)*, and then drains into the vortex veins. The lumen diameter of the vessels through which the aqueous humor passes increases along the path.

If retinal ganglion cell (RGC) death occurs, this elevation in IOP is termed glaucoma. Elevation in IOP with no detectable loss of RGC is called ocular hypertension.

The IOP measured with a Tonopen applanation tonometer (Medtronics, Jacksonville, Fla) in the horse ranges from 7 to 37 mm Hg, with a mean IOP of 23.3 ± 6.9 mm Hg (Fig. 8-5).[4] This normally elevated IOP is unusual in land animals. Horses appear more tolerant of ocular hypertension than other species. Some anecdotal reports indicate that IOP can remain high (>50 mm Hg) for several days and horses can retain vision, unlike dogs and other species. Horses that are anesthetized and "tipped" in the Trendelenburg position while insufflated with carbon dioxide (CO_2) for orthopedic laparoscopic surgery can have an IOP >70 mm Hg for more than 1 hour with no apparent effects on vision. (Lassaline, Unpublished data, 2003). Although the horse does not seem to experience significant diurnal changes in IOP, in one study, IOP in the afternoon was slightly higher than IOP in the morning.[5] Failure to use auriculopalpebral nerve blocks during tonometry may result in slight overestimates of IOP but is recommended in fractious horses. Horses who require sedation for ocular examination may show dramatic decreases in IOP, as illustrated by a study in which xylazine decreased IOP by 23% to 27%.[5]

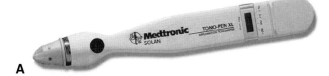

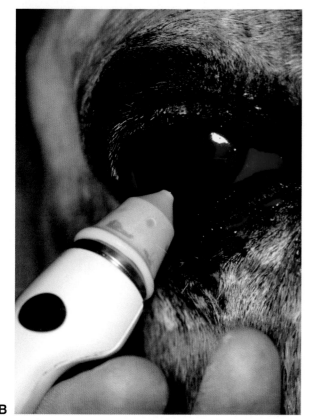

B

Fig. 8-5 The Tonopen applanation tonometer is necessary for the diagnosis of elevated intraocular pressure (IOP) and serial measurements of IOP in response to therapy. **A,** Tonopen XL tonometer **B,** Tonopen tonometer in use on a horse. (Photograph [A] courtesy Medtronic Solan, Jacksonville, Fla.)

Tonography is tonometry measured over 4 minutes. It measures the ease or facility of the exit of aqueous humor from the eye. Tonography demonstrates a very high facility of conventional outflow in horses compared with other species (0.88 ± 0.65 µl in horses; 0.32 ± 0.16 µl in dogs; 0.28 ± 0.01 µl in humans). [6]

Retinal Ganglion Cells and the Equine Optic Nerve

The horse has a very large retinal sensory surface area, vast numbers of photoreceptors, a massive population of RGCs with large cell bodies, a large optic disc area and optic nerve cross-sectional area (15.7 mm² vs 5.17 mm² in humans), high total optic nerve axon counts (1.076 × 10⁶ vs 1.159 × 10⁶ in humans), large

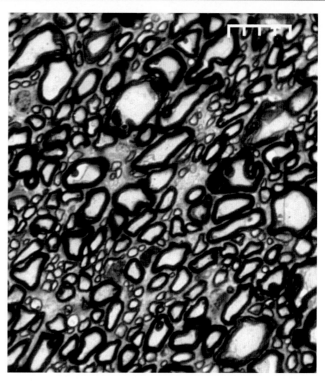

Fig. 8-6 Large myelinated axons predominate in the optic nerve of the healthy horse. (Toluidine blue stain. Bar equals 2 µm.)

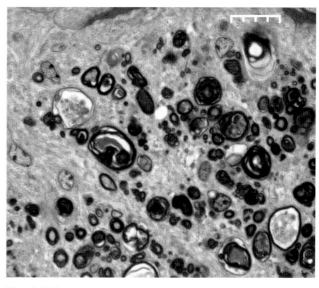

Fig. 8-7 Few axons remain in the optic nerve of a horse with chronic glaucoma. (Toluidine blue stain. Bar equals 2 µm.)

mean individual optic nerve axon cross-sectional areas (3.11 vs 1.75 µm² in humans), and 4.4 times the percentage of optic nerve axons >2 µm in diameter compared with humans (35.5% in horses vs 8.0% in humans).[7] The comparatively low density of axons in the horse optic nerve (62,800 axons/mm² in horses vs 175,000 axons/mm² in humans) undoubtedly reflects a low tissue density of RGCs, because the ratio of ganglion cells to optic nerve axons is 1:1 (Figs. 8-6 and 8-7).[7]

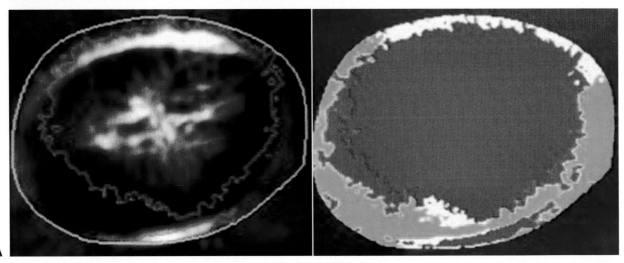

A   B

Fig. 8-8 Scanning laser tomography of the oval optic nerve head *(ONH)* of this healthy horse consists of a confocal laser tomographic, extended focus, reflectance/intensity image **(A)** and a stereometric topography analysis image in pseudocolor **(B)**. Red indicates areas below the retinal surface, and green, areas above the retinal surface. The white areas are caused by irregularities in the disc surface. Note the posterior excavation of the neuroretinal rim and the 6 o'clock position. The scanning laser tomographic measurements indicate that the equine neuroretinal rim area is smallest at the superior and inferior rims and largest at the nasal and temporal rims. The disc area is 17.6 mm², the cup area is 14.6 mm², and the cup-to-disc area ratio is 0.83 in this horse.

The prelaminar optic nerve is known as the optic disc, optic nerve head (ONH), or optic papilla and is surrounded by the white, peripapillary scleral ring of Elschnig noted at the 6 o'clock position in the horse ONH. Myelin extends anterior to the equine lamina cribrosa to cover the surface of the optic disc. The myelinated axons generally stop at the edge of the scleral canal, although myelinated axons in the retinal nerve fiber layer are noted in the horizontal retinal quadrants of some horses. The equine ONH is oval with the horizontal axis longer. Scanning laser ophthalmoscopy of the equine ONH indicates that the neuroretinal rim area is smallest at the superior and inferior rims of the horse optic disc and larger at the nasal and temporal rims (Fig. 8-8). The intrapapillary region of the ONH is the area inside Bruch's membrane at the scleral canal and consists of the neuroretinal rim and the optic cup (Figs. 8-9 and 8-10). The optic cup is defined on the basis of contour.

ONH cup enlargement or "cupping" is associated with advanced glaucoma in the horse (Fig. 8-11). Optic nerve "cupping" occurs as a result of axonal loss, laminar plate compression (Fig. 8-12), rotation of the scleral insertion zone posteriorly, outward bowing of the lamina cribrosa, and a widening of the scleral canal behind Bruch's membrane. The associated enlargement of the ONH cup with these laminar and axonal changes is unique to glaucoma and is not found in other optic neuropathies. The neuroretinal rim is the intrapapillary equivalent to the nerve fiber layer. The neuroretinal rim becomes narrowed, because RGCs and axons are lost in glaucoma. The ratio of the cup-to-disc area is used to evaluate progression of glaucomatous optic

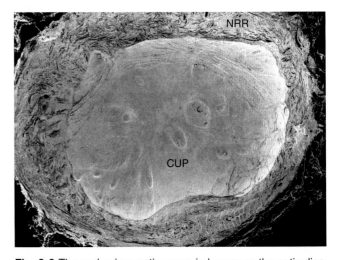

Fig. 8-9 The prelaminar optic nerve is known as the optic disc, optic nerve head (ONH), or optic papilla. The equine ONH is oval with the horizontal axis longer. The intrapapillary region of the ONH consists of the narrow neuroretinal rim *(NRR)* and the large central optic cup. This scanning electron micrograph illustrates the NRR and optic cup *(CUP)*.

nerve damage in humans. Enlargement of the cup-to-disc ratio indicates optic nerve axonal loss and is associated with deterioration in visual fields.

Large RGCs have large-diameter optic nerve axons, overlapping retinal receptive fields, and provide rapid transfer of visual input for detection of moving objects, an advantage for an animal such as the horse. The marked proportion of large-diameter ganglion cells in the horse retina may be an adaptation to cover a large retinal sensory surface area with a relatively low population density of ganglion cells.[7]

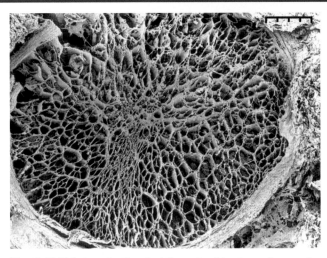

Fig. 8-10 This trypsin digest of the scleral lamina cribrosa of a horse reveals the many laminar pores through which optic nerve axon bundles exit the eye to go to the brain. (Bar equals 690 μm.)

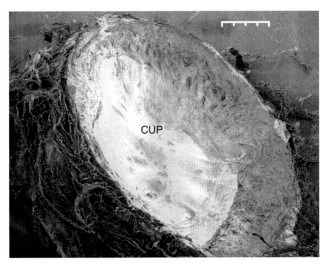

Fig. 8-11 This scanning electron micrograph demonstrates the optic nerve head cup *(CUP)* enlargement that is associated with advanced glaucoma in the horse. Optic nerve "cupping" occurs as a result of axonal loss, laminar plate compression, and posterior bowing of the lamina cribrosa. The neuroretinal rim narrows because retinal ganglion cells and axons are lost in glaucoma. The ratio of the cup-to-disc area is used to evaluate progression of glaucomatous optic nerve damage. (Bar equals 690 μm.)

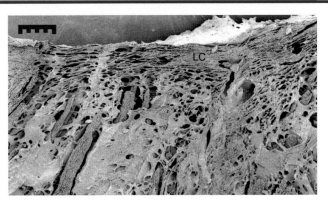

Fig. 8-12 Glaucoma causes compression of the anterior laminar beams of the lamina cribrosa *(LC)* in this trypsin digest of the optic nerve head of a horse with glaucoma. (Bar equals 500 μm.)

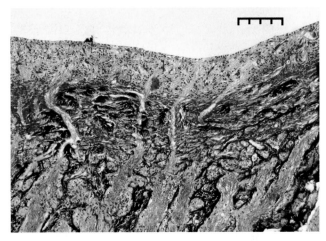

Fig. 8-13 This histologic section of a equine optic nerve has the neural axon bundles (pink) passing through the plates of the scleral lamina cribrosa (collagen is blue). (Gomori's trichrome stain. Bar equals 2.3 μm.)

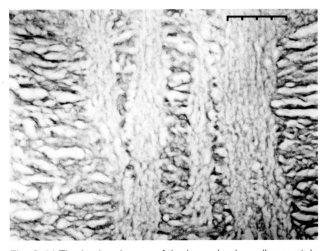

Fig. 8-14 The laminar beams of the horse lamina cribrosa stain for collagen type I in this histologic section. (Bar equals 15 μm.)

RGC axons of the retinal nerve fiber layer become arranged into optic nerve fiber bundles by astrocytes in the choroidal lamina cribrosa. The scleral lamina cribrosa is a specialized extracellular matrix of the central nervous system that spans the scleral canal as a complex, multilayered set of collagenous plates (Fig. 8-13).[8] The multiple plates of the scleral lamina cribrosa contain a hydrodynamic extracellular matrix of elastic and collagen fibers (types I, III, and VI), astrocytes, and capillaries (Fig. 8-14). The optic nerve axons are insulated from the surrounding extracellular matrix by tubes of astrocytes through the entire length of the scleral lamina cribrosa.

The intralaminar optic nerve of horses with glaucoma contains a significantly larger total number of laminar pores, pores of significantly smaller individual area, and pores that are rounder than those in the intralaminar optic nerve of healthy horses.[8] The intralaminar optic nerves of horses with glaucoma contain a higher percentage of connective tissue (74%) than the optic nerves of healthy horses (67%).[7,8] These differences may represent an anatomic variation found in horses predisposed to develop glaucoma, as well as changes resulting from IOP-induced radial stress forces causing stretching of the scleral lamina cribrosa.

The scleral lamina cribrosa is a transition zone of high to low hydrostatic tissue pressure caused by the prominent pressure gradient formed by the IOP and intraorbital pressure. The axoplasmic flow in the optic nerve axons is subjected to this abrupt change in tissue pressure.[9] The elevated IOP found in glaucoma exacerbates this pressure gradient and is associated with posterior displacement of the lamina cribrosa and disruption of optic nerve axon axoplasmic flow (Figs. 8-12, 8-13, and 8-14). The lamina cribrosa is thus an active and compliant structure in the horse whose movement during normal and abnormal fluctuations in IOP can both protect and obstruct optic nerve axoplasmic flow.[8]

GLAUCOMA

The glaucomas are a group of diseases resulting from reductions in aqueous humor outflow that cause an IOP increase above that which is compatible with normal function of the retina and optic nerve. All glaucomas consist of five stages: (1) an initial event or series of events that progressively reduce function of the aqueous humor outflow system; (2) morphologic alterations of the aqueous outflow system that eventually lead to obstruction of aqueous humor outflow and IOP elevation; (3) elevated IOP that is too high for normal RGC and optic nerve axon function; (4) RGC and optic nerve axon degeneration; and (5) progressive visual deterioration that eventually leads to blindness.[10] True glaucoma was thought to be a variant of ERU and an uncommon ocular problem in horses.[11-14]

EQUINE GLAUCOMA

The suspected low prevalence of glaucoma in the horse is surprising (0.07% in the United States),[9,13] given the horse's propensity for ocular injury and marked intraocular inflammatory responses, which might be expected

to lead to secondary glaucoma. There were estimated to be 6.9 million horses in the United States in 1996.[15] The calculated prevalence of glaucoma in horses would indicate that 4830 horses have glaucoma, which seems an overestimate. The infrequency of diagnosis in the horse may be due, in part, to the limited availability of tonometers in equine practice, but also to the fact that large diurnal fluctuations in IOP, even in chronic ERU cases, may make documentation of elevated IOP difficult. Equine glaucoma is not easily recognized in the early stages of the disease because of the subtle nature of the clinical signs.[13,14] This may be explained by the prominent role of uveoscleral aqueous humor outflow in the horse, which may be higher than that in other species, and by microanatomic differences in the aqueous humor outflow pathways in horses compared with those in other species.[1-3]

Types of Equine Glaucoma

The glaucomas of horses are frequently categorized into primary, secondary, and congenital types. The terms may not be completely relevant because all glaucomas are secondary to some causative mechanism. Primary glaucomas have a bilateral and heritable potential, have no overt ocular abnormality to account for the increase in IOP, and have not been conclusively reported in the horse. The secondary glaucomas in horses have an identifiable cause such as iridocyclitis, lens luxation, or intraocular neoplasia. Iris and ciliary body neoplasms can obstruct aqueous humor outflow to cause secondary glaucoma. Congenital glaucoma caused by developmental anomalies of the ICA (goniodysgenesis) has been reported in foals (Table 8-1).[16-19]

Risk Factors for Progression of Equine Glaucoma

Horses with active or quiescent uveitis, aged horses (>15 years old), and Appaloosas are at increased

Table 8-1	Glaucoma Types
Types of Glaucoma	**Causes**
Primary	Possibly heretible
Secondary	Severe iridocyclitis
	Lens luxation
	Intraocular neoplasia
	Intraocular infection
Congenital	Goniodysgenesis

risk for the development of glaucoma.[6,7,9,13,14] Glaucoma has also been reported in the American paint, Standardbred, Morgan, Trakehner, Percheron, mule, Paso Fino, Quarter horse, Tennessee Walking horse, Thoroughbred, Arabian, pony (Americas, Connemara, Shetland), American Saddlebred, and Warmblood.[6,7,9,13,14] Congenital glaucoma has been reported in Thoroughbred, Arabian, and Standardbred foals. [16-19]

Elevated IOP is clearly the primary risk factor for rapid progression of optic nerve damage and blindness in the horse, but iridocyclitis is the primary risk factor for development of glaucoma.[13,18,20]

Pathogenesis of Intraocular Pressure Elevation

Physical obstruction of the aqueous humor outflow pathways can occur as result of contraction of pre-iridal postinflammatory membranes; clogging of the ICA with inflammatory debris; and posterior synechia causing pupillary block, iris bombe, and trabecular compression and angle closure.[18,21] Postinflammatory uveal atrophy may predispose the ICA to collapse. Anterior lens luxation and vitreal prolapse appear common in Appaloosas and Rocky Mountain horses and may obstruct the pupil or the ICA. ICA obstruction by melanoma or other tumor cells can also occur.[14,18,21] Infectious endophthalmitis can cause secondary glaucoma.

IOP-induced, compressive conformational distortion within the scleral lamina cribrosa in glaucoma results in rotation, misalignment, and collapse of the laminar pores and laminar channels such that optic nerve axoplasmic flow is reduced and eventually blocked to cause RGC death. Glaucoma in the horse results in extensive and diffuse optic nerve damage, and the optic nerve axon density in horses with glaucoma is reduced by 65%.[7] Gliosis is dramatic, with primarily glial cells remaining in the severely atrophied optic nerves. The median individual optic nerve axon cross-sectional areas were smaller in glaucomatous eyes than in normal eyes (1.60 vs 1.35 μm^2), indicating that horses with glaucoma lose optic nerve axons of large individual cross-sectional area more rapidly than medium- and small-sized axons.[7]

DIAGNOSIS AND CLINICAL SIGNS OF GLAUCOMA

The diagnosis of equine glaucoma is made with the documentation of elevated IOP and the presence of clinical signs specific to glaucoma (Table 8-2). The IOP in horses with glaucoma and horses with ERU does not remain consistently elevated because large diurnal fluctuations in IOP can occur.[13] Frequent tonometric IOP measurements during the day may be necessary to detect transient IOP spikes. This wide variation in IOP not only interferes with the diagnosis of glaucoma but also complicates the monitoring of the response to therapy. The IOP will eventually decrease in buphthalmic globes as the ciliary body atrophies.

Equine glaucoma may not be easily recognized in the early stages of the disease because of the subtle clinical signs. Veterinarians generally have a low index of suspicion of glaucoma in horses with eye problems because the pupils are often only slightly dilated, and overt discomfort is uncommon. Afferent pupillary light reflex deficits, linear band opacities, mild corneal edema, decreased vision, lens luxations, mild iridocyclitis, and optic nerve atrophy/cupping may also be found in eyes of horses with glaucoma (Table 8-2). Linear "band opacities" are thinned areas of Descemet's membrane that resemble Haab striae but do not display the typical curling of the ruptured elastic basement membrane on histologic examination.[18,22] The band opacities in horses may be associated with edema in early stages and with fibrosis if glaucoma is chronic. They may also be found in normotensive eyes after traumatic corneal injury and in apparently "normal" eyes. Congenital glaucoma of foals may be bilateral. Corneal edema, corneal stria, mild buphthalmos, lens luxation, lens coloboma, absent corpora nigra, iris hypoplasia, retinal degeneration, and optic nerve cupping may also be found (Figs. 8-15 to 8-28).[16-19]

Fixed and dilated pupils are observed in horses with glaucoma. Positive dazzle and menace reflexes may remain in many eyes with glaucoma. The pupils may be miotic, and posterior synechia and iris bombe may be present in ERU cases. Some eyes may have subluxated or luxated lenses (Fig. 8-29).

Table 8-2	Clinical Signs of Glaucoma
Acute Glaucoma	**Chronic Glaucoma**
Mydriasis	Corneal edema may be
Corneal edema: mild	permanent
to severe	Extensive synechia in some
Lens subluxation to luxation	Lens luxation
Iridocyclitis: synechia, flare	Retinal degeneration
Linear band opacities:	Optic nerve atrophy with
normotensive eyes and	exposure of the
hypertensive eyes	lamina cribrosa
Blepharospasm: mild to severe	Buphthalmos
	Blindness

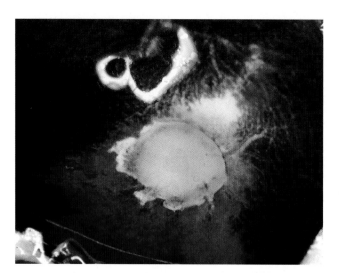

Fig. 8-15 This tissue photograph is of a pale, glaucomatous optic nerve and nontapetal depigmentation in a horse.

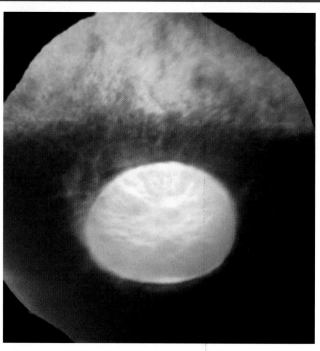

Fig. 8-16 This fundus photograph shows optic nerve atrophy caused by glaucoma. The anterior lamina cribrosa is seen as reticulated lines caused by loss of myelin and axons.

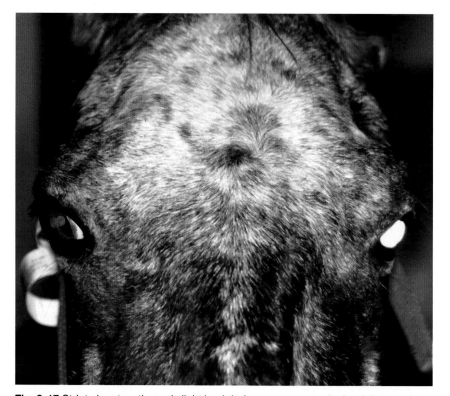

Fig. 8-17 Striate keratopathy and slight buphthalmos are present in the right eye of this Appaloosa with glaucoma.

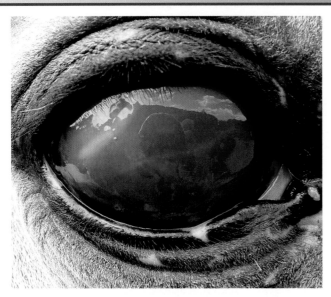

Fig. 8-18 Generalized corneal edema is present in this glaucomatous equine eye.

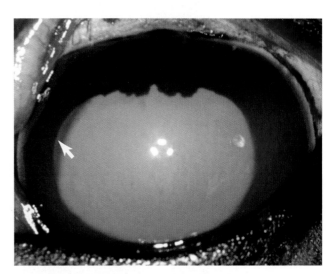

Fig. 8-20 The pupil is dilated and the cornea slightly edematous in this Thoroughbred mare with an intraocular pressure of 80 mm Hg. An aphakic crescent is noted nasally *(arrow)*.

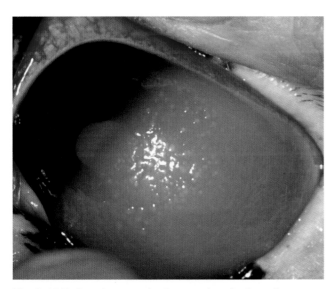

Fig. 8-19 Bullous keratopathy from profound edema is present in this glaucomatous globe in a horse.

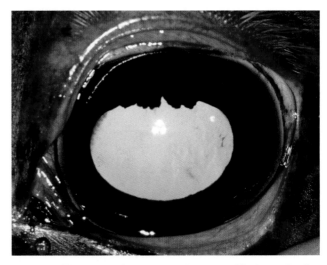

Fig. 8-21 The intraocular pressure is 20 mm Hg 1 month after transscleral cyclophotocoagulation in the eye shown in Fig. 8-20.

ONH cupping/degeneration will be present in advanced cases of equine glaucoma (Fig. 8-15). Areas of retinal degeneration may be present in some cases (Fig. 8-16). Buphthalmos will occur in eyes with end-stage glaucoma, and enucleation may be necessary (Fig. 8-17). Corneal edema and vascularization, buphthalmos, blindness caused by optic nerve atrophy, and pain in some cases characterize chronic glaucoma in the horse. An ulcerative exposure keratitis may also develop.

Glaucoma in the horse results in early peripheral retinal and optic nerve damage with progression to generalized retinal and optic nerve atrophy (Figs. 8-6 and 8-7). The equine eye seems to tolerate elevations in IOP that would quickly blind a dog; however, blindness is the result. The marked number of axons in the optic nerve of the horse may act as an anatomic reservoir of axons, which provides some early protection against total loss of vision despite very high IOP.

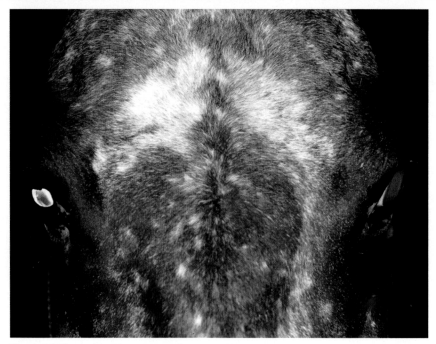

Fig. 8-22 The intraocular pressure is 65 mm Hg, the pupil is fixed and dilated, and the cornea is edematous in this buphthalmic left eye of an Appaloosa mare.

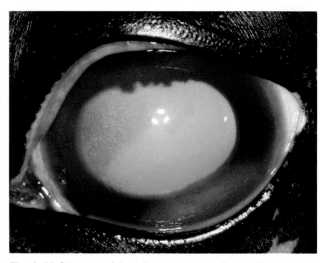

Fig. 8-23 Close-up of the left eye shown in Fig. 8-22.

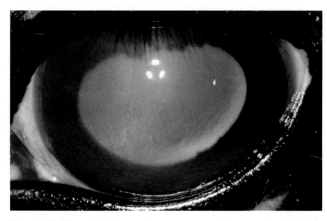

Fig. 8-24 Elevated intraocular pressure, edema, and mydriasis persist 10 days after initiation of medical therapy in the horse from Fig. 8-22.

Horses with glaucoma also appear to lose large optic nerve axons more rapidly than medium and small axons. Large RGCs are involved in motion detection, stereopsis, and sensitivity to dim light, but the consequences of the loss of such axons to the visual capabilities of the horse in early glaucoma are not known. The progressive, sustained elevation in IOP found in glaucoma in the horse is associated with optic nerve cupping, atrophy, and blindness (see Figs. 8-7, 8-15, and 8-16).

Hypertensive Iridocyclitis

Classic iridocyclitis in ERU is associated with hypotony caused by decreased production of aqueous humor by the ciliary body and increased absorption of aqueous humor by the iris, ciliary body, and trabecular meshworks. Some cases of "glaucoma" in horses may actually be eyes with iridocyclitis (ERU) that are in a phase of ocular hypertension or elevated IOP.[11] This might explain the cases of "glaucoma" that resolve with therapy and

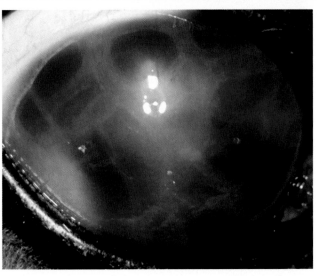

Fig. 8-25 Large band opacities or striae are present in this glaucomatous equine eye.

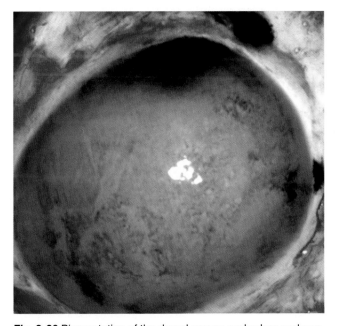

Fig. 8-26 Pigmentation of the dorsal cornea and sclera and generalized corneal edema are found in an eye with glaucoma caused by an intraocular melanoma.

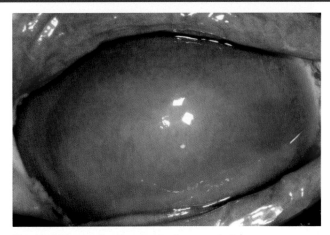

Fig. 8-27 Generalized corneal edema and glaucoma are present in an eye that had some unknown "trauma."

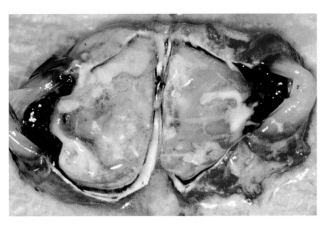

Fig. 8-28 Suppurative endophthalmitis from a gram-negative rod infection caused the glaucoma in the eye from Fig 8-27.

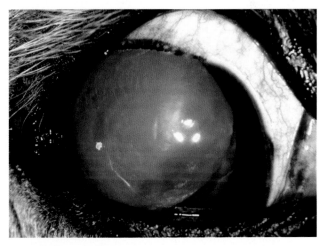

Fig. 8-29 Anterior lens luxation and secondary glaucoma in a 21-year-old Arabian mare.

appear to have no effect on vision. Differentiating true glaucoma cases from uveitic ocular hypertension in horses is not possible at present. Both equine glaucoma and ERU are associated with RGC death.[7,18,23]

MEDICAL TREATMENT

The events and mechanisms that lead to obstruction of aqueous humor outflow and increased IOP in the horse are not well understood, which makes it very difficult to institute effective therapy. Medical management of equine glaucoma follows the same general guidelines as that for glaucoma in other species, with the aims of therapy being reduction of IOP and suppression of iridocyclitis (Table 8-3). The initial response to

IOP-reducing medical therapy in early cases of equine glaucoma is usually good, but the long-term prognosis for maintaining vision with medical therapy alone is guarded. However, partial vision may be retained for extended periods, despite dramatically high IOP, in some horses. Glaucoma is particularly aggressive and difficult to control in the Appaloosa.

The goals of therapy in glaucoma are to reduce the IOP to levels that are compatible with the health of the retina and optic nerve by decreasing production of aqueous humor by the ciliary body and increasing outflow of aqueous humor through the conventional and unconventional outflow systems. Iridocyclitis must be vigorously suppressed if it is present. Various combinations of drugs and surgery may be needed to reduce the IOP to selected target levels that are compatible with preservation of vision in horses with glaucoma. A target IOP of <20 mm Hg is a reasonable goal in the glaucomatous equine eye. Control of IOP can improve vision in horses with decreased vision through resolution of marked corneal edema and improvement of vascular perfusion.

The β-adrenergic blocker timolol maleate (0.5%) can decrease the IOP in the equine eye by 17% (4.2 mm Hg) if it is administered topically twice a day.[24] β-Blockers interfere with the production of cyclic adenosine monophosphate by the enzyme adenyl cyclase to reduce aqueous humor production. The maximum effect is in the afternoon and occurs 4.5 days after administration. A decrease in pupil size has also been observed in one study, but there were no other adverse effects.[24]

Aqueous humor production can also be reduced if 99% of the carbonic anhydrase enzyme in the ciliary body is inhibited. The carbonic anhydrase inhibitor dorzolamide (2%) alone or in combination with timolol maleate is effective in lowering IOP by 10% (2 mm Hg)

when administered topically twice a day in horses.[25] Once-a-day use actually increased IOP in horses.[24]

Acetazolamide, dichlorphenamide, and methazolamide are systemically administered carbonic anhydrase inhibitors used for short-term IOP reduction in horses. They can aid the patient because they bring IOP "spiking" under control. When acetazolamide is given orally, it is absorbed rapidly and has somewhat lower bioavailability, but it is eliminated more slowly than when it is administered intravenously.[26] A dose of 2 to 3 mg/kg, administered orally two to four times a day, "may be useful" for lowering IOP.[26] Both dichlorphenamide (1 mg/kg twice a day) and methazolamide (0.25 mg/kg) are administered orally. Administration of systemic carbonic anhydrase inhibitors should be accompanied by electrolyte supplementation because of presumed potassium loss.

Direct and indirect acting parasympathomimetic drugs increase the facility of aqueous outflow in many mammals by constricting the ciliary muscles to open the trabecular meshworks. These drugs also inhibit unconventional outflow. Pilocarpine (2% every 6 hours) has been used to treat glaucoma in horses, but it does not significantly decrease IOP in horses and may exacerbate iridocyclitis. Pilocarpine is irritating to the eye, causes miosis, and may cause elevations (~24%) in IOP in some eyes.[27] Acetylcholinesterase inhibitors such as demecarium bromide have effects similar to those of pilocarpine. The use of these drugs in horses with glaucoma is no longer recommended.

Prostaglandin analogues are members of a new class of ocular hypotensive drugs developed for treatment of glaucoma in humans. Latanoprost (0.005%) is an analogue of prostaglandin F_{2a} that increases uveoscleral outflow, induces miosis, and has a small effect on IOP in the equine eye if administered once a day.[28] It lowered IOP by 1 mm Hg in geldings (5%) and 3 mm Hg in mares (17%). Prostaglandin-induced adverse effects included conjunctival hyperemia, epiphora, and blepharospasm. Synthetic prostaglandins dramatically potentiate the clinical signs of uveitis and should be used cautiously in horses with glaucoma and quiescent uveitis. They should not be used in glaucomatous eyes with mild or active iridocyclitis[29] because phthisis bulbi can result from severe hypotony induced by the prostaglandin. The newer prostaglandin derivatives may exacerbate the elevation in IOP in some horses with glaucoma.

Atropine has been recommended as possible therapy for equine glaucoma.[2,14] It was once thought to reduce the incidence of glaucoma in horses with uveitis but should be used cautiously in horses with glaucoma because it may cause IOP spikes and does not appear to have the benefit of lowering IOP as once proposed. Atropine, administered once a day, had no effect on

Table 8-3	Topically Applied Medications for Equine Glaucoma		
Medication	**Type**	**Dose**	
Timolol maleate 0.5%	β-Blocker	0.2 ml bid	
Dorzolamide 2%*	CAI	0.2 ml bid	
Latanoprost 0.005%†	Prostaglandin	0.2 ml qd‡	
Atropine 1%	Anticholinergic	0.2 ml bid§	
Prednisolone acetate 1%	Corticosteroid	0.2 ml tid	

bid, Twice a day; tid, three times a day.
*Cosopt (combination of timolol and dorzolamide), Merck & Co., Whitehouse Station, NJ.
†Xalatan, Pharmacia and Upjohn, Kalamazoo, Mich.
‡Not recommended unless close tonometric monitoring is available.
§Selected cases with strict intraocular pressure tonometric monitoring.

IOP but caused mydriasis.[30] Atropine administered twice a day caused an 11% reduction in IOP in treated eyes of 10 horses and an increase in IOP in one horse.[31] Use of topically administered atropine for the specific purpose of IOP reduction is no longer recommended unless the horse can be closely monitored with a tonometer.

Antiinflammatory therapy consisting of topically administered corticosteroids such as prednisolone acetate and systemically administered nonsteroidal antiinflammatory drugs such as phenylbutazone and flunixin meglumine are beneficial in the control of the iridocyclitis inducing the elevation in IOP. A topical nonsteroidal antiinflammatory drug such as diclofenamic acid and systemically administered dexamethasone may also be used.

SURGICAL TREATMENT

When medical therapy is inadequate, surgery should be performed to control IOP and preserve vision in the horse with glaucoma. The surgical options for a visual eye include transscleral laser cyclophotoablation and gonioimplant filtration procedures in the equine patient with glaucoma that has some vision. Cyclocryoablation, ciliary body ablation, placement of intrascleral prostheses, and enucleation are indicated for blind, chronically painful, and buphthalmic eyes.

Transscleral Cyclophotocoagulation

When IOP cannot be controlled with medical therapy, Nd:YAG or diode laser cyclophotocoagulation or ablation may be a viable alternative for long-term IOP control (Fig. 8-30). Transscleral laser cyclophotoablation involves the use of laser energy to preferentially destroy the ciliary body epithelium and stroma of the pars plicata, thereby reducing aqueous humor production. Of the various laser sources available, the Nd:YAG laser and semiconductor diode laser have been used most commonly for cyclophotoablation in veterinary ophthalmology. Contact transscleral laser cyclophotocoagulation (TSCPC) is effective in controlling IOP and maintaining vision in the horse (Figs. 8-31 to 8-33). Laser cyclophotocoagulation is least efficacious in lowering IOP and maintaining vision in equine eyes that are atropine responsive, suggesting that these eyes are utilizing their unconventional aqueous humor outflow pathways.

A mean drop of 17 mm Hg can be expected during the first few days after Nd:YAG laser TSCPC in the glaucomatous equine eye. The IOP-lowering effects occur 2 to 4 weeks after diode laser cyclophotocoagualtion. The IOP was 25 mm Hg less at 20 weeks after laser cyclophotocoagulation.[32] Forty to 60 sites 4 to 6 mm posterior to the limbus, except nasally, should be targeted with the laser.[32-34] Accurate anatomic positioning of TSCPC optimizes therapeutic outcomes.[33] The settings for the Nd:YAG laser are 10 W, 0.4 sec.[32]

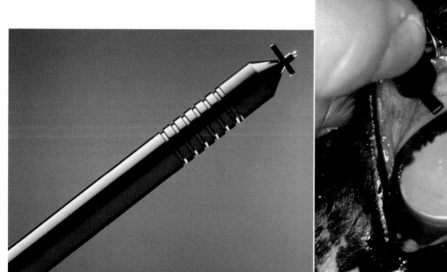
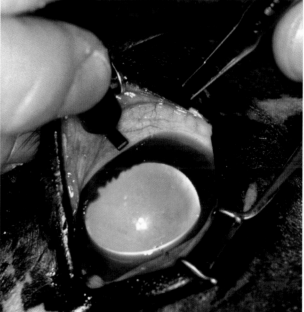

Fig. 8-30 A diode laser is used for transscleral cyclophotocoagulation of the eye shown in Fig. 8-23. **A,** Tip of the diode laser glaucoma probe. **B,** Placement of the laser probe on the equine eye.

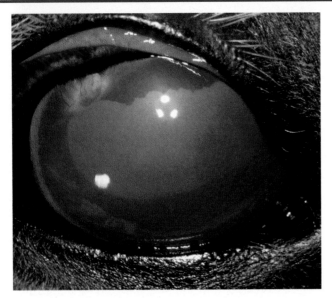

Fig. 8-31 Generalized corneal edema and mydriasis are present in the glaucomatous eye of a Paso Fino stallion. Intraocular pressure is 55 mm Hg.

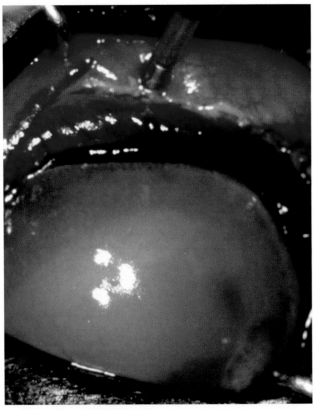

Fig. 8-32 Nd:YAG laser transscleral cyclophotocoagulation is performed on the eye shown in Fig. 8-31.

The settings for the diode laser are 1500 mW power, 1500-msec duration (2.25 J/site).[33,34] Too little laser energy (0.75 J/site) does not cause sufficient coagulative necrosis to the pars plicata, whereas too much laser energy (4 J/site) will cause too much collateral normal tissue damage.[34]

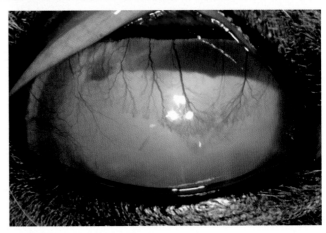

Fig. 8-33 The intraocular pressure is 20 mm Hg, and the is eye stable and quiet 5 months after laser cyclophotocoagulation in the eye shown in Fig. 8-31.

Uveitis and corneal edema will increase initially after TSCPC. Medical therapy must be maintained until the iridocyclitis is reduced and the IOP diminished after laser cytophotocoagulation. Laser therapy should not be performed until any uveitis or corneal edema present is controlled with corticosteroids. The corneal edema of the horse with glaucoma appears to be due more to uveitis than to increased IOP, and this corneal edema may become permanent after laser cyclophotocoagulation as a result of increased uveitic damage to the corneal endothelium.

Superficial corneal ulcers may develop as a result of corneal desensitization from the TSCPC or exposure during the procedure.

Gonioimplants

Gonioimplant filtration surgeries to bypass the obstructed ICA and direct the outflow of aqueous humor to the subconjunctival spaces are experimental in the horse (Fig. 8-34) but have been successful.[35] They have a short lifespan because of fibrosis of the drainage tube and/or filtration bleb.

Cyclocryosurgery

Blind, buphthalmic eyes can benefit from nitrous oxide–induced cryodestruction of the ciliary body, or cyclocryotherapy. A 3-mm–diameter cryoprobe is placed on the conjunctiva/sclera 6 mm posterior to the limbus for a 1-minute freeze-thaw cycle in six locations. Cyclocryotherapy is associated with severe postoperative iridocyclitis and should only be used in blind eyes.[36] The IOP-lowering effects may only last 6 weeks, and cyclocryotherapy may need to be repeated.

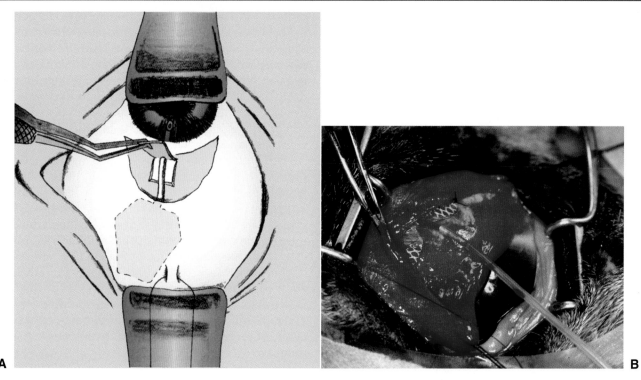

A   **B**

Fig. 8-34 Implantation of a gonioimplant for treatment of glaucoma. **A,** Schematic of placement of a gonioimplant. **B,** A gonioimplant is placed in the eye of an Appaloosa with glaucoma that was not responsive to medical therapy.

Ciliary Body Ablation

Intravitreal injection of intravenous gentamicin (25 mg with 1 mg of dexamethasone) can induce phthisis bulbi in a blind equine eye to result in varying degrees of pain reduction. A single injection is typically sufficient for pain reduction, but a second may be necessary in some cases. After sedation, frontal nerve block, instillation of topical anesthetic and phenylephrine (2.5% to vasoconstrict conjunctival vessels), and with appropriate restraint, the ciliary body ablation is performed with a 20-gauge needle attached to a 3-ml syringe. The needle is positioned dorsolaterally, approximately 7 mm posterior to the limbus at a 45-degree angle (toward the optic nerve and away from the lens). Before the gentamicin/dexamethasone is injected, an equal volume (or greater) of vitreous is aspirated. If no vitreous can be aspirated, an aqueous paracentesis can be performed to decrease the intraocular volume and thereby temporarily decrease IOP. Progressive increases in globe size (buphthalmos) may be prevented. Equal volumes of dexamethasone may minimize discomfort from the injection.

Salvage Procedures

Eyes with glaucoma caused by infection or intraocular tumors and eyes with painful lens luxations should

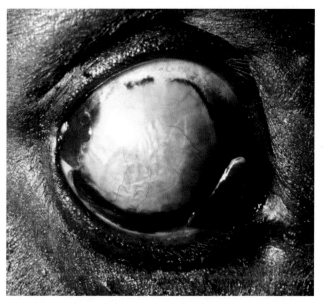

Fig. 8-35 An intraocular silicone prosthesis 1 year after evisceration of the eye because of chronic glaucoma. Although the cornea was scarred, the horse appeared comfortable and received no therapy.

be enucleated. Chronically painful and blind eyes and severely buphthalmic globes should be enucleated or have intrascleral prostheses implanted. A 34- to 44-mm–diameter intrascleral silicone implant can provide a cosmetic alternative to enucleation (Fig. 8-35).[37] Intraorbital silicone implants can minimize the pitting of the skin after enucleation (for more information, see the discussion of diseases of the globe and orbit in Chapter 2).

WHY IS EQUINE GLAUCOMA AN "ENIGMA"?

Glaucoma in the horse consists of many conflicting "facts" and clinical anecdotes. The true nature of equine glaucoma remains a puzzle. Glaucoma in horses results in the death of a neuron, the RGC, and causes persistent elevations in IOP. Ganglion cells also die in ERU.[37] ERU is also associated with "hypertensive" phases of IOP. The relationship between these two eye diseases of horses is quite similar and parallel.

Despite a large population of large-diameter optic nerve axons, the horse can maintain functional vision in spite of elevated IOP. This occurs despite the fact that the critical collapsing pressure of large-diameter axons is lower than that of small-diameter axons.[7] Such large axons must be under severe stresses during glaucomatous episodes. Does the equine eye have a reservoir of RGCs and axons that allows for some vision despite the progressive glaucoma damage, or do these axons not collapse until late in the disease?

Tonographic values indicate a large functioning conventional outflow system, and the structure of the ICA indicates an apparent prominence of the unconventional outflow system. It thus appears that the equine eye has both outflow pathways available. Is this why glaucoma is rarely diagnosed in the early stages? Uveoscleral outflow is independent of IOP and morphologically prominent in the horse. Does this correlate to a safety mechanism for preventing complete aqueous humor obstruction? Or does the unconventional outflow system not work in the horse, as suggested by the microanatomy? The optic nerve axons can only tolerate high IOP if the IOP is balanced by an increase in the ophthalmic artery pressure. Is this ocular perfusion pressure gradient elevated in the equine eye and thus more important than IOP?

Pilocarpine contracts the weak ciliary muscles and reduces the intercellular spaces in the supraciliary space of the horse but does not lower IOP.[2,27] Pilocarpine acts by inducing the ciliary musculature to contract and

pull on the "scleral spur" in human eyes. In horses, neither of these structures is well developed, so it makes sense that pilocarpine would have little effect on aqueous outflow. The IOP is not responsive to atropine in most equine glaucomatous eyes, although it may decrease IOP by a small percentage in healthy horses.[31] Considering the prominence of the two types of aqueous drainage pathways in the horse, these results are surprising and somewhat confusing.

Many "glaucoma" cases in horses may actually be eyes with "hypertensive uveitis" from ERU, thus displaying less RGC degeneration and able to maintain sight once the IOP and uveitis are controlled. This "glaucoma" may even be "cured." Eyes with "hypertensive uveitis" can have a resolution of their clinical signs, but eyes with true glaucoma will progress to blindness.

Haab striae in normotensive and nonbuphthalmic equine globes are not "breaks" or "ruptures" in Descemet's membrane, as is the case in dogs.[13,14,18,22] How do these thinned areas occur in nonbuphthalmic eyes? Is the elasticity of Descemet's membrane in horses unique?

Glaucomatous globes in horses respond to TSCPC better than those in other species.[33] TSCPC damages the supraciliary spaces and ciliary body, but the IOP eventually declines in most horses.

FUTURE STUDY

There is much that is not understand in the pathogenesis of equine glaucoma. Until better knowledge of the disease processes is available, controlling the disease will be difficult. Understanding why the horse maintains vision despite chronically high IOP may also assist in the management of canine glaucoma. Furthermore, the relationship between ERU and glaucoma remains poorly understood.

ACKNOWLEDGMENTS

Drs. Michael Boeve, Sheila Crispin, Raine Karpinski, Derek Knottenbelt, Margie Neaderland, and Andy Matthews assisted us in writing this chapter.

REFERENCES

1. Samuelson D A, Smith P J, Brooks DE: Morphologic features of the aqueous humor drainage pathways in horses, *Am J Vet Res* 50:720-727, 1989.
2. Smith PJ et al: Unconventional aqueous humor outflow of microspheres perfused into the equine eye, *Am J Vet Res* 47: 2445-2453, 1986.
3. DeGeest JP et al: The morphology of the equine iridocorneal angle: a light and scanning electron microscopic study, *Equine Vet J Suppl* 3:30-35, 1990.
4. Miller PE, Pickett JP, Majors LJ: Evaluation of two applanation tonometers in horses, *Am J Vet Res* 51:935-937, 1990.
5. Van Der Woerdt A et al: Effect of auriculopalpebral nerve block and intravenous administration of xylazine on intraocular pressure and corneal thickness in horses, *Am J Vet Res* 56:155-158, 1995.
6. Smith PJ et al: Tonometric and tonographic studies in the normal pony eye, *Equine Vet J Suppl* 3:36-38, 1990.

7. Brooks DE et al: Histomorphometry of the optic nerves of normal horses and horses with glaucoma, *Vet Comp Ophthalmol* 5:193-210, 1995.

8. Brooks DE et al: Immunohistochemistry of the extracellular matrix of the normal equine lamina cribrosa, *Vet Ophthalmol* 3:127-132, 2000.

9. Yablonski ME, Asamoto A: Hypothesis concerning the pathophysiology of optic nerve damage in open angle glaucoma, *J Glaucoma* 2:119-127, 1993.

10. Brooks DE, Komaromy AM, Kallberg ME: Comparative optic nerve physiology: implications for glaucoma, neuroprotection and neuroregeneration, *Vet Ophthalmol* 2:13-26, 1999.

11. Nicolas E: Veterinary and comparative ophthalmology. London, 1925, H & W Brown Publishers, pp 399-406. (Translated by H Gray).

12. Carter HE: Incurable blindness in horses: a nineteenth-century view, *Vet Int* 1:47-52, 1992.

13. Miller TR et al: Equine glaucoma: clinical findings and response to treatment in 14 horses, *Vet Comp Ophthalmol* 5:170-182, 1995.

14. Brooks DE: Equine glaucoma. In Robinson NE, editor: *Current therapy in equine medicine* ed 5, Philadelphia, 2003, WB Saunders, pp 486-488.

15. USA Horse Population Data: *The economic impact of the horse industry in the United States,* Washington, DC, 1996, American Horse Council Foundation.

16. Gelatt KN: Glaucoma and lens luxation in a foal, *Vet Med Small Anim Clin* 68:261-263, 1973.

17. Barnett KC et al: Buphthalmos in a Thoroughbred foal, *Equine Vet J* 20:132-135, 1988.

18. Wilcock BP, Brooks DE, Latimer CA: Glaucoma in horses, *Vet Pathol* 28:74-78, 1991.

19. Halenda RM et al: Congenital equine glaucoma: clinical and light microscopic findings in two cases, *Vet Comp Ophthalmol* 7:105-116, 1997.

20. Pickett JP, Ryan J: Equine glaucoma: a retrospective study of 11 cases from 1988 to 1993, *Vet Med* 88:756-763, 1993.

21. Barnett KC et al: *Color atlas of equine ophthalmology*, London, 1995, Mosby-Wolfe, pp 142-145.

22. Heusser H: Ueber flecken und vascularization der Hornhaut des pferdes, *Graefes Arch Ophthalmol* 106: 10-62, 1921.

23. Deeg CA et al: Immunopathology of recurrent uveitis in spontaneously diseased horses, *Exp Eye Res* 75:127-133, 2002.

24. Van Der Woerdt A et al: Effect of single- and multiple-dose 0.5% timolol maleate on intraocular pressure and pupil size in female horses, *Vet Ophthalmol* 3:165-168, 2000.

25. Willis AM et al: Effect of topical administration of 2% dorzolamide hydrochloride or 2% dorzolamide hydrochloride-0.5% timolol maleate on intraocular pressure in clinically normal horses, *Am J Vet Res* 62:709-713, 2001.

26. Alberts MK et al: Pharmacokinetics of acetazolamide after intravenous and oral administration in horses, *Am J Vet Res* 61: 965-968, 2000.

27. Van Der Woerdt A et al: Normal variation in, and effect of 2% pilocarpine on, intraocular pressure and pupil size in female horses, *Am J Vet Res* 59:1459-1462, 1998.

28. Davidson HJ et al: Effect of topical ophthalmic latanoprost on intraocular pressure in normal horses, *Vet Ther* 3:72-80, 2002.

29. Willis AM et al: Effects of topical administration of 0.005% latanoprost solution on eyes of clinically normal horses, *Am J Vet Res* 62:1945-1951, 2001.

30. Mughannam AJ, Buyukmihci NC, Kass PH: Effect of topical atropine on intraocular pressure and pupil diameter in the normal horse eye, *Vet Ophthalmol* 2:213-215, 1999.

31. Herring IP et al: Effect of topical 1% atropine sulfate on intraocular pressure in normal horses, *Vet Ophthalmol* 3:139-143, 2000.

32. Whigham HM et al: Treatment of equine glaucoma by transscleral neodymium:yttrium aluminum garnet laser cyclophotocoagulation: a retrospective study of 23 eyes of 16 horses, *Vet Ophthalmol* 2:243-250, 1999.

33. Miller TL et al: Description of ciliary body anatomy and identification of sites for transscleral cyclophotocoagulation in the equine eye, *Vet Ophthalmol* 4:183-190, 2001.

34. Morreale R, Wilkie DA, et al: The effect of varying laser energy on semiconductor diode laser transscleral cyclophotocoagulation (TSCP) in the normal equine eye. Proceedings of the American College of Veterinary Ophthalmology, Denver, Colo, October 9-13, 2002, p 31 (abstract).

35. Kellner SJ: Glaukom beim Pferd-2. Teil. [Glaucoma in the horse. Part II.] *Pferdeheilkunde* 10:261-266, 1994.

36. Frauenfelder HC, Vestre WA: Cryosurgical treatment of glaucoma in a horse, *Vet Med Small Anim Clin* 76:183-186, 1981.

37. Meek LA: Intraocular silicone prosthesis in a horse, *J Am Vet Med Assoc* 193:343-345, 1988.

9 Diseases of the Ocular Posterior Segment

David A. Wilkie

Evaluation of the posterior segment of the equine eye is an essential part of an ophthalmic, pre-purchase, and general physical examination. Initial examination includes a history with respect to vision, determination of menace and pupillary light responses, and evaluation of clarity of transmitting media (cornea, aqueous, lens, vitreous). The resting pupil size and direct and consensual pupillary light response are evaluated. Menace response should be evaluated in various visual fields: anterior, central, and posterior. Although it is possible to examine portions of the fundus without dilation, for proper examination of the posterior segment of the equine eye, mydriasis, a darkened environment, and proper equipment are essential. Diagnostic mydriasis is achieved by using topical 1% tropicamide (Mydriacyl), which has an onset of action of 15 to 25 minutes and a duration of action of 8 to 12 hours. As a solution, 0.2 ml of tropicamide is easily applied with a tuberculin syringe and the hub of a 25-gauge needle and sprayed on the cornea. If required, sedation and nerve blocks can be performed to facilitate examination. Blocking of the auriculopalpebral nerve will facilitate examination by allowing the clinician to elevate the superior eyelid (see Chapter 1).

Both direct and indirect ophthalmoscopy should be used for examination of the equine posterior segment. Indirect examination is performed initially for an overview of the fundus, and direct ophthalmoscopy is preferred for detailed examination of the optic nerve and retinal blood vessels. Indirect examination with a 20-diopter (D) condensing lens and a Finoff transilluminator will provide a more panoramic but less magnified view of the fundus with lateral and axial magnifications of ×0.79 and ×0.84, respectively.[1] Indirect examination provides better visualization of the peripheral retina. Indirect examination can also be performed by using an indirect headset that provides stereopsis and leaves the examiner a free hand to elevate the superior eyelid (Figs. 9-1 and 9-2). Indirect examination allows visualization of the fundus through cloudy transmitting media, such as aqueous flare or lenticular sclerosis, which is often not possible with direct examination. To perform indirect examination, the examiner holds the light at arm's length from the horse's eye. A tapetal reflection is obtained, and a condensing lens is placed 2 to 8 cm in front of the horse's eye. A virtual, upside down, reversed image is created. If a headset is used, it will provide the examiner with illumination and stereopsis. Alternately, a device called a PanOptic ophthalmoscope (Welch Allyn, Skaneateles Falls, NY) can be used. This is an indirect, monocular ophthalmoscope that provides an erect image with a field of view greater than that provided by direct examination (for more information, see Chapter 1).

Direct examination provides the greatest magnification with lateral and axial magnifications of ×7.9 and ×8.4, respectively (Fig. 9-3).[1] Direct ophthalmoscopy should be used for detailed examination of the optic nerve, retinal blood vessels, and peripapillary region. For examination of the posterior segment, the direct ophthalmoscope is set to 0 D, and the ophthalmoscope is held approximately 2 cm from the horse's eye (Fig. 9-4). The optic nerve should be in focus for most examiners at this setting. Changing the diopter settings will allow the clinician to focus vitread or more posterior to determine whether an abnormality is elevated or depressed, respectively. The image obtained with a direct ophthalmoscope is upright and magnified (Fig. 9-5). Abnormalities of the cornea, aqueous, lens, and vitreous make direct examination difficult. In such instances, indirect examination should be performed.

Biomicroscopy should also be used for examination of not only the anterior segment but also the anterior third of the vitreous for vitreous syneresis, asteroid hyalosis, debris, membranes, vascular remnants, and hyalites (see Chapter 1 for more information).

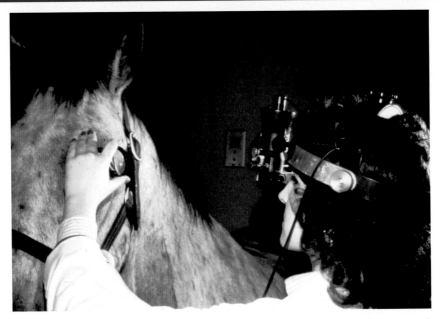

Fig. 9-1 Indirect ophthalmoscopic examination with a 20-diopter condensing lens and a headset.

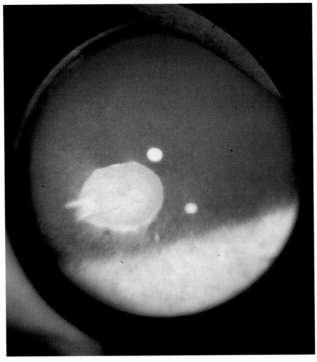

Fig. 9-2 View of the equine posterior segment as seen through a 20-diopter indirect lens. The image is upside down and reversed. A proliferation lesion is present on the optic nerve.

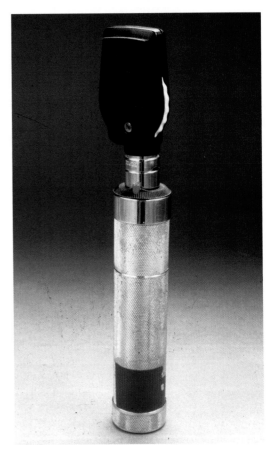

Fig. 9-3 Welch-Allyn direct ophthalmoscope.

During examination of the posterior segment, what the clinician sees is dependent on color and thickness of the three concentric tunics—the retina, choroid, and sclera—that comprise the posterior eye wall. The neurosensory retina (NSR) has the optical consistency of wax or tissue paper, rendering tissues below it less reflective and dull. A loss of retinal tissue will therefore increase the reflectivity and color of the underlying tissue. This is called hyperreflectivity in the tapetal fundus. Alternately, thickening of the retina (e.g., edema, cells, dysplasia) will obscure and dull the underlying tissue. The outermost layer of the retina is the monolayer, or retinal pigment epithelium (RPE),

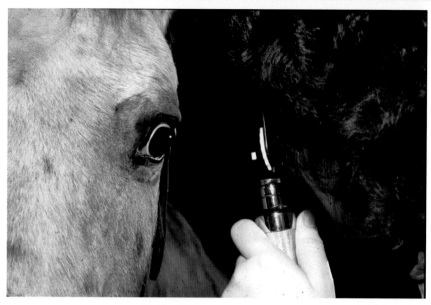

Fig. 9-4 Technique of direct ophthalmoscopy in the horse.

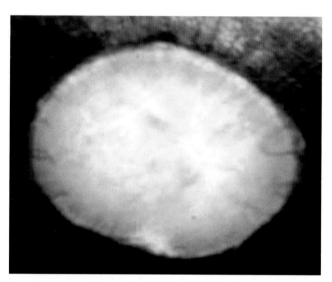

Fig. 9-5 Image of an equine optic nerve as seen by direct examination.

which is pigmented in the ventral nontapetal retina and nonpigmented over the tapetum in most horses. The choroid is composed of melanin-containing cells, blood vessels, and dorsally, the fibrous tapetum. The outermost tunic, the sclera, appears white. The color of the horse, amount of melanin, and thickness of the tapetum all influence the normal appearance on fundic examination. Normal variations are common, and the clinician must be familiar with these before being able to interpret and understand abnormalities.

Posterior segment examination should include evaluation of the vitreous, tapetal and nontapetal fundus, retina, retinal blood vessels, and optic nerve. Variations in the normal equine fundus are common, and familiarity with these variations is essential.[2-9]

Additional diagnostic tests may include ocular ultrasonography, computed tomography, electroretinography (ERG), and visual evoked potential (VEP).

Ultrasonography is indicated when opacities of the transmitting media prevent examination of the posterior segment. Typically, cataracts and hyphema are the most common indications for ultrasound examination of the posterior aspect of the globe.[10] A 5.0- to 20.0-MHz ultrasound probe will provide diagnostic images of the posterior globe. The 5.0-MHz probe provides less near-field resolution and greater penetration of the orbit, whereas the 20-MHz probe provides excellent resolution of the anterior segment, but the posterior eye wall is the limit of its penetration in the equine eye. Direct corneal contact with the use of petroleum jelly is the technique of choice, provided that the cornea is intact. Imaging can be performed through the eyelid if the cornea is compromised (see Chapter 1 for more information).

Evaluation of the orbit and optic nerve can be done by means of computed tomography with the horse under general anesthesia. A computed tomography scan is indicated for horses with suspected traumatic optic neuropathy or orbital and optic nerve mass lesions. ERG and VEPs are generally performed after general anesthesia has been induced, although the procedures can be done with sedation alone.[5] ERG is used to assess the overall health of the rod and cone photoreceptors, as well as the inner retina, whereas a VEP is used to evaluate transmission along the optic nerve and signal reception by the visual cortex. Normal values for both the ERG and VEP have been reported in the horse.[5]

Abnormalities on fundic examination include vitreous degeneration; membranes; inclusions and vascular remnants; changes in size, shape, and color of the optic nerve and retinal vessels; elevation or depression of the optic nerve; retinal dysplasia, detachment, and hemorrhage; changes in tapetal reflectivity (hyperreflective and hyporeflective); and changes in pigmentation. Most abnormalities are identified in the peripapillary region and can be visually significant because this area has a greater concentration of retinal axons. Abnormalities that are hyperreflective indicate thinning or loss of retinal tissue and are observed in the tapetal fundus. Hyperreflective changes include retinal atrophy or degeneration, retinal tears, and retinal detachment. Hyporeflective changes can indicate an increase in tissue thickness resulting from cellular infiltrates, edema, or folding of the retina as seen in retinal dysplasia. Hyporeflective changes appear dull gray or white, depending on the background (tapetal vs nontapetal). In addition, the retina may appear elevated. Inflammation can result in depigmentation and pigment clumping in the nontapetal fundus and hyperpigmentation in the tapetal fundus. These changes must be differentiated from normal variations in pigmentation of the RPE.

Posterior segment abnormalities can be congenital or acquired and include both primary ophthalmic and systemic diseases. When present, posterior segment abnormalities must be assessed with respect to current and future visual impact and importance with respect to usefulness and safety of the horse. The clinician should remember that much of what is examined by ophthalmoscopy is a direct extension of the brain and central nervous system. In addition, it is the only area where arterioles and venules can be viewed directly. This is, in reality, clinical histopathology. Lesions adjacent to the optic nerve or involving the area centralis will have a greater impact on vision than those that are more peripheral. The menace response in various visual fields and maze testing can be used to assess current vision. In addition, evidence of anterior segment disease or inflammation and the possibility of progression and future inflammatory episodes should be considered. Use of the animal must also be considered because a barrel horse or competitive jumper requires greater vision than a brood mare or halter show horse. The possibility that a lesion is inherited or breed-related should also be considered if the animal is to be used for breeding.

Despite the significance of the retina and choroid to vision, little is known about posterior segment diseases in the horse as compared with diseases of the anterior or posterior segment in other species. This may be a result of fewer inherited abnormalities and fewer infectious and hematogenous diseases because of the horse's paurangiotic retina, or it may simply reflect a lack of examination of the equine posterior segment by veterinarians.

CLINICAL ANATOMY AND PHYSIOLOGY

The posterior segment of the eye includes the vitreous, retina, choroid, sclera, and optic nerve. The anteriormost extent of the posterior segment is the ora ciliaris retinae. The anterior extension of the ora ciliaris varies by quadrant of the eye and is important because it has significance for glaucoma and vitreoretinal surgery.[11] The ora is located more anteriorly in the nasal and ventral quadrants and further posterior in the dorsal and temporal quadrants.[11] This makes the dorsal and temporal locations the areas of choice for surgical approaches to the posterior segment.

The vitreous body is predominately composed of type II collagen fibrils, hyaluronic acid, and water. It is divided into cortical, intermediate, and central zones and has a volume of approximately 28 ml in the adult horse.[12] Normally, the vitreous is transparent and uniform in appearance. Abnormalities of the vitreous generally result in loss of uniformity with debris, membranes, and collagen fibrils appearing to float and swirl in a liquid medium. In addition, changes in vitreous color are often noted as a result of inflammation. On ultrasonography, the vitreous is normally anechoic with increased vitreous echogenicity, indicating degeneration, inflammation, hemorrhage, mass lesions, or retinal detachment.

The horse has a paurangiotic (partially vascularized) retina with 30 to 60 small retinal vessels radiating from the margin of an elliptical optic disc. These vessels are visible for a distance of 1 to 2 disc diameters but are less prominent dorsal and ventral to the optic nerve (Fig. 9-6). The remainder of the equine retina is avascular, being supplied from the underlying choroid. The thickness of the NSR varies from 250 μm medial to the optic disc to 80 μm at the ora ciliaris.[13] The majority of the equine retina is <130 μm in thickness to allow for oxygen diffusion from the underlying choroid.[13] The choroidal or vascular tunic is external to the NSR. It is composed of the larger choroidal vessels, the tapetum, choriocapillaris, and melanocytes. In the equine eye, the choroid is responsible for the majority of retinal nutrition because the retina is paurangiotic.

The fundus is divided into the dorsal tapetal and ventral nontapetal regions. The fibrous tapetum is situated in the dorsal choroid and is responsible for the characteristic yellow-green color of this portion of the fundus. Variations in tapetal color are related to iris and coat color and include yellow, orange, and blue-green.[3,6,8] Dark bay and brown horses usually have a blue-green tapetum with a dark nontapetal region (Figs. 9-7 and 9-8). Lighter chestnuts and palominos may have a yellow tapetum with a less pigmented nontapetal region (Figs. 9-9 and 9-10). Gray and white horses generally have a yellow tapetum with a lightly

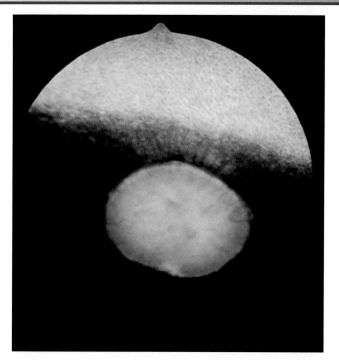

Fig. 9-6 Normal optic nerve and peripapillary fundus. Note the notch at the 6 o'clock optic nerve and the decrease in the number of retinal vessels in this region.

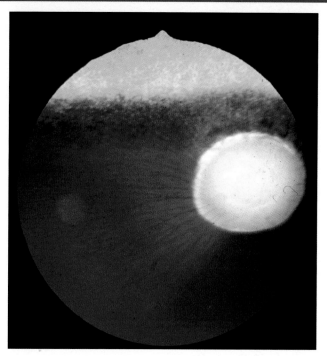

Fig. 9-8 Normal fundus with a green tapetum.

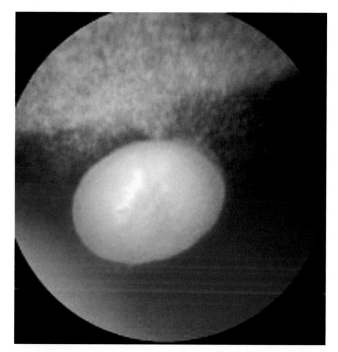

Fig. 9-7 Normal fundic photograph of a dark bay horse with a blue tapetum.

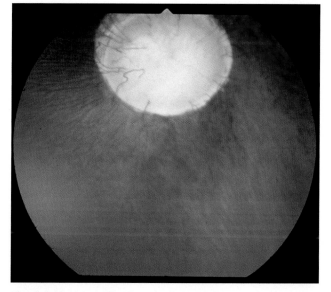

Fig. 9-9 Nontapetal fundus of a light-colored horse. An area of choroidal hypopigmentation is present, allowing visualization of the choroidal vasculature.

pigmented or nonpigmented nontapetal fundus. This may allow visualization of the choroidal vasculature and sclera. Finally, in color-dilute horses, the tapetum may be hypoplastic or absent.[14-16] Tapetal hypoplasia can be generalized or confined to a portion of the

tapetum, most often immediately dorsal to the optic disc (Fig. 9-11). Color and thickness of the tapetum and choroidal pigment vary not only between horses but also within horses from right to left eyes. Near the periphery of the tapetum, it is not unusual to see focal

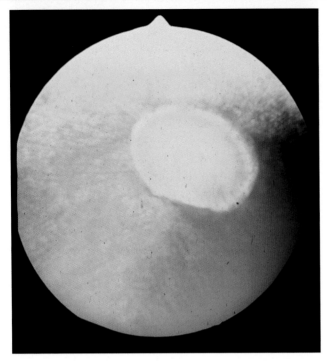

Fig. 9-10 Normal fundus of a palomino horse, demonstrating a yellow tapetum and area of choroidal hypopigmentation.

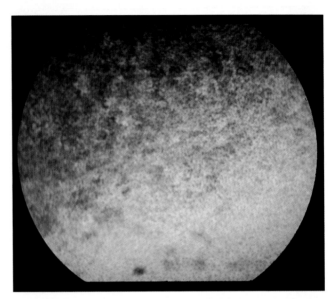

Fig. 9-12 Dorsal tapetum with areas of retinal pigment epithelium pigmentation obscuring the underlying green tapetum. This is a normal variation.

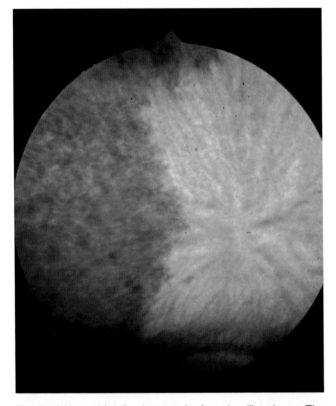

Fig. 9-11 Normal fundic photograph of a color-dilute horse. The edge of the optic nerve is visible ventrally. The tapetum is absent in half of the dorsal fundus, allowing visualization of the choroidal vasculature and sclera.

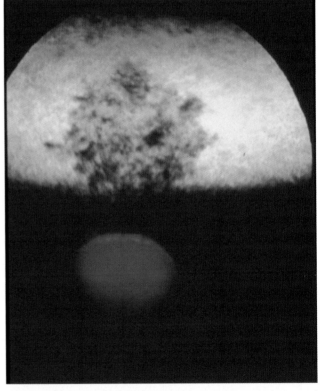

Fig. 9-13 Retinal pigment epithelium pigmentation over the tapetal retina dorsal to the optic nerve. This is a normal variation.

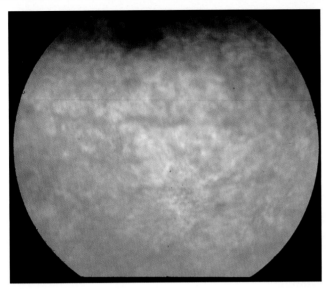

Fig. 9-14 Normal nontapetal fundus of a color-dilute horse. The underlying choroidal vasculature can be seen.

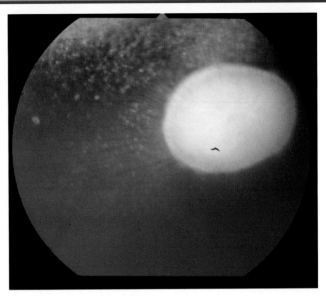

Fig. 9-15 Peripapillary pigment variation. Multifocal areas of hypopigmentation are noted. The overlying retinal vessels are normal.

areas of RPE pigmentation obscuring the underlying tapetum (Fig. 9-12). In addition, random foci of RPE pigmented freckles or nevi may appear throughout the tapetum (Fig. 9-13). These must be differentiated from postinflammatory hyperpigmentation or choroidal melanoma. The tapetum of the horse is penetrated by small choroidal arterioles, which serve to supply the retina via the choriocapillaris. These vessels are seen end-on on fundic examination and appear as uniformly distributed dark dots in the tapetum, called the stars of Winslow. The function of the tapetum is to enhance vision in low-light conditions by allowing reflected light the opportunity to stimulate the photoreceptors a second time. However, although the tapetum improves the threshold of light detection, it also causes glare and thereby decreases visual acuity in bright light.[14]

The ventral, nontapetal fundus is generally dark brown or black but can appear lighter or nonpigmented, depending on coat color.[6,8] In color-dilute horses the tapetum may be hypoplastic or absent, and the choroid and RPE may demonstrate partial or complete albinism. This can affect one or both eyes and can even be observed to vary within an eye. Choroidal vasculature and vortex veins may be visible, especially in association with tapetal hypoplasia and ocular albinism (Fig. 9-14).[3] These vessels may appear as radiating, dark striae seen through a normal tapetum or as red vessels in a subalbinotic to albinotic eye.

Focal areas of nonpigmentation or depigmentation are often observed in the peripapillary nontapetal fundus (Fig. 9-15). These are often normal variations, but because previous intraocular inflammation can also result in depigmentation, a complete ophthalmic examination should be performed to rule out prior disease. In addition, infection with equine herpesvirus-1 (EHV-1)

has been reported to result in focal white chorioretinal lesions in the nontapetal fundus (see discussion of chorioretinitis).[17]

The retina consists of the NSR and RPE. The photoreceptors, rods and cones, are located in the sensory retina. The rods predominate and are responsible for achromatic low-light vision, whereas the cones are responsible for vision in bright light and color vision. The horse lacks a fovea but has an area centralis, which serves as the area of maximum visual acuity and has an increased density of retinal ganglion cells. The equine area centralis is a horizontal band of 1 mm by 22 mm and is located approximately 3 mm dorso-temporal to the optic nerve.[18,19] The concentration of ganglion cells in the area centralis is 6000 cells/mm^2 as compared with <500 cells/mm^2 in the dorsal and ventral retina.[20] The horse has dichromatic vision with a short wavelength cone (spectral peak of 425 nm) and a middle wavelength cone (spectral peak of 540 nm).[21] This translates into a blue-gray and yellow-green visual spectrum. The visual field of the horse is approximately 350 degrees with a small area, 65 to 70 degrees, of binocular overlap.[5]

The optic disc is normally oval, salmon pink, and situated slightly temporal and ventral in the nontapetal fundus. The optic nerve will fill the view of a direct ophthalmoscope; it measures 3 to 5 mm vertically and has a horizontal diameter of 5 to 8 mm.[14] The optic nerve in foals may appear more round. The surface of the optic nerve is often irregular and honeycombed as a result of the axons exiting at the fibrous lamina cribrosa. Ventrally, the optic nerve may appear notched (Fig. 9-6). The equine optic nerve is composed of approximately 1 million axons, with larger axons found at the periphery of the optic nerve as compared with the central portion.[19,22] These large axons are

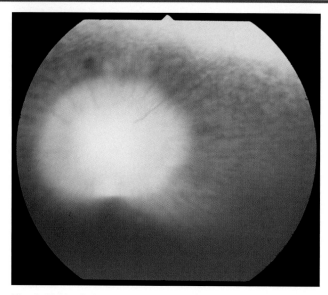

Fig. 9-16 Myelin is seen radiating from the optic nerve along the nerve fiber layer axons in an aged horse.

preferentially lost in equine glaucoma.[22] Although the optic nerve is myelinated, myelin does not typically extend to the intraocular portion of the nerve. If myelin does extend into the eye, it is most often associated with retinal vessels. Myelin extending along the nerve fiber layer axons appears as light gray striations and is more common in aged horses (Fig. 9-16). Radiating from the margin of the optic nerve are 30 to 60 small arterioles and venules. They cannot be distinguished from one another and may be absent at the 6 o'clock region of the nerve. These retinal vessels travel 1 to 2 optic disc diameters into the retina before they disappear. Occasionally, a small vessel may be seen to emerge from the central optic nerve and course across its surface. The margin of the optic nerve may have a peripapillary ring associated with changes in thickness of the tapetum or pigmentation of the RPE or choroid. This circumpapillary ring can be dark or hypopigmented. This is a normal variation, provided that the overlying retinal vessels do not deviate or attenuate while crossing this region. Changes in vessel direction or thickness suggest a coloboma or degeneration.

IMPACT OF DISEASE OF THE OCULAR POSTERIOR SEGMENT ON THE EQUINE INDUSTRY

The significance of posterior segment disease to an individual horse and the equine industry is difficult to quantitate. Equine recurrent uveitis (ERU) affects 5% to 15% of the equine population and is the most common cause of posterior segment abnormalities. As a result of ERU, secondary glaucoma, retinal detachment, and retinal and optic nerve degeneration may affect vision and thus function. These changes are generally observed by owners and can be quantitated. However, more subtle lesions may go unnoticed, resulting in poor performance and affecting use without the owner being aware of the reason. In addition, posterior segment abnormalities noted on a pre-purchase examination may result in a loss of value. Finally, horses with posterior segment lesions significant enough to result in visual disturbance may present a safety concern for the owner with respect to riding, driving, or behavior. The impact of posterior segment disease is significantly greater than has been appreciated, and veterinarians are strongly encouraged to make examination of the posterior segment a routine part of a physical examination.

CONGENITAL DISEASES

Congenital abnormalities of the equine posterior segment are uncommon. They can be seen alone or in association with multiple congenital anomalies such as anterior segment dysgenesis, congenital megaloglobus, the Rocky Mountain horse (RMH) syndrome, and other such ocular anomalies. In one study, the incidence of congenital ocular abnormalities was 0.5% of all equine cases presented.[23]

Subretinal and intraretinal hemorrhages may be noted in neonatal foals.[24] In one study of 167 neonatal Thoroughbred foals, 27 (16%) were found to have retinal hemorrhages.[24] Most hemorrhages were bilateral, and females were more commonly affected than males.[24] Hemorrhages were punctate in 36% and "splash-like" in 56%; the number of hemorrhages per eye ranged from 1 to 20.[24] Such hemorrhages may be the result of intraocular vascular hypertension with capillary rupture during parturition.[14] Hemorrhages will resolve over a few weeks with no visual or residual abnormalities.[24]

Colobomas

Colobomas are absences of or defects in normal ocular tissue and typically occur in the area of the embryonic optic fissure, which is ventral to slightly ventronasal; if colobomas are noted elsewhere, they are considered atypical. Colobomas can be unilateral or bilateral and can affect the iris, ciliary body, lens, retina, choroid, optic disc, and sclera.[3,15,16,25-27] They can occur alone or in association with multiple congenital ocular anomalies.

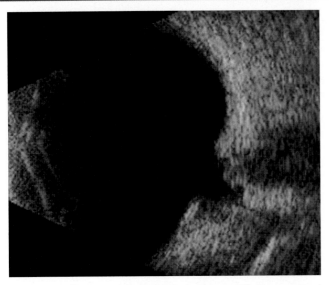

Fig. 9-17 Ultrasound examination of a posterior segment coloboma. The posterior eye wall extends posteriorly toward the orbit in the area of the optic nerve.

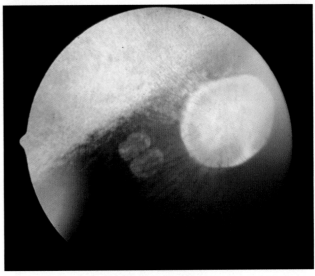

Fig. 9-18 Two "window defects" or retinal pigment epithelium colobomas are noted adjacent to the optic nerve.

One report of a Thoroughbred with bilateral optic disc colobomas also included mention of microphthalmos, microcornea, and iris and lens abnormalities.[28] Posterior segment colobomas have been found to affect the optic disc in horses, most commonly the Quarter horse.[25-27] Others report a predisposition in the Appaloosa.[14] Optic nerve colobomas accounted for 1.8% of all congenital ocular anomalies in one study.[23] Small colobomas must be distinguished from the small 6 o'clock notch and peripapillary ring that can be normal in some horse optic nerves (Fig. 9-6).[14] Severe colobomas involving the optic disc have been associated with vision deficits, specifically in the Quarter horse (Fig. 9-17).[25-27]

Clinical Appearance and Diagnosis

Colobomas can involve other areas of the fundus and appear white (complete absence of choroid) or orange and white (some choroidal vasculature present). Involvement of the area centralis will have a more significant impact on vision, although most horses with colobomas are asymptomatic. On ophthalmoscopic examination, the edges of the coloboma may appear recessed below the surrounding tissue.

Additionally, a "window defect" involving the RPE has been described as an RPE coloboma (Fig. 9-18).[3,14] The abnormality occurs most commonly in the nontapetal fundus adjacent to the optic disc and appears as a sharply demarcated focal area of decreased pigmentation. Such an abnormality has no known visual or genetic significance.

Treatment

There is no treatment for colobomas.

Long-Term Prognosis and Inheritability Information

Given the predisposition of colobomas in Quarter horses, breeding of affected animals and their sires and dams should be avoided.

Optic Nerve Hypoplasia

Optic nerve hypoplasia can be unilateral or bilateral and is a rare congenital abnormality.[29] Optic nerve hypoplasia accounted for 0.9% of all congenital ocular anomalies in one study.[23]

Clinical Appearance and Diagnosis

In optic nerve hypoplasia, the optic nerve appears pale, is smaller than normal, and may be depressed or recessed; retinal vessels are difficult to visualize.[14,30] Numbers of retinal ganglion cells are reduced, the pupil is dilated, and the pupillary light response is reduced or absent.[14] Nystagmus and decreased to absent vision are also observed.

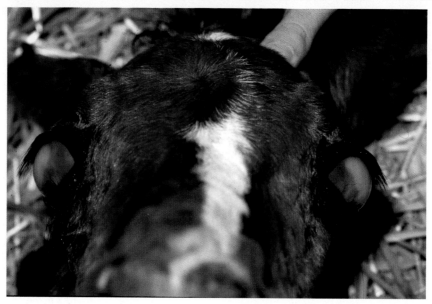

Fig. 9-19 Gross photograph of a foal with bilateral congenital megaloglobus and corneal opacities.

Treatment

There is no treatment for optic nerve hypoplasia.

Long-Term Prognosis and Inheritability Information

The cause is not known, visual loss depends on severity, and affected horses should not be used for breeding.

Retinal Dysplasia

Retinal dysplasia is a congenital malformation of the retina with the formation of folds or rosettes that appear clinically as retinal folds or larger areas of geographic dysplasia. Retinal dysplasia can be developmental or occur as a result of inflammation. Retinal dysplasia accounted for 3.5% of all congenital ocular anomalies in one study.[23]

Clinical Appearance and Diagnosis

On ophthalmoscopic examination, dysplasia can appear as gray or hyperpigmented areas caused by retinal disorganization and RPE proliferation, respectively. Histologically, the NSR is folded and disorganized, often forming rosettes. The rosettes can be single or multiple and unilateral or bilateral. Retinal folds can be associated with in utero infections and have been attributed to various viral infections. In other species they are also seen in association with multiple congenital ocular anomalies, which are inherited. One example of multiple congenital anomalies with associated retinal dysplasia in the horse is the RMH syndrome.[31] In addition, congenital megaloglobus has been seen with associated severe retinal dysplasia. The retinal dysplasia in one case was associated with a cartilaginous choristoma of the choroid (Wilkie D. Unpublished data). (Figs. 9-19, 9-20, and 9-21).

Treatment

Retinal folds are nonprogressive, and no treatment is required.

Long-Term Prognosis and Inheritability Information

Although one author states that retinal dysplasia is not inheritable,[5] not all veterinarians share this opinion. Others comment that the Thoroughbred may be predisposed to retinal dysplasia.[14] Breeding of horses with severe retinal dysplasia and/or multiple congenital ocular anomalies should be discouraged.

Congenital Retinal Detachment

Congenital retinal detachment can be an isolated finding or can be associated with the anterior segment dysgenesis of the RMH; severe retinal dysplasia;

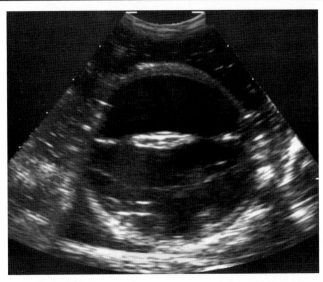

Fig. 9-20 Ultrasound examination of the right eye of the foal in Fig. 9-19. Congenital megaloglobus with microphakia, vitreous dysplasia, and retinal detachment are confirmed histologically because retinal dysplasia with nonattachment is present.

or multiple congenital defects such as coloboma, microphakia, microphthalmos, and lens luxation.[15] Retinal detachment accounted for 6.2% of all congenital ocular anomalies in one study.[23] One proposed cause is a failure of attachment of the NSR to the underlying RPE, which occurs as a result of incomplete invagination of the optic vesicle.[14]

Clinical Appearance and Diagnosis

The affected eye is blind with dilated nonresponsive pupils. Clinically, a veil of gray tissue radiating forward from the optic nerve is observed. If the retina is torn from the ora and falls ventral, tapetal hyperreflection will be noted. Hyphema, cataract, and secondary glaucoma may occur as a result of chronic retinal detachment.

Treatment

There is no treatment for congenital retinal detachment, and affected animals should not be used for breeding.

Long-Term Prognosis and Inheritability Information

A predilection for the Standardbred and Thoroughbred has been suggested.[14-16] Hyphema, cataract, and secondary glaucoma may occur as a result of chronic retinal detachment.

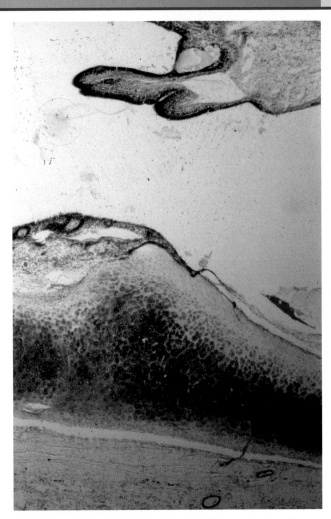

Fig. 9-21 Histopathologic examination of the posterior globe of the horse in Fig. 9-19. The retina is nonattached with retinal dysplasia and a cartilaginous choristoma of the retinal pigment epithelium or choroid.

Rocky Mountain Horse Multiple Ocular Abnormalities

Multiple, congenital anterior and posterior segment abnormalities have been described in the RMH, Kentucky Saddle horse, and Mountain Pleasure horse breeds.[14,31] The abnormalities are associated with coat color, and horses with chocolate coat color and a white mane and tail are more severely affected.[31]

Clinical Appearance and Diagnosis

The abnormalities can affect the cornea, iris, ciliary body, lens, and retina. With respect to the posterior segment, temporal peripheral retinal cysts, retinal dysplasia, RPE proliferation, and retinal detachment have been described in affected horses.[31] Cysts can involve the posterior iris, ciliary body, or peripheral retina and are always located temporally. Cysts can be unilateral or bilateral and affect 48% of RMHs examined.[11] Retinal dysplasia appears as linear folds, most commonly in the temporal retina; affects 24% of the horses examined; and is only found in association with retinal or ciliary body cysts (Fig. 9-22).[31] These lesions have been confirmed by histologic examination as retinal dysplasia, hypoplasia, rosette formation, and RPE proliferation. Proliferation of the RPE appears as pigmented, curvilinear streaks that originate and terminate at the ora and extend toward the optic disc. These pigmented streaks are believed to indicate previous retinal detachment (Fig. 9-23).[31] Retinal detachments appear to be associated with peripheral retinal cysts and thus occur temporally. Rhegmatogenous detachments were also observed in 16% of horses examined.[31]

Treatment

There is no treatment, and affected animals should not be used for breeding.

Long-Term Prognosis and Inheritability Information

The anterior segment dysgenesis of the RMH is inherited as a recessive trait with incomplete penetrance.[31]

Congenital Stationary Night Blindness

Congenital stationary night blindness has been reported in the Appaloosa and the Quarter horse.[32-35] This condition is similar to congenital stationary night blindness in humans.[35] It has also been noted in Thoroughbreds, Paso Finos, and Standardbreds.[16] Affected horses have a defect in neural transmission between the photoreceptors and the inner retina, perhaps at the level of the bipolar cells.[35] Congenital stationary night blindness accounted for 3.5% of congenital ocular anomalies in one study.[23]

Clinical Appearance and Diagnosis

Affected horses have severely compromised vision in low-light conditions (nyctalopia) and may have some decreased function in day vision as well.[33,36] Owners may notice a reluctance to enter darkened areas such as barns or difficulty riding in evening conditions. Findings on posterior segment examination are normal. Some affected horses also exhibit microphthalmia, dorso-medial strabismus, nystagmus, and an unusual gaze associated with head elevation, which has been termed star gazing (Fig. 9-24). It has also been suggested that abnormalities in daylight vision, head elevation, and strabismus may relate to concurrent myopia.[10,14]

There are no histologic or ultrastructural differences between affected and normal equine retinas. Diagnosis can be confirmed by ERG in which a normal a wave but a decreased photopic and absent scotopic b wave are noted.[33,35]

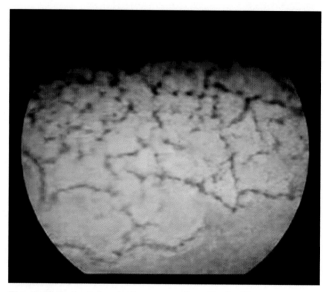

Fig. 9-22 Retinal dysplasia as seen in a Rocky Mountain horse. (Photograph courtesy Dr. David Ramsey.)

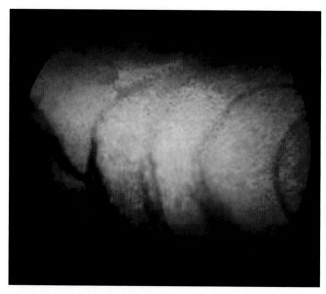

Fig. 9-23 Pigment streaks of retinal pigment epithelium extending outward from the ora. These are suggestive of previous retinal detachment. (Photograph courtesy Dr. David Ramsey.)

Treatment

As indicated by the name, the condition is congenital and nonprogressive. There is no treatment, and affected animals should not be used for breeding.

Long-Term Prognosis and Inheritability Information

The abnormality is thought to be inherited in a recessive or sex-linked recessive pattern with the defect located on the X chromosome.[5,33]

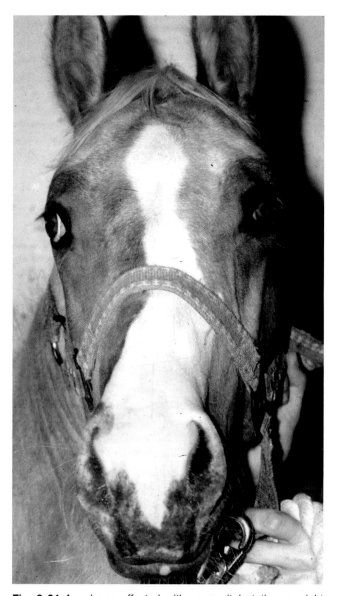

Fig. 9-24 Appaloosa affected with congenital stationary night blindness, demonstrating dorsomedial strabismus and an unusual gaze associated with head elevation termed star gazing.

Persistent Hyaloid Artery

The hyaloid artery travels from the optic nerve anteriorly to the posterior lens capsule, where it connects with the posterior portion of the tunica vasculosa lentis. This vascular network generally disappears before or at the time of birth.[12,16]

Clinical Appearance and Diagnosis

Persistence of the hyaloid vasculature is uncommon in the horse compared with other domestic animals. It can be seen as an isolated finding or in association with other congenital anomalies such as posterior lenticonus, cataract, retinal dysplasia, coloboma, microphthalmia, or retinal detachment. If a posterior, axial cataract is noted, it should be monitored for progression.

Treatment

No treatment is indicated.

Long-Term Prognosis and Inheritability Information

Most instances of an isolated persistent hyaloid artery will spontaneously regress by 6 to 9 months of age.[12] There is no known genetic component to this disease.

ACQUIRED DISEASES

Ocular Trauma

The equine eye is often subject to severe traumatic injury, perhaps as a result of its prominent position in the head. Traumatic injuries are divided according to the tissues involved and the severity of the injury: contusions (overlying tissue is intact), penetrating injuries (tissue is abraded or partially cut), and perforating injuries (tissue is cut completely). Blunt trauma—whether contusive, penetrating, or perforating—generally results in more severe ocular damage than injury caused by a sharp object. Unfortunately, most ocular trauma in the horse is blunt in nature. In contrast to sharp perforating injuries, blunt trauma results in a rapid increase in intraocular pressure, an explosive rupture from the inside outward, and the expulsion of the intraocular contents (Fig. 9-25). The resulting rent in the fibrous tunic is often large and irregular, and portions of the cornea or sclera

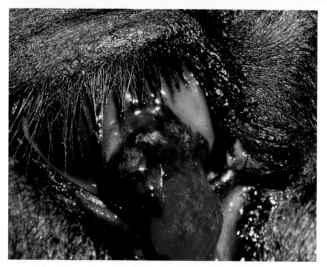

Fig. 9-25 Traumatic rupture of the cornea with expulsion of the intraocular contents as a result of blunt force trauma.

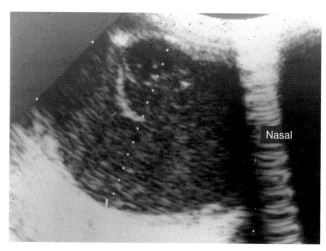

Fig. 9-27 Ultrasound examination of a globe after acute, traumatic hyphema. Vitreous hemorrhage and rupture of the posterior lens capsule are noted.

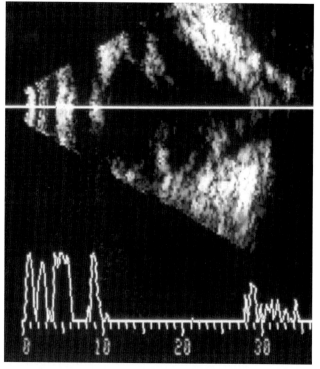

Fig. 9-26 Ultrasound examination of a globe with acute blunt trauma. The posterior eye wall has been ruptured.

may be lost. The typical wound is one that originates at the limbus and extends forward into the cornea and posterior into the sclera. However, the posterior portion of the eye may rupture, and the horse may be presented with hyphema and decreased intraocular pressure. Ocular ultrasound examination is required for an accurate diagnosis and determination of prognosis (Fig. 9-26).

Clinical Appearance and Diagnosis

Vitreous hemorrhage, lens luxation, retinal tears, retinal hemorrhage, retinal and choroidal detachment, and optic nerve damage are all associated with blunt trauma to the eye and orbit.[16,37]

If the hyphema is complete and precludes the evaluation of intraocular structures, ocular ultrasound examination is indicated to assess the lens position, vitreous, retina, and posterior eye wall. The greatest resolution of the ocular tissues of interest is achieved with a 7.5-MHz, or preferably, a 10-MHz probe. If the cornea is intact, the probe can be placed directly on it; if the cornea is compromised, imaging can be performed through the eyelid or an offset device. Evaluation for lens rupture or luxation, vitreous hemorrhage, retinal and choroidal detachment, and posterior eye wall rupture should be performed (Fig. 9-27).

Treatment

Repair of these explosive ruptures is difficult, and the treatment of choice is often enucleation. If cosmetic repair is important, an intraocular silicone prosthesis can be used in some patients, provided there is sufficient tissue left to close the fibrous tunic. This procedure should be performed as soon as possible after injury. If the injury is chronic and atrophy of the globe has occurred, placement of an intraocular prosthesis is not possible. The only cosmetic alternative in these horses is an orbital implant with a cosmetic corneoscleral prosthesis.[38] This requires multiple procedures and referral to an ophthalmologist and ocularist to achieve an acceptable cosmetic outcome.

Long-Term Prognosis

In general, damage to the posterior segment, especially in association with hemorrhage, carries a grave prognosis.

Head Trauma

Trauma to the head of the horse has been associated with acute unilateral or bilateral blindness without associated compromise of the globe. The pupil in the affected eye will be dilated, but the remainder of the findings on ophthalmic examination may be normal initially. Occasionally, retinal hemorrhage and papilledema are present. Fundic examination several weeks later may reveal optic nerve pallor, indicating optic nerve atrophy (Fig. 9-28). The cause of this lesion is hypothesized to be stretching of the optic nerve or trauma from bony fractures adjacent to the optic nerve. A small number of horses with head trauma may benefit from systemic antiinflammatory therapy in the acute phase. However, the prognosis is guarded, and treatment is usually unrewarding. For more information, see the discussion of traumatic optic neuropathy.

Chorioretinitis

Chorioretinitis, inflammation of the choroid and retina, may be the result of ERU or may be a manifestation of systemic disease. Chorioretinitis is the most common abnormality identified on examination of the equine fundus. The reader should refer to Chapters 6, 7, and 12 for complete discussions of uveitis, ERU, and ocular manifestations of systemic disease.

Clinical Appearance and Diagnosis

The appearance of chorioretinitis on fundic examination depends on whether the lesions are active or old. Active lesions are characterized by edema, cellular infiltrate, and hemorrhage or retinal detachment; and they often appear gray, white, or hazy. The retina may be elevated by subretinal fluid and inflammatory cells (Figs. 9-29 and 9-30). Inactive lesions, or chorioretinal scars, appear as hyperreflective or hyperpigmented in the tapetal fundus and may appear to be depigmented or to have pigment clumping in the nontapetal fundus (Fig. 9-31). If the retina was elevated during the active phase of the disease, it may re-attach in a wrinkled or folded fashion, appearing as gray linear folds.

These folds are most commonly seen radiating from the optic nerve. Chorioretinitis lesions can be focal or diffuse and unilateral or bilateral and are most commonly seen in the peripapillary region. The "classic" inactive chorioretinal scar is seen circumpapillary and is termed a butterfly lesion (Fig. 9-32). This is an area

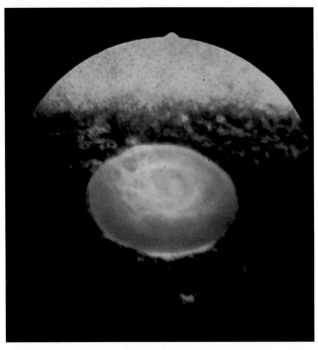

Fig. 9-28 Optic nerve degeneration caused by head trauma. The optic nerve is pale with retinal vascular attenuation.

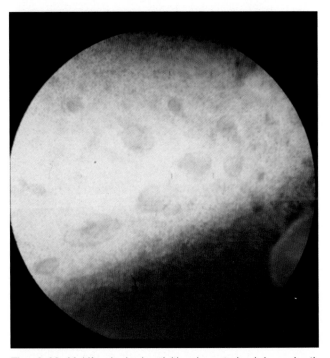

Fig. 9-29 Multifocal chorioretinitis characterized by subretinal edema and tapetal hyporeflectivity. (Photograph courtesy Dr. Brian Gilger.)

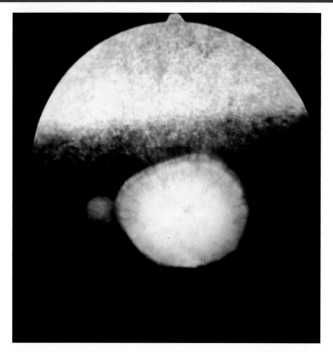

Fig. 9-30 Focal area of retinitis with cellular infiltrate seen as a gray-white lesion adjacent to the optic nerve. (Photograph courtesy Dr. Brian Gilger.)

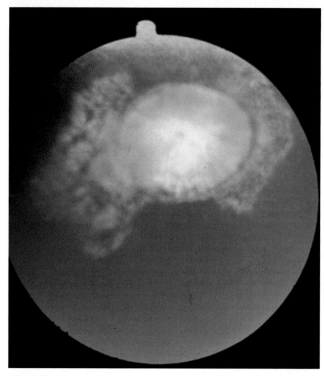

Fig. 9-32 Peripapillary chorioretinal scar, also called a butterfly lesion.

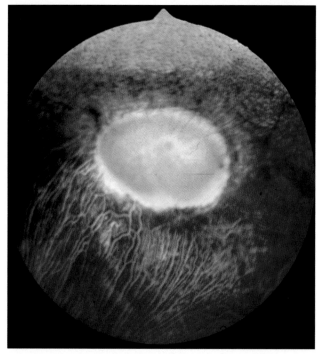

Fig. 9-31 Choroidal depigmentation and degeneration of the ventral optic nerve after inflammation.

of depigmentation and pigment clumping that radiates nasally and temporally from the optic nerve. Lesions can be confined to one side of the optic nerve. During the active phase of the disease, the peripapillary retina may be elevated; soft or hard exudates may be present; and retinal vasculitis, seen as indistinct margins and vascular cuffing, may be observed.[16] This lesion can be associated with ERU, but the anterior segment often appears normal. The prevalence of peripapillary chorioretinal lesions in otherwise normal eyes has been reported to be 5% to 8%.[4,39] Posterior segment changes, in the absence of anterior segment disease, can and do occur with ERU; however, any optic neuritis or peripapillary chorioretinitis could result in similar changes.

Immunohistochemical examination of the retinas from horses with naturally occurring ERU and from ponies with experimental *Leptospira*-induced uveitis demonstrated a range of findings.[40] Minimal to severe retinal changes were observed and were characterized by major histocompatibility complex class II antigen-expressing cells and T lymphocytes, suggesting an immunologic cause of retinal damage.[40] Ponies with *Leptospira*-induced uveitis demonstrated B lymphocytes that were seroreactive for *Leptospira interrogans* serovar *pomona*.[40] Additional studies have confirmed chorioretinal changes in horses with ERU that are characterized by T-lymphocyte infiltration and destruction of photoreceptor outer segments and inner retina.[41] T-cell–rich lymphoid follicle formation was noted in the iris and choroid.[41] Analysis of vitrectomy samples from horses with ERU demonstrates immunoglobulin G antibodies and autoreactive T lymphocytes specific for retinal antigens, which provides support for the

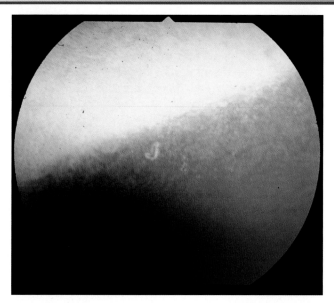

Fig. 9-33 Focal "bullet" lesion at the tapetal-nontapetal junction.

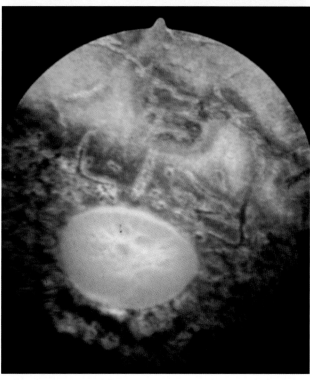

Fig. 9-34 Retinal and optic nerve degeneration caused by severe blood loss.

possibility of a local autoimmune-mediated disease involving the posterior segment.[42] For a complete discussion, see Chapter 7.

In experimental infection with EHV-1, chorioretinal lesions have been produced 6 to 8 weeks after intranasal infection.[17,43] On the basis of findings from fluorescein angiography, it is hypothesized that EHV-1 infection can result in infarction of the choroidal vasculature and subsequent focal loss of RPE. Clinically, this appears as multifocal white lesions in the peripapillary nontapetal fundus.[17]

Focal chorioretinopathy, termed bullet-hole chorioretinitis, has been described.[5,15,16] Lesions are generally multifocal, appear ventral to the optic disc, and are white with a pigmented center (Fig. 9-33). They are small and do not appear raised or depressed. On histologic examination, a loss of normal retinal architecture with RPE hyperplasia and migration of RPE cells into the retina can be observed.[12] It has been suggested that these lesions may be the result of previous chorioretinitis and may have a viral cause.[15] An association with respiratory disease in foals has been suggested.[16] Lesions are similar in appearance to those described in experimental EHV-1 infection.[17] These lesions have been seen in many horses of all age-groups (Wilkie D. Unpublished data). One report suggests that 10% to 20% of horses are affected with bullet-hole scars.[16] They are nonprogressive, and although they may be postinflammatory lesions, are best considered incidental findings.

A more diffuse chorioretinitis has been described in which lesions are vermiform, circular, or band-shaped and are hyperreflective in the tapetum and depigmented in the nontapetal region (Fig. 9-34).[16] Similar lesions have occurred in association with severe blood loss. Optic nerve degeneration may be present in some instances. Vision is generally decreased, especially if the optic nerve is affected. Trauma and vascular infarction are also possible causes.[16]

Chorioretinitis or panuveitis may also be a manifestation of systemic disease and has been documented with equine infectious anemia,[44] adenovirus,[45,46] West Nile virus,[47,48] neonatal septicemia,[49] *Rhodococcus equi*,[46,50] *Streptococcus equi* var *equi*,[51,52] Lyme disease,[46,50] brucellosis,[53] *Leptospira interrogans pomona*, equine granulocytic ehrlichiosis,[54] toxoplasmosis,[55] *Halicephalobus gingivalis* (*H. deletrix*),[56,57] and onchocerciasis.[58] In general, any infectious or parasitic agent that is hematogenously disseminated, is capable of causing vasculitis, or exhibits aberrant migration could result in anterior or posterior uveitis. Neonatal foals with septicemia or bacteremia are often presented with anterior uveitis, which may occasionally extend to the posterior segment as a panuveitis. For a complete discussion, see Chapter 12.

Treatment

Treatment is directed at the underlying cause, but there is no specific medical or surgical therapy for focal or diffuse chorioretinitis.

Long-Term Prognosis

Focal lesions are usually of no significance. Although it is hypothesized that numerous or diffuse lesions could result in visual changes, clinically, these lesions appear to have no detectable effect on vision. However, vision should be assessed in affected animals, and attention should be paid to the purpose of each animal and the effect vision loss may have on function. In cases of peripapillary depigmentation, the veterinarian should perform a careful examination of the anterior segment, looking for subtle atrophy of the corpora nigra, pigment on the anterior lens capsule, and yellowing of the lens or vitreous—all of which suggest previous inflammation and support a diagnosis of ERU.

Retinal Detachment

A retinal detachment is the separation of the NSR from the outer RPE. The retina is normally supported in place by the vitreous and the RPE, which has metabolic pumps that maintain an osmotic gradient that keep the NSR in apposition with the RPE. The retina can detach as a result of fluid accumulation between the NSR and RPE, a retinal tear and migration of fluid from the vitreous into the intraretinal space, blunt force trauma, or traction toward the vitreous secondary to resolution of vitreal hemorrhage or after hyalitis. Accumulation of fluid between the NSR and RPE is most commonly the result of inflammation, with ERU being the most common cause. This is termed a bullous detachment, and re-attachment can occur if the inflammation is resolved and the RPE is able to pump the fluid out of the intraretinal space. The retina may re-attach with folds or wrinkles, most commonly radiating outward from the optic nerve. Such folds indicate previous bullous detachment.

Retinal detachments associated with a retinal tear are termed rhegmatogenous detachments. In such cases, fluid migrates from the vitreous side of the retina, through the tear, forcing the NSR from the RPE. Dorsal tears are more likely to progress as gravity works to pull the retina down. Trauma, rupture of peripheral retinal cysts, and anomalies of the RMH are all associated with rhegmatogenous detachments.

Clinical Appearance and Diagnosis

Clinically, a retinal detachment can be partial or complete (Fig. 9-35). Partial detachments are not associated with detectable vision loss in most instances. They are most often discovered on a pre-purchase examination or during examination of an eye for anterior

segment disease. A focal bullous detachment appears as an elevated, hazy area of retina with subretinal fluid. Bullous detachments may occur as a result of systemic disease (see the discussion of chorioretinitis).

With a complete detachment, the retina appears as a gray, floating veil of tissue extending into the vitreous toward the lens (Fig. 9-36). If it is displaced far enough

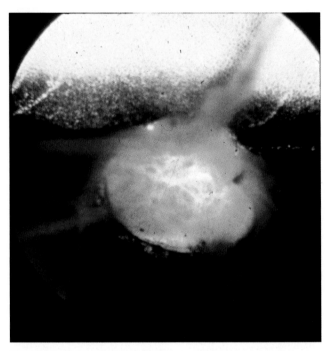

Fig. 9-35 The peripapillary retina is detached, appearing as a gray veil of tissue over and around the optic nerve.

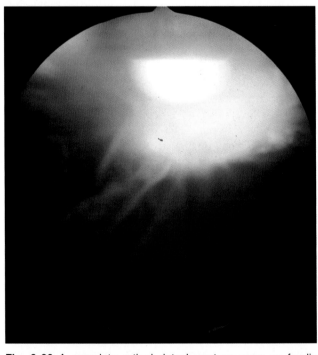

Fig. 9-36 A complete retinal detachment as seen on fundic examination.

anteriorly, the retina may be visible by penlight examination. The retina is normally attached at the optic nerve and ora ciliaris retinae. As a consequence of a retinal detachment, the retina may tear at the ora and fall ventrally, obscuring the optic nerve (Fig. 9-37). This is called a giant tear. Once a retinal detachment has progressed to this stage, little treatment can be offered.

Traction detachments occur after intravitreal hemorrhage or inflammation, termed hyalitis. Trauma, ERU, and extension of chorioretinitis can result in vitreous

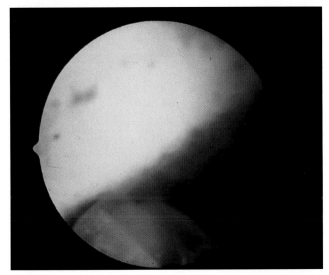

Fig. 9-37 A complete retinal detachment with a giant tear. The retina has avulsed from the dorsal ora and fallen ventrally over the optic nerve. The tapetum appears hyperreflective.

hemorrhage and hyalitis. Traction bands may form, appearing as tan to gray strands in the vitreous. These may attach to the inner retina and undergo contracture, elevating the retina and leading to a retinal detachment. Treatment of traction retinal detachments consists of a vitrectomy and severing of the traction bands, but concurrent intraocular disease generally prevents this as a viable option.

Retinal detachment may also be noted in horses presented for examination because of a congenital or juvenile cataract or a cataract caused by chronic uveitis. An ocular ultrasound examination is indicated to evaluate the posterior segment in horses with a mature or hypermature cataract (Figs. 9-38 and 9-39).

Treatment

The underlying cause of inflammation needs to be managed, and if management is successful, a bullous detachment may re-attach if the inflammation is resolved and the RPE is able to pump the fluid out of the intraretinal space.

If detected early, retinal tears (rhegmatogenous detachments) can be isolated and prevented from progressing by laser retinopexy. The technique consists of delivering laser energy across the pupil through an indirect ophthalmoscope and a condensing lens.

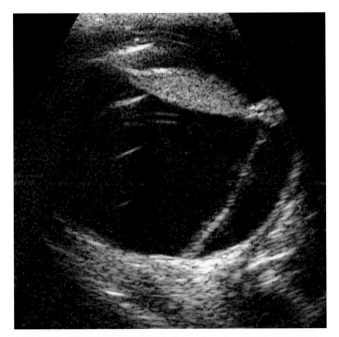

Fig. 9-38 Ultrasound examination of a horse presented for cataract. The retina is partially detached with a hyperechoic line present in the vitreous extending from the optic nerve posteriorly to the ora anteriorly.

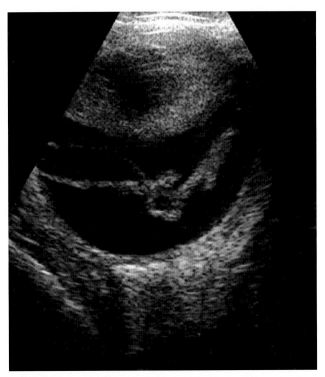

Fig. 9-39 Complete retinal detachment with a mature cataract.

The diode laser is the instrument of choice, delivering a wavelength of 810 nm, which is preferentially absorbed by melanin. The energy is transformed into heat, resulting in thermal coagulation and a focal scar. Multiple scars are created to surround and isolate the tear, preventing progression of the detachment.

Treatment of traction retinal detachments consists of a vitrectomy and severing of the traction bands, but concurrent intraocular disease generally prevents this as a viable option.

Long-Term Prognosis

The prognosis for a retinal detachment depends on the severity, underlying cause, and chronicity of the lesions.

Retinal Degeneration

Retinal degeneration is far less common as a primary disease in horses than in dogs and cats. Primary retinal degeneration or progressive retinal atrophy will be bilateral and progressive, and Thoroughbreds may be predisposed.[14,16] Affected horses show progressive vision loss with areas of nontapetal depigmentation and hyperpigmentation, and in the later stages, optic nerve atrophy.[16] Similar changes can occur in association with aging and are referred to as senile retinal degeneration.[14,59] In one study of 83 geriatric horses, 35 animals and 64 eyes were noted to have senile retinopathy or retinal degeneration.[60] The prevalence of senile retinal degeneration increases with age.[60]

Clinical Appearance and Diagnosis

Retinal degeneration appears as hyperreflective changes in the tapetal retina and as multifocal depigmentation and hyperpigmentation in the nontapetal retina (Fig. 9-40).[14] The optic nerve becomes pale, and the peripapillary retinal vessels are attenuated. Vision loss may begin with nyctalopia (night blindness) and progress to day vision loss. In one study, most cases of senile retinal atrophy observed were bilateral and most common in the peripapillary region.[60] Some of these cases were confirmed histologically by a variable loss of inner and outer retinal layers and retinal gliosis.[60] In other cases, a focal peripheral retinal degeneration associated with age has been described.[13] Peripheral cystoid retinal degeneration has also been noted in some geriatric eyes.[13,29,60] Peripheral cystoid retinal degeneration occurs at the ora and is observed

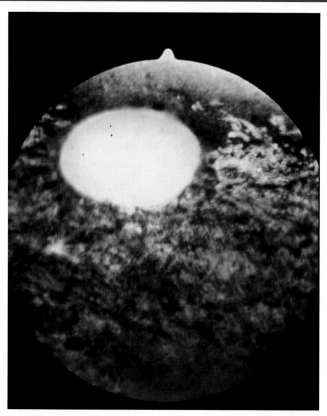

Fig. 9-40 Retinal and optic nerve degeneration. Optic nerve pallor, pigment clumping, and depigmentation are all present.

in many species. Although generally an incidental finding, it can predispose to rhegmatogenous retinal detachment if a cyst ruptures. Unilateral retinal degeneration can be associated with glaucoma, trauma, or vascular ischemia.

A lysosomal storage disease, neuronal ceroid lipofuscinosis, has also been described in three horses that demonstrated neurologic symptoms and vision loss in one instance.[61] Clinical symptoms were noted by 1 year of age, and euthanasia was performed by 1.5 years of age. Eosinophilic, autofluorescent material was found in the perikarya of neurons in the brain, spinal cord, retina, and mesenteric ganglia.[61] Immunohistochemistry confirmed the diagnosis as ceroid lipofuscinosis.

Treatment

There is no treatment for retinal degeneration, and affected animals should not be used for breeding.

Long-Term Prognosis

The long-term prognosis for retinal degeneration in general is good, because the lesion is usually mild and slowly progressive; however, the prognosis depends

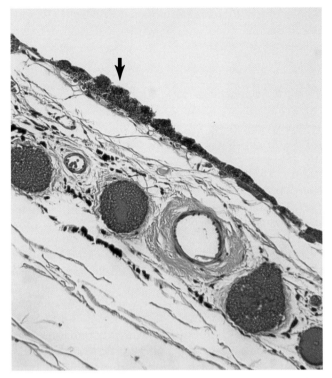

Fig. 9-41 Histopathologic examination of the choroid and retinal pigment epithelium (RPE) of a horse with equine motor neuron disease. Note the accumulation of ceroid-lipofuscin in the RPE *(arrow).*

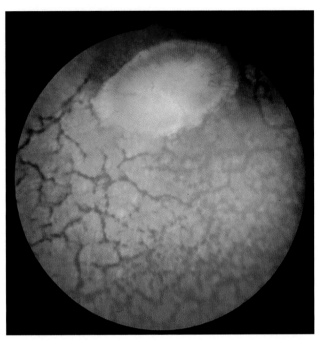

Fig. 9-42 Optic nerve and nontapetal fundus of a horse with equine motor neuron disease. Note the honeycomb pattern of pigment deposits in the retinal pigment epithelium.

on severity and the underlying cause. Neuronal ceroid lipofuscinosis is an inherited neurodegenerative disorder, and affected horses and their parents and siblings should not be used for breeding.

Equine Motor Neuron Disease

Equine motor neuron disease is a neurodegenerative disease that occurs as a result of a chronic dietary deficiency of the antioxidant, vitamin E.[62,63] Ceroid-lipofuscin subsequently accumulates in the RPE in the tapetal and nontapetal fundus (Fig. 9-41).[62]

Clinical Appearance and Diagnosis

On examination with an ophthalmoscope, equine motor neuron disease appears as an irregular, reticulated, or honeycomb pattern of accumulations of pigment in the tapetal and nontapetal retina (Figs. 9-42 and 9-43). Although vision impairment is inconsistent, a 50% reduction in the electroretinogram b-wave amplitude has been documented.[62] The ophthalmoscopic findings are used in conjunction with the musculoskeletal signs to make a diagnosis of equine motor neuron disease.

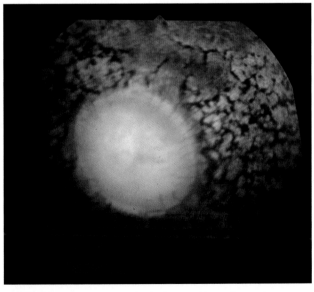

Fig. 9-43 Tapetal photograph of a horse with equine motor neuron disease.

Treatment

Supplementation with vitamin E and provision of fresh forage may stabilize the neurologic signs but do not appear to reverse the RPE changes. See Chapter 12 for further information.

Long-Term Prognosis

The prognosis depends on severity of disease and response to therapy.

Photic Head Shaking

A condition of head shaking or head tossing induced by exposure to light and eliminated by blindfolding, darkened environment, and contact lenses has been reported in the horse.[64,65] The problem is usually seen in the spring and summer, is exacerbated by exercise, and may be accompanied by sneezing, snorting, and nasal rubbing.[64]

Clinical Appearance and Diagnosis

Differential diagnoses for photic head shaking include middle ear disorders, ear mites, guttural pouch mycosis, other ocular disorders such as vitreous floaters, and nasal and dental disease.[64] Findings on ophthalmic examination in animals with photic head shaking are normal. It is hypothesized that an optic-trigeminal response is occurring, with optic stimulation resulting in referred stimulation in areas innervated by the trigeminal nerve.[64]

Treatment

Oral administration of cyproheptadine (0.3 mg/kg) (Sidmark Laboratories Inc., East Hanover, NJ) every 12 hours has been effective in several horses.[64,65] Cyproheptadine is an antihistamine (H_1 blocker) and a serotonin antagonist and is hypothesized to alleviate photic head shaking by moderating the trigeminal nerve sensation, having a central effect on melatonin, or inducing anticholinergic activity.[64] Bilateral infraorbital neurectomy has also been used for medically refractive cases. Before surgery, an infraorbital nerve block is performed to determine whether this procedure alleviates clinical signs and is warranted.[64,65]

Long-Term Prognosis

Prognosis depends on severity of the condition and the response to treatment.

Optic Nerve Degeneration or Atrophy

Atrophy of the optic nerve occurs as a result of trauma, inflammation, glaucoma, ischemia, and compression.

Acute blood loss has also been implicated in optic nerve degeneration with or without retinal degeneration (see Fig. 9-34).[29,66]

Clinical Appearance and Diagnosis

In many instances, on examination shortly after the onset of sudden blindness, peripapillary exudates are observed. Regardless of the cause, optic nerve pallor, visualization of the lamina cribrosa, and peripapillary vascular attenuation are common end points. If inflammation has been present, peripapillary depigmentation and pigment clumping may be present. Orbital mass lesions can result in compression of the optic nerve and are often also associated with exophthalmos (Fig. 9-44). Orbital masses can be inflammatory or neoplastic. Lymphosarcoma and extraadrenal paraganglioma are the most common equine orbital neoplasms. Glaucoma in the horse is typically caused by intraocular inflammation and ERU. Chronic glaucoma will result in buphthalmia, corneal edema, lens luxation, and retinal and optic nerve degeneration.[22] In one study of 83 geriatric horses, optic nerve atrophy was observed in seven eyes of four horses.[60]

Treatment

There is no treatment for optic nerve atrophy.

Long-Term Prognosis

The prognosis for vision is poor.

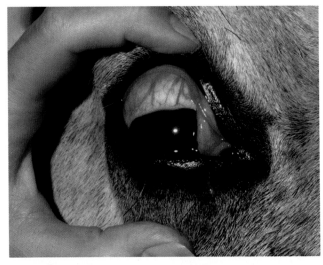

Fig. 9-44 Exophthalmos and strabismus caused by orbital lymphosarcoma.

Traumatic Optic Neuropathy

Blunt trauma to the head can result in sudden unilateral or bilateral blindness.[37,67-69] Trauma may include rearing or falling backward; striking the poll; or blunt injury to the side of the face caused by a kick, twitch handle, or other blunt device. The trauma may result in fracture of the basisphenoid bone and compression or hemorrhage in the intracanalicular area of the optic nerve. Additionally, motion of the brain away from the fixed intracanalicular portion of the optic nerve may result in neuropraxia of the retinal ganglion cell axons.

Clinical Appearance and Diagnosis

The pupil is fixed and dilated with absent menace response in the affected eye. Initially, the optic nerve appears normal on fundic examination. Papilledema, focal hemorrhages, and accumulations of axoplasmic materials may occur in the first 24 to 48 hours but are not seen in all cases. Within 2 to 4 weeks, the optic nerve becomes pale, and the fibers of the lamina cribrosa become apparent as the axons of the retinal ganglion cells disappear (Fig. 9-28). Over time, atrophy of the NSR and hypertrophy of the RPE—which appears clinically as vascular attenuation, tapetal hyperreflectivity, and areas of hyperpigmentation—will be observed on histologic examination.[67]

Treatment

Immediate treatment with antiinflammatory agents such as systemic corticosteroids, nonsteroidal antiinflammatory drugs, and dimethyl sulfoxide is advised but appears to be of little benefit.

Long-Term Prognosis

The prognosis for vision after traumatic optic nerve neuropathy is poor. If vision has not returned within 2 weeks, the prognosis is grave.

Ischemic Optic Neuropathy

Ischemic optic neuropathy is caused by sudden hypoxemia of the optic nerve as a result of acute hypovolemia, thromboembolic disease, or surgical occlusion of the internal or external carotid artery.[14,70]

Ligation or occlusion of the internal or external carotid artery is used as treatment for guttural pouch mycosis to prevent epistaxis associated with vascular invasion by fungal plaques.[70] With arterial occlusion, the affected eye will be on the side ipsilateral to the surgical site.

Clinical Appearance and Diagnosis

Initially, the affected optic nerve appears normal, but the affected eye is blind. The nerve becomes edematous and hyperemic within 24 hours. Focal peripapillary hemorrhages and accumulation of axoplasmic material may be observed in 24 to 48 hours (Fig. 9-45). This appears as white material extending vitread from the optic nerve (Fig. 9-46). Optic nerve degeneration, characterized by pallor and vascular attenuation, becomes apparent in 2 to 4 weeks.

Treatment

There is no treatment for ischemic optic neuropathy.

Long-Term Prognosis

Prognosis for vision is grave.

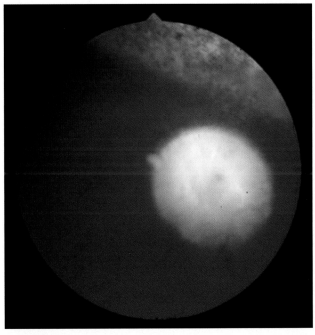

Fig. 9-45 Twenty-four hours after occlusion of the vascular supply to the optic nerve, the nerve is edematous, and white axoplasmic material is seen at the margin of the optic nerve.

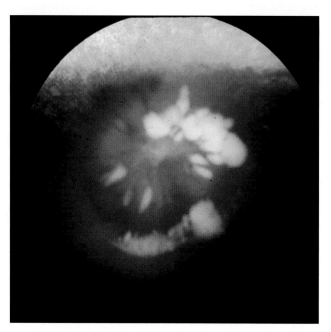

Fig. 9-46 Several days after vascular occlusion, peripapillary hemorrhages, optic nerve hyperemia, and accumulation of axoplasmic materials are observed.

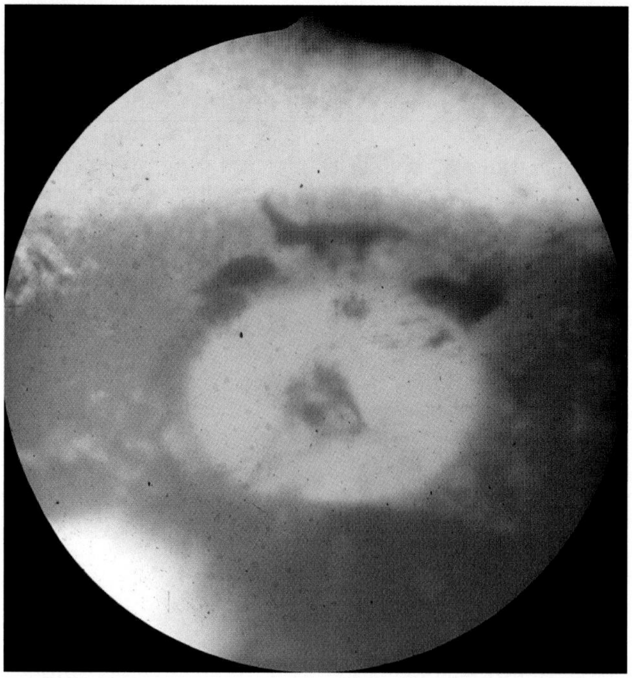

Fig. 9-47 Optic neuritis is observed, along with hemorrhage, peripapillary edema, and cellular exudates.

Optic Neuritis

The optic nerve is an anterior extension of the central nervous system, and as such, is subject to diseases that result from inflammation, edema, infection, parasitism, and neoplasia of the central nervous system.

Clinical Appearance and Diagnosis

Clinically, the optic nerve appears hazy and edematous, often with white exudates and hemorrhage (Fig. 9-47). The peripapillary retina may be elevated. Vision is generally decreased to absent, and the papillary light response will be slow to absent with a dilated pupil.

Parasites, such as *Halicephalobus gingivalis (H. deletrix)*, have been demonstrated to result in chorioretinitis and optic neuritis.[56,57] These are typically disseminated with lesions in multiple organ systems. Optic neuritis can also occur with ERU. Borna disease, a viral encephalomyelitis exotic to North America, has also been reported to cause optic neuritis.[16,29]

Treatment

Treatment for optic neuritis is directed at the underlying cause.

Long-Term Prognosis

Prognosis for vision is dependent on the severity of disease and response to treatment.

Proliferative and Exudative Optic Neuropathy

Exudative optic neuritis has been described in older horses and may result in acute-onset bilateral blindness.[14,15,29] It must be distinguished from benign exudative/proliferative optic neuropathy, which occurs in aged horses (>15 years) and is generally an incidental finding.[16] Proliferative lesions may enlarge with time and can result in some vision or behavior changes if they become large enough to obscure portions of the retina.[16] In one study of 83 geriatric horses, proliferative optic neuropathy was noted in two animals and was unilateral in both.[60]

Clinical Appearance and Diagnosis

Exudative optic neuropathy appears as a white to gray material obscuring the optic nerve, which, if visible, is edematous with or without hemorrhages (Figs. 9-48 and 9-49). The cause is not known, but it is hypothesized to be an ocular response to a variety of

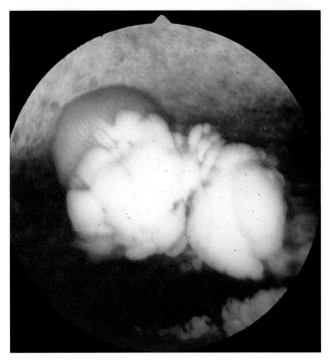

Fig. 9-48 Exudative optic neuropathy.

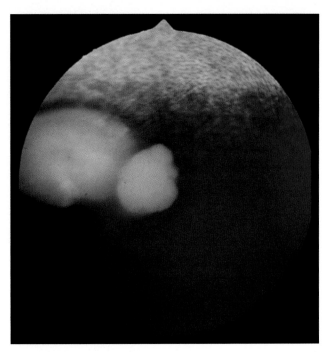

Fig. 9-50 Proliferative optic neuropathy.

findings on examination (Fig. 9-50).[14,15,16,29,71] On histologic examination, the lesion resembles a schwannoma.[72] Optic nerve neoplasia, traumatic optic neuropathy, and ischemic optic neuropathy are also differential diagnoses.

Treatment

There is no treatment for either condition.

Long-Term Prognosis

The prognosis for vision with exudative optic neuropathy is generally poor; however, the prognosis for vision with benign proliferative optic neuropathy is excellent, because these lesions are usually incidental findings.

OTHER MISCELLANEOUS POSTERIOR SEGMENT DISEASE IN THE HORSE

Neoplasia

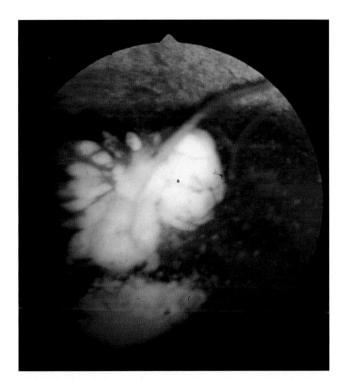

Fig. 9-49 Exudative optic neuropathy with associated retinal detachment.

systemic diseases such as infection with *Streptococcus equi* or *Actinobacillus equuli*, septicemia, EHV-1, and possibly ERU.[14] This must be distinguished from benign exudative/proliferative optic neuropathy, a condition of white or gray material anterior to the optic nerve in a visual eye with otherwise normal

Primary neoplasia of the equine posterior segment is rare. Teratoid medulloepitheliomas are seen in young horses and appear as white masses in the vitreous (Figs. 9-51, 9-52, and 9-53).[73,74] These can be rapidly growing, and enucleation is indicated and usually curative. Astrocytomas, gliomas, and schwannomas may

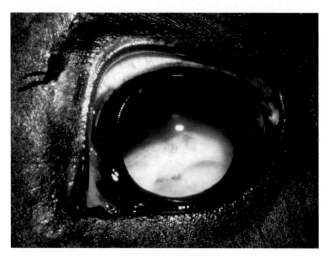

Fig. 9-51 Gross photograph of a foal with leukocoria caused by a teratoid medulloepithelioma of the posterior globe.

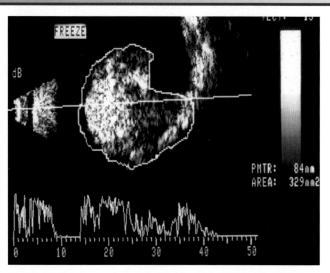

Fig. 9-53 Ultrasound examination of the teratoid medulloepithelioma seen in Fig. 9-51. The mass measures 84 mm over the surface.

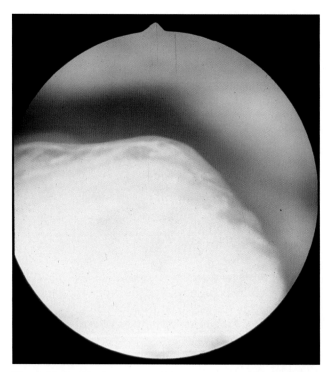

Fig. 9-52 Fundic photograph of the teratoid medulloepithelioma seen in Fig. 9-51.

occur and are typically benign (Fig. 9-54).[75] Choroidal melanoma is also a possible primary tumor of the posterior globe, and enucleation is advised. Metastatic tumors can also occur, with lymphosarcoma being most common. In general, metastatic tumors are associated with more significant inflammation and hemorrhage than are primary tumors. Retinal detachment,

hyphema, glaucoma, blindness, and pain may be observed with metastatic neoplasia.

Hyalitis

Hyalitis or inflammation of the vitreous can be seen with ERU or as an extension of chorioretinitis. In Europe, hyalitis appears to be a common manifestation of ERU. In evaluation of 130 vitreous samples from 117 European horses affected with ERU, which were collected during vitrectomy, leptospires were isolated in 35 samples (26.9%).[76] The most common serovar was *grippotyphosa*.[76] In addition, 92 vitreous samples (70.7%) were positive for leptospiral antibodies.[76] Results of other similar studies have also confirmed the presence of leptospires in the vitreous of horses with ERU with an additional finding of *Leptospira interrogans* in the vitreous of 52% of horses with ERU, but not in any control eyes.[77-79] Further, it has been demonstrated that horses with ERU have an increase in vitreous IgA as compared with serum IgA, suggesting a local immunologic reaction to antigens within the eye.[80]

With hyalitis, the vitreous will take on a yellow-green appearance as a result of serum pigments. Vitreous debris, fibrin, and inflammatory cells in the vitreous and on the posterior lens capsule and vitreous collagen are often seen to float and swirl in the vitreous as the tissue-water components of the vitreous separate, leaving free water, which contains products of inflammation. Posterior cortical cataract and retinal detachment may occur as a result of hyalitis.

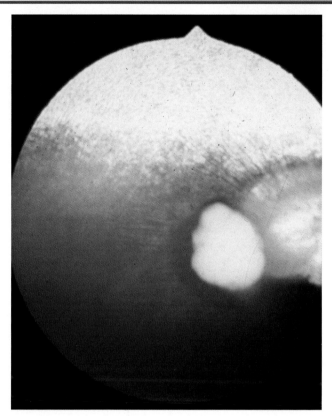

Fig. 9-54 Astrocytoma of the optic nerve.

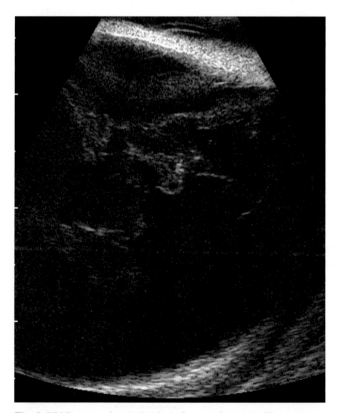

Fig. 9-55 Ultrasound examination of an equine eye with a cataract and vitreous degeneration. Echogenic material is observed in the mid to anterior vitreous and is seen to move when evaluated in real time.

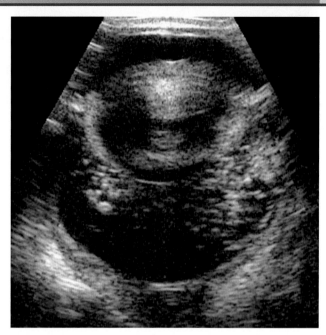

Fig. 9-56 Ultrasound examination of an equine eye with a cataract and asteroid hyalosis.

Vitreous Degeneration or Syneresis

Vitreous degeneration or syneresis is more common in aged horses and in such cases is a benign condition. Vitreous syneresis can also be a pathologic change associated with inflammation.[12] In one study of 83 geriatric horses, vitreous degeneration was the most common abnormality, being present in 38 animals and 72 eyes.[60] The prevalence of vitreous degeneration increased with age.[60] With syneresis may come vitreous floaters that can affect behavior, causing shying or head shaking (Fig. 9-55). Although examination for vitreous floaters in horses with the complaint of head shaking is an essential part of the ophthalmic examination, seldom are these the cause (Wilkie. Unpublished data). Evaluation for photic head shaking, refractive errors, ear or nasal disease, or various behavior concerns is more likely to result in a diagnosis.

Asteroid hyalosis, deposits of calcium-phosphate crystals in the vitreous, also occurs in horses (Fig. 9-56). This is an incidental finding and is more common in aged horses.

Vitrectomy and Vitreous Surgery

Surgical management of ERU with vitrectomy has been described.[76,77,81] This appears more accepted among European veterinary ophthalmologists, and a large number of horses have been treated with this technique. ERU in European horses may differ in its manifestation as a posterior segment disease with marked hyalitis, and therefore this technique has received more widespread recognition in Europe. The anatomy for surgical entry into the vitreous through the pars plana has been described.[11] In addition to vitrectomy, insertion of a sustained-release cyclosporine implant into the vitreous or suprachoroidal space has been described for prolonged management of ERU.[82,83] For a more detailed discussion, see Chapter 7.

REFERENCES

1. Murphy CJ, Howland HC: The optics of comparative ophthalmology, *Vis Res* 27:599-607, 1987.
2. Crispin SM, Matthews AG, Parker J: The equine fundus. I. examination, embryology, structure and function, *Equine Vet J Suppl* 22:42-49, 1990.
3. Matthews AG, Crispin SM , Parker J: The equine fundus. II. Normal anatomical variants and colobomata, *Equine Vet J Suppl* 22:50-54, 1990.
4. Matthews AG, Crispin SM , Parker J: The equine fundus. III. Pathological variants. *Equine Vet J Suppl* 22:55-61, 1990.
5. Brooks DE: Equine ophthalmology. In Gelatt KN, editor: *Veterinary ophthalmology*, ed 3, Philadelphia, 1991, Lippincott, Williams and Wilkins, pp 1053-1116.
6. Riis RC: Equine ophthalmology. In Gelatt KN, editor: *Veterinary ophthalmology*, Philadelphia, Lea and Febiger, 1981, 586-592.
7. Davidson MG: Equine ophthalmology. In Gelatt KN, editor: *Veterinary ophthalmology*, ed 2, Philadelphia, Lea and Febiger, 1991;576-610.
8. Munroe GA, Barnett KC: Congenital ocular disease in the foal, *Vet Clin North Am Large Anim Pract* 6:519-537, 1984,
9. Gelatt KN: Ophthalmoscopic studies in the normal and diseased ocular fundi of horses, *J Am Anim Hosp Assoc* 7:158-163, 1971.
10. Scotty NC et al: Diagnostic ultrasonography of equine lens and posterior segment, *Vet Ophthalmol* 7:127-139, 2004.
11. Miller TL et al: Description of ciliary body anatomy and identification of sites for transscleral cyclophotocoagulation in the equine eye, *Vet Ophthalmol* 4:183-190, 2001.
12. Barnett KC et al: *Equine ophthalmology: an atlas and text*, London, 2004, Elsevier Limited, pp 201-246.
13. Ehrenhofer MCA et al: Normal structure and age-related changes of the equine retina, *Vet Ophthalmol* 5:39-47, 2002.
14. Cutler TJ et al: Diseases of the equine posterior segment, *Vet Ophthalmol* 3:73-82, 2000.
15. Rebhun WC: Equine retinal lesions and retinal detachments, *Equine Vet J Suppl* 2:86-90, 1983.
16. Rebhun WC: Retinal and optic nerve diseases, *Vet Clin North Am Equine Pract* 8:587-608, 1992.
17. Slater JD et al: Fluorescein angiographic appearance of the normal fundus and of focal chorioretinal lesions in the horse, *Invest Ophthalmol Vis Sci* 36:S779, 1995.
18. Hebel R: Distribution of retinal ganglion cells in five mammalian species (pig, sheep, ox, horse, dog), *Anat Embryol (Berl)* 150:45-51, 1976.
19. Brooks DE, Komaromy AM, Kallberg ME: Comparative retinal ganglion cell and optic nerve morphology, *Vet Ophthalmol* 2:3-11, 1999.
20. Duke-Elder SS: *System of ophthalmology, vol 1, The eye in evolution*, London, 1958, Henry Kimpton, pp 446-504.
21. Carroll J et al: Cone photopigment spectral sensitivities in the horse, *Vet Ophthalmol* 2:257-262, 1999.
22. Brooks DE et al: Histomorphometry of the optic nerves of normal horses and horses with glaucoma, *Vet Comp Ophthalmol* 5:193-210, 1995.
23. Roberts SM: Congenital ocular anomalies, *Vet Clin North Am Equine Pract* 8:459-478, 1992.
24. Munroe G: Survey of retinal hemorrhages in neonatal thoroughbred foals, *Vet Rec* 146:95-101, 2000.
25. Wheeler CA, Collier LL: Bilateral colobomas involving the optic discs in a quarterhorse, *Equine Vet J Suppl* 10:39-41, 1990.
26. Bildfell R et al: Bilateral optic disc colobomas in a Quarter horse filly, *Equine Vet J* 35:325-327, 2003.
27. Schuh CL: Bilateral colobomas in a horse, *J Comp Pathol* 100:331-335, 1989.
28. Williams DL, Barnett KC: Bilateral optic disc colobomas and microphthalmos in a thoroughbred horse, *Vet Rec* 132:101-103, 1993.
29. Rubin LF: *Atlas of veterinary ophthalmoscopy,* Philadelphia, 1974, Lea & Febiger.
30. Gelatt KN, Leipold HW, Coffman JR: Bilateral optic nerve hypoplasia in a colt, *J Am Vet Med Assoc* 155:627-631, 1969.
31. Ramsey DT et al: Congenital ocular abnormalities of Rocky Mountain horses, *Vet Ophthalmol* 2:47-59, 1999.
32. Rebhun WC et al: Clinical manifestations of night blindness in the Appaloosa horse, *Comp Contin Educ Pract (Vet)* 6:S103-S106, 1984.
33. Witzel DA et al: Night blindness in the Appaloosa: sibling occurrence. *J Equine Med Surg* 1:383-386, 1977.
34. Witzel DA, Joyce JR, Smith EL: Electroretinography of congenital night blindness in an Appaloosa filly, *J Equine Med Surg* 1:226-229, 1977.
35. Witzel DA et al: Congenital stationary night blindness: an animal model, *Invest Ophthalmol Vis Sci* 17-788-795, 1978.
36. Gelatt KN: Congenital and acquired ophthalmic diseases in the foal, *Anim Eye Res* 2:15-27, 1993.
37. Millichamp NJ: Ocular trauma, *Vet Clin North Am Equine Pract* 8:521-536, 1992.
38. Gilger BC et al: Use of a hydroxyapatite orbital implant in a cosmetic corneoscleral prosthesis after enucleation in a horse, *J Am Vet Med Assoc* 222:343-345, 2003.
39. Roberts SR: Fundus lesions in equine periodic ophthalmia, *J Am Vet Med Assoc* 141:229-239, 1962.
40. Kalsow CM, Dwyer AE: Retinal immunopathology in horses with uveitis, *Ocul Immunol Inflamm* 6:239-251, 1998.
41. Deeg CA et al: Immunopathology of recurrent uveitis in spontaneously diseased horses, *Exp Eye Res* 75:127-133, 2002.
42. Deeg CA et al: Immune responses to retinal autoantigens and peptides in equine recurrent uveitis, *Invest Ophthalmol Vis Sci* 42:393-398, 2001.
43. Slater JD et al: Chorioretinopathy associated with neuropathology following infection with equine herpesvirus-1, *Vet Rec* 131:237-239, 1992.
44. Hahn CN, Mayhew IG, MacKay RJ: Diseases of multiple or unknown sites. In Colahan PT et al, editors: *Equine medicine and surgery, vol 1*, St Louis, 1999, Mosby, pp 884-903.
45. McChesney AE, England JJ, Rich LJ: Adenoviral infection in foals, *J Am Vet Med Assoc* 162:545-549, 1973.
46. Stiles J: Ocular manifestations of systemic disease. Part 3. The Horse. In Gelatt KN, editor: *Veterinary ophthalmology*, ed 3, Philadelphia, 1999, Lippincott Williams and Wilkins, pp 1473-1492.
47. Anninger WV et al: West Nile virus-associated optic neuritis and chorioretinitis, *Am J Ophthalmol* 136:1183-1185, 2003.

48. Kuchtey RW et al: Uveitis associated with West Nile virus infection, *Arch Ophthalmol* 121:1648-1649, 2003.

49. Rebhun WC: Diseases of the uvea. In Mayhew IG, editor: *Equine medicine and surgery, vol 2,* St Louis, 1999, Mosby, pp 1253-1260.

50. Lavach JD: Ocular manifestations of systemic diseases, *Vet Clin North Am Equine Practice* 8:627-636, 1992.

51. Barratt-Boyes SM et al: *Streptococcus equi* infection as a cause of panophthalmitis in a horse, *Equine Vet Sci* 11:229-231, 1991.

52. Roberts SR: Chorioretinitis in a band of horses, *J Am Vet Med Assoc* 158:2043-2046, 1971.

53. Jones TDC: The relation of brucellosis to periodic ophthalmia in Equidae, *Am J Vet Res* 1:54-57, 1940.

54. Pusterla N et al: Digenetic trematodes, *Acanthatrium* sp. and *Lecithodendrium* sp., as vectors of *Neorickettsia risticii*, the agent of Potomac horse fever, *J Helminthol* 77:335-339, 2003.

55. McDonald DR, Cleary DJ: Toxoplasmosis in the equine, *Southwest Vet* 23:213-214, 1970.

56. Rames DS, et al: Ocular *Halicephalobus* (syn. *Micronema*) *deletrix* in a horse, *Vet Pathol* 32:540-542, 1995.

57. Kinde H et al: *Halicephalobus gingivalis (H. deletrix)* infection in two horses in southern California, *J Vet Diagn Invest* 12:162-165, 2000.

58. Lavach JD: Parasitic diseases. In Lavach JD, editor: *Large animal ophthalmology*, St Louis, 1990, Mosby, pp 252-269.

59. Barnett KC: The ocular fundus of the horse, *Equine Vet J* 4:17-20, 1971.

60. Chandler KJ, Billson FM, Mellor DJ: Ophthalmic lesions in 83 geriatric horses and ponies, *Vet Rec* 153:319-322, 2003.

61. Url A et al:. Equine neuronal ceroid lipofuscinosis, *Acta Neuropathol* 101:410-414, 2001.

62. Riis RC et al: Ocular manifestations of equine motor neuron disease, *Equine Vet J* 31;99-110, 1999.

63. Riis RC, Divers TJ: Effect of vitamin E deficiency on horse retinas, *Vet Ophthalmol* 3:254-259, 2000.

64. Madigan JE et al: Photic headshaking in the horse: 7 cases, *Equine Vet J* 27:306, 1995.

65. Wilkins PA: Cyproheptadine: medical treatment for photic headshakers, *Comp Contin Educ Pract (Vet)* 19:98-102, 1997.

66. Platt H et al: Degenerative lesions of the optic nerve in Equidae, *Equine Vet J Suppl* 2:91-97, 1983.

67. Matz K, et al: Bilateral blindness after injury in a riding horse, *Tierarztl Prax* 21:225-232, 1993.

68. Reppas GP et al: Trauma-induced blindness in two horses, *Aust Vet J* 72:270-272, 1995.

69. Martin L, Kaswan R, Chapman W: Four cases of traumatic optic nerve blindness in the horse, *Equine Vet J* 18:133-137, 1986.

70. Hardy J, Wilkie DA, Robertson J: Ischemic optic neuropathy and blindness after arterial occlusion for treatment of guttural pouch mycosis in two horses, *J Am Vet Med Assoc* 196:1631-1634, 1990.

71. Saunders LZ, Bistner SI, Rubin LF: Proliferative optic neuropathy in horses, *Vet Pathol* 9:368-378, 1972.

72. Riis RC, Rebhun WC: Proliferative optic neuropathy in a horse caused by a granular cell tumor, *Equine Vet J Suppl* 10:69-72, 1990.

73. Ueda Y et al: Ocular medulloepithelioma in a Thoroughbred, *Equine Vet J* 25:558-561, 1993.

74. Eagle RC Jr, Font RL, Swerczek TW: Malignant medulloepithelioma of the optic nerve in a horse, *Vet Pathol* 15:488-494, 1978.

75. Dugan SJ: Ocular neoplasia, *Vet Clin North Am Equine Pract* 8:609-626, 1992.

76. Brem S et al: 35 *Leptospira* isolated from the vitreous body of 32 horses with recurrent uveitis (ERU), *Berl Munch Tierarztl Wochenschr* 112:390-393, 1999.

77. Brem S et al: Demonstration of intraocular *Leptospira* in 4 horses suffering from equine recurrent uveitis (ERU), *Berl Munch Tierarztl Wochenschr* 111:415-417, 1998.

78. Wollanke B, Rohrbach BW, Gerhards H: Serum and vitreous humor antibody titers in and isolation of *Leptospira interrogans* from horses with recurrent uveitis, *J Am Vet Med Assoc* 219:795-800, 2001.

79. Wollanke B et al: Intraocular and serum antibody titers to *Leptospira* in 150 horses with equine recurrent uveitis (ERU) subjected to vitrectomy, *Berl Munch Tierarztl Wochenschr* 11:134-139, 1998.

80. Wagner B et al: Demonstration of immunoglobulin isotypes in the vitreous body as a contribution to the etiology of recurrent equine uveitis, *DTW Dtsch Tierarztl Wochenschr* 104:467-470, 1997.

81. Fruhauf B et al: Surgical management of equine recurrent uveitis with single port pars plana vitrectomy, *Vet Ophthalmol* 1:137-151, 1998.

82. Gilger BC et al: Effect of an intravitreal cyclosporine implant on experimental uveitis in horses, *Vet Immunol Immunopathol* 76:239-255, 2000.

83. Gilger BC et al: Long-term effect on the equine eye of an intravitreal device used for sustained release of cyclosporine A, *Vet Ophthalmol* 3:105-110, 2000.

10 Equine Vision: Normal and Abnormal

Paul E. Miller
Christopher J. Murphy

An understanding of equine vision is important for many reasons, not the least of which is that for millennia humans have depended on the horse's visual abilities for their livelihood, personal safety, and sometimes very survival. Equine practitioners are also often asked to judge the suitability of a particular horse for specific uses, ranging from the visually demanding (e.g., identification and isolation of a calf in the case of a cutting horse) to those that can be performed by nearly blind animals, such as a broodmare walking in an enclosed pasture without injuring herself. In 1999 the Guide Horse Foundation was created for the purpose of providing Miniature horses as an alternative to guide dogs for visually impaired people (http://www.guidehorse.org). Additionally, although preservation of vision is the driving force in the treatment of most ocular disorders, lack of familiarity with these abilities may make it difficult to give the horse owner an accurate prognosis or to select the treatment option that will most likely provide the best outcome in terms of visual performance.

Ophthalmic disorders add another layer of complexity to estimation of a horse's visual capabilities. Some ocular diseases do not alter vision at all, whereas others have such a profound impact that even the ability to perceive light is lost. Furthermore, the externally apparent severity of the disease or size of an opacity does not always correlate with the impact the disorder has on the animal's vision. For example, eyes with copious ocular discharge or a large cataract in the periphery of the lens may retain essentially normal visual performance, whereas the presence of a small, axial, opacity in the posterior nucleus of the lens may degrade visual acuity significantly. In other instances, the clinician may be asked to examine a horse to determine whether an ocular disorder is the root cause of undesirable behaviors such as shying from objects or head shaking. Therefore in this chapter, the normal visual abilities of the horse and the impact that select ocular abnormalities may have on equine vision and behavior are discussed.

"SEEING"

The act of seeing is a complex process that depends on (1) light from the outside world falling onto the eye, (2) the eye efficiently transmitting and properly focusing images of objects on the retina where they are detected, (3) the transmission of this information to the brain, and (4) the brain processing this information to make it useful.[1] The act of vision is not simply a faithful recording of every feature of a scene, as a camera would do, because that would quickly overwhelm the visual system with massive amounts of information that may not be pertinent to the horse's survival or lifestyle. For example, in bright light, billions of photons interact with more than 100 million photoreceptors in each eye every second, which in turn converge on one million ganglion cells before passing to the brain.[2-5] Given that the photoreceptors and intervening neurons may refine the information that they pass along to the ganglion cells as often as 30 to 60 times per second[6-8] and that the ganglion cells, in turn, may process this further to send a new volley of information to the brain three times per second,[1] it is clear that the optic nerves are flooding the brain with massive amounts of information, much like a large telephone cable serving a major metropolitan area simultaneously carries millions of phone conversations. The brain does not, and cannot, consciously "listen" to all of these "conversations" at the same time, but instead categorizes the information into specific "topics," which are channeled to specific areas of the brain for further processing.[9-12] In addition, unlike a camera, the brain compares this input with previous images, images from the other eye, and input from other senses such as hearing, smell, and touch. Once this is completed, only the information

371

that is relevant to the task at hand or the horse's survival rises to the level of conscious attention. Therefore the act of seeing depends not only on the function and health of the eye but also on the cognitive processes in the brain that decide what information merits conscious attention and what is to remain subconscious or discarded.

On a more detailed level, the information carried from the eye is packaged into many discrete "topics," including an object's brightness, size, location of its edges, its "internal" features such as texture and contrast, the direction in which it is moving, its velocity, its overall orientation as represented on the retinal surface, its shape, its color, and many others. However, a critical aspect of vision is that an object (a wolf, for example) is identified as separate from its surroundings (dense vegetation). Because this distinction is so important for survival, animals (including humans) with normal vision, can "see" an object if it differs sufficiently from its surroundings in any *one* of five different aspects: luminance ("brightness"), motion, texture, binocular disparity (depth), or color.[9] In general, objects are differentiated on the basis of their motion, texture, depth, and luminance roughly equally well; but separations based on color are less easily made.[9-12] In this chapter the normal subunits of equine vision are described, including the ability to perceive light, motion, and contrast; visual perspective and field of view; depth perception; visual acuity; and color vision. However, in reality, a complete description of how well a horse sees requires not only an understanding of each of these subunits of vision but also an understanding of how the brain synthesizes these constituent parts into a unified perception of the world. Unfortunately, the horse's higher visual pathways are understood only in broad strokes, and hence, understanding of equine vision has significant gaps.

SENSITIVITY TO LIGHT

The ability to perceive light is a fundamental aspect of vision, although the eyes of most mammals, including horses and humans, are capable of detecting photons that are located in only a tiny portion of the electromagnetic spectrum—typically between 380 and 760 nm.[8,13,14] Even in this *visible spectrum,* not all photons are detected equally well, and so light perception depends not only on the number of photons "raining" onto the retina but also on the sensitivity of the eye to that particular wavelength.[8,14] The term luminance (sometimes called value by artists) is the perceived "lightness" of an object.[9,15] Luminance is not purely a physical phenomenon because a dim-appearing "blue" light and a bright-appearing "yellow" light

may comprise exactly the same number of photons; instead, luminance depends on how sensitive the retinal photoreceptors are to the wavelength of light that is striking the retina.[12,15] Therefore a yellow leaf may appear "brighter" than a green leaf under viewing conditions favoring photoreceptor subtypes most sensitive to yellow, whereas under dim lighting conditions, the same green leaf may now appear "brighter," or more luminous, than the yellow one. This phenomenon, called the Purkinje shift, is the result of the eye shifting between rod and cone vision as light intensity varies; this also explains why blue objects appear lighter and red ones appear darker in twilight versus daylight.[16] Another way of appreciating the difference between luminance and color is to remove all the color information with a computer program and look at a scene in shades of gray.[15] When this is done, it becomes obvious that many objects can be differentiated on the basis of their luminance alone and that color is a less important clue. Luminance is important because the perception of depth, three-dimensionality, movement (or lack thereof), and spatial organization are all carried by a part of the visual system that responds only to luminance differences and is insensitive to color.[10,11,15,17]

Humans, and presumably horses, are largely unaware of the enormous variation in light intensity in the real world. A major challenge confronting both species is to adapt to light intensities that vary from the dimmest star to bright sunlight on snow, a factor of as much as 40 billion.[4] One mechanism for adjusting to this wide range is to switch back and forth between two different types of photoreceptors: the rods and cones, each of which has been optimized to perform best at different ends of the intensity spectrum.[4,12] In both humans and horses, the overall ratio of rod to cone photoreceptors is approximately 20 to 1[2,18] (humans have about 5 million cones and 100 million rods), but the distribution of these cells is quite different between the two species. In humans, the cones are densely packed in the central retina (fovea) and rapidly fall off to low numbers just 1 to 2 mm away from the fovea,[2] whereas in horses, the distribution of cones is believed to be more uniform across the retina with perhaps an increase in the temporal region of the visual streak.[19,20] Rod photoreceptors can reliably respond to a single photon of light[21] and are the primary receptors used when the light levels range from virtually complete darkness to those found at dawn and twilight.[4] In humans, rods achieve their peak response to light when they are continuously illuminated by about 500 photons/sec, or by a sudden flash of about 100 photons.[4] This means that by midmorning on a sunny day, the rods have become saturated by light, and that in order for useful vision to be maintained, the eye must shift over to using primarily cones. Although cones can also detect a single photon, this interaction typically generates very little response, and the effective lower threshold for cone vision is about 3 photons/sec. The cones also support color vision, but humans do not begin to appreciate color until the light intensity rises to about 10 photons/sec.[4] In contrast to rods, the cones' response to a steady background light does not saturate, and cones can increase in responsiveness to light intensities as high as 1,000,000 photons/sec (a level so high that it can essentially "cook" the cell).[4] By comparison, bright sunlight on snow at high altitude has an intensity of about 300,000 photons/sec.[4] In a sense, switching between rod and cone photoreceptors is similar to a photographer switching between use of a slow-speed, "fine-grain" film designed to produce highly detailed color images in bright light and use of a fast-speed, "coarse-grain" black-and-white film designed for less detailed gray-scale images in low light. However, as the eye shifts from rod to cone photoreceptors, what is lost in terms of sensitivity to light is replaced by improved color vision and visual acuity.

In addition to switching between rod and cone photoreceptor subtypes, there are several other mechanisms for adjusting to the wide range of lighting intensities that occur in the real world. Changing pupil size can rapidly alter the amount of light that reaches the retina, but this mechanism limits the range of light intensities only by about 10-fold in humans[4] and probably only by a few fold more in horses according to their range of pupillary excursions.[22] Another relatively rapid but more robust mechanism involves changing neural processing by the retinal bipolar and ganglion cells. This pathway can facilitate adaptation over a range of about 1000- fold.[4] The major but slower mechanism for adjusting to varying light intensity is to chemically alter the sensitivity of the photoreceptors to light.[12,23] Light chemically disassociates the retinal photopigments into their constituent parts, and this depletion (photoreceptor bleaching) leads to a proportional increase in the amount of light required to trigger a response by the photoreceptor.[4,12,23] Conversely, when an animal is placed in darkness, the photopigment is reconstituted into its active form, and the eye becomes more sensitive to light. This light and dark adaptation occurs over a period of minutes (5 minutes for cones and 20 to 30 minutes for rods) and can easily be appreciated by simply walking into and out of a dark barn on a bright sunny day.[4,12] In humans, these photochemical changes can provide a range of adaptation to light intensity that varies on the order of 100 million–fold.[4] Hence, vision is maintained over an enormous range of light intensities by making relatively slow but massive changes in photoreceptor sensitivity and then "fine-tuning" the intensity by faster alterations in pupil size and retinal processing.

In addition to these mechanisms, horses have a number of other adaptations that humans do not, which improve vision in dim light (Fig. 10-1). The horse has one of the largest eyes among the terrestrial vertebrates,[24-26] and this allows more light to enter the eye. Admission of light to the eye is further enhanced by horizontal elongation of the cornea and pupil[27,28] and by the equine pupil's ability to dilate to an area six times larger than that of a human pupil (3 to 3.5 times greater than cat's or dog's) to allow even more light to

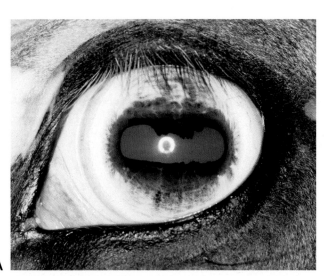

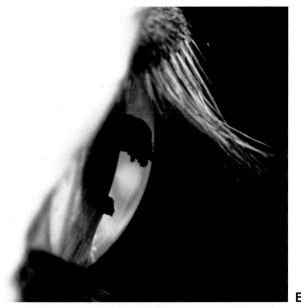

A

B

Fig. 10-1 A, A normal equine eye demonstrating several adaptations to vision in dim and bright light including an large elongated cornea, a horizontal rectangular pupil, and corpora nigra. **B,** Note how the superior corpora nigra functions as an "awning" and shields the retina from bright light originating from above. Similarly, the inferior corpora nigra may partially shield the retina from rays reflected off the ground.

reach the retina.[22,29,30] An elongated slit-like pupil is common in species that are active at night and daytime because in bright light this shape closes more completely than a round pupil, thereby better protecting a highly light-sensitive retina from very bright light.[31,32] The horizontally elongated, roughly rectangular shape of the horse's pupil in daylight also provides it with a wider view of the horizon than it would obtain with a circular pupil with identical surface area.[31] This allows the horse to scan the visual horizon while at the same time reducing the variations in luminosity the retina must cope with between the usually brighter sky and the usually darker ground. The equine version of the rod photopigment, rhodopsin, also differs somewhat from that of humans,[33] and like that of dogs and other species adapted for vision in dim light, it may continue to increase in sensitivity to light for a longer period when the animal is placed in the dark.[34-36]

The horse's vision in dim light is also improved by a large, superiorly located, roughly triangular, reflective tapetum lucidum that provides the photoreceptors a second chance to capture each photon (Fig. 10-2).[37-44] However, this improved ability to capture light comes at the price of reducing the potential visual acuity of the eye because the retina is not able to determine whether the photon hit the photoreceptor on the first pass or whether it was reflected there from a slightly different point in space. In horses, the tapetal reflection is accomplished by the regular spacing of uniform diameter collagen fibrils in the choroid.[40,43,44] The color of the tapetum as seen with an ophthalmoscope is the result of the physical interaction of light with the fibrous

tapetum, and not the result of colored pigments in the tapetum.[40,43,44] Yellow or green tapetal reflections represent regions where these fibrils are more numerous, whereas deep blue to purple reflections represent thinner tapetal domains. In contrast to the fibrous tapetum of most mammalian herbivores, in many carnivores, modified cellular constituents are used as a tapetum.[37,40-42] Although the equine tapetum is not as efficient a reflector as the cellular tapetum of some nocturnal carnivores such as the cat (which can reflect up to 130 times more light than the human fundus),[41] it is undoubtedly superior to the human eye, which lacks a tapetum altogether. The presence of a tapetum suggests that the horse's lower limit for vision in dim light is much less than that for humans but not as low as that for cats (which is 5.5 to 7 times less than that for humans[45]) and perhaps that for certain other predators with a tapetum. The modification of different constituents (collagen, cells, or even crystals in some species) to create a reflective layer in the fundus and thereby improve vision in dim light suggests that the tapetum has evolved separately on a number of occasions and that it represents an evolutionary "arms race" between various predator and prey combinations in which each is seeking a distinct survival advantage over the other.[37-44]

Although the equine visual system appears to have evolved to function best in dim lighting circumstances, it also has several features that improve vision in bright light, suggesting that the horse is adapted for an arrhythmic photic lifestyle. For example, the nuclear region of the equine lens contains yellow pigments (Fig. 10-3),[46] as do human lenses and those of other highly diurnal species such as squirrels.[47,48] These pigments filter out shorter (blue) wavelengths of light, much as yellow-tinted sunglasses do for humans, thereby reducing glare in bright light and improving the contrast of some objects against their background because blue wavelengths of light are scattered 16 times more easily than red wavelengths.[47,48] This pigment also filters out higher-energy rays that are more likely to damage the retina, thereby protecting the delicate photoreceptors in bright daylight.[47,48] The large corpora nigra on the central, superior border of the iris also improves vision in bright light by augmenting pupillary constriction and acting as an "internal visor," which blocks direct sunlight exposure of the inferior retina, thereby further reducing glare and improving vision in bright light. The much smaller corpora nigra on the inferior pupillary border may behave in a similar way to reduce the impact of light reflected off the ground. In fact, in very bright light, the horse's pupil may constrict to such a degree that the superior corpora nigra apposes the inferior iris, effectively dividing the pupil into two segments. The impact of this on the animal's vision is

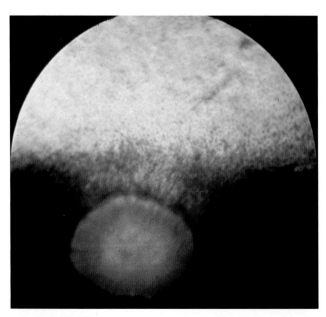

Fig. 10-2 The fibrous tapetum of horses reflects light to enhance vision in dim light. However, this reflection may also scatter light and reduce visual acuity.

unclear, but two pupils oriented in the same plane as the visual streak on the retina may improve the animal's vision in bright light[31] (see discussion of optical consequences of pupil shape). In a sense, the horse has evolved to be a "visual generalist" in which it has some degree of vision under all lighting circumstances, unlike humans who tend to function best in bright light and cats who function well in dim light.

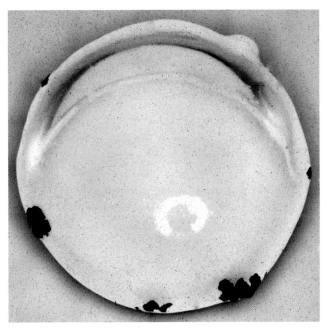

Fig. 10-3 Yellow pigments present in the equine lens may filter out blue light, thereby reducing glare and improving contrast in bright light.

SENSITIVITY TO MOTION

Another fundamental component of vision is determining whether an object is moving, because moving objects are more likely to demand some form of a response than static objects. Motion detection is relatively easy if the horse itself is stationary because any change in the position of an object on the retina represents motion. However, detecting motion in real life is complicated because movement may occur on the part of the object, the horse, or both. Therefore if the horse is also moving, it must closely coordinate the movements of its eyes, head, neck, and entire body to prevent the retinal image from "bouncing" in such a jerky manner (like the image captured on a video camera when the operator is running) that the animal would be functionally blind.[4] When a horse is trotting, some of these compensatory mechanisms can be seen at work by observing that the head (and therefore the eyes) bob only slightly because of a series of reflexive counterbalancing motions by the body and neck (Fig. 10-4).

Images are stabilized on the retina in virtually all mammals, including the horse, by several systems, including a stabilization (fixation) system, a vestibulo-ocular reflex system, and an optokinetic system.[49-51] Some prey species with laterally placed eyes, wide fields of view, and no fovea (such as the rabbit and goldfish) use these three systems almost exclusively.[49] Such animals tend to have relatively small extraocular muscles and rely on panoramic vision for the early detection and avoidance of danger. Predators who have forward-looking eyes, comparatively smaller fields of view,

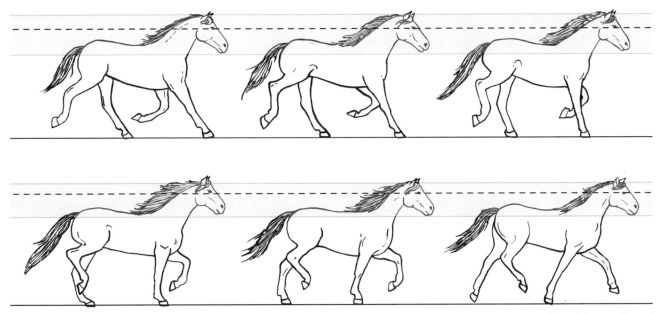

Fig. 10-4 When trotting the image on the retina remains relatively stationary during movement through a series of carefully coordinated movements of the head and neck.

relatively well-developed extraocular muscles, a fovea (or at least a localized central region with heightened photoreceptor density such as the area centralis in cats), and improved binocular vision for catching prey have an additional set of more complicated eye movements, including saccades, smooth pursuit movements, and vergence eye movements.[49-51] These movements allow the region of the retina with the greatest visual acuity to be aimed at, and track, an object, especially while both the pursuer and pursued are moving. However, the relative contribution of the later set of eye movements to equine vision is unclear because although the horse has laterally placed eyes and no true fovea, it has very well-developed extraocular muscles and a degree of binocular overlap and visual acuity that rivals, if not exceeds, that of many predators, including wolves.

The fixation system attempts to maintain an object of interest in a relatively stable position on the area of the retina with the greatest visual acuity. However, no image is ever truly stationary on the retina because the eyes of all animals "drift" to a minor degree as a result of involuntary tremors of the head and neck, respiratory movements, and cardiac pulse. In fact, for unknown reasons, at the level of the brain, if the image is held completely stable on the retina, humans' (and undoubtedly the horse's) ability to perceive the image rapidly fades.[52] In humans, this spontaneous drift is up to four times greater in the dark than in the light because, to some extent, in the light the drift is counteracted by an image stabilization system in which photoreceptors with large receptive fields generate an "error signal" and redirect the eyes back toward the target.[49] These redirecting movements, as well as other types of eye movements, generally follow two fundamental laws. *Sherrington's law of reciprocal innervation* proposes that whenever an extraocular muscle receives a neural impulse to contract, its antagonistic muscle receives a signal to relax. For example, if the lateral rectus muscle of the right eye contracts to redirect the animal's gaze to the right, the medial rectus muscle of the right eye relaxes. *Hering's law of motor correspondence* refers to movements that allow the two eyes to act like "yoked" pairs and move in a coordinated fashion. Hence, if the lateral rectus muscle of the right eye contracts to redirect the animal's gaze to the right, the medial rectus muscle of the left eye also contracts so as to move the two eyes toward the same point in space. However, compensatory eye movements created by the fixation system are relatively slow because they depend on the speed at which the retina can process an image, and hence, this system cannot be used to maintain vision if the object, horse, or both are moving quickly.

Two, even faster, reflexive eye movement systems also stabilize an image on the retina. These pathways work to cancel out motion of an object across the retina when the horse itself is moving (the vestibulo-ocular reflex or "doll's eye reflex") or when object is moving across the horse's visual field (optokinetic nystagmus). Of all the types of movements, head movements have the greatest potential to disrupt vision because visual processing cannot even begin to match the speed at which images can sweep across the retina when the head moves.[49] For the purpose of reducing the impact of head movements, signals from the motion-detecting semicircular canals of the vestibular system direct the eyes to rotate in the direction opposite that in which the head is moving so as to maintain the visual axes relatively fixed in space. The eye movements of the vestibulo-ocular reflex consist of a slow phase in the direction opposite that in which the head is moving (compensatory smooth eye movement) to steady the image on the retina—and if head movement continues past a certain point—a rapid, "quick phase" (involuntary saccade) in which the eye "jumps" ahead to preview the upcoming scene.[49-51] This form of vestibular nystagmus is normal and compensates for most head movements, allowing the horse to move and see at the same time. Lateral-eyed, afoveate animals with large fields of view, such as the rabbit, tend to rely heavily on this type of eye movement; whereas forward-looking predators can either use the vestibulo-ocular reflex or override it so that during a chase their eyes can remain locked onto the target ahead of them rather than remaining locked on a fixed point in space.[49] Although it is unclear why, a horse seems to exhibit quick phase eye movements to a greater degree when the head is moving in a horizontal plane than when it is moving in a vertical plane. This may be because horses, like humans, generate a horizontal saccade by using input from only one side of the brain; a vertical saccade would require simultaneous activity from both sides of the brain.[51]

As the head continues to rotate at the same speed, the fluid in the vestibular canals soon begins moving at or near the same rate as the head, and therefore it can no longer direct the compensatory eye movements. However, the image is still "slipping" across large regions of the retina, and now the phylogenetically old optokinetic nystagmus system takes over and uses this visual stimulus to continue to direct the eye movements and keep the image stationary on the retina.[49-51] It is also possible to "trick" the brain into activating the optokinetic nystagmus system by keeping the animal stationary and making the surrounding environment appear to rotate around it. The latter "trick" has been used to estimate an animal's visual acuity because this type of nystagmus occurs only if the animal is actually able to distinguish the object in question as separate from the background.[53] However, this is a less-than-ideal method, because the stimulus for the optokinetic reflex is the image "slipping" on large regions of the retina, rather than the fine details of the object as viewed by the visual streak or fovea.[49-51] Hence, the estimates of visual acuity obtained in this manner are not likely to represent peak visual acuity because that depends on the performance of the visual streak or fovea. Nevertheless, the vestibulo-ocular reflex and the opto-kinetic system can be thought of as a single system that uses two different sensory signals, vestibular and visual, to help solve the same problem: maintaining retinal image stability during self-rotation and movement.

The need for an optokinetic system has been questioned because, in contrast to most animals, it is rudimentary to absent in humans,[49] and few land animals run in a circle for 10 to 20 seconds or more. It might be of value to a reining horse that whirls on its rear quarters for up to 8 to 10 revolutions. More likely, however, the purpose of the optokinetic system is to respond to cyclical, sustained, relatively low-velocity head movements such as those that occur during walking, trotting, and the like. The clinician can exploit these types of visually guided ocular rotations when examining a horse. If the horse's head is rotated downward, for example, the eye rotates upward, thereby allowing examination of particular regions of the cornea or anterior segment that may otherwise be covered by the eyelids.

In addition to these three involuntary stabilizing reflexes, many species also have voluntary eye movements such as saccades and smooth pursuit movements that keep images directed on important regions of the retina.[49-51] Saccades are rapid (0.02 to 0.1 second) voluntary movements that quickly shift the eyes to keep a moving or new image on the area of the retina with the greatest visual acuity. These movements may be quite large, covering up to 100 degrees in humans.[49] When the head is stationary, some species such as the rabbit and goldfish, do not make saccades for all practical purposes.[49] These species have little need to do so because their laterally placed eyes already provide them with a large field of view, and their horizontally oriented visual streak allows them to scan the horizon without moving the globe. The involuntary rapid eye movements seen in the vestibulo-ocular reflex and optokinetic systems in these species are often referred to as quick phases rather than true saccades, although their amplitude, duration, and velocity are essentially the same as those of a voluntary saccade.[49-51] When a rabbit (and under certain conditions, a horse) makes a voluntary head movement, a saccade in the direction in which the head is turning is initiated simultaneously with or just before the head movement.[49] This causes the gaze to "jump ahead," and while the head is moving, the eye holds its new position by means of the vestibulo-ocular reflex until the head catches up and the gaze is again properly aligned.[49] Humans and animals with a central area of particularly acute vision (area centralis), such as dogs and cats, can also make voluntary saccadic eye movements without moving the head. Although the horse also has laterally placed eyes and a large field of view, it also appears to be capable of making saccades without moving its head, especially when it is apprehensive; but it does not seem to make these movements as often as animals with more frontally located eyes.

Because the eye rapidly "skips ahead" during a saccade, there is no time for the retina to process the intervening visual information or for the brain to correct or refine the movement during the shift. In effect, the eye is functionally blind during a saccade, and the target may be slightly undershot or overshot.[49-51] If the eye is shifting a large distance, the initial saccade moves the eye about 90% of the distance, and one or more smaller corrective saccades make up the remainder. The "smearing" of the image on the retina during a saccade is generally not consciously appreciated, and even though the eye has moved a large distance, the external world is perceived to be stable.[49-51] This is another way that the eye differs from a camera because when a camera moves, the external world also appears to move. Once the image stabilizes on the retina at the end of a saccade, the new information overpowers that which may have started during the saccade, and higher visual pathways "backward mask" the old information, thereby smoothing the image and rendering the animal unaware of the rapid, large shift that occurred.[49] It is tempting to speculate that because the horse has a large field of view, it needs to make fewer saccades and that this improves its vision (at least to a minor degree) by virtue of a reduction in the image smearing that occurs during these movements.

In many species, once the image has been captured on the visual streak by a saccade and any small "catch-up" saccades have been made, relatively voluntary, smooth-pursuit eye movements track a moving object so that its image remains on the retinal area with the greatest visual acuity (fovea or area centralis).[49-51] Like the saccadic system, smooth pursuit evolved with the development of retinal areas of greater resolution and is most well developed in species equipped with this type of retinal architecture. Under normal conditions, the stimulus for smooth pursuit is similar to that for the optokinetic system, for example, movement of the image across the retina (retinal slip).[49,50] However, smooth pursuit is different in that the movement of the object is the point of interest, whereas with the optokinetic system, the drive is to follow the background that is moving in the opposite direction. Smooth-pursuit movements are driven by images that stimulate the fovea or area centralis and are usually small and relatively slow, whereas the slow phases of the optokinetic system are induced by large patterns that stimulate large areas of the retina.[51] To be effective, smooth-pursuit eye movements must override not only the fixation maintenance system, which tries to keep the eyes fixated on the same point in space, but also the optokinetic system, which tries to follow the massively slipping background images instead of the target.[49] Additionally, if the horse's head is also moving, the vestibulo-ocular reflex also needs to be cancelled out if smooth-pursuit movements are to allow the image to be examined more closely. [49]

Stationary objects are also viewed with smooth-pursuit eye movements because there is always slight motion of the image on the retina as the muscles of the head, neck, and body attempt to maintain a steady posture.[4,49-51] Because smooth-pursuit eye movements track an image by using "retinal slip," the image on the retina is always moving to some degree. This is another way in which the visual system differs from a camera because, in effect, it requires movement to function properly. Although the image of the object being observed may seem to be stationary, this is purely a perceptual phenomenon and is the result of higher visual pathway processing of the image. Animals with visual streaks (such as horses) typically do not show smooth-pursuit movements when an object moves horizontally along the direction of the streak[4] but appear to do so when an object moves vertically across the streak.

Saccadic and smooth-pursuit movements result in the two eyes moving equally in a synchronous (conjugate) fashion, and the viewing angle between the two eyes remains the same. Typically, these movements are elicited when the object of interest is moving from side to side or up and down. If the object of interest is moving toward or away from the viewer, convergent or divergent "vergence" eye movements, respectively, are used to change the viewing angle between the two eyes to keep the object in proper focus. Convergence is also usually accompanied by accommodation (adjusting the focal power of the lens so that near objects are seen more clearly) and miosis that optically increases the animal's depth of field, thereby enhancing the animal's depth perception and the visualization of near objects.[54] These three responses—convergence, accommodation, and miosis—are neurologically distinct, but because they generally occur simultaneously, they are referred to as the near response.[54] Vergence eye movements are typically fairly slow (taking up to 1 second in humans),[51] and as during a saccade, visual sensitivity is markedly reduced during the movement itself. The extent to which horses perform vergence eye movements has not been carefully investigated, but the relatively large area of binocular overlap and certain behaviors (see discussion of depth perception) suggest that they are readily capable of performing these types of movements. However, the comparably slower rate of pupillary constriction of horses versus that of humans suggests that horses may perform vergence movements more slowly than humans do.

Horses, like humans, detect moving objects more easily than stationary ones. This is especially true for objects in the horse's peripheral visual field, which has a visual acuity so low that it may permit only "movingness" and "brightness," rather than discrete objects, to be seen.[24] This poor peripheral visual acuity, coupled with a "prey mentality," may explain why horses often shy from even innocuous objects located in their peripheral visual field. Although the peripheral retina has often been described as subserving motion detection, it is erroneous to infer that animals with large peripheral visual fields are better at motion detection than those with better-developed, central visual areas such as a fovea. The peripheral retina does have a greater number of the ganglion cell subtypes devoted to motion detection (the magnocellular pathway and the retinal amacrine cells, which subserve movement and directional sensitivity of the retina),[3,55] but the central retina has more densely packed photoreceptors and a lower threshold for motion detection. In one study, the more densely packed human fovea had a 10- to 12-fold lower threshold for detecting motion than that of a cat.[56,57] Because horses have significantly better visual acuity than cats, it is likely that horses are better at detecting motion than cats but not quite as good at it as humans. However, it remains to be determined whether there are differences between the peripheral retina and central retina of horses that would render their peripheral field of view more sensitive to objects moving at specific speeds, objects moving in certain directions, or objects with features that make them more "attention grabbing" for some reason. Like many aspects of the equine visual system, there are many unknowns in how horses detect motion. It is possible that a much greater degree of processing of the image may occur at the level of the retina than is currently appreciated and that novel mechanisms for motion detection may be discovered with more careful investigation in the future.

VISUAL PERSPECTIVE AND FIELD OF VIEW

The horse's visual perspective can vary greatly and depends to a large extent on whether the head is down and the animal is grazing or whether the head is up and the animal is scanning the horizon. Furthermore, breed differences can result in the same environment being perceived quite differently. For example, a field of tall grass may appear to be a dense, impenetrable brush to a Miniature horse, but a wide-open savanna to a Clydesdale (Fig. 10-5).

The lateral position of the eyes in the skull affords the horse a wide, panoramic view (Fig. 10-6).[19,24,32] Additionally, the nasal extension of the retina and

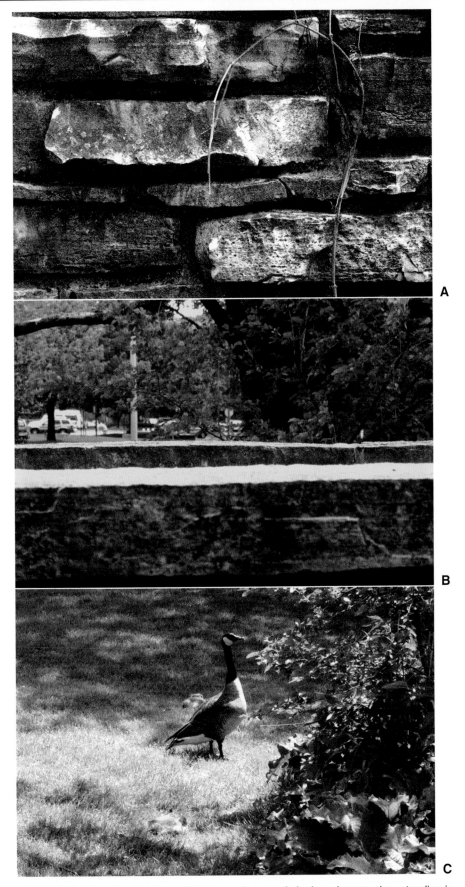

Fig. 10-5 The visual perspective of horses varies greatly by breed, even when standing in the same location. **A,** Miniature horse. **B,** Arabian. **C,** Belgian Draft horse.

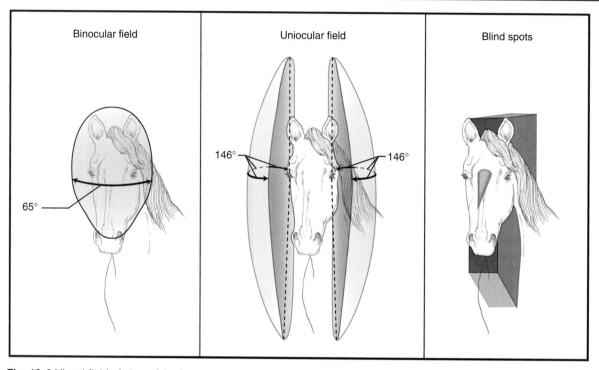

Fig. 10-6 Visual field of view of the horse.

comparatively greater vertical width of the pupil nasally than temporally further enhances the horse's temporal peripheral visual field. On the basis of anatomic relationships, the horse is believed to have a total monocular visual field in the horizontal meridian (i.e., the portion of the horizon that can be seen by an eye when fixed on one point) of approximately 190 to 195 degrees, and up to 178 degrees in the vertical (superior to inferior) meridian. When the visual fields of the two eyes are combined, the total horizontal visual field is up to 350 degrees, and the horse has virtually a complete sphere of vision around its body with only a few minor "blind spots." [24,32,19] These blind spots are small and located superior and perpendicular to the forehead, directly below the nose, in a small oval region in the superior visual field where light strikes the optic nerve itself, and the width of the animal's head directly behind it. Clearly, this extensive visual field makes it very difficult for a predator or human handler to "sneak up" on a horse.

The visual fields of the two eyes overlap anteriorly and below the nose for 55 to 65 degrees, although some authors suggest the overlap may be as great as 70 to 80 degrees.[19] This degree of binocular overlap rivals or exceeds that of domestic dogs, which ranges from 30 to 60 degrees, depending on breed.[24,25,58,59] This would seem to challenge the generally accepted view that predators have binocular vision superior to that of prey species. In reality, however, depth perception also plays a significant role in "breaking the camouflage" of an object (e.g., a wolf) against its background, and so this would also be of distinct advantage to prey species.[60] It is also possible that, as has been described for certain bird species, the animal's lifestyle and the extent of the binocular field do not necessarily predict the quality of its stereoscopic vision.[61,62]

DEPTH PERCEPTION

Stereopsis (binocular depth perception) results when the two eyes view the world from slightly different vantage points and the images from the overlapping visual fields are fused into one.[60] If the relatively disparate images on the two retinas were not blended, viewing a scene with both eyes would simply result in double vision (diplopia), and depth perception would actually be impaired. The new information that stereopsis provides is as qualitatively important to the overall sense of vision as is the perception of motion, color, or contrast. The ability to perceive depth varies greatly between individual humans[63,64] and cats,[65] and although similar work has not been done with horses, some horses undoubtedly are better than others at detecting depth. How these differences may affect their usefulness for certain types of work is uncertain because horses with one eye can often still function well as jumpers or barrel racers, even though these tasks would seem to demand a fairly sophisticated degree of depth perception. Also, several horses with only one functional

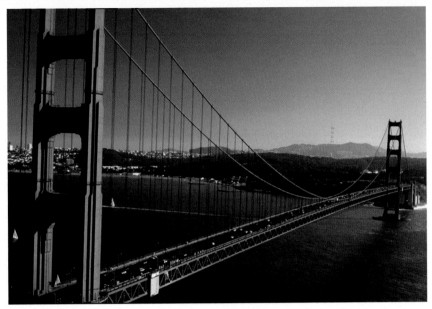

Fig. 10-7 Several cues allow depth to be perceived with one eye or in a two-dimensional photograph. These cues include apparent size (the left tower appears closer because it is larger than the right), looming (cars moving toward the viewer appear to become progressively larger), interposition (near objects, such as the bridge, overlay the more distant hills), aerial perspective (water vapor and dust in the air make the more distant hills less distinct and relatively color-desaturated), shading (shadows on the tower suggest depth), perspective (the parallel roadways appear to converge toward the horizon), relative velocity (the nearer cars appear to move faster than the more distant ones), and motion parallax (if the eye is fixed on the center of the bridge, the images of near objects appear to move opposite the direction in which the observer moves his or her head, whereas distant objects move in the same direction as the head).

eye have performed well in top-tier races such as the Kentucky Derby.[66]

As any artist can attest, animals and humans use several monocular clues to perceive depth. These include relative brightness (brighter objects tend to be closer), size (larger objects are closer or objects progressively increasing in size are getting closer), contour and areas of light and shadows (the gradation in the intensity of a shadow on a curved object makes it appear to be projecting away from or toward the observer), object overlay (closer objects block distant ones), linear perspective (parallel lines like those of a railroad track converge onto a vanishing point at distance), aerial perspective (water vapor, dust, and smoke in the atmosphere make distant objects indistinct and relatively color-desaturated), density of optical texture (the fine details of the surface of an object become less apparent the farther away it is), relative velocity (near objects appear to move faster than distant ones), and motion parallax (objects at different distances appear to move at different speeds or in different directions, depending on the observer's point of fixation [Fig. 10-7]).[60] There is good evidence that horses are able to use at least some of these static monocular clues to recognize depth in two-dimensional photographs, and it appears that they are even susceptible to some of the pictorial visual illusions to which humans are susceptible.[67,68] Because of their huge monocular visual fields, it is clearly advantageous for horses to be able to use monocular clues to estimate depth.

Nevertheless, two eyes are better than one, because the binocular threshold for depth perception in horses is five times better than the monocular threshold.[69] Although the two eyes of horses are farther apart than those of humans (resulting in a greater relative disparity between the two retinal images and theoretically better depth perception), humans still have better depth perception than horses. From 2 m away, humans can detect a few millimeters' difference in depth, whereas from the same distance, horses can detect only a 9-cm difference (a 10- to 20-fold poorer performance).[69] The latter value approximates that of cats.[70,71] The latter difference may have some biologic relevance because it is also approximately the same difference in depth between grass in a pasture and the ground under it. The familiar behavior of a horse rotating its nose upward to better observe distant objects may be an attempt to exploit its improved binocular depth perception, because binocular overlap is oriented down the nose in horses, rather than straight ahead as it is in humans.[24,72]

86. Studdert MJ, Blackney MH: Isolation of an adenovirus antigenically distinct from equine adenovirus type 1 from diarrheic foal feces, *Am J Vet Res* 43:543-544, 1982.

87. McChesney AE, England JJ, Rich LJ: Adenoviral infection in foals, *J Am Vet Med Assoc* 162:545-549, 1973.

88. Chirnside E, Sinclair R, Mumford JA: Respiratory viral diseases. In Reed SM, Bayly WM, editors: *Equine internal medicine*, Philadelphia, 1998, Saunders, pp 93-106.

89. Hannant D, Mumford JA, Jessett DM: Duration of circulating antibody and immunity following infection with equine influenza virus, *Vet Rec* 122:125-128, 1988.

90. Townsend HG et al: Efficacy of a cold-adapted, intranasal, equine influenza vaccine: challenge trials, *Equine Vet J* 33:637-643, 2001.

91. Centers for Disease Control and Prevention: West Nile virus activity—United States. *MMWR Morb Mortal Wkly Rep* 2003; 52:1132, 2001.

92. Bender K, Thompson FEJ: West Nile virus: a growing challenge, *Am J Nurs* 103:32-39, 2003.

93. Deubel V et al: Variations in biological features of West Nile viruses, *Ann N Y Acad Sci* 951:195-206, 2001.

94. Davis BS et al: West Nile virus recombinant DNA vaccine protects mouse and horse from virus challenge and expresses in vitro a noninfectious recombinant antigen that can be used in enzyme-linked immunosorbent assays, *J Virol* 75:4040-4047, 2001.

95. Porter MB et al: West Nile virus encephalomyelitis in horses: 46 cases (2001), *J Am Vet Med Assoc* 222:1241-1247, 2003.

96. Solomon T et al: Natural and nosocomial infection in a patient with West Nile encephalitis and extrapyramidal movement disorders, *Clin Infect Dis* 36:E140-E145, 2003.

97. Autorino GL et al: West Nile virus epidemic in horses, Tuscany region, Italy, *Emerg Infect Dis* 8:1372-1378, 2002.

98. Anninger WV et al: West Nile virus-associated optic neuritis and chorioretinitis, *Am J Ophthalmol* 136:1183-1185, 2003.

99. Kuchtey RW et al: Uveitis associated with West Nile virus infection, *Arch Ophthalmol* 121:1648-1649, 2003.

100. Ostlund EN et al: Equine West Nile encephalitis, United States, *Emerg Infect Dis* 7:665-669, 2001.

101. Davis JL, Jones SL: Equine primary immunodeficiencies, *Compend Contin Educ Pract Vet* 25:548-556, 2003.

102. Ng T et al: Equine vaccine for West Nile virus, *Dev Biol* 114: 221-227, 2003.

103. Rebhun WC: Diseases of the uvea. In Mayhew IG, editor: *Equine medicine and surgery*, vol 2, St. Louis, 1999, Mosby, pp 1253-1260.

104. Barratt-Boyes SM et al: *Streptococcus equi* infection as a cause of panophthalmitis in a horse, *Equine Vet Sci* 11:229-231, 1991.

105. Roberts SR: Chorioretinitis in a band of horses, *J Am Vet Med Assoc* 158:2043-2046, 1971.

106. De Lahunta A, Cummings JF: Neuro-ophthalmologic lesions as a cause of visual deficit in dogs and horses, *J Am Vet Med Assoc* 150:994-1011, 1967.

107. Sweeney CR et al: Description of an epizootic and persistence of *Streptococcus equi* infections in horses, *J Am Vet Med Assoc* 194:1281-1286, 1989.

108. Fintl C et al: Endoscopic and bacteriological findings in a chronic outbreak of strangles, *Vet Rec* 147:480-484, 2000.

109. Spoormakers TJ et al: Brain abscesses as a metastatic manifestation of strangles: symptomatology and the use of magnetic resonance imaging as a diagnostic aid, *Equine Vet J* 35:146-151, 2003.

110. Pusterla N et al: Purpura haemorrhagica in 53 horses, *Vet Rec* 153:118-121, 2003.

111. Freeman DE et al: A large frontonasal bone flap for sinus surgery in the horse, *Vet Surg* 19:122-130, 1990.

112. Morris DD: Disease of the hemolymphatic system, In Reed SM, Bayly WM, editors: *Equine internal medicine*, Philadelphia, 1998, Saunders; pp 564-566.

113. Roberts MC, Kelly WR: Renal dysfunction in a case of purpura haemorrhagica, *Vet Rec* 110:114-116, 1982.

114. Ainsworth DM: Rhodococcal infections in foals, *Equine Vet Educ* 11:191-198, 1999.

115. Johnson JA, Prescott JF, Markham RJF: The pathology of experimental *Corynebacterium equi* infection in foals following intragastric challenge, *Vet Pathol* 20:450-459, 1983.

116. Davis JL et al: Pharmacokinetics of azithromycin in foals after i.v. and oral dose and disposition into phagocytes, *J Vet Pharmacol Ther* 25:99-104, 2002.

117. Martens RJ et al: *Rhodococcus equi* foal pneumonia: protective effects of immune plasma in experimentally infected foals, *Equine Vet J* 21:249-255, 1989.

118. Ainsworth DM et al: Lack of residual lung damage in horses in which *Rhodococcus equi*-induced pneumonia had been diagnosed, *Am J Vet Res* 54: 2115-2120 1993.

119. Burgess EC, Gillette D, Pickett P: Arthritis and panuveitis as a manifestation of *Borrelia burgdorferi* in a Wisconsin pony, *J Am Vet Med Assoc* 190:1340-1342, 1986.

120. Burgess EC, Mattison M: Encephalitis associated with *Borrelia burgdorferi* infection in a horse, *J Am Vet Med Assoc* 191:1457-1458, 1987.

121. Magnarelli LA et al: Serologic confirmation of *Ehrlichia equi* and *Borrelia burgdorferi* infections in horses from the northeastern United States, *J Am Vet Med Assoc* 217:1045-1050, 2000.

122. Cohen ND et al: Seroprevalence of antibodies to *Borrelia burgdorferi* in a population of horses in central Texas, *J Am Vet Med Assoc* 201:1030-1034, 1992.

123. Madigan JE: Equine ehrlichiosis, *Vet Clin North Am Equine Pract* 9:423-428, 1993.

124. Sorenson K et al: Lyme disease antibodies in Thoroughbred broodmares correlating to early pregnancy failure, *J Equine Vet Sci* 10:166-168, 1990.

125. Jones TDC: The relation of brucellosis to periodic ophthalmia in Equidae, *Am J Vet Res* 1:54-57, 1940.

126. Cohen ND, Carter GK, McMullan WC: Fistulous withers in horses: 24 cases (1984-1990), *J Am Vet Med Assoc* 201:121-124, 1992.

127. Kowalski JJ: Bacterial and mycotic infections. In Reed SM, Bayly WM, editors: *Equine internal medicine*, Philadelphia, 1998, Saunders , pp 61-93.

128. Gaughan EM, Fubini SL, Dietze A: Fistulous withers in horses: 14 cases (1978-1987), *J Am Vet Med Assoc* 193:964-966, 1988.

129. Gilger BC: Equine recurrent uveitis. In Robinson NE, editor: *Current therapy in equine medicine*, ed 5, Philadelphia, 2003, Saunders pp 468-473.

130. Bernard WV: Leptospirosis, *Vet Clin North Am Equine Pract* 9:435-444, 1993.

131. Divers TJ, Byars TD, Shin SJ: Renal dysfunction associated with infection of *Leptospira interrogans* in a horse, *J Am Vet Med Assoc* 201:1391-1392, 1992.

132. Frazer ML: Acute renal failure from leptospirosis in a foal, *Aust Vet J* 77:499-500, 1999.

133. Hodgin EC, Miller DA, Lozano F: *Leptospira* abortion in horses, *J Vet Diagn Invest* 1:283-287, 1989.

134. van den Ingh TS, Hartman EG, Bercovich Z: Clinical *Leptospira interrogans* serogroup *Australis* serovar *lora* infection in a stud farm in The Netherlands, *Vet Q* 11:175-182, 1989.

135. Nervig RM, Garrett LA: Use of furosemide to obtain bovine urine samples for leptospiral isolation, *Am J Vet Res* 40:1197-1200, 1979.

136. Theirmann AB: Isolation of leptospires in diagnosis of leptospirosis, *Mod Vet Pract* 65:758-759, 1984.

137. Maurin M, Bakken JS, Dumler JS: Antibiotic susceptibilities of *Anaplasma (Ehrlichia) phagocytophilum* strains from various geographic areas in the United States, *Antimicrob Agents Chemother* 47:413-415, 2003.

138. Pusterla N et al: Digenetic trematodes, *Acanthatrium* sp. and *Lecithodendrium* sp., as vectors of *Neorickettsia risticii*, the agent of Potomac horse fever, *J Helminthol* 77:335-339, 2003.

139. Ziemer EL, Keenan DP, Madigan JE: *Ehrlichia equi* infection in a foal, *J Am Vet Med Assoc* 190:199-200, 1987.

140. Nyindo MB et al: Immune response of ponies to experimental infection with *Ehrlichia equi*, *Am J Vet Res* 39:15-18, 1978.

141. Gribble DH: Equine ehrlichiosis, *J Am Vet Med Assoc* 155: 462-469, 1969.

142. Sippel WL, Cooperrider DE, Gainer JH: Equine piroplasmosis in the United States, *J Am Vet Med Assoc* 141:694-698, 1962.

143. Bruning A: Equine piroplasmosis an update on diagnosis, treatment and prevention, *Br Vet J* 152:139-151, 1996.

144. de Waal DT: Equine piroplasmosis: a review, *Br Vet J* 148:6-14, 1992.

145. Kuttler KL, Zaugg JL, Gipson CA: Imidocarb and parvaquone in the treatment of piroplasmosis (*Babesia equi*) in equids, *Am J Vet Res* 48:1613-1616, 1987.

146. Zaugg JL, Lane VM: Efficacy of buparvaquone as a therapeutic and clearing agent of *Babesia equi* of European origin in horses, *Am J Vet Res* 53:1396-1399, 1992.

147. Dubey JP et al: Serologic prevalence of *Toxoplasma gondii* in horses slaughtered for food in North America, *Vet Parasitol* 86:235-238, 1999.

148. Dubey JP: Persistence of encysted *Toxoplasma gondii* in tissues of equids fed oocysts, *Am J Vet Res* 46:1753-1754, 1985.

149. McDonald DR, Cleary DJ: Toxoplasmosis in the equine, *Southwest Vet* 23:213-214, 1970.

150. Chhabra MB, Gautam OP: Antibodies to *Toxoplasma gondii* in equids in north India, *Equine Vet J* 12:146-148, 1980.

151. Alexander CS, Keller H: Atiologie und Vorkommen der periodischen augenentzundung des pferdes iim Raum Berlin, *Tierarztl. Prax* 18:623-627, 1990.

152. Chadna VK et al: Localized subcutaneous cryptococcal granuloma in a horse, *Equine Vet J* 25:166-168, 1993.

153. Riley CB et al: Cryptococcosis in seven horses, *Aust Vet J* 69: 135-139, 1992.

154. Steckel RR et al: Antemortem diagnosis and treatment of cryptococcal meningitis in a horse, *J Am Vet Med Assoc* 180:1085-1089, 1982.

155. Blanchard PC, Filkins M: Cryptococcal pneumonia and abortion in an equine fetus, *J Am Vet Med Assoc* 201:1591-1592, 1992.

156. Scott EA, Duncan JR, McCormack JE: Cryptococcosis involving the postorbital area and frontal sinus in a horse, *J Am Vet Med Assoc* 165:626-627, 1974.

157. Beech J: Cytology of tracheobronchial aspirates in horses, *Vet Pathol* 12:157-164, 1975.

158. Ryan MJ, Wyand DS: Cryptococcus as a cause of neonatal pneumonia and abortion in two horses, *Vet Pathol* 18:270-272, 1981.

159. al-Ani FK: Epizootic lymphangitis in horses: a review of the literature, *Rev Sci Tech* 18:691-699, 1999.

160. Brown C: Diseases affecting the glandular and tubular lymphatic system: epizootic lymphangitis. In Mayhew IG, editor: *Equine medicine and surgery, vol 2,* St Louis, 1999, Mosby, pp 2057-2058.

161. Soliman R et al: Ocular histoplasmosis due to *Histoplasma farciminosum* in Egyptian donkeys, *Mycoses* 34:261-266, 1991.

162. Cook WR: The clinical features of guttural pouch mycosis in the horse. *Vet Rec* 83:336-345, 1968.

163. Cook WR: The pathology and aetiology of guttural pouch mycosis in the horse. *Vet Rec* 83:422-428, 1986.

164. Whitley RD, Gelatt KN: Mycotic encephalitis associated with a guttural pouch mycosis. In Gelatt KN, editor: *Veterinary ophthalmology*. Philadelphia, 1978, Lea and Febiger.

165. Hatziolos BS, Sass B, Albert TF: Blindness in a horse probably caused by gutturomycosis, *Zentralbl Veterinarmed* 22:362-371, 1975.

166. Hatziolos BS, Sass B, Albert TF: Ocular changes in a horse with gutturomycosis, *J Am Vet Med Assoc* 167:51-54, 1975.

167. Sweeney CR, Habacker PL: Pulmonary aspergillosis in horses: 29 cases (1974-1997), *J Am Vet Med Assoc* 214:808-811, 1999.

168. Schmallenbach KH et al: Studies on pulmonary and systemic *Aspergillus fumigatus*-specific IgE and IgG antibodies in horses affected with chronic obstructive pulmonary disease (COPD), *Vet Immunol Immunopathol* 66:245-256, 1998.

169. Sweeney CR: Fungal pneumonia. In Smith BP, editor: *Large animal internal medicine*, St. Louis, 1996, Mosby–Year Book, pp 576-577.

170. Roffey SJ et al: The disposition of voriconazole in mouse, rat, rabbit, guinea pig, dog, and human, *Drug Metab Dispos* 31:731-741, 2003.

171. Schmidt GM et al: Equine onchocerciasis: lesions in the nuchal ligament of midwestern U.S. horses, *Vet Pathol* 19:16-22, 1982.

172. Lloyd S, Soulsby EJ: Survey for infection with *Onchocerca cervicalis* in horses in eastern United States, *Am J Vet Res* 39:1962-1963, 1978.

173. Schmidt GM et al: Equine ocular onchocerciasis: histopathologic study, *Am J Vet Res* 43:1371-1375, 1982.

174. Lavach JD: Parasitic diseases. In Lavach JD, editor: *Large animal ophthalmology*, St. Louis, 1990, Mosby, pp 252-269.

175. Pollitt CC et al: Treatment of equine onchocerciasis with ivermectin paste, *Aust Vet J* 63:152-156, 1986.

176. Moore CP: Eyelid and nasolacrimal disease, *Vet Clin North Am Equine Pract* 8:499-519, 1992.

177. Pusterla N et al: Cutaneous and ocular habronemiasis in horses: 63 cases (1988-2002), *J Am Vet Med Assoc* 222:978-982, 2003.

178. Mohamed FH et al: Cutaneous habronemiasis in horses and domestic donkeys (*Equus acinus acinus*), *Rev Ele Med Vet Pays Trop* 42:535-540, 1990.

179. Fadock VA: Parasitic skin diseases of large animals, *Vet Clin North Am* 6:3-26, 1984.

180. Campbell WC, Benz GW. Ivermectin: a review of efficacy and safety, *J Vet Pharmacol Ther* 7:1-16, 1984.

181. Wijesundera WS, Chandrasekharan NV, Karunanayake EH: A sensitive polymerase chain reaction based assay for the detection of *Setaria digitata*: the causative organism of cerebrospinal nematodiasis in goats, sheep and horses, *Vet Parasitol* 81:225-233, 1999.

182. Frauenfelder HC, Kazacos KR, Lichtenfels JR: Cerebrospinal nematodiasis caused by a filaricide in a horse, *J Am Vet Med Assoc* 177:359-362, 1980.

183. Levine ND: *Nematode parasites of domestic animals and of man*, Minneapolis, 1980, Burgess.

184. Jemelka ED: Removal of *Setaria digitata* from the anterior chamber of the equine eye, *Vet Med Small Anim Clin* 71:673-675, 1976.

185. Thurman JD, Johnson BJ, Lichtenfels JR: Dirofilariasis with arteriosclerosis in a horse, *J Am Vet Med Assoc* 185:532-533, 1984.

186. Moore CP et al: Equine ocular parasites: a review, *Equine Vet J Suppl* 2:76-85, 1983.

187. Rezabek GB, Giles RC, Lyons ET: *Echinococcus granulosus* hydatid cysts in the livers of two horses, *J Vet Diagn Invest* 5:122-125, 1993.

188. Barnett KC, Cottrell BD, Rest JR: Retrobulbar hydatid cyst in the horse, *Equine Vet J* 20:136-138, 1988.

189. Bryan RT, Schantz PM: Echinococcosis (hydatid disease), *J Am Vet Med Assoc* 195:1214-1217, 1989.

190. Spalding MG, Greiner EC, Green SL: *Halicephalobus (Micronema) deletrix* infection in two half-sibling foals, *J Am Vet Med Assoc* 196:1127-1129, 1990.

191. Kinde H et al: *Halicephalobus gingivalis* (*H. deletrix*) infection in two horses in southern California, *J Vet Diagn Invest* 12:162-165, 2000.

192. Rames DS et al: Ocular *Halicephalobus (Micronema) deletrix* infection in a horse, *Vet Pathol* 32:540-542, 1995.

193. Jose-Cunilleras E: Verminous encephalomyelitis. In Reed SM, Bayly WM, Sellon DC, editors: *Equine internal medicine*, St Louis, 2004, Saunders, pp 659-665.
194. Dunn DG et al: Nodular granulomatous posthitis caused by *Halicephalobus* (syn. *Micronema*) sp. in a horse, *Vet Pathol* 30:207-208, 1993.
195. Theon AP: Radiation therapy in the horse, *Vet Clin North Am Equine Pract* 14:673-688, 1998.
196. Theon AP: Intralesional and topical chemotherapy and immunotherapy, *Vet Clin North Am Equine Pract* 14:659-671, 1998.
197. Lunn DP, Horohov DW: Immunodeficiency. In Reed SM, Bayly WM, Sellon DC, editors: *Equine internal medicine*, St Louis, 1994, Saunders, pp 37-52.
198. Bowling AT, Byrns G, Spier SJ: Evidence for a single pedigree source of the hyperkalemic periodic paralysis susceptibility gene in Quarter horses, *Anim Genet* 27:279-281, 1996.
199. Naylor JM: Selection of Quarter horses affected with hyperkalemic periodic paralysis by show judges, *J Am Vet Med Assoc* 204:926-928, 1994.
200. Rudolph JA et al: Periodic paralysis in Quarter horses: a sodium channel mutation disseminated by selective breeding, *Nat Genet* 2:144-147, 1992.
201. Naylor JM: Equine hyperkalemic periodic paralysis: review and implications, *Can Vet J* 35:279-285, 1994.
202. Naylor JM: Hyperkalemic periodic paralysis, *Vet Clin North Am Equine Pract* 13:129-144, 1997.
203. Carr EA et al: Laryngeal and pharyngeal dysfunction in horses homozygous for hyperkalemic periodic paralysis, *J Am Vet Med Assoc* 209:798-803, 1996.
204. Donoghue S et al: Vitamin A nutrition of the equine: growth, serum biochemistry and hematology, *J Nutr* 111:365-374, 1981.
205. Greiwe-Crandell KM et al: Seasonal vitamin A depletion in grazing horses is assessed better by the relative dose response test than by serum retinol concentration, *J Nutr* 125:2711-2716, 1995.
206. Lewis LD: *Vitamins for horses, and plant poisoning of horses*, Baltimore, 1995, Williams & Wilkins.
207. Howell CE, Hart GH, Ittner NR: Vitamin A deficiency in horses, *Am J Vet Res* 2:60-74, 1941.
208. Geor RJ et al: Systemic lupus erythematosus in a filly, *J Am Vet Med Assoc* 197:1489-1492, 1990.
209. Rees CA: Disorders of the skin. In Reed SM, Bayly WM, Sellon DC, editors: *Equine internal medicine*, ed 2, St Louis, 2004 Saunders, pp 667-720.
210. Kimyai-Asadi A, Jih MH: Paraneoplastic pemphigus, *Int J Dermatol* 6:367-372, 2001.
211. Fadok VA: An overview of equine dermatoses characterized by scaling and crusting, *Vet Clin North Am Equine Pract* 11:43-51, 1995.
212. Grassnickel W: Pemphigus and pemphigoid disease in the horse, *Monatshefte Veterinarmed* 15:735-739, 1960.
213. Power HT, McEvoy EO, Manning TO: Use of a gold compound for the treatment of pemphigus foliaceus in a foal, *J Am Vet Med Assoc* 180:400-403, 1982.
214. Bailey E: Prevalence of anti-red blood cell antibodies in the serum and colostrums of mares and its relationship to neonatal isoerythrolysis, *Am J Vet Res* 43:1917-1921, 1982.
215. Traub-Dargatz JL et al: Neonatal isoerythrolysis in mule foals, *J Am Vet Med Assoc* 206:67-70, 1995.
216. Becht JL, Semrad SD: Hematology, blood typing, and immunology of the neonatal foal, *Vet Clin North Am Equine Pract* 1:91-116, 1985.
217. McCue PM: Cushing's disease, *Vet Clin North Am Equine Pract* 18:533-543, 2002.
218. Love S: Equine Cushing's disease, *Br Vet J* 149:139-153, 1993.
219. Donaldson MT et al: Treatment with pergolide or cyproheptadine of pituitary pars intermedia dysfunction (equine Cushing's disease), *J Vet Intern Med* 16:742-746, 2002.
220. Hillyer MH et al: Diagnosis of hyperadrenocorticism in the horse, *Equine Vet Educ* 4:131-134, 1992.
221. Dybdal NO et al: Diagnostic testing for pituitary pars intermedia dysfunction in horses, *J Am Vet Med Assoc* 204:627-632, 1994.
222. Millichamp NJ: Ocular trauma, *Vet Clin North Am Equine Pract* 8:521-536, 1992.
223. Martin CL, Kaswan R, Chapman W: Four cases of traumatic optic nerve blindness in the horse, *Equine Vet J* 18:133-137, 1986.
224. Firth EC: Vestibular disease, and its relationship to facial paralysis in the horse: a clinical study of 7 cases, *Aust Vet J* 53:560-565, 1977.
225. Ragle CA: Head trauma, *Vet Clin North Am Equine Pract* 9:171-183, 1993.
226. Sinha AK, Hendrickson DA, Kannegieter NJ: Head trauma in two horses, *Vet Rec* 128:518-521, 1991.
227. Hirono I et al: Reproduction of progressive retinal degeneration (bright blindness) in sheep by administration of ptaquiloside contained in bracken, *J Vet Med Sci* 55:979-983, 1993.
228. Shahin M, Smith BL, Prakash AS: Bracken carcinogens in the human diet, *Mutat Res* 443:69-79, 1999.
229. Curran JM, Sutherland RJ, Peet RL: A screening test for subclinical liver disease in horses affected by pyrrolizidine alkaloid toxicosis, *Aust Vet J* 74:236-240, 1996.
230. Hintz HF: Molds, mycotoxins, mycotoxicosis, *Vet Clin North Am Equine Pract* 6:410-431, 1990.

13 Practical Management of Blind Horses

Ann Dwyer

A variety of equine ophthalmic diseases may eventually cause horses to lose their sight. In many cases, the attending veterinarians have provided proper treatment and the caretakers have followed medication schedules, but blinding sequelae still occur. Recurrent uveitis is the most common cause of blindness; but corneal disease, accidents, trauma, tissue degeneration, and infection also have the potential to cause vision loss (Fig. 13-1). Data on the incidence of blindness in horses are scant, but field experience suggests that at least 1% to 2% of horses lose sight in one or both eyes during their lifetime.

The following is a list of several facts relating to the size and temperament of horses that are of concern if vision loss is imminent.

1. Horses have a natural history as grazing animals hunted by predators. This gives them a wary temperament. They are prone to display sudden fight-or-flight responses. When cornered, horses may kick, strike, or run.

2. Horses are herd animals that follow a strict social hierarchy. Visual cues are paramount in establishing the dominance order of the group. Individual animals that ignore the visual cues of their herd mates are often bitten, shoved, or kicked by dominant individuals.

3. Horses are large creatures, usually weighing more than 1000 pounds. However, their lower legs have a diameter as slim as that of a baseball bat and are relatively fragile. Horses trapped in fences or other hazards often panic. The result can be fractured extremity bones and other severe injuries.

Given these truths of equine anatomy, social life, and behavior, how do horses cope with the loss of their primary orienting sense? Remarkably, they may adapt well as long as they have steady temperaments and dedicated owners who are commited to the challenge of providing a safe and predictable home.

ADAPTATION TO BLINDNESS

Although blindness can occur suddenly, onset in most horses is gradual. Caretakers of horses with failing vision usually notice progressive uncertainty, especially in low-light situations. Typically, horses may bump into walls or fences and show reluctance to walk over terrain that is unfamiliar. Often, herd behavior changes, even among horses that have been pastured together for years. Horses that are ridden may shy frequently, refuse to obey simple commands, and show reluctance to move forward. Some horses go through a period of fear when complete blindness occurs, showing anxious behavior.[1] Rapid circling, "freezing" in place, prolonged neighing, spooking, and aggressive body motions (e.g., crashing into walls, running over a handler) may be observed. Other horses do not show a dramatic behavior change but may traumatize themselves by running into unfamiliar obstacles. Initially, the balance of blind horses may be altered. They may show a head tilt or postural change and may walk in circles. As time goes on, acceptance of vision loss occurs, and the behavior of individual animals becomes more settled and predictable. Owners of blind horses report that the adjustment period takes anywhere from a few weeks to a few months.

Safe adaptation to blindness is highly dependent on the temperament of the individual horse.[1] Many horses exhibit little change in behavior, quickly orient themselves to their environment, and accept blindness without incident. However, horses that show excessive fear during the adaptation period can be dangerous. Frantic behavior (e.g., circling in a stall, calling to herd mates, ignoring restraint attempts with lead ropes or ties) can cause injury to the horse or handler. Generally, horses that have very high-strung, nervous dispositions are most challenged. Animals with calmer demeanors may adapt well.

Owners and other handlers can help horses through the adaptation phase by providing a safe environment

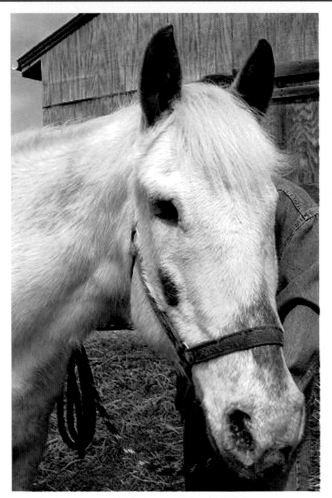

Fig. 13-1 Jake, a 25-year-old Appaloosa gelding. Jake has been blind since the age of 16 as a result of insidious uveitis; both eyes were enucleated to resolve recurrent calcific keratopathy. Jake is used regularly for trail riding. (Photograph courtesy Lisa and Greg Weren, Hilton, NY.)

had sight. These people usually provide the training of a newly blind horse, and this interaction is a key factor in the transition phase. Adaptive lessons are learned as long as the trainer gives consistent cues and is relaxed and nonthreatening. The initial training generally consists of essential verbal cues such as "whoa," "step up," "step down," and "stand." As training goes on, the horse may learn to pick up nonverbal cues as well by responding to the trainer's touch, footfalls, and body position. People working with newly blind horses should be patient, because some lessons take longer to learn than others. Owners who have chosen to maintain blind horses benefit from talking to others who have gone through similar experiences.

No matter how gentle an individual horse is, any horse that has lost its vision may change its behavior quickly if it senses that a nearby person is anxious, afraid, or hostile. A blind horse may also spook if an outside stimulus (e.g., honking automobile, loose dog underfoot, snow sliding off a roof) suddenly scares it. Signage should be posted on stalls or paddocks of blind horses to alert visitors to the animal's handicap. Strangers should be cautioned about approaching horses that are in the early phases of adapting to vision loss. Regular handlers should stand near a blind horse's shoulder when working with it, because this is the safest position from which to take evasive action if the horse reacts suddenly.

COPING IN THE DARK

Experience is the cane of the blind.

Popular Haitian saying

Over and over, owners of blind horses recite inspiring stories of the navigational skills of their "dark-adapted" animals. Many say that their blind horses travel their home terrain with such confidence that outside observers mistake them for sighted animals.

Horses that have lost vision appear to have the ability to construct a "mental map" of their environment and are capable of knowing the perimeter of several different paddocks or large pastures, as well as their stalls. Blind horses often run and play in their fenced enclosures, halting with confidence just short of the boundary. No one knows whether horses gain this geographic knowledge by "memorizing" the stride distance between fences, by feeling subtle alterations in ground topography, or by some other perceptive ability. People who confine horses in electrically charged wire enclosures speculate that the horses may be able sense the presence of the electric current running through the wire.

Blind horses demonstrate increased use of their remaining special senses, especially hearing. Their ears

and spending time with the horse after vision has been lost. Identifying the stressors that cause anxiety (primarily confinement and separation from other horses) is important. Although blind horses have been known to "map" and adapt to a wide variety of stalls, sheds, and pastures, common sense dictates that the ideal initial environment should be a treeless paddock with a board fence and a stall or run-in shed with smooth, solid walls. Some horses benefit from the presence of a calm, sighted companion in their paddock or barn. Others fare better if they are kept alone during the transition period. All horses with recent loss of vision benefit from steady handling, regular grooming, and predictable schedules for meals and turnout (Table 13-1).

Blind horses appear to be settled by the voices, smell, and touch of people they knew and trusted when they

Table 13-1	Methods to Help Horses Adapt to Blindness	
Categories	**Initial Adjustment to Blindness (0-3 to 6 m)**	**Long-Term Adjustment to Blindness (>3 to 6 mo)**
Behavioral	Identify and eliminate things that cause anxiety in each individual horse (e.g., confinement, separation from other horses).	Talk to blind horses often when near them. Reinforce compliant behavior.
Environment	Treeless paddock with board fence. Stall or run-in shed with smooth, solid walls. Tape up bucket handle hooks, cover sharp nails, and remove wire in stalls and paddocks.	Remove hazards from pastures (e.g., low tree branches). Use board or smooth fencing; maintain a safe stall or shed. Demonstrate the boundaries of any new enclosure. Encourage the horse to touch fences, gates, and water sources with its muzzle.
Companion(s)	With or without presence of a calm, sighted companion in paddock and/or barn.	Choose turnout companions that are nonthreatening. If a guide horse emerges, consider putting a bell on its halter.
Horsemanship	Steady handling. Predictable feed and turnout schedules. Regular grooming. Speak to the horse when approaching and working with it. Use consistent phrases and inflections when teaching voice commands. Approach the shoulder area initially. Stay near it when working around the horse.	Do not clip the whiskers on the muzzle. Practice loading on and off a trailer. Keep feed and water in the same location. Handle bilaterally blind horses from both sides of their bodies. For horses with unilateral blindness, avoid initiating alarming sensations (such as injections) on the blind side. Approach the shoulder area initially. Stay near it when working around the horse.

may move often, collecting sound waves like satellite dishes. They act as if their hearing is several times more acute than that of the average horse and appear to orient themselves in their environment on the basis of the loudness and direction of the sounds they hear. The sense of smell also appears enhanced, and horses are often seen scenting the ground or air, moving their noses toward perceivable smells as they search for other horses, food piles, or water.

Horses use their sense of touch, specifically their muzzles, to map their environment. The muzzle is one of the most richly innervated regions of the horse's body. The density of sensory nerves in the equine lip and nose region is similar to the concentration of sensory nerves in the human hand. A blind horse running its nose over a pasture fence or stall gathers information about the world in much the same way that a blind person reading Braille does with his or her fingertips. Blind horses should be encouraged to explore their surroundings and touch new people and things with their muzzles. The long whiskers of the lower face and lips should not be clipped because these structures help the horse "map" and understand the environment.

Blind horses with even temperaments often modify the fight-or-flight behavior that can be so hazardous to the health of a sighted horse. Many anecdotes demonstrate that these animals can choose to override their natural tendency to panic when faced with a situation in which they are stuck or trapped. Caretakers tell stories of blind horses that were tangled in fences or farm machinery calmly waiting for assistance, and as a result, the horses experienced minimal injury. A sighted horse in a similar situation would be expected to thrash and struggle and sustain severe trauma. Still, not all blind horses show such good sense. Some sustain serious injuries if they wander into hazards such as tree branches, holes, ponds, ditches, insecure fencing, or farm equipment; therefore the environment of the blind horse should always be made as safe as possible.

"BULLIES AND BUDDIES": SOCIAL INTERACTIONS BETWEEN BLIND AND SIGHTED HORSES

Social interaction between blind and sighted horses is variable and highly dependent on the innate temperaments of the individuals that are pastured together. Some dominant sighted horses take advantage of a blind horse, chasing the handicapped individual away from feed sources, bullying, biting, and pushing it around. When this kind of social structure prevails, blind horses fail to thrive. They keep to themselves and hang back when the hostile herd members gather. They may lose weight because of poor access to food and may fail to come up to the turnout gate when other horses are being brought in. They lack confidence and may adopt a skittish attitude.

Fortunately, the opposite often occurs. One or more protective individuals from a group of horses will form a "buddy relationship" with the blind individual (Fig. 13-2). Horses that act as "seeing eyes" will lead their unsighted companions over unfamiliar terrain and guide them around obstacles. Sometimes the guidance is in the form of a nose-to-tail physical presence. Other times, the paired off horses will not physically touch, but the blind horse will listen and scent for subtle clues that define the location of the buddy. The guide horse appears to make an effort to stay clear of all obstacles that could be harmful. Vocal contact is frequent, with both individuals calling back and forth to each other. In some cases the sighted horse wears a bell on its halter, which jingles as the horse moves, and the sound cues provide guidance. Observers have seen buddy horses actually appear to purposely lead blind partners through lanes and gates.

Conscientious owners spend time observing herd interactions to identify both bully and buddy alliances. The best management is to turn blind horses out only with friendly guide horses or neutral, nondominant individuals. Hostile dominant horses should be housed in separate enclosures. Blind horses gain reassurance if their pasture friends are housed in adjacent stalls in the home stable. They often project very confident behavior when their guide horses are nearby.

BLIND MARES WITH FOALS

Blind mares that deliver foals deserve special mention. They are as maternal as sighted mares and show strong protective behavior toward their offspring, especially in the first few weeks of the foal's life. They need to know that their foal is nearby and are often more relaxed if the foal wears a halter with a bell (Fig. 13-3). Like sighted mares, they show signs of panic if separated from their offspring. A blind mare that is stressed by separation and trying to reach her foal can be dangerous, because she will be heedless of people or obstacles in her path. Farm employees and veterinarians working on blind broodmares or their foals should always take care to restrain the pair in such a way that the mare is aware that the foal is near. This usually means holding the foal close to the mare's front end where she can swing her head and touch, hear, or smell the foal.

SPECIAL PARTNERSHIPS

The biggest factor that determines the success of adapting a formerly sighted horse to a life of blindness is the

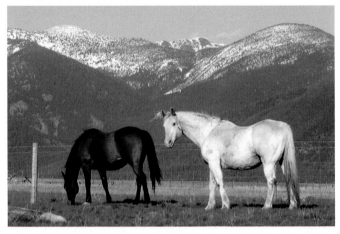

Fig. 13-2 Shasta, a blind Appaloosa (light-colored horse with head raised), pastured with a sighted mare. Blueberry, the visual horse, acts as a guide horse and companion. Shasta has adapted fully to the pasture and knows the location of the boundary sheep wire fence. (Photograph courtesy Steve Smith, Rolling Dog Ranch Animal Sanctuary, Ovando, Montana.)

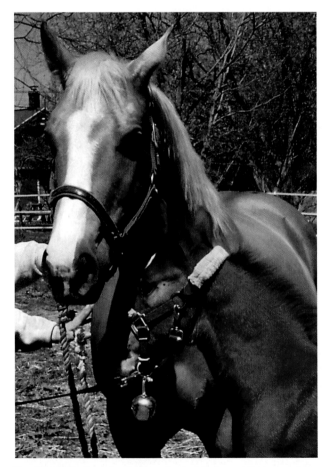

Fig. 13-3 A bell on the halter of a foal helps a blind mare know the location of the foal. Bell in photograph is larger than those normally used. (Photograph courtesy Rocking Horse Equestrian Center, Penfield, NY.)

dedication of the owner.[1] The owner must commit to the responsibility of providing a good environment for the horse and must assume the role of visual guide. The best human partners create a new handling, and sometimes a new riding, vocabulary.

Responsible caretakers use consistent pronunciation of commands and inflections that are high, low, or mid range in pitch to teach blind horses the meaning of cues such as "step up," "step down," "whoa," "stand," and "come." Some horses respond to instructions to turn left or turn right as well. Communication is often quite refined, especially in horses that are used for dressage or other riding purposes (Fig. 13-4). Trainers, riders, and owners often speak of the rewards of working with blind horses, citing heightened awareness of their own special senses and a deep and satisfying sense of partnership with their animals with special needs.

COMMON SENSE TIPS FOR MANAGING BLIND HORSES

Table 13-1 outlines methods to help horses adapt to vision loss. Veterinarians can also provide the following list of tips to owners of blind horses.

1. Blind-proof the environment. Tape up bucket handle hooks, cover sharp nails, and take down pieces of wire in stalls and paddocks (Fig. 13-5). Cut down low hanging tree branches. Consider board fencing for paddocks.

2. Do not clip the whiskers on the muzzle because these are helpful sensing structures.

3. Demonstrate the boundaries of any enclosure to the horse. Encourage the horse to touch fences, gates, and water sources with its muzzle.

4. Talk to blind horses often when in their presence. Use reassuring tones and keep the pitch consistent, especially when issuing commands. Avoid any voice tones that communicate anxiety. Repeat commands to reinforce understanding. Reinforce compliant behavior.

5. Practice loading on and off a trailer. The experience of stepping up onto a ramp or step trailer may help the horse learn ground voice commands.

6. Monitor herd interactions and choose turnout combinations that isolate the blind horse from dominant bullies. If a guide horse emerges, consider putting a bell on its halter (Fig. 13-3).

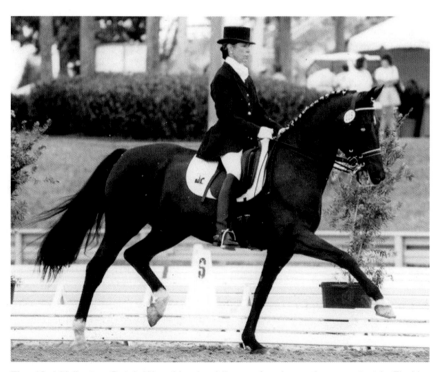

Fig. 13-4 Valiant, a Dutch Warmblood gelding performing a dressage test in Florida. Bilaterally blind since the age of 6, this horse has been trained for upper level dressage since he lost his sight. His rider, Jeanette Sassoon, provides performance cues or "aids" by subtle shifts in the position, pressure, and balance of her hands, legs, and body. (Photograph courtesy Dr. Dennis Brooks and Jeanette Sassoon.)

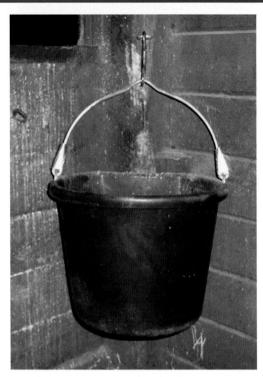

Fig. 13-5 Stalls in which blind horses live should be free of hazards. Bucket handle hooks should be covered with tape to prevent trauma to the globe and lids.

7. Make any environmental changes slowly. Try to keep feed and water in the same location.

8. Handle bilaterally blind horses from both sides of their bodies. For horses that are sighted in one eye, avoid initiating alarming sensations (e.g., injections) on the blind side. Approach the shoulder area initially, and use this region as a base location for most handling and leading.

9. Be aware that blind broodmares do not know what time of day it is and may deliver foals in broad daylight. It may be helpful to hang a bell on the halter of the foal in the first weeks of life (see Fig. 13-3).

10. Set limits and expectations for behavior and reinforce them. Spoiling a blind horse is *never* a good idea.

LIVES THAT BLIND HORSES LEAD

A veterinarian cannot make recommendations that blind horses be ridden, because each horse's circumstances are unique, and safety considerations must take priority in any choice of equestrian activity. However, some comments can be made about the various ways blind horses are managed.

Many blind horses are kept as simple "pasture pets." They may or may not be ridden but are treasured family members. Their owners enjoy caring for them and are happy to provide them basic shelter, feed, and handling in return for their affection and companionship. If the horse has a calm and gentle temperament and has successfully adapted to blindness, it may provide a steadying influence in the form of company for flighty young stock or older sighted horses who do not tolerate solitude. Enucleated or phthisical blind animals have a "different" appearance that is at first a bit startling. When these horses are kept as pasture pets, they often teach children and adult family members valuable lessons in tolerance and acceptance.

Other blind horses are used as trail horses. These animals generally have a strong bond with their riders and are highly cued to riding aids and voice commands. Mileage on unfamiliar trails cements the trust between horse and rider, because the horse depends on the rider for guidance and avoidance of hazards. Blind trail horses are taught to step over logs and small obstacles in their path in response to voice or tactile cues. Anecdotal reports indicate that many blind horses adopt a very confident attitude on the trail if their partnership with a rider is strong. Some horses like to take the dominant "lead" position if riding is done in a group; others prefer to follow sighted horses. Most owners who maintain blind trail horses report that these animals are eager to go out on rides, willing to enter and exit trailers, and very agreeable companions on the trail. Like blind people who travel with guide dogs, these horses seem to enjoy an outing using the rider as a pair of "seeing eyes."

Many mares that go blind are used as broodmares. Their breeding behavior is similar to that of sighted mares. However, lacking photoreceptors, they do not respond to artificial light treatment for inducing estrus early in the year when the natural photoperiod is short. Most cycle normally by April and thus can be bred relatively early in the year. Their gestational issues are exactly the same as those of sighted horses, and they should be placed on the same schedule for nutrition, deworming, and vaccination as other mares on the farm. If a mare became blind as a result of leptospirosis-associated uveitis, then serologic testing is recommended for other broodmares on the farm, because leptospiral infection is well documented as a cause of abortion. Most sighted mares foal in the middle of the night, but blind broodmares can foal at any time of day or night, so extra vigilance is warranted when these mares near their due dates.

A few blind male horses have been used as breeding stallions. With proper handling, breeding these horses can be successful. However, a veterinary consult is advised if a blind mare or stallion is under consideration for breeding. In some instances (e.g., Appaloosas with insidious uveitis or German Warmbloods with certain equine leukocyte antigen [ELA] haplotypes), there may be a genetic predisposition to blindness (Antczak DF et al. Unpublished data, 1989).[2] These animals should not be used for breeding.

A few blind horses have gone on to celebrated careers as high-level athletes. Dressage is an equestrian discipline practiced by many well-adapted blind horses (Fig. 13-4). The sport involves a high level of precise communication between horse and rider. The signals that are used are primarily tactile because the rider uses subtle changes in the position and pressure of the hands, legs, seat, and body balance to tell the horse to change gait, speed, rhythm, and direction. Unlike other equestrian sports that involve obstacles (jumping), high speed (racing and polo), carriages (driving), or interaction with cows, poles, or barrels (western events), dressage takes place in a level arena at fairly low speeds and thus poses fewer hazards for a blind animal. The rider tells the horse where the boundaries of the ring are by changes in his or her weight and body position and turns corners as part of the test pattern. Blind horses have been trained to Olympic dressage standards by skilled and empathetic trainers and have competed against sighted animals at a variety of levels.

HORSES WITH UNILATERAL LOSS OF SIGHT

Most of this chapter addresses the special issues of horses that have no vision at all. However, many horses lose vision in one eye for a variety of reasons, retaining normal vision in the fellow eye. Horses that lose vision in just one eye usually adapt very well. They may show a head tilt for a short time after surgery if an eye has been enucleated, but generally revert quickly to a normal head carriage. Because they cannot see people or objects that approach on the blind side, they may be skittish when approached on that side. As a result, horses that see on one side are often led and approached on that side. Painful or unpleasant stimuli such as injections are best administered on the sighted side. When the horse is handled on the blind half of the body, the handler should talk to the horse in a reassuring tone and keep a hand on the horse's body to steady the horse.

Veterinary ophthalmologists are not able to calibrate acuity or depth perception in either one- or two-eyed horses with certainty. Horses that have unilateral blindness have only half the visual field of a fully sighted horse, so obvious safety questions arise when athletic use of these animals is debated. For this reason, owners are usually advised to use one-eyed horses as sport horses with caution. This is prudent because riding accidents can be dangerous to both horses and riders, and horses with half a visual field may be riskier to ride than others. However, a survey of the world of equestrian competition shows that unilaterally blind horses can be found leading just about every type of sporting life that fully sighted horses lead. Half-blind horses have run in the Kentucky Derby and other premiere stakes races, have competed in international events, have won championships in western events, and have had storied careers as polo, driving, harness, dressage, and show horses. Riders often comment that these horses approach jumps with confidence and appear to gauge distance well.

FINAL COMMENTS ON MANAGING BLIND HORSES

Working with horses that have lost a special sense such as vision is a humbling and powerful learning experience. The adaptive abilities of blind horses teach lessons of perception and persistence. Athletic accomplishments of blind horses testify to the mysterious mental telepathy that develops between horses and riders. The fact that some sighted horses choose social roles as guides for blind animals shows that the virtues of generosity and kindness can occur in the animal kingdom. A person who helps disentangle a blind horse that is trapped in a fence is reminded that patience and common sense can prevail in the most difficult situations.

Blind horses can be an inspiration to children and adults who live with mental or physical disabilities. They can also be beloved pets that teach lessons of tolerance and acceptance of diversity. They are living proof that communication and connection between species occurs on many levels and in many ways. Few sights are more heartwarming than watching blind horses enjoy a good roll and a playful buck in a pasture on a sunny summer afternoon. These horses are telling us that life is sweet and full of value even when it is not perfect.

However, as stated in the beginning of this chapter, horses, even sighted ones, are large and unpredictable creatures that are often their own worst enemies. Working with blind animals can be hazardous. Even the gentlest horse with the steadiest behavior can spook if provoked or startled. Some high-strung horses never adapt well to blindness and pose constant risk to themselves and their handlers.

The decision regarding how to manage a horse without vision is a highly personal one. Although special value and emotional rewards can be part of the experience of housing and caring for a blind horse, serious injury can result as well. Sometimes hard choices must be made, and some blind horses are euthanized. Rarely is this decision made lightly, but sometimes it is the best alternative for both the horse and the people involved. In other instances, blind horses are maintained for many years as valued individuals and treasured friends. Owners weighing the difficult decision of what to do with a horse that has lost sight may be helped by the thoughts of John Milton, the blind poet who wrote these words more than 400 years ago:

> *To be blind is not miserable; not to be able to bear blindness, that is miserable.*
>
> *John Milton, blind British poet.*
> *Second Defence 1654*

Ultimately, individual circumstances dictate choices of management of blind horses.

REFERENCES

1. Hillenbrand L: Leading the blind, *Equus* 229:70-80, 1996.
2. Deeg CA et al: Equine recurrent uveitis is strongly associated with the MHC class I haplotype ELA-A9, *Equine Vet J* 36:73-75, 2004.

Index